Student Quick Tips

Use this Student Quick Tips guide for a quick and eas⸏⸏⸏⸏⸏⸏⸏⸏⸏⸏raw-Hill Connect. You'll get valuable tips on registering, doing assignmei⸏⸏⸏⸏⸏⸏ᴜ accessing resources, as well as information about the support center hours.

Getting Started

TIP: To get started in Connect, you will need the following:

- Your instructor's Connect Web Address

  Sample of Connect Web Address:

  http://www.mcgrawhillconnect.com/class/instructorname_section_name

- Connect Access Code

TIP: If you do not have an access code or have not yet secured your tuition funds, you can click "Free Trial" during registration. This trial will provide temporary Connect access (typically three weeks) and will remind you to purchase online access before the end of your trial.

Registration and Sign In

1. Go to the Connect Web Address provided by your instructor
2. Click on **Register Now**
3. Enter your email address

TIP: If you already have a McGraw-Hill account, you will be asked for your password and will not be required to create a new account.

4. Enter a registration code or choose **Buy Online** to purchase access online

connect™

5. Follow the on-screen directions

TIP: Please choose your Security Question and Answer carefully. We will ask you for this information if you forget your password.

6. When registration is complete, click on **Go to Connect Now**

7. You are now ready to use **Connect**

Trouble Logging In?

* Ensure you are using the same email address you used during registration

* If you have forgotten your password, click on the "Forgot Password?" link at your Instructor's Connect Course Web Address

* When logged into Connect, you can update your account information (e.g. email address, password, and security question/answer) by clicking on the *"My Account"* link located at the top-right corner

Home (Assignments)

TIP: If you are unable to begin an assignment, verify the following:

* The assignment is available (start and due dates)

* That you have not exceeded the maximum number of attempts

* That you have not achieved a score of 100%

* If your assignment contains questions that require manual grading, you will not be able to begin your next attempt until your instructor has graded those questions

TIP: Based on the assignment policy settings established by your Instructor, you may encounter the following limitations when working on your assignment(s):

- Ability to Print Assignment

- Timed assignments – once you begin a *"timed assignment,"* the timer will not stop by design

TIP: *"Save & Exit"* vs. *"Submit"* button

- If you are unable to complete your assignment in one sitting, utilize the *"Save & Exit"* button to save your work and complete it at a later time

- Once you have completed your assignment, utilize the *"Submit"* button in order for your assignment to be graded

Library

TIP: The *Library* section of your Connect account provides shortcuts to various resources.

- If you purchased ConnectPlus, you will see an *eBook* link, which can also be accessed from the section information widget of the *Home* tab

- *Recorded Lectures* can be accessed if your instructor is using *Tegrity Campus* to capture lectures. You may also access recorded lectures when taking an assignment by clicking on the projector icon in the navigation bar

- Many McGraw-Hill textbooks offer additional resources such as narrated slides and additional problems, which are accessible through the *Student Resources* link

Reports

TIP: Once you submit your assignment, you can view your available results in the *Reports* tab.

- If you see a dash (-) as your score, your instructor has either delayed or restricted your ability to see the assignment feedback

- Your instructor has the ability to limit the amount of information (e.g. questions, answers, scores) you can view for each submitted assignment

Need More Help?

CONTACT US ONLINE

Visit us at:

www.mcgrawhillconnect.com/support

Browse our support materials including tutorial videos and our searchable Connect knowledge base. If you cannot find an answer to your question, click on "Contact Us" button to send us an email.

GIVE US A CALL

Call us at:

1-800-331-5094

Our live support is available:

Mon-Thurs:	9 am – 12 pm ET
Friday:	9 am – 7 pm ET
Sunday:	7 pm – 12 pm ET

	Lifestyle physical activity	Moderate exercise program	Vigorous exercise program
Description	Moderate physical activity (150 minutes per week; muscle-strengthening exercises 2 or more days per week)	Cardiorespiratory endurance exercise (20–60 minutes, 3–5 days per week); strength training (2–3 nonconsecutive days per week) and stretching exercises (2 or more days per week)	Cardiorespiratory endurance exercise (20–60 minutes, 3–5 days per week); interval training; strength training (3–4 nonconsecutive days per week); and stretching exercises (5–7 days per week)
Sample activities or program	• Walking to and from work, 15 minutes each way • Cycling to and from class, 10 minutes each way • Doing yard work for 30 minutes • Dancing (fast) for 30 minutes • Playing basketball for 20 minutes • Muscle exercises such as push-ups, squats, or back exercises	• Jogging for 30 minutes, 3 days per week • Weight training, 1 set of 8 exercises, 2 days per week • Stretching exercises, 3 days per week	• Running for 45 minutes, 3 days per week • Intervals: running 400 m at high effort, 4 sets, 2 days per week • Weight training, 3 sets of 10 exercises, 3 days per week • Stretching exercises, 6 days per week
Health and fitness benefits	Better blood cholesterol levels, reduced body fat, better control of blood pressure, improved metabolic health, and enhanced glucose metabolism; improved quality of life; reduced risk of some chronic diseases Greater amounts of activity can help prevent weight gain and promote weight loss	All the benefits of lifestyle physical activity, plus improved physical fitness (increased cardiorespiratory endurance, muscular strength and endurance, and flexibility) and even greater improvements in health and quality of life and reductions in	All the benefits of lifestyle physical activity and a moderate exercise program, with greater increases in fitness and somewhat greater reductions in chronic disease risk Participating in a vigorous exercise

...rrent topics covered ...de financial wellness, ...l networking, hooking up, ...net addiction, caffeinated ...olic beverages, obesity, ...etes, medical marijuana, ...and cancer, cell phones ...adiation, distracted ...ng, health care reform, ...many more. New On the ...ronment boxes help ...ents connect with the ...onment and make ...ronmentally responsible ...es.

ON THE ENVIRONMENT

Environmental Hazards and Reproductive Health: Endocrine Disruptors

For many years, scientists have known that certain chemicals in the environment can have a significant impact on the reproductive health of animals. One of the best-known examples is DDT, a pesticide that nearly caused the extinction of the bald eagle and many other species before its use was banned in the United States in 1972. Another well-known example is DES (diethylstilbestrol), a drug given to women between about 1940 and 1970 to prevent miscarriage. DES was subsequently found to cause reproductive cancers and other adverse effects in the women's daughters, sons, and possibly even grandchildren.

DDT and DES are examples of endocrine-disrupting chemicals (EDCs), substances that act like hormones and disrupt normal hormone activity, particularly activity related to reproduction and development. The most studied EDCs are environmental estrogens, which mimic the female sex hormone estrogen and can duplicate or exaggerate its effects. Other EDCs can block estrogen, mimic or block androgens (male sex hormones), or otherwise alter hor-

levels of testosterone and females having excessive levels of estrogen. Such outcomes have been replicated in laboratory animals, confirming the role of EDCs in disrupting normal sexual and reproductive development, particularly from prenatal exposure. The effects of EDCs on humans are less clear. At high doses, as in the case of DES, they clearly affect reproductive development and physiology, but at low doses, like those found in the environment, no adverse health effects have been definitively documented. However, according to a 2009 Endocrine Society Scientific Statement, the evidence for adverse reproductive outcomes in humans, including infertility and anatomical malformations, is strong.

The widespread use of EDCs began in the late 1930s and 1940s, when the chemical and plastics industries were taking off. They include industrial solvents and lubricants, plastics, pesticides, flame retardants, and pharmaceuticals. These chemicals are so ubiquitous in our environment and food supply today that their residues have been found as part of the "body burden" of virtually every animal or human who is tested.

in the environment long after they are no longer produced and bioaccumulate in the food chain. EDCs also occur naturally as phytoestrogens in plants such as soybeans.

The effects of EDCs include the following:

• DDT, a pesticide still used as an anti-malaria insecticide in Africa and Southeast Asia, inhibits development of female reproductive organs, causes decreased female fertility, and may increase the risk of childhood obesity.

CONNECT CORE CONCEPTS IN
HEALTH

TWELFTH EDITION
BRIEF

PAUL INSEL
STANFORD UNIVERSITY

WALTON ROTH
STANFORD UNIVERSITY

VALUE EDITION for

BOROUGH OF MANHATTAN COMMUNITY COLLEGE

with Connect Plus Access

Boston   Burr Ridge, IL   Dubuque, IA   New York   San Francisco   St. Louis
Bangkok   Bogotá   Caracas   Lisbon   London   Madrid
Mexico City   Milan   New Delhi   Seoul   Singapore   Sydney   Taipei   Toronto

Connect Core Concepts in Health, Twelfth Edition Brief
Value Edition for Borough of Manhattan Community College
with Connect Plus Access

1 2 3 4 5 6 7 8 9 0 BOM BOM 13 12 11

ISBN-13: 978-0-07-757172-6
ISBN-10: 0-07-757172-X

Learning Solutions Representative: Nicole Schmitt
Production Editor: Nichole Birkenholz
Printer/Binder: BookMasters, Inc.

CONTENTS

Preface   *xiv*

1 TAKING CHARGE OF YOUR HEALTH   1

WELLNESS: NEW HEALTH GOALS   1
The Dimensions of Wellness   1
New Opportunities for Taking Charge   3
Promoting Health and Preventing Disease   5
The Healthy People Initiative   6
Health Issues for Diverse Populations   7

CHOOSING WELLNESS   12
Factors That Influence Wellness   12

REACHING WELLNESS THROUGH LIFESTYLE MANAGEMENT   14
Getting Serious About Your Health   14
Building Motivation to Change   15
Enhancing Your Readiness to Change   17
Dealing with Relapse   17
Developing Skills for Change: Creating a Personalized Plan   17
Putting Your Plan into Action   20

BEING HEALTHY FOR LIFE   20
Tips for Today and the Future   20
Connect to Your Choices   21
Summary   21
For More Information   21
Selected Bibliography   22

2 STRESS: THE CONSTANT CHALLENGE   24

WHAT IS STRESS?   24
Physical Responses to Stressors   25
Emotional and Behavioral Responses to Stressors   27

STRESS AND HEALTH   28
The General Adaptation Syndrome   28
Allostatic Load   29
Psychoneuroimmunology   30
Links Between Stress and Specific Conditions   30

COMMON SOURCES OF STRESS   32
Major Life Changes   32
Daily Hassles   32
College Stressors   32
Job-Related Stressors   32
Social Stressors   32
Other Stressors   33

MANAGING STRESS   34
Social Support   34
Communication   36
Exercise   36

Nutrition   36
Sleep   36
Time Management   38
Striving for Spiritual Wellness   38
Confiding in Yourself Through Writing   38
Cognitive Techniques   38
Relaxation Techniques   39
Counterproductive Coping Strategies   42

CREATING A PERSONAL PLAN FOR MANAGING STRESS   43
Identifying Stressors   43
Designing Your Plan   43
Getting Help   44
Behavior Change Strategy   44
Tips for Today and the Future   44
Connect to Your Choices   45
Summary   45
For More Information   45
Selected Bibliography   46

3 PSYCHOLOGICAL HEALTH   47

DEFINING PSYCHOLOGICAL HEALTH   47
Positive Psychology   47
What Psychological Health Is Not   49

MEETING LIFE'S CHALLENGES   50
Growing Up Psychologically   50
Achieving Healthy Self-Esteem   51
Being Less Defensive   53
Being Optimistic   53
Maintaining Honest Communication   54
Dealing with Loneliness   54
Dealing with Anger   54

PSYCHOLOGICAL DISORDERS   55
Anxiety Disorders   56
Mood Disorders   58
Schizophrenia   61

SUICIDE   61

GETTING HELP   63
Self-Help   63
Peer Counseling and Support Groups   64
Professional Help   65
Tips for Today and the Future   65
Connect to Your Choices   66
Summary   66
Behavior Change Strategy   67
For More Information   68
Selected Bibliography   68

4 INTIMATE RELATIONSHIPS AND COMMUNICATION 70

DEVELOPING INTIMATE RELATIONSHIPS 70
Self-Concept and Self-Esteem 70
Friendship 71
Love, Sex, and Intimacy 72
Challenges in Relationships 73
Unhealthy Relationships 75
Ending a Relationship 75

COMMUNICATION 75
Nonverbal Communication 75
Communication Skills 76
Gender and Communication 76
Conflict and Conflict Resolution 77

PAIRING AND SINGLEHOOD 78
Choosing a Partner 78
Dating 80
Living Together 81
Same-Sex Partnerships 82
Singlehood 82

MARRIAGE 84
Benefits of Marriage 84
Issues in Marriage 84
The Role of Commitment 85
Separation and Divorce 85

FAMILY LIFE 86
Becoming a Parent 86
Parenting 86
Single Parents 87
Stepfamilies 87
Successful Families 88
Connect to Your Choices 88
Tips for Today and the Future 88
Summary 88
For More Information 89
Selected Bibliography 90

5 SEXUALITY, PREGNANCY, AND CHILDBIRTH 91

SEXUAL ANATOMY 91
Female Sex Organs 91
Male Sex Organs 92

HORMONES AND THE REPRODUCTIVE LIFE CYCLE 95
Differentiation of the Embryo 95
Female Sexual Maturation 95
Male Sexual Maturation 98
Aging and Human Sexuality 99

SEXUAL FUNCTIONING 100
Sexual Stimulation 100
The Sexual Response Cycle 100
Sexual Problems 101

SEXUAL BEHAVIOR 103
Sexual Orientation 103
Varieties of Human Sexual Behavior 103

Atypical and Problematic Sexual Behaviors 105
Commercial Sex 105
Responsible Sexual Behavior 106

UNDERSTANDING FERTILITY 107
Conception 107
Twins 108
Infertility 108

PREGNANCY 109
Changes in the Woman's Body 110
Fetal Development 111
The Importance of Prenatal Care 115
Complications of Pregnancy and Pregnancy Loss 118

CHILDBIRTH 119
Choices in Childbirth 119
Labor and Delivery 120
The Postpartum Period 122
Connect to Your Choices 122
Tips for Today and the Future 123
Summary 123
For More Information 123
Selected Bibliography 124

6 CONTRACEPTION AND ABORTION 125

PRINCIPLES OF CONTRACEPTION 125

REVERSIBLE CONTRACEPTION 126
Oral Contraceptives: The Pill 126
Contraceptive Skin Patch 128
Vaginal Contraceptive Ring 129
Contraceptive Implants 129
Injectable Contraceptives 130
Intrauterine Devices (IUDs) 130
Male Condoms 131
Female Condoms 132
The Diaphragm with Spermicide 133
FemCap 134
The Contraceptive Sponge 134
Vaginal Spermicides 135
Abstinence, Fertility Awareness, and Withdrawal 135
Combining Methods 137

PERMANENT CONTRACEPTION 138
Male Sterilization: Vasectomy 138
Female Sterilization 139

WHICH CONTRACEPTIVE METHOD IS RIGHT FOR YOU? 140

THE ABORTION ISSUE 142
Legal Status of Abortion 142
Public Opinion 144
Personal Considerations 145
Abortion Statistics 145
Methods of Abortion 146
Complications of Abortion 148
Tips for Today and the Future 149
Connect to Your Choices 149
Summary 149
For More Information 150
Selected Bibliography 150

7 THE USE AND ABUSE OF PSYCHOACTIVE DRUGS 152

ADDICTIVE BEHAVIOR 152
What Is Addiction? 152
Characteristics of Addictive Behavior 153
The Development of Addiction 153
Characteristics of People with Addictions 154
Examples of Addictive Behaviors 154

DRUG USE, ABUSE, AND DEPENDENCE 155
Drug Abuse and Dependence 155
Who Uses Drugs? 156
Why Do People Use Drugs? 158
Risk Factors for Dependence 158
Other Risks of Drug Use 158

HOW DRUGS AFFECT THE BODY 159
Changes in Brain Chemistry 159
Drug Factors 159
User Factors 160
Social Factors 160

REPRESENTATIVE PSYCHOACTIVE DRUGS 161
Opioids 161
Central Nervous System Depressants 161
Central Nervous System Stimulants 164
Marijuana and Other Cannabis Products 167
Hallucinogens 168
Inhalants 169

DRUG USE: THE DECADES AHEAD 170
Drugs, Society, and Families 170
Legalizing Drugs 170
Drug Testing 170
Treatment for Drug Dependence 172
Preventing Drug Abuse 173
Behavior Change Strategy 174
Connect to Your Choices 174
Tips for Today and the Future 174
Summary 175
For More Information 175
Selected Bibliography 176

8 ALCOHOL AND TOBACCO 177

THE NATURE OF ALCOHOL 177
Alcoholic Beverages 177
Absorption 178
Metabolism and Excretion 178
Alcohol Intake and Blood Alcohol
    Concentration 178

ALCOHOL AND HEALTH 180
The Immediate Effects of Alcohol 180
Drinking and Driving 182
The Effects of Chronic Use 183
The Effects of Alcohol Use During Pregnancy 184
Possible Health Benefits of Alcohol 185

ALCOHOL ABUSE AND DEPENDENCE 185
Abuse Versus Dependence 185
Binge Drinking 186
Alcoholism 186

Gender and Ethnic Differences 188
Helping Someone with an Alcohol Problem 190

WHO USES TOBACCO? 190

WHY PEOPLE USE TOBACCO 191
Nicotine Addiction 191
Social and Psychological Factors 191
Why Start in the First Place? 192

HEALTH HAZARDS 193
Tobacco Smoke: A Toxic Mix 193
The Immediate Effects of Smoking 194
The Long-Term Effects of Smoking 194
Other Forms of Tobacco Use 196

THE EFFECTS OF SMOKING ON THE NONSMOKER 198
Environmental Tobacco Smoke 198
Smoking and Pregnancy 199

WHAT CAN BE DONE? 199
Action at Many Levels 199
Individual Action 200

HOW A TOBACCO USER CAN QUIT 200
The Benefits of Quitting 200
Options for Quitting 201
Connect to Your Choices 202
Tips for Today and the Future 202
Summary 202
Behavior Change Strategy 203
For More Information 204
Selected Bibliography 205

9 NUTRITION BASICS 206

NUTRITIONAL REQUIREMENTS: COMPONENTS OF A HEALTHY DIET 206
Proteins—The Basis of Body Structure 207
Fats—Essential in Small Amounts 208
Carbohydrates—An Ideal Source of Energy 209
Fiber—A Closer Look 212
Vitamins—Organic Micronutrients 213
Minerals—Inorganic Micronutrients 215
Water—Vital but Often Ignored 216
Other Substances in Food 216

NUTRITIONAL GUIDELINES: PLANNING YOUR DIET 217
Dietary Reference Intakes (DRIs) 217
Dietary Guidelines for Americans 218
General Guidelines 218
USDA's MyPyramid 221
The Vegetarian Alternative 224
Dietary Challenges for Special Population Groups 225

A PERSONAL PLAN: MAKING INFORMED CHOICES ABOUT FOOD 227
Reading Food Labels 227
Dietary Supplements 227
Protecting Yourself Against Foodborne Illness 229
Organic Foods 229
Guidelines for Fish Consumption 231
Additives in Food 231

Food Irradiation *232*
Genetically Modified Foods *232*
Food Allergies and Food Intolerances *234*

Tips for Today and the Future *234*
Connect to Your Choices *234*
Behavior Change Strategy *235*
Summary *235*
For More Information *236*
Selected Bibliography *237*

10 EXERCISE FOR HEALTH AND FITNESS *241*

WHAT IS PHYSICAL FITNESS? *241*
Cardiorespiratory Endurance *241*
Muscular Strength *242*
Muscular Endurance *242*
Flexibility *242*
Body Composition *243*
Skill-Related Components of Fitness *243*

PHYSICAL ACTIVITY AND EXERCISE FOR HEALTH AND FITNESS *243*

THE BENEFITS OF EXERCISE *244*
Reduced Risk of Premature Death *244*
Improved Cardiorespiratory Functioning *244*
More Efficient Metabolism and Improved Cell Health *244*
Improved Body Composition *244*
Disease Prevention and Management *244*
Improved Psychological and Emotional Wellness *245*
Improved Immune Function *246*
Prevention of Injuries and Low-Back Pain *246*
Improved Wellness for Life *246*

DESIGNING YOUR EXERCISE PROGRAM *246*
First Steps *248*
Cardiorespiratory Endurance Exercises *250*
Developing Muscular Strength and Endurance *251*
Flexibility Exercises *253*
Training in Specific Skills *254*
Putting It All Together *254*

GETTING STARTED AND STAYING ON TRACK *255*
Selecting Instructors, Equipment, and Facilities *255*
Eating and Drinking for Exercise *255*
Managing Your Fitness Program *256*

Tips for Today and the Future *259*
Connect to Your Choices *259*
Behavior Change Strategy *260*
Summary *260*
For More Information *261*
Selected Bibliography *261*

11 WEIGHT MANAGEMENT *263*

BASIC CONCEPTS OF WEIGHT MANAGEMENT *263*
Body Composition *263*
Energy Balance *264*
Evaluating Body Weight and Body Composition *265*
Excess Body Fat and Wellness *266*
What Is the Right Weight for You? *269*

FACTORS CONTRIBUTING TO EXCESS BODY FAT *269*
Genetic Factors *269*
Physiological Factors *269*
Lifestyle Factors *269*
Psychosocial Factors *270*

ADOPTING A HEALTHY LIFESTYLE FOR SUCCESSFUL WEIGHT MANAGEMENT *271*
Diet and Eating Habits *271*
Physical Activity and Exercise *271*
Thinking and Emotions *272*
Coping Strategies *272*

APPROACHES TO OVERCOMING A WEIGHT PROBLEM *272*
Doing It Yourself *272*
Dietary Supplements and Diet Aids *272*
Weight-Loss Programs *273*
Prescription Drugs *274*
Surgery *274*

BODY IMAGE *275*
Severe Body Image Problems *275*
Acceptance and Change *275*

EATING DISORDERS *275*
Anorexia Nervosa *276*
Bulimia Nervosa *276*
Binge-Eating Disorder *278*
Borderline Disordered Eating *278*
Treating Eating Disorders *278*

Behavior Change Strategy *279*
Tips for Today and the Future *280*
Connect to Your Choices *280*
Summary *280*
For More Information *280*
Selected Bibliography *281*

12 CARDIOVASCULAR DISEASE AND CANCER *282*

THE CARDIOVASCULAR SYSTEM *282*

RISK FACTORS FOR CARDIOVASCULAR DISEASE *283*
Major Risk Factors That Can Be Changed *283*
Contributing Risk Factors That Can Be Changed *287*
Major Risk Factors That Can't Be Changed *287*
Possible Risk Factors Currently Being Studied *289*

MAJOR FORMS OF CARDIOVASCULAR DISEASE *291*
Atherosclerosis *291*
Heart Disease and Heart Attack *292*
Stroke *294*
Congestive Heart Failure *296*
Other Forms of Heart Disease *296*

PROTECTING YOURSELF AGAINST CARDIOVASCULAR DISEASE *296*
Eat Heart-Healthy *296*
Exercise Regularly *297*
Avoid Tobacco *297*

Know and Manage Your Blood Pressure *297*
Know and Manage Your Cholesterol Levels *298*
Develop Effective Ways to Handle Stress and Anger *298*

WHAT IS CANCER? *298*
Tumors *298*
Metastasis *298*
Types of Cancer *299*
The Incidence of Cancer *299*

COMMON CANCERS *300*
Lung Cancer *300*
Colon and Rectal Cancer *301*
Breast Cancer *301*
Prostate Cancer *302*
Cancers of the Female Reproductive Tract *304*
Skin Cancer *306*
Head and Neck Cancers *307*
Testicular Cancer *308*

THE CAUSES OF CANCER *309*
The Role of DNA *309*
Tobacco Use *309*
Dietary Factors *309*
Inactivity and Obesity *310*
Carcinogens in the Environment *310*

DETECTING, DIAGNOSING, AND TREATING CANCER *310*
Detecting Cancer *310*
Diagnosing and Treating Cancer *311*
Connect to Your Choices *313*
Tips for Today and the Future *313*
Summary *313*
Behavior Change Strategy *314*
For More Information *315*
Selected Bibliography *315*

13 IMMUNITY AND INFECTION *317*

THE CHAIN OF INFECTION *317*

THE BODY'S DEFENSE SYSTEM *318*
Physical and Chemical Barriers *318*
The Immune System *318*
Epidemics and Pandemics *321*
Immunization *321*
Allergy: The Body's Defense System Gone Haywire *321*

PATHOGENS AND DISEASE *323*
Bacteria *323*
Viruses *325*
Fungi *326*
Protozoa *327*
Parasitic Worms *327*
Prions *327*
Emerging Infectious Diseases *328*
Other Immune Disorders: Cancer and Autoimmune Diseases *329*

SUPPORTING YOUR IMMUNE SYSTEM *329*

THE MAJOR STDS *329*
HIV Infection and AIDS *329*
Chlamydia *336*

Gonorrhea *337*
Pelvic Inflammatory Disease *338*
Human Papillomavirus *338*
Genital Herpes *339*
Hepatitis B *340*
Syphilis *341*
Other STDs *341*

WHAT YOU CAN DO *342*
Education *342*
Diagnosis and Treatment *342*
Prevention *342*
Connect to Your Choices *343*
Tips for Today and the Future *343*
Summary *343*
For More Information *344*
Selected Bibliography *344*

14 ENVIRONMENTAL HEALTH *346*

ENVIRONMENTAL HEALTH DEFINED *346*

POPULATION GROWTH AND CONTROL *347*

AIR QUALITY AND POLLUTION *348*
Air Quality and Smog *349*
The Greenhouse Effect and Global Warming *349*
Thinning of the Ozone Layer *350*
Energy Use and Air Pollution *350*
Indoor Air Pollution *350*
Preventing Air Pollution and Conserving Energy *351*

WATER QUALITY AND POLLUTION *353*
Water Contamination and Treatment *353*
Water Shortages *353*
Sewage *353*
Protecting the Water Supply *353*

SOLID WASTE POLLUTION *354*
Solid Waste *354*
Reducing Solid Waste *355*

CHEMICAL POLLUTION AND HAZARDOUS WASTE *356*
Asbestos *356*
Lead *356*
Pesticides *357*
Mercury *357*
Other Chemical Pollutants *357*
Preventing Chemical Pollution *358*

RADIATION *358*
Medical Uses of Radiation *359*
Cell Phones and Radon *359*
Avoiding Radiation *359*

NOISE POLLUTION *359*

YOU AND THE ENVIRONMENT *359*
Tips for Today and the Future *360*
Connect to Your Choices *360*
Summary *360*
For More Information *360*
Selected Bibliography *361*

15 CONVENTIONAL AND COMPLEMENTARY MEDICINE 362

SELF-CARE 362
Self-Assessment 362
Knowing When to See a Physician 363
Self-Treatment 363

PROFESSIONAL CARE 364

CONVENTIONAL MEDICINE 366
Premises and Assumptions of Conventional Medicine 366
The Providers of Conventional Medicine 368
Choosing a Primary Care Physician 369
Getting the Most Out of Your Medical Care 370

COMPLEMENTARY AND ALTERNATIVE MEDICINE 371
Alternative Medical Systems 372
Mind-Body Medicine 373
Natural Products 374
Manipulative and Body-Based Methods 375
Other CAM Practices 377
Evaluating Complementary and Alternative Therapies 378

PAYING FOR HEALTH CARE 379
The Current System 379
Health Insurance 380
Health Care Reform 380
Tips for Today and the Future 382
Connect to Your Choices 382
Summary 382
For More Information 383
Selected Bibliography 383

16 PERSONAL SAFETY 384

DIFFERENTIATING INJURIES 384

UNINTENTIONAL INJURIES 384
What Causes an Injury? 385
Motor Vehicle Injuries 385
Home Injuries 389
Leisure Injuries 391
Work Injuries 392

VIOLENCE AND INTENTIONAL INJURIES 393
Factors Contributing to Violence 394
Assault 395
Homicide 395
Gang-Related Violence 395
Hate Crimes 395
School Violence 396
Workplace Violence 396
Terrorism 396
Family and Intimate Violence 397
Sexual Violence 399
What You Can Do About Violence 402

PROVIDING EMERGENCY CARE 403
Connect to Your Choices 404
Tips for Today and the Future 404
Summary 404
Behavior Change Strategy 405

For More Information 405
Selected Bibliography 406

17 THE CHALLENGE OF AGING 407

GENERATING VITALITY AS YOU AGE 407
What Happens as You Age? 407
Life-Enhancing Measures: Age-Proofing 408

DEALING WITH THE CHANGES OF AGING 410
Planning for Social Changes 410
Adapting to Physical Changes 411
Handling Psychological and Mental Changes 412

AGING AND LIFE EXPECTANCY 413
America's Aging Minority 413
Family and Community Resources for Older Adults 414
Government Aid and Policies 415

WHAT IS DEATH? 415
Defining Death 416
Learning About Death 416
Denying Versus Welcoming Death 416

PLANNING FOR DEATH 417
Making a Will 417
Considering Options for End-of-Life Care 418
Deciding to Prolong Life or Hasten Death 418
Completing an Advance Directive 420
Becoming an Organ Donor 420
Planning a Funeral or Memorial Service 420

COPING WITH DYING 421
The Tasks of Coping 422
Supporting a Dying Person 422

COPING WITH LOSS 423
Experiencing Grief 423
Supporting a Grieving Person 424

COMING TO TERMS WITH DEATH 424
Connect to Your Choices 426
Tips for Today and the Future 426
Summary 426
For More Information 427
Selected Bibliography 427

APPENDIX

NUTRITION RESOURCES A-1

Credits C-1

Index I-1

BOXES

 IN THE NEWS
Health Care Reform 11
Coping After Violence on Campus 34
Antidepressant Use in Young People 60

Same-Sex Marriage and Civil Unions *83*
Sex Addiction *106*
Emergency Contraception *137*
Key Abortion Decisions and Legislation *144*
Prescription Drug Abuse Among American Teenagers *163*
Caffeinated Alcoholic Beverages: The Dangers of Being "Drunk
    and Wide Awake" *181*
Reducing Your Trans Fat Intake *220*
Drugs and Supplements for Improved Athletic
    Performance *253*
Are Diet Sodas Bad for You? *270*
HPV and Cancer *305*
The 2009 H1N1 Flu Pandemic *322*
The Gulf Oil Spill of 2010 *351*
Evidence Mounting for CAM Therapies *367*
The Human Dimension in Antiterrorism Efforts *398*
Profound Trauma and Loss *425*

ON THE ENVIRONMENT

The Environmental Challenge *13*
The Green Way to Manage Stress *40*
ADHD and Exposure to Nature *64*
Environmental Hazards and Reproductive Health *96*
Environmental Hazards and Miscarriage *143*
Meth and the Environment: A Toxic Impact *166*
Tobacco Use and the Environment *199*
Organic Farming, Organic Foods *232*
Bottled Water and the Environment *257*
Cancer and the Environment *311*
Environmental Health Checklist *347*
Medicine and Drugs from Nature *375*
Extreme Weather and Personal Safety *387*
Green Burials *421*

MIND/BODY/SPIRIT

Financial Wellness *4*
Altruism: Is Doing Good Good for Your Health? *35*
Are Intimate Relationships Good for Your Health? *84*
Spirituality and Drug Abuse *158*
Tobacco Use and Religion: Global Views *192*
Anger, Hostility, and Heart Disease *288*
Stress and Genital Herpes *340*
The Health Benefits of Expressive Writing *364*
The Power of Belief: The Placebo Effect *374*
In Search of a Good Death *422*

TAKE CHARGE

Meditation and the Relaxation Response *41*
Realistic Self-Talk *52*
Strategies for Enhancing Support in Relationships *74*
Guidelines for Effective Communication *76*
Hooking Up *81*
Communicating About Sexuality *107*

Physical Activity During Pregnancy *117*
Talking with a Partner About Contraception *141*
If Someone You Know Has a Drug Problem . . . *173*
Dealing with an Alcohol Emergency *180*
Drinking Behavior and Responsibility *189*
Setting Intake Goals for Protein, Fat, and Carbohydrate *211*
Choosing More Whole-Grain Foods *212*
Eating for Healthy Bones *216*
Judging Portion Sizes *223*
Eating Strategies for College Students *226*
Safe Food Handling *231*
Making Time for Physical Activity *245*
Determining Your Target Heart Rate Range *250*
What to Do in Case of a Heart Attack, Stroke, or Cardiac
    Arrest *293*
How to Perform a Breast Self-Exam *303*
Testicle Self-Examination *309*
Preventing STD Infection *336*
Preventing Date Rape *401*
Staying Safe on Campus *403*

CRITICAL CONSUMER

Evaluating Sources of Health Information *15*
Choosing and Evaluating Mental Health Professionals *66*
Home Pregnancy Tests *109*
Smoking Cessation Products *201*
Using Food Labels *228*
Using Dietary Supplement Labels *230*
Choosing Exercise Footwear *256*
Is Any Diet Best for Weight Loss? *273*
Choosing and Using Sunscreens and Sun-Protective
    Clothing *308*
Getting an HIV Test *334*
How to Be a Green Consumer *355*
Evaluating Health News *369*
Avoiding Health Fraud and Quackery *372*
Choosing a Bicycle Helmet *390*

DIMENSIONS OF DIVERSITY

Health Disparities Among Ethnic Minorities *10*
Diverse Populations, Discrimination, and Stress *33*
Ethnicity, Culture, and Psychological Disorders *57*
Interfaith and Intrafaith Partnerships *79*
Genital Alteration *94*
Ethnicity and Genetic Diseases *114*
Contraceptive Use Among American Women *140*
Drug Use and Ethnicity: Risk Factors and Protective
    Factors *171*
Metabolizing Alcohol: Our Bodies Work Differently *179*
Exercise for People with Special Health Concerns *247*
Ethnicity and CVD *290*
HIV/AIDS Around the World *330*
Poverty and Environmental Health *356*
Health Care Reform: Who's Left Out? *381*

Violence and Health: A Global View *397*
El Día de los Muertos: The Day of the Dead *417*

GENDER MATTERS

Women's Health/Men's Health *8*
Women, Men, and Stress *29*
Depression, Anxiety, and Gender *63*
Gender and Communication *77*
Pregnancy Tasks for Fathers *112*
Men's Involvement in Contraception *142*
Gender Differences in Drug Use *157*
Gender and Tobacco Use *196*
How Different Are the Nutritional Needs of Women and Men? *225*
Gender Differences in Muscular Strength *252*
Gender, Ethnicity, and Body Image *277*
Women and CVD *289*
Women Are Hit Hard by STDs *337*
Gender and Environmental Health *357*
Injuries Among Young Men *386*
Why Do Women Live Longer? *414*

IN FOCUS

Headaches: A Common Symptom of Stress *31*
Does Exercise Improve Mental Health? *59*
Online Relationships *80*
The Adoption Option *146*
Drug Use Among College Students *156*
Club Drugs *164*
College Binge Drinking *186*
Core Training *254*
Diabetes *268*
Exercise and CVD Risk *299*
Renewable Energy *352*
Herbal Remedies: Are They Safe? *378*
Cell Phones, Texting, and Distracted Driving *388*
Repetitive Strain Injury *393*
Can Exercise Delay the Effects of Aging? *409*

TOPICS OF SPECIAL CONCERN TO WOMEN

Aging among women, *410–411, 412, 414*
Alcohol metabolism in women, *178–179*
Alcohol use, special risks for women, *184–185*
Alcoholism, patterns among women, *189*
Amenorrhea, *269*
Anxiety disorders, *63*
Arthritis, *329*
Body composition, *263–264*
Body image, negative, *277*
Breast cancer, *301–302*
Breast self-examinations, *302, 303*
Cancer and women, *300, 301–302, 304–306*

Cardiovascular disease, risk among women, *288, 289*
Caregiving for older adults, *414*
Carpal tunnel syndrome, *392, 393*
Causes of death among women, *397*
Cervical cancer, *304, 305*
Communication styles among women, *76–77*
Contraception, female methods, *126–130, 132–135, 137–138, 139–140*
Depression, risk among women, *63, 122*
Dietary recommendations for women, *211, 223, 225*
Drug use, rates and special risks for women, *157*
Eating disorders, *275–278*
Ectopic pregnancy, *118*
Environmental health risks, *357*
Family violence, *397–399*
Female athlete triad, *269*
Financial planning for retirement, *410–411*
Folic acid, *297*
Gender roles, *28, 71*
Health concerns and status, general, *7–9*
Heart attack risk among women, *288, 289*
HIV infection rates and transmission, *332*
Hormone replacement therapy, *99*
Hormones, female, *95, 289*
Infertility, female, *108–109*
Life expectancy of women, *414*
Marital status, *84*
Menopause, *99, 412*
Menstrual cycle, *95–97*
Migraine, *31*
Muscular strength, development of, *252*
Osteoporosis, *216, 412*
Ovarian cancer, *306*
Pap tests and pelvic exams, *128, 304*
Parenting, single, by women, *87*
Pelvic inflammatory disease, *101, 131, 338*
Post-traumatic stress disorder, *31, 63*
Poverty rates among older women, *410–411, 414*
Pregnancy and childbirth, *107–124*
Premenstrual syndrome and premenstrual dysphoric disorder, *98*
Psychological disorders among women, *63*
Rape, *400–401*
Sexual anatomy, female, *91–92*
Sexual functioning, female, *100–101*
Sexual harassment, *402, 403*
Sexual health problems and dysfunctions, female, *101–103*
Sexually transmitted diseases and pregnancy, *332, 335, 337, 339, 340–341*
Sexually transmitted diseases, symptoms and special risks among women, *330, 337*
Stalking and cyberstalking, *398–399*
Sterilization, female, *139*
Stressors and responses to stress among women, *28–29*
Tobacco use, rates and special risks among women, *196*
Uterine cancer, *306*
Violence against women, *397–402*

TOPICS OF SPECIAL CONCERN TO MEN

Aging among men, *414*
Alcohol abuse and dependence, patterns among men, *189*
Alcohol metabolism in men, *178–179*
Body composition, *263–264*
Body image, negative, *277*
Cancer and men, *300, 302–304, 308*
Cardiovascular disease risk among men, *288, 289*
Causes of death among men, *397*
Cigars and pipes, *197*
Circumcision, *93, 94*
Cluster headaches, *31*
Communication styles among men, *76–77*
Contraception, male methods, *131–132, 136, 138–139*
Dietary recommendations for men, *211, 223, 225*
Drug use, rates of, *157*
Environmental health risks, *357*
Family violence, *397–399*
Firearm-related injuries, *394, 395, 396*
Gambling, *154*
Gender roles, *28, 71*
Health concerns and status, general, *7–9*
Heart attack risk among men, *288, 289*
HIV infection rates and transmission, *332*
Homicide, rates among men, *395*
Hormones, male, *29, 95, 99–100*
Infertility, male, *108–109*
Injuries, rates of, *386*
Life expectancy of men, *414*
Marital status, *84*
Motor vehicle injuries, *385–386*
Motorcycle and motor scooter injuries, *389*
Muscular strength, development of, *252*
Oral cancer, *197*
Parenting, single, by men, *87*
Poverty rates among older men, *411*
Pregnancy, men's roles, *112*
Prostate cancer, *302–304*
Psychological disorders among men, *63*
Rape, *400–401*
Schizophrenia, *61*
Sexual anatomy, male, *92–93*
Sexual functioning, male, *100–101*
Sexual harassment, *402, 403*
Sexual health problems and dysfunctions, male, *101–103*
Sexually transmitted diseases, symptoms and special risks among men, *104, 337*
Spit tobacco, *196–197*
Stalking and cyberstalking, *398–399*
Sterilization, male, *138–139*
Stressors and responses to stress among men, *28, 29*
Suicide, *61–62, 63*
Testicular cancer, *101, 308, 309*
Testicular self-examination, *309*
Tobacco use, rates and special risks among men, *196*
Violent behavior among men, *394*
Violent deaths of men, *394, 395, 396*

Note: The health issues and conditions listed here include those that disproportionately influence or affect women or men. For more information, see the Index under gender, women, men, and any of the special topics listed here.

DIVERSITY TOPICS RELATED TO ETHNICITY

Alcohol metabolism, *179*
Alcohol use and abuse patterns, *189–190*
Asthma, *356*
Body image, *277*
Cancer, rates and risk, *303–304, 306, 308*
Cardiovascular disease patterns and risks, *290*
Contraceptive use, patterns of, *140*
Cystic fibrosis, *114*
Death, attitudes toward, *417*
Diabetes, *268*
Dietary patterns and considerations, *219*
Discrimination and health, *10, 33*
Drug use, risk and protective factors, *171*
Environmental health, *356*
Genetic disorders, *114*
Glaucoma, *410*
Hate crimes, *395–396*
Health disparities, general, *10*
Health insurance status, *379–380*
Health status and concerns, general, *9–10*
Heart disease, *290*
Hemochromatosis, *114*
HIV/AIDS rates, *332*
Homicide rates, *395*
Hypertension, *219*
Lactose intolerance, *114*
Lead poisoning, *356–357*
Marketing, targeted, *191, 198, 200*
Metabolic syndrome, *289–290*
Osteoporosis, *412*
Overweight/obesity, rates and trends, *270, 277*
Poverty rates among older adults, *411*
Prostate cancer, *302–304*
Psychological disorders, symptoms and rates, *57*
Sickle cell disease, *114*
Single-parent families, *87*
Smoking rates, *190*
Stress and discrimination, *33*
Suicide rates, *62*
Tay-Sachs disease, *114*
Thallasemia, *114*
Tobacco use, *190, 194*
Violence, rates of, *395–396*

Note: The health issues and conditions listed here include those that disproportionately influence or affect specific U.S. ethnic groups or for which patterns may appear along ethnic lines. For more information, see the Index under ethnicity, culture, names of specific population groups, and any of the topics listed here.

PREFACE

A Personal Plan for Learning

Raising students' awareness about health risks is one critical step toward motivating them to change their health behaviors.

- The most trusted text in personal health for more than 30 years, *Connect Core Concepts in Health* provides students with accurate, scientifically based health information and informs them about the behaviors that promote health and the behaviors that put their health at risk. With up-to-date coverage of topics ranging from financial literacy to heart health to the latest nutritional and physical activity guidelines, *Connect Core Concepts in Health* help students master the science of health as a basis for healthy life choices.

- Now, a new online adaptive diagnostic tool provides students with a personal plan for learning. Using this tool, students discover what they already know and what they don't know yet. By following an individualized learning path, students are able to study more efficiently and effectively and master the key concepts of the course.

- *Connect Core Concepts in Health* also supports students' learning with a wealth of print and online features. In addition to feature boxes highlighting current topics in the news and issues related to diversity, gender, mind-body health, and consumer health, the twelfth edition focuses attention on environmental issues with new "On the Environment" boxes. Also new to this edition are two vibrant color transparency sections called "Touring Lifestyle Behaviors" and "Touring the Cardiorespiratory System," designed to engage students and reinforce learning, especially for visual learners.

Explore . . . Learn . . . Live

A Personal Approach to Behavior Change

Connect Core Concepts in Health empowers students to approach topics and issues in health as an opportunity to explore, evaluate, and apply what they learn to their own lives.

- *Connect Personal Health* equips students with an online toolkit of assignable activities that promote behavior change, including self-assessments, video activities, practice quizzes with immediate feedback, a fitness and nutrition journal, and behavior change tools, tips, and strategies. *Connect Personal Health* also helps instructors personalize their course material to maximize student learning and to reach their teaching goals.

- A new text-online feature called "Connect to Your Choices" challenges students to explore their inner motivations for their health choices and reflect on their options.

Connect to your Choices

Have you ever thought about why you approach emotional and psychological problems the way you do? Many factors can influence the choices we make about psychological health, some not as obvious as others. Do you hold in your feelings and hide them from others because that's what was modeled in your family? Do you drink or use drugs when you feel depressed or anxious because you aren't aware of any other options? Do you think getting professional help for a psychological problem is a sign that you're weak or crazy?

What are the external factors that influence your choices about psychological health? What are your inner motivations and core values, and how do they affect your choices? Based on what you learned in this chapter, will you make some different choices in the future? If so, what will they be?

Go online to Connect to complete this activity. www.mcgraw-hillconnect.com

- Proven features like Take Charge, Tips for Today and the Future, and Ask Yourself: Questions for Critical Thinking and Reflection help students see how to put personal responsibility to themselves and their world into practice.

Explore . . .
your health behaviors, motivations, and goals.

Learn . . .
what you need to know about the science of health.

Live . . .
your healthiest, most fulfilling life.

OTHER KEY FEATURES AND LEARNING AIDS

- Boxes with the "*Connect* **Activity**" icon feature a student activity in *Connect*. Instructors can assign the activity to ensure that their students are getting the most from the boxes.

- **Behavior Change Strategies** in selected chapters offer specific behavior management/modification plans related to the chapter topic.

- **Quick Stats** marginal notations focus attention on particularly striking statistics related to the topic at hand. Quick Stats alternate with highlighted **quotes from the text,** designed to reinforce key concepts.

- **Vital Statistics** tables and figures highlight important facts and figures in formats that may be more immediately accessible by some learners.

- Chapter-opening learning objectives labeled **Looking Ahead** prepare students for the upcoming chapter content.

- A **running glossary** and terms in boldface type help students handle new vocabulary.

- **Chapter summaries** give students a concise review of key concepts.

- **For More Information** sections point students toward recommended books, newsletters, organizations, hot lines, and Web sites. **Selected Bibliographies** provide reference information for each chapter, and a complete **Index** includes references to glossary terms in boldface type.

- The **Nutrition Resources Appendix** helps students access nutritional information online, including nutritional information from popular fast-food restaurants.

NEW FEATURES AND CHANGES TO THE TWELFTH EDITION

The twelfth edition of *Connect Core Concepts in Health* has been **updated throughout** with the most current health information available. (A list of content revisions by chapter follows.) In addition, the text has been **streamlined for accessibility and readability,** new headings have been inserted, and key data have been chunked into lists, charts, tables, and figures. These improvements allow students to locate, interpret, and retain important information more easily. New and updated images and graphics heighten the book's visual appeal.

New to this edition are two vibrant **color transparency sections** called "Touring Lifestyle Behaviors" and "Touring the Cardiorespiratory System," inserted in Chap-

ters 8 and 12, respectively. In addition to illustrations of the cardiorespiratory system, the heart and lungs, and the process of atherosclerosis, the inserts include representations of the effects of tobacco use, the stages of alcohol intoxication, and the effects of exercise, as well as visual explanations of diabetes and the greenhouse effect. Designed to engage students, especially visual learners, the illustrations are linked to learning objectives.

Also new to this edition is a feature series called "**On the Environment.**" Included in selected chapters, these boxes helps students see their interconnections with the environment and empower them to take responsibility for their environmental health and for the health of the planet. Topics range from "nature deficit disorder" to the effects of endocrine-disrupting chemicals on human reproductive health to the environmental benefits of organic farming.

Content Revisions by Chapter

Chapter 1: New Mind/Body/Spirit box added, "Financial Wellness"; new In the News box added, "Health Care Reform," and chapter updated with new health care reform information; new On the Environment box added, "The Environmental Challenge"; mortality statistics updated throughout (Figure 1.1 showing leading causes of death in the United States and Figure 1.3 showing leading causes of death for young adults), with latest data from the National Center for Health Statistics; new coverage of *Healthy People 2020* added and selected *Healthy People 2010* objectives updated.

Chapter 2: New On the Environment box added, "The Green Way to Manage Stress"; In the News box updated, "Coping After Violence on Campus"; new Mind/Body/Spirit box added, "Altruism: Is Doing Good Good for Your Health?"; statistics on stress updated throughout, with data from the 2009 American Psychological Association's annual "Stress in America" survey; statistics on sleep updated throughout, with data from the National Sleep Foundation; discussion of sleep expanded and new Figure 2.4 added, illustrating sleep apnea; new information added on affirmations as a cognitive technique for managing stress.

Chapter 3: Discussion of psychological health expanded, with more information on positive psychology, emotional intelligence, self-esteem, and optimism; section on suicide expanded; Table 3.1 updated, showing defense and coping mechanisms; new On the Environment box added, "ADHD and Exposure to Nature"; In the News box "Antidepressant Use in Young People" updated.

Chapter 4: Demographic statistics updated throughout, with data from the U.S. Census Bureau, the National Center for Health Statistics, the American College Health Association, and others; discussion of friendship expanded, with new surveys on social networks; discussion of social networking updated and expanded; discussion of love, intimacy, and coupling updated; In Focus box "Online Relationships" updated; new In Focus box added, "Hooking Up"; In the News box "Same-Sex Marriage and Civil Unions" updated; discussion of sexual orientation and gender identity updated.

Chapter 5: Statistics on sexual behavior updated, with data from the American College Health Association and the CDC; new Dimensions of Diversity box added, "Genital Alteration"; new On the Environment box added, "Environmental Hazards and Reproductive Health: Endocrine Disruptors"; discussion of prenatal hormones expanded; discussion of ovulation timing clarified; discussion of female and male sexual development expanded; discussion of common sexual health problems expanded; discussion of common sexual dysfunctions expanded; discussion of gender roles and gender identity expanded and clarified to include cisgender, transgender, and intersex; new section added, "Why People Have Sex," based on a recent survey; new discussion of sexting added; new In the News box added, "Sex Addiction"; new Critical Consumer box added, "Home Pregnancy Tests"; new Take Charge box added, "Physical Activity During Pregnancy"; discussion of prenatal nutrition expanded with latest recommendations from the U.S. Department of Health and Human Services.

Chapter 6: New information added on injectable contraceptives and on a variety of oral contraceptives; In the News box updated, "Emergency Contraception"; Table 6.3 updated with statistics on the effectiveness/failure rates of all types of contraceptive methods; section "Which Contraceptive Method Is Right for You?" expanded; information about the legal status of abortion updated; statistics about abortion rates and methods updated; new On the Environment box added, "Environmental Hazards and Miscarriage."

Chapter 7: Statistics on drug use and abuse updated, with data from the Minding the Future Survey, the National Survey on Drug Use and Health, the Youth Risk Behavior Survey, and others; new In the News box added, "Prescription Drug Abuse Among American Teenagers"; Table 7.1, "Drug Use Among Americans," updated; discussion of the legal status of medical marijuana updated; new On the Environment box added, "Meth and the Environment: A Toxic Impact."

Chapter 8: Statistics on alcohol use and abuse updated, with data from the Minding the Future Survey, the National Survey on Drug Use and Health, the Youth Risk Behavior Survey, and others; statistics on alcohol-related accidents, injuries, deaths, and arrests updated; new In the News box added, "Caffeinated Alcoholic Beverages: The Dangers of Being 'Drunk and Wide Awake'"; discussion of health effects of alcohol expanded, with new information on breast cancer; statistics on tobacco use updated, with data from the National Survey on Drug Use and Health, the Youth Risk Behavior Survey, the American Cancer Society, and others; new On the Environment box added, "Tobacco Use and the Environment"; discussion updated of recent court rulings on cigarette labeling; new section added on electronic cigarettes.

Chapter 9: New recommendations added from 2010 Dietary Guidelines Advisory Committee Report; overview of nutrients expanded; new On the Environment box added, "Organic Farming, Organic Foods"; new recommendations included on sodium intake; discussion of dietary supplements expanded; Table 9.1 updated, "Types of Fatty Acids and Their Possible Effects on Health"; In the News box "Reducing Your Trans Fat Intake" updated.

Chapter 10: Latest ACSM exercise recommendations for strength training and flexibility exercise added; latest physical activity recommendations included from the 2008 *Physical Activity Guidelines for Americans*; new On the Environment box added, "Bottled Water and the Environment"; new In Focus box added, "Core Training."

Chapter 11: Statistics on overweight and obesity updated throughout, with data from the National Center for Health Statistics and the CDC; new Table 11.1 added, "Obesity Prevalence, by Age and Sex, of American Adults, 2007–2008"; discussion of BMI updated; discussion of dietary supplements and diet aids updated; discussion of diabetes updated.

Chapter 12: Statistics on heart disease updated throughout, with data from the American Heart Association's *Heart Disease and Stroke Statistics, 2010*; new In Focus box added, "Exercise and CVD Risk"; discussion of hormone replacement therapy updated; Table 12.3, "Defining Characteristics of Metabolic Syndrome," updated; Take Charge box "What to Do in Case of a Heart Attack, Stroke, or Cardiac Arrest" updated with latest information from the American Heart Association; heart-healthy dietary recommendations updated with information from the report of the 2010 Dietary Guidelines Advisory Committee; statistics on cancer updated throughout, with data from the American Cancer Society's *Cancer Facts and Figures, 2010*; discussion of cancer development expanded; new On the Environment box added, "Cancer and the Environment"; new In the News box added, "HPV and Cancer"; Take Charge box updated, "How to Perform a Breast Self-Exam," with latest information from the American Cancer Society; Table 12.4 updated, "Screening Guidelines for the Early Detection of Cancer in Average-Risk Asymptomatic People," with latest guidelines from the American Cancer Society.

Chapter 13: Statistics on disease incidence updated throughout; new section added on epidemics and pandemics; new In the News box added, "The 2009 H1N1 Flu Pandemic"; statistics on STDs updated throughout, with data from the CDC, WHO, Guttmacher Institute, and others; Dimensions of Diversity box "HIV/AIDS Around the World" updated.

Chapter 14: Statistics updated throughout, with data from the World Health Organization, World Wildlife Fund, United Nations, and others; new On the Environment box added, "Environmental Health Checklist"; information on climate change updated, with information about the 2009 Copenhagen Climate Change Conference; discussion of e-waste updated; new In Focus box added, "Renewable Energy"; new In the News box added, "The Gulf Oil Spill of 2010"; discussion of radiation expanded to include concerns about cell phones; new information on "carbon footprints" added.

Chapter 15: Discussion of prescription medications expanded; discussion of complementary and alternative medicine updated with new categories and latest information from the NCCAM; discussion of naturopathy added; new On the Environment box added, "Medicine and Drugs from Nature"; Table 15.1 updated, "Use of Complementary and Alternative Therapies by Adults"; new In the News box added, "Evidence Mounting for Alternative Therapies"; information added on the *Exercise Is Medicine* initiative; new Dimensions of Diversity box added, "Health Care Reform: Who's Left Out?"; discussion of health care, health insurance, and paying for health care updated with information on the health care reform legislation of 2010.

Chapter 16: Statistics updated throughout with data from the National Safety Council, Federal Bureau of Investigation, CDC, WHO, and others; Table 16.1 updated with new data from the National Safety Council; new In Focus box added, "Repetitive Strain Injuries'"; new In the News box added, "The Human Dimension in Antiterrorism Efforts"; discussion of distracted driving and cell phone use updated; new On the Environment box added, "Extreme Weather and Personal Safety."

Chapter 17: Statistics on life expectancy and quality of life updated; recommendations for physical activity for older adults updated, with information from the 2008 *Physical Activity Guidelines Advisory Committee Report;* new In Focus box added, "Can Exercise Delay the Effects of Aging?"; statistics on death rates, mortality, organ donation, and suicide/assisted suicide updated; discussion of hospice care expanded with new information and statistics; new On the Environment box added, "Green Burials."

TEACHING AND LEARNING TOOLS: AN INTEGRATED LEARNING SYSTEM

McGraw-Hill *Connect,* a new web-based assignment and assessment platform, connects students with their coursework and with their instructors. With **Connect Personal Health,** students gain access to a wealth of online content, including self-assessments, video activities, a fitness and nutrition journal, practice quizzes with immediate feedback, and a media-rich eBook. *Connect Personal Health* meets students online, where they live, bringing the text to life and enhancing its usefulness as a practical guide.

Connect Personal Health now includes an intelligent learning system that diagnoses students' knowledge of a subject and then creates an individualized learning path to help them gain mastery of the material. This **adaptive diagnostic tool** helps students discover what they know already and what they don't know yet. Whether the system is assigned by you or used independently by students as a study tool, the results can be recorded in an easy-to-use grade report that allows you to measure student progress and coach your students to success. Your students will lean faster, study more efficiently, and retain more knowledge when using this innovative tool.

The *Connect Core Concepts in Health* **Online Learning Center (www.mhhe.com/inselbrief12e)** provides many resources for instructors:

- **Course Integrator Guide**
- **Test bank**
- **PowerPoint slides**
- **Image bank**
- **Transparency masters and student handouts**
- **Web links**

Blackboard and McGraw-Hill Higher Education have teamed up! Now, all McGraw-Hill content (text, tools, and homework) can be accessed directly from within your Blackboard course—all with a single sign-on. McGraw-Hill's content is seamlessly woven within your Blackboard course. *Connect* assignments within Blackboard automatically (and instantly) feed grades directly to your Blackboard grade center. No more keeping track of two grade books! Even if your institution is not currently using Blackboard, McGraw-Hill has a solution for you. Ask your sales representative for details.

Classroom Performance System (CPS) brings interactivity into the classroom or lecture hall. CPS is a wireless response system that gives instructors immediate feedback on polling or quiz questions from the entire class.

Tegrity Campus is a service that captures audio and computer screen shots from your lectures, allowing students to review class material when studying or completing assignments. Lectures are captured in a searchable format so that students can replay any part of any class across an entire semester of class recordings. With classroom resources available all the time, students can study more efficiently and learn more successfully.

CourseSmart, the largest provider of eTextbooks, offers students the option of receiving *Connect Core Concepts in Health* as an eBook. At CourseSmart your students can take advantage of significant savings off the cost of a print textbook, reduce their impact on the environment, and gain access to powerful web tools for learning. CourseSmart eTextbooks can be viewed online or downloaded to a computer. The eTextbooks allow students to do full text searches, add highlighting and notes, and share notes with classmates. Visit www.CourseSmart.com to learn more and to try a sample chapter.

 McGraw-Hill Create allows you to create a customized textbook or eBook tailored to your course and syllabus. You can search through thousands of McGraw-Hill texts, rearrange chapters, combine material from other content sources, and include your own content or teaching notes. Create even allows you to personalize your book's appearance by selecting the cover and adding your name, school, and course information. To register and to get more information, go to http://create.mcgraw-hill.com.

Student Resources available with *Connect Core Concepts in Health* include the following:

- Wellness Worksheets help students become more involved in their wellness and better prepared to implement successful behavior change. They include assessment tools, Internet activities, and knowledge-based reviews of key concepts. They are available in *Connect.*

- NutritionCalc Plus 3.2, a dietary analysis program, is available on CD-ROM or in an Internet version.

- The *Daily Fitness and Nutrition Journal* helps students plan and track their fitness programs. It is available in Connect.

- The Health and Fitness Pedometer allows students to count their daily steps and track their physical activity level.

ACKNOWLEDGMENTS

Connect Core Concepts in Health has benefited from the thoughtful commentary, expert knowledge, and helpful suggestions of many people. We are deeply grateful for their participation in the project.

Academic Contributors

Melissa Bernstein, Ph.D., R.D., L.D.,
Rosalind Franklin University of Medicine and Science
Nutrition Basics

Thomas D. Fahey, Ed.D.,
California State University, Chico
Exercise for Health and Fitness

James Freeman, M.D., M.P.H.,
Stanford University
Cardiovascular Health and Cancer

Michael Hoadley, PhD.,
Assistant Vice-President for Academic Affairs, Center for Academic Technology Support, Eastern Illinois University
Personal Safety

Paul M. Insel, Ph.D.,
Stanford University
Taking Charge of Your Health

Mary Iten, PhD.,
University of Nebraska at Kearney
The Challenge of Aging

Robert Jarski, Ph.D.,
Professor of Health Sciences
Director, Complementary Medicine and Wellness Program, Oakland University
Conventional and Complementary Medicine

Nancy Kemp, M.D.
Sexuality, Pregnancy, and Childbirth; Contraception and Abortion; Immunity and Infection

John Kowalczyk, Ph.D.,
University of Minnesota, Duluth
Environmental Health

Inna Landres, M.D.,
Stanford Hospital and Clinics
Contraception and Abortion

Javier Lopez-Zetina,
Associate Professor, Health Science Department, California State University, Long Beach
The Use and Abuse of Psychoactive Drugs

Amy McMullen, M.D.,
Stanford University
Cardiovascular Health and Cancer

Jacob W. Roth, Ph.D.,
Chief of Adult Psychiatry, Kaiser Permanente San Jose Medical Center; Adjunct Clinical Faculty, Stanford University
The Challenge of Aging

Walton T. Roth, M.D.,
Stanford University
Stress: The Constant Challenge; Psychological Health

Judith Sharlin, Ph.D., R.D.,
Department of Nutrition, Simmons College
Weight Management

Rachel Stern,
M.S., R.D., Nutrition Consultant
Alcohol and Tobacco

Philip Takakjian, Ph.D.
Intimate Relationships and Communication

Sarah Waller, M.D.,
Stanford University
Sexuality, Pregnancy, and Childbirth

Patrick Zickler,
Senior Health and Science Writer, Circle Solutions, Inc.
Alcohol and Tobacco

Martha Zuniga, Ph.D.,
University of California, Santa Cruz
Immunity and Infection

Academic Advisors and Reviewers of the Twelfth Edition

Marshina Baker, Bowie State University
Martha Beagle, Berea College
Linda Beatty, McLennan Community College
William Bock, Ball State University
Jeff Bolles, University of North Carolina at Pembroke
Christine Derr, California State University, Monterey Bay
Lisa Dukes, Iowa State University
Karen Edwards, University of Delaware
Brian Goslin, Oakland University
Karen Helmick, Finger Lakes Community College
Lorie Henley, Finger Lakes Community College
Robert Hess, Community College of Baltimore
Leslie Hickcox, Portland Community College, Cascade Campus
Tom Hicks, El Camino College
Kimberly D. Hieftje, Indiana University, Bloomington
Jon Hisgen, Carroll University

Harold Horn, Lincoln Land Community College
Colleen Maloney-Hinds, Crafton Hills College
Andi Milburn, San Diego City College
Richard Morris, Rollins College, Winter Park
David Oster, Jefferson College
Lesley Rennis, Borough of Manhattan Community College
Cynthia Smith, Central Piedmont Community College
Jeffery Waddy, South Suburban College
Bonnie Young, Georgia Perimeter College, Dunwoody
Kara Zografos, California State University, Fresno

Personal Health Symposia Participants

Dede Bodnar, San Diego City College
Christine Bouffard, Waubonsee Community College
Jennifer Fay, Arizona State University
Gabrielle Floyd, Texas Southern University
Kathy Gilbert, Indiana University
Christine Gorman, Kean University
Kris Jankovitz, California Polytech State University
Raeann Koerner, Ventura College
Jennifer Langeland, Western Michigan University
Grace Lartey, Western Kentucky University
Randy Maday, Butte College
Craig Newton, Middle Georgia College
Kay Perrin, University of South Florida
Karla Rues, Ozarks Technical Community College
Cindy Shelton, University of Central Arkansas
Jake Silvestri, Hudson Valley Community College
Gayle Truitt-Bean, Clarion University of Pennsylvania
Jae Westfall, The Ohio State University

Finally, we are grateful to the *Connect Core Concepts in Health* book team at McGraw-Hill, without whose efforts the book could not have been published. Thanks to all!

Paul M. Insel
Walton T. Roth

LOOKING AHEAD...

After reading this chapter, you should be able to:

- Describe the dimensions of wellness
- Identify major health problems in the United States today
- Describe the influence of gender, ethnicity, income, disability, family history, and environment on health
- Explain the importance of personal decision making and behavior change in achieving wellness
- List some available sources of health information and explain how to think critically about them
- Describe the steps in creating a behavior management plan to change a health-related behavior

Taking Charge of Your Health

1

A college sophomore sets the following goals for herself:

- To join new social circles and make new friends whenever possible
- To exercise every day
- To clean up trash and plant trees in blighted neighborhoods in her community

These goals may differ, but they have one thing in common. Each contributes, in its own way, to this student's health and well-being. Not satisfied merely to be free of illness, she wants more. She has decided to live actively and fully—not just to be healthy, but to pursue a state of overall wellness.

WELLNESS: NEW HEALTH GOALS

Generations of people have viewed health simply as the absence of disease. That view largely prevails today. The word **health** typically refers to the overall condition of a person's body or mind and to the presence or absence of illness or injury. **Wellness** is a relatively new concept that expands our idea of health. Beyond the simple presence or absence of disease, wellness refers to optimal health and vitality—to living life to its fullest.

Enhanced wellness involves making conscious decisions to enhance your health and to control **risk factors** that contribute to illness or injury. Some risk factors, such as genetic predisposition to a particular disease or condition, are beyond the control of the individual. Other risk factors, such as the kinds of food you eat, are well within individual control. People of every age can reduce their health risks and pursue wellness by choosing healthy behaviors, such as exercising, not smoking, and managing stress.

The Dimensions of Wellness

Experts have defined six dimensions of wellness, which are listed in Table 1.1. These dimensions are interrelated; each has an effect on the others. Further, the process of achieving wellness is continuing and dynamic (Figure 1.1), involving change and growth. Wellness is not static. Ignoring any dimension of wellness can have harmful effects on your life. But that is the encouraging aspect of wellness: You can actively pursue it.

CORE CONCEPTS IN HEALTH

Mc Graw Hill **connect**™

|PERSONAL HEALTH

www.mcgrawhillconnect.com/personalhealth

Table 1.1 — Examples of Qualities and Behaviors Associated with the Dimensions of Wellness

PHYSICAL	EMOTIONAL	INTELLECTUAL	INTERPERSONAL	SPIRITUAL	ENVIRONMENTAL
• Eating well • Exercising • Avoiding harmful habits • Practicing safer sex • Recognizing symptoms of disease • Getting regular checkups • Avoiding injuries	• Optimism • Trust • Self-esteem • Self-acceptance • Self-confidence • Ability to understand and accept one's feelings • Ability to share feelings with others	• Openness to new ideas • Capacity to question • Ability to think critically • Motivation to master new skills • Sense of humor • Creativity • Curiosity • Lifelong learning	• Communication skills • Capacity for intimacy • Ability to establish and maintain satisfying relationships • Ability to cultivate support system of friends and family	• Capacity for love • Compassion • Forgiveness • Altruism • Joy • Fulfillment • Caring for others • Sense of meaning and purpose • Sense of belonging to something greater than oneself	• Having abundant, clean natural resources • Maintaining sustainable development • Recycling whenever possible • Reducing pollution and waste

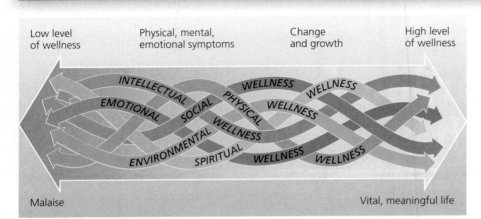

FIGURE 1.1   The wellness continuum. The concept of wellness includes vitality in six interrelated dimensions, all of which contribute to overall wellness.

Physical Wellness   Your physical wellness includes not just your body's overall condition and the absence of disease but your fitness level and your ability to care for yourself. The higher your fitness level is, the higher your level of physical wellness will be. Similarly, as you develop the ability to take care of your own physical needs, you ensure greater physical wellness. To achieve optimum physical wellness, you need to make choices that will help you avoid illnesses and injuries.

Emotional Wellness   Your emotional wellness relates to your mental health and reflects your ability to understand and deal with your feelings. Emotional wellness involves the ability to live a full and creative life and the flexibility to deal with life's challenges. Indications of healthy mental and emotional functioning are characteristics such as a person's sense of worth, sense of control, emotional awareness and coping skills, problem-solving skills, stress-management skills, beliefs, creativity, sense of humor, and cultural identity. Achieving emotional wellness means finding solutions to emotional problems, with professional help if necessary.

Intellectual Wellness   Those who enjoy intellectual wellness constantly challenge their minds. An active mind is essential to wellness because it detects problems, finds solutions, and directs behavior. People who enjoy intellectual wellness never stop learning; they try to learn new things throughout their lifetime. They seek out new experiences and challenges.

Interpersonal Wellness   Your interpersonal (or social) wellness is defined by your ability to develop and maintain satisfying and supportive relationships. Such relationships are essential to physical and emotional health. Social wellness requires participating in and contributing to your community and to society.

Spiritual Wellness   To enjoy spiritual wellness is to possess a set of guiding beliefs, principles, or values that give meaning and purpose to your life, especially in difficult times. The spiritually well person focuses on the positive aspects of life and finds spirituality to be an antidote for negative feelings such as cynicism, anger, and pessimism. Organized religions help many people develop spiritual health. Religion, however, is not the only source or form of spiritual wellness. Many people find meaning and purpose in their lives on their own—through nature, art, meditation, or good works—or with loved ones.

TERMS

health   The overall condition of body or mind and the presence or absence of illness or injury.

wellness   Optimal health and vitality, encompassing all the dimensions of well-being.

risk factor   A condition that increases one's chances of disease or injury.

Table 1.2   Leading Causes of Death in the United States, 2007

RANK	CAUSE OF DEATH	NUMBER OF DEATHS	PERCENT OF TOTAL DEATHS*	DEATH RATE†	LIFESTYLE FACTORS
	All causes	2,423,712	100.0	760.2	
1	Heart disease	616,067	25.4	190.9	D I S A
2	Cancer	562,875	23.2	178.4	D I S A
3	Stroke	135,952	5.6	42.2	D I S A
4	Chronic lower respiratory diseases	127,924	5.3	40.8	S
5	Unintentional injuries (accidents)	123,706	5.1	40.0	I S A
6	Alzheimer's disease	74,632	3.1	22.7	
7	Diabetes mellitus	71,382	2.9	22.5	D I S
8	Influenza and pneumonia	52,717	2.2	16.2	S
9	Kidney disease	46,448	1.9	14.5	D I S A
10	Septicemia (systemic blood infection)	34,828	1.4	11.0	A
11	Intentional self-harm (suicide)	34,598	1.4	11.3	A
12	Chronic liver disease and cirrhosis	29,165	1.2	9.1	A
13	Hypertension (high blood pressure)	23,965	1.0	7.4	D I S A
14	Parkinson's disease	20,058	0.8	6.4	
15	Assault (homicide)	18,361	0.8	6.1	A
	All other causes	451,034	18.6		

Key   D   Diet plays a part   S   Smoking plays a part
        I   Inactive lifestyle plays a part   A   Excessive alcohol use plays a part

NOTE: Although not among the overall top 15 causes of death, HIV/AIDS (11,295 deaths in 2007) is a major killer. In 2007, HIV/AIDS was the 13th leading cause of death for Americans aged 15–24 years and the 6th leading cause of death for those aged 25–44 years.

*Percentages may not total 100% due to rounding.

†Age-adjusted death rate per 100,000 persons.

SOURCE: National Center for Health Statistics. 2010. Deaths: Final data for 2007. *National Vital Statistics Report* 58(19).

Environmental Wellness   Your environmental wellness is defined by the livability of your surroundings. Personal health depends on the health of the planet—from the safety of the food supply to the degree of violence in society. Your physical environment either supports your wellness or diminishes it. To improve your environmental wellness, you can learn about and protect yourself against hazards in your surroundings and work to make your world a cleaner and safer place.

Other Aspects of Wellness   Many experts consider occupational wellness and financial wellness to be additional important dimensions of wellness. *Occupational wellness* refers to the level of happiness and fulfillment you gain through your work. An occupationally well person truly likes his or her work, feels a connection to others in the workplace, and has opportunities to be challenged and gain recognition. To achieve occupational wellness, try to set career goals that reflect your personal values.

Financial wellness refers to your ability to live within your means and manage your money in a way that gives you peace of mind. For more on this topic, see the box "Financial Wellness."

New Opportunities for Taking Charge

Wellness is a fairly new concept. A century ago, Americans considered themselves lucky just to survive to adulthood. A child born in 1900, for example, could expect to live only about 47 years. **Morbidity** and **mortality rates** (rates of illness and death, respectively) from common **infectious diseases** (such as pneumonia, tuberculosis, and diarrhea) were much higher than Americans experience today.

Since 1900, life expectancy has nearly doubled, due largely to the development of vaccines and antibiotics to fight infections and to public health measures, such as water purification and sewage treatment, to improve living conditions. But even though life expectancy has increased, poor health will limit most Americans' activities during the last 15% of their lives, resulting in some sort of impaired life (Figure 1.2). Today, a different set of diseases has emerged as our major health threat, and heart disease, cancer, and stroke are now the three leading causes of death for Americans (Table 1.2). Treating such **chronic diseases** is costly and difficult.

morbidity rate   The relative incidence of disease among a population.

mortality rate   The number of deaths in a population in a given period of time; usually expressed as a ratio, such as 75 deaths per 1000 members of the population.

infectious disease   A disease that can spread from person to person; caused by microorganisms such as bacteria and viruses.

chronic disease   A disease that develops and continues over a long period of time, such as heart disease or cancer.

TERMS

With the news full of stories of home mortgage foreclosures, credit card debt, and personal bankruptcies, it has become painfully clear that many Americans do not know how to manage their finances. Are such stressful experiences inevitable in today's world? Not at all. You can avoid them by developing the skills that contribute to financial wellness. These skills include knowing how to manage your money, using self-discipline to live within your means, using credit cards wisely, staying out of debt, meeting your financial obligations, having a long-range financial plan, and saving. They also include managing your emotional relationship with money and being in charge of your financial decisions. If you haven't developed these skills yet, now is the time to start.

Learn to Budget

Having a budget is a way of tracking where your money goes and making sure you're spending it on the things that are most important to you. Basic budgeting worksheets are available online, but you can also just use a notebook with lined paper. On one page, list your monthly income by source, and on another, list your expenditures. If you're not sure where you spend your money, track your expenditures for a few weeks or a month. Then organize them into categories, such as housing, food, transportation, entertainment, services, personal care, clothes, books and school supplies, health, credit card/loan payments, and miscellaneous.

Now total your income and expenditures. Are you taking in more than you spend, or are you spending more than you're taking in? Are you spending your money where you want to spend it, or are you surprised by your spending patterns? Use what you find out to set guidelines and goals for yourself. If your expenditures exceed your income, identify where you can begin to make some cuts.

Be realistic about what you can cut, but also realize that you may have to adjust your mind-set about what you can afford. Once you have a balance between income and expenses, don't stop there—try to have a little left over each month for an emergency fund or savings.

Be Wary of Credit Cards

College students are prime targets for credit card companies, and most undergraduates have at least one card. A 2009 report found that college students use credit cards to live beyond their means, not just for convenience. The average outstanding balance on undergraduate credit cards was more than $3000.

The best way to avoid credit card debt is to have just one card, to use it only when necessary, and to pay off the entire balance every month. Make sure you understand terms like *APR* (annual percentage rate—the interest you're charged on your balance), *credit limit* (the maximum amount you can borrow at any one time), *minimum monthly payment* (the smallest payment your creditor will accept each month), *grace period* (the number of days you have to pay your bill before interest, late fees, or other penalties are charged), and *over-the-limit* and *late fees* (the amount you'll be charged if your payment is late or you go over your credit limit).

Get Out of Debt

If you do have credit card debt, stop using your cards and start paying them off. If you can't pay the whole balance, try to at least pay more than the minimum payment each month. Most people are surprised by how long it will take to pay off a loan by making only the minimum

payments. For example, to pay off a credit card balance of $2000 at 10% interest with monthly payments of $20 would take 203 months—17 years. To see for yourself, check out an online credit card calculator like http://www.bankrate.com/calculators/credit-cards/credit-card-payoff-calculator.aspx. By carrying a balance and incurring finance charges, you are also paying back much more than your initial loan—money you could be putting to other uses.

Start Saving

The same miracle of compound interest that locks you into years of credit card debt can work to your benefit if you start saving early (for an online compound interest calculator, visit http://www.moneychimp.com/calculator/compound_interest_calculator.htm). Experts recommend "paying yourself first" every month—that is, putting some money into savings before you start paying your bills, depending on what your budget allows. If you work for a company with a 401(k) retirement plan, contribute as much as you can every pay period.

Become Financially Literate

Although modern life requires financial literacy—which includes everything from basics like balancing a checkbook to more sophisticated endeavors like developing a long-term financial plan—most Americans have not received any kind of education in financial skills. The U.S. government has established the Financial Literacy and Education Commission (www.MyMoney.gov) to help Americans develop financial literacy and learn how to save, invest, and manage their money better.

Make it a priority to achieve financial wellness, and start now. Money may not buy you love, but having control over your money can buy you a lot of peace of mind.

SOURCES: Federal Deposit Insurance Corporation. 2010. *Money Smart: A Financial Education Program* (http://www.fdic.gov/consumers/consumer/moneysmart/young.html; retrieved October 28, 2010.); Plymouth State University. 2009. *Financial Wellness* (http://www.plymouth.edu/finaid/wellness/index.html; retrieved October 28, 2010); U.S. Financial Literacy and Education Commission. 2009. *Do You Want to Learn How to Save, Manage, and Invest Your Money Better?* (http://www.mymoney.gov; retrieved October 28, 2010).

Table 1.3	Key Contributors to Death Among Americans	
	NUMBER OF DEATHS PER YEAR	PERCENT OF TOTAL DEATHS PER YEAR
Tobacco	440,000	18.1
Obesity*	112,000	4.6
Alcohol consumption	85,000	3.5
Microbial agents	75,000	3.1
Toxic agents	55,000	2.3
Motor vehicles	43,000	1.8
Firearms	29,000	1.2
Sexual behavior	20,000	0.8
Illicit drug use	17,000	0.7

NOTE: The factors listed here are defined as lifestyle and environmental factors that contribute to the le ading killers of Americans. Microbial agents include bacterial and viral infections like influenza and pneumonia; toxic agents include environmental pollutants and chemical agents such as asbestos.

*The number of deaths due to obesity is an area of ongoing controversy and research. Recent estimates have ranged from 112,000 to 365,000.

SOURCES: Centers for Disease Control and Prevention. 2005. *Frequently Asked Questions About Calculating Obesity-Related Risk* (http://www.cdc.gov/PDF/ Frequently_Asked_Questions_About_Calculating_Obesity-Related_Risk.pdf; retrieved May 6, 2010); Mokdad, A. H., et al. 2005. Correction: Actual causes of death in the United States, 2000. *Journal of the American Medical Association* 293(3): 293–294; Mokdad, A. H., et al. 2004. Actual causes of death in the United States, 2000. *Journal of the American Medical Association* 291(10): 1238–1245.

The good news is that people have some control over whether they develop chronic diseases. People make choices every day that increase or decrease their risks for such diseases. Each of us can take personal responsibility for **lifestyle choices** that include behaviors such as smoking, diet, exercise, and alcohol use. As Table 1.3 makes clear, lifestyle factors contribute to many deaths in the United States, and people can influence their own health risks.

The need to make good choices is especially true for teens and young adults. For Americans age 15–24, for example, the top three causes of death are unintentional injuries (accidents), homicide, and suicide (Table 1.4).

Promoting Health and Preventing Disease

People are a nation's most important resource. The creativity, vitality, and prosperity of a country depend on the health of its people. Governments as well as communities find it in their long-term interests to promote health and prevent disease. The World Health Organization (WHO) defines **health promotion** as "the process of enabling people to increase control over their health and its determinants, and thereby improve their health." The primary means of promoting health are public health policies and agencies that identify and discourage unhealthy and high-risk behaviors and that encourage and provide incentives for judicious health behaviors. Many college campuses have health promotion programs or activities.

In the United States, the National Institutes of Health (NIH) and the Centers for Disease Control and Prevention (CDC) are federal agencies charged with promoting the public's health. NIH is the primary federal agency for conducting and supporting medical research. NIH scientists investigate ways to prevent disease as well as the causes, treatments, and cures for common and rare diseases. Composed of 27 institutes and centers, the NIH provides leadership and financial support to researchers in every state and around the world. The NIH translates research results into interventions and communicates research findings to patients, health care providers, and the public.

Disease prevention is a major focus of public health promotion. Working at disease prevention, the CDC

lifestyle choice A conscious behavior that can increase or decrease a person's risk of disease or injury; such behaviors include smoking, exercising, eating a healthy diet, and others.

health promotion The process of enabling people to increase control over their health and its determinants, and thereby improve their health.

disease prevention The process of providing tools that people and communities need to protect their health by reducing risks; promoting health; preventing disease, injury, and disability; and preparing for new health threats.

TERMS

Table 1.4	Leading Causes of Death Among Americans Ages 15–24		
RANK	CAUSE OF DEATH	NUMBER OF DEATHS	PERCENT OF TOTAL DEATHS
1	Accidents:	15,897	46.8
	Transport	10,928	32.2
	Nontransport	4,969	14.6
2	Homicide	5,551	16.3
3	Suicide	4,140	12.2
4	Cancer	1,653	4.8
5	Heart disease	1,369	4.0
	All causes	33,982	

SOURCE: National Center for Health Statistics. 2010. Deaths: Final data for 2007. *National Vital Statistics Report* 58(19).

collaborates with partners throughout the nation and the world to provide tools that people and communities need to protect their health through health promotion; prevention of disease, injury, and disability; and preparedness for new health threats. Prevention research focuses on identifying risk factors and protective factors for diseases, disorders, and injuries; identifying high-risk behaviors; and developing, managing, and evaluating preventive interventions.

The Healthy People Initiative

The national Healthy People initiative aims to prevent disease and improve Americans' quality of life. Healthy People reports, published each decade since 1980, set national health goals based on 10-year agendas. The initiative's most recent iteration, *Healthy People 2020,* was developed in 2008–2009 and released to the public in 2010. *Healthy People 2020* envisions "a society in which all people live long, healthy lives" and proposes the eventual achievement of the following broad national health objectives:

- Eliminate preventable disease, disability, injury, and premature death. This objective involves activities such as taking more concrete steps to prevent diseases and injuries among individuals and groups, promoting healthy lifestyle choices, improving the nation's preparedness for emergencies, and strengthening the public health infrastructure.

- Achieve health equity, eliminate disparities, and improve the health of all groups. This objective involves identifying, measuring, and addressing health differences between individuals or groups that result from a social or economic disadvantage.

- Create social and physical environments that promote good health for all. This objective involves the use of health interventions at many different levels (such as anti-smoking campaigns by schools, workplaces, and local agencies), improving the situation of undereducated and poor Americans by providing

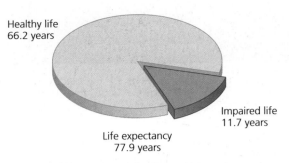

Healthy life 66.2 years

Impaired life 11.7 years

Life expectancy 77.9 years

VITAL STATISTICS

FIGURE 1.2 Quantity of life versus quality of life. Years of healthy life as a proportion of life expectancy in the U.S. population.

SOURCES: National Center for Health Statistics. 2010. Deaths: Final data for 2007. *National Vital Statistics Reports* 58(19); National Center for Health Statistics. *Healthy People 2010.* Midcourse Review. Hyattsville, Md.: Public Health Service.

a broader array of educational and job opportunities, and actively developing healthier living and natural environments for everyone.

- Promote healthy development and healthy behaviors across every stage of life. This objective involves taking a cradle-to-grave approach to health promotion by encouraging disease prevention and healthy behaviors in Americans of all ages.

In a shift from the past, *Healthy People 2020* emphasizes the importance of health determinants—factors that affect the health of individuals, demographic groups, or entire populations. Health determinants are social (including factors such as ethnicity, education level, and economic status) and environmental (including natural and human-made environments). Thus, one goal is to improve living conditions in ways that reduce the impact of negative health determinants.

Examples of individual health promotion goals from the most recent version of Healthy People for which goals have been published (*Healthy People 2010*), along with estimates of how well Americans are tracking toward achieving those goals, appear in Table 1.5.

Table 1.5	Selected *Healthy People 2010* Objectives		
OBJECTIVE		ESTIMATE OF CURRENT STATUS (%)	GOAL (%)
Increase the proportion of adults who engage regularly in moderate physical activity.		32	50
Increase the proportion of people who consume at least 3 daily servings of vegetables.		4	50
Increase the prevalence of healthy weight among people age 20 and older.		32	60
Reduce the proportion of adults 18 and older who use cigarettes.		21	12
Reduce the proportion of college students reporting binge drinking during the past 2 weeks.		41	20
Increase the proportion of adults who take protective measures to reduce the risk of skin cancer.		73	85
Increase the use of safety belts by motor vehicle occupants.		83	89
Increase the number of residences with a functioning smoke alarm on every floor.		90	100
Increase the proportion of persons with health insurance.		83	100

SOURCE: National Center for Health Statistics. 2010. *DATA 2010: The Healthy People 2010 Database, January 2010 Edition* (http://wonder.cdc.gov/data2010/obj.htm; retrieved May 6, 2010).

College students face a variety of wellness challenges, from stress to sleep deprivation to unhealthy food options. But many students make healthy lifestyle choices and enjoy a high level of wellness.

Based on the Healthy People initiative but designed specifically for college students, the Healthy Campus program assists colleges in developing plans to improve student health. The American College Health Association's manual for the program, titled *Healthy Campus: Making It Happen,* is a companion to *Healthy People 2010.* The Healthy Campus program was developed through a broad consultation process built on scientific consensus.

Healthy Campus 2010 provides planning guidelines and more than 200 health-related objectives. Using baselines and targets for meeting these objectives, schools can customize their health programs. For example, a school might choose goals such as increasing the proportion of students who exercise at least 3 days a week or increasing the proportion of students who follow responsible sexual practices. *Healthy Campus 2020* is currently under development.

Health Issues for Diverse Populations

Americans are a diverse people. Our ancestry is European, African, Asian, Pacific Islander, Latin American, and Native American. We live in cities, suburbs, and rural areas and work at every imaginable occupation.

When it comes to health, most differences among people are insignificant; most health issues concern us all equally. We all need to eat well, exercise, manage stress, and cultivate satisfying personal relationships. We need to know how to protect ourselves from heart disease, cancer, sexually transmitted diseases, and injuries. We need to know how to use the health care system.

But some of our differences, as individuals and as members of groups, have important implications for health.

Some of us, for example, have a genetic predisposition for developing certain health problems, such as high cholesterol. Some of us have grown up eating foods that raise our risk of heart disease or obesity. Some of us live in an environment that increases the chance that we will smoke cigarettes or abuse alcohol. These health-related differences among individuals and groups can be biological—determined genetically—or cultural—acquired as patterns of behavior through daily interactions with our families, communities, and society. Many health conditions are a function of biology and culture combined. A person can have a genetic predisposition for a disease, for example, but won't actually develop the disease itself unless certain lifestyle factors are present, such as stress or a poor diet.

Health-related differences among groups can be identified and described in the context of several different dimensions. Those highlighted by the Healthy People initiative are gender, ethnicity, income and education, disability, geographic location, and sexual orientation.

Sex and Gender   Sex and gender profoundly influence wellness. The WHO defines **sex** as the biological and physiological characteristics that define men and women. These characteristics are related to chromosomes and their effects on reproductive organs and the functioning of the body. Menstruation in women and the presence of testicles in men are examples of sex-related characteristics. **Gender** is defined as roles, behaviors, activities, and attributes that a given society considers appropriate for men and women. A person's gender is rooted in biology and physiology, but it is shaped by experience and environment—how society responds to individuals based on their sex. Examples of gender-related characteristics that affect wellness include higher rates of smoking and drinking among men and lower earnings among women (compared with men doing similar work).

Both sex and gender have important effects on wellness, but they can be difficult to separate (see the box "Women's Health/Men's Health"). For example, more

*1 in 3 American men and 1 in 5 American women have **no regular health care provider.***

sex   The biological and physiological characteristics that define men and women.

gender   The roles, behaviors, activities, and attributes that a given society considers appropriate for men and women.

TERMS

Women's Health/Men's Health

In terms of their health, women and men differ in many ways. They have different life expectancies, for one thing, and suffer from various diseases at different rates. Men and women tend to differ in some health-related behaviors, and they respond in dissimilar ways to some medications and medical treatments. The following table highlights some of the gender differences that can affect wellness.

Health Issues	Women	Men
Life expectancy	On average, live about 5 years longer but have higher rates of disabling health problems such as arthritis, osteoporosis, and Alzheimer's disease	Have a shorter life expectancy but lower rates of disabling health problems
Height and weight	Shorter on average, with a lower proportion of muscle; tend to have a "pear" shape with excess body fat stored in the hips; obesity is more common in women than men	Taller on average, with a higher proportion of muscle; tend to have an "apple" shape with excess body fat stored in the abdomen
Skills and fluencies	Score better on tests of verbal fluency, speech production, fine motor skills, and visual and working memory	Score better on tests of visual-spatial ability (such as the ability to imagine the relationships between shapes and objects when rotated in space)
Heart attacks	Experience heart attacks about 10 years later than men, on average, with a poorer 1-year survival rate; more likely to experience atypical heart attack symptoms (such as fatigue and difficulty breathing) or "silent" heart attacks that occur without chest pain	Experience heart attacks about 10 years earlier than women, on average, with a better 1-year survival rate; more likely to have "classic" heart attack symptoms (such as chest pain)
Stroke	More likely to have a stroke or die from one, but also more likely to recover language ability after a stroke that affects the left side of the brain	Less likely to die from a stroke, but also more likely to suffer permanent loss of language ability after a stroke that affects the left side of the brain
Immune response	Stronger immune systems; less susceptible to infection by certain bacteria and viruses, but more likely to develop autoimmune diseases such as lupus	Weaker immune systems; more susceptible to infection by certain bacteria and viruses, but less likely to develop autoimmune diseases
Smoking	Lower rates of smoking than men, but higher risk of lung cancer at a given level of exposure to smoke	Higher rates of smoking and spit tobacco use
Alcohol	Become more intoxicated at a given level of alcohol intake	Become less intoxicated at a given level of alcohol intake, but are more likely to use or abuse alcohol or to develop alcoholism
Stress	More likely to react to stress with a "tend-and-befriend" response that involves social support; may have a longevity advantage because of a reduced risk of stress-related disorders	More likely to react to stress with aggression or hostility; this pattern may increase the rate of stress-related disorders
Depression	More likely to suffer from depression and to attempt suicide	Lower rates of depression than women and less likely to attempt suicide, but four times more likely to succeed at suicide
Headaches	More commonly suffer migraines and chronic tension headaches	More likely to suffer from cluster headaches
Sexually transmitted diseases (STDs)	More likely to be infected with an STD during a heterosexual encounter; more likely to suffer severe, long-term effects from STDs, such as chronic infection and infertility	Less likely to be infected with an STD during a heterosexual encounter

women began smoking with changes in culturally defined ideas about women's behavior (a gender issue). Because women are more vulnerable to the toxins in tobacco smoke (a sex issue), cancer rates also increased.

Ethnicity   Compared with the U.S. population as a whole, American ethnic minorities have higher rates of death and disability from many causes. These disparities result from a complex mix of genetic variations, environmental factors, and health behaviors.

Some diseases are concentrated in certain gene pools, the result of each ethnic group's relatively distinct history. Sickle-cell disease is most common among people of African ancestry. Tay-Sachs disease afflicts people of Eastern European Jewish heritage and French Canadian heritage. Cystic fibrosis is more common among Northern Europeans. In addition to biological differences, many cultural differences occur along ethnic lines. Ethnic groups may vary in their traditional diets; their family and interpersonal relationships; their attitudes toward tobacco, alcohol, and other drugs; and their health beliefs and practices. All of these factors have implications for wellness. (See the box "Health Disparities Among Ethnic Minorities" for more information.)

The federal government collects population and health information on five broad ethnic minority groups in American society. Each group has some specific health concerns:

• *Latinos* are a diverse group, with roots in Mexico, Puerto Rico, Cuba, and South and Central America. Many Latinos are of mixed Spanish and American Indian descent or of mixed Spanish, Indian, and African American descent. Latinos on average have lower rates of heart disease, cancer, and suicide than the general population, but higher rates of infant mortality and a higher overall birth rate; other areas of concern include gallbladder disease and obesity. At current rates, about 1 in 2 Latinas will develop diabetes in her lifetime.

• *African Americans* have the same leading causes of death as the general population, but they have a higher infant mortality rate and lower rates of suicide and osteoporosis. Health issues of special concern for African Americans include high blood pressure, stroke, diabetes, asthma, and obesity. African American men are at significantly higher risk of prostate cancer than men in other groups, and early screening is recommended for them.

• *Asian Americans* include people who trace their ancestry to countries in the Far East, Southeast Asia, or the Indian subcontinent, including Japan, China, Vietnam, Laos, Cambodia, Korea, the Philippines, India, and Pakistan. Asian Americans have a lower death rate and a longer life expectancy than the general population. They have lower rates of coronary heart disease and obesity. However, health differences exist among these groups. For example, Southeast Asian men have higher rates of smoking and lung cancer, and

Vietnamese American women have higher rates of cervical cancer.

• *American Indians and Alaska Natives* typically embrace a tribal identity, such as Sioux, Navaho, or Hopi. American Indians and Alaska Natives have lower death rates from heart disease, stroke, and cancer than the general population, but they have higher rates of early death from causes linked to smoking and alcohol use, including injuries and cirrhosis. Diabetes is a special concern for many groups; for example, the Pimas of Arizona have the highest known prevalence of diabetes of any population in the world.

• *Native Hawaiian and Other Pacific Islander Americans* trace their ancestry to the original peoples of Hawaii, Guam, Samoa, and other Pacific Islands. Pacific Islander Americans have a higher overall death rate than the general population and higher rates of diabetes and asthma. Smoking and obesity are special concerns for this group.

Income and Education   Inequalities in income and education underlie many of the health disparities among Americans. In fact, poverty and low educational attainment are far more important predictors of poor health than any ethnic factor. Income and education are closely related, and groups with the highest poverty rates and least education have the worst health status. These Americans have higher rates of infant mortality, traumatic injury and violent death, and many diseases, including heart disease, diabetes, tuberculosis, HIV infection, and some cancers. They are more likely to eat poorly, be overweight, smoke, drink, and use drugs. They are exposed to more day-to-day stressors and have less access to health care services (see the box "Health Care Reform").

Disability   People with disabilities have activity limitations, need assistance, or perceive themselves as having a disability. About 1 in 5 people in the United States has some level of disability, and the rate is rising, especially among younger segments of the population. People with disabilities are more likely to be inactive and overweight. They report more days of depression than people without disabilities. Many also lack access to health care services.

Geographic Location   About 1 in 4 Americans currently lives in a rural area—a place with fewer than 10,000 residents. People living in rural areas are less likely to be physically active, to use safety belts, or to obtain screening tests for preventive health care. They have less access to timely emergency services and much higher rates of some diseases and injury-related death than people living in urban areas. They are also more likely to lack health insurance. Children living in dangerous neighborhoods—rural or urban—are four times more likely to be overweight than children living in safer areas.

Sexual Orientation   The 1–5% of Americans who identify themselves as homosexual or bisexual make up a

DIMENSIONS OF DIVERSITY

Among America's ethnic groups, striking disparities exist in health status, access to and quality of health care, and life expectancy.

For example, the estimated life expectancy of black Americans (73.6) is nearly 5 years shorter than that of whites (78.4). Blacks also have the highest age-adjusted death rate (958 per 100,000 population) of any ethnic group. Whites have the second-highest death rate (749), followed by Native Americans/Alaska Natives (627), Hispanics (531), and Asian Americans/Pacific Islanders (415).

In studying the underlying causes of health disparities, it is often difficult to separate the many potential contributing factors.

Income and Education

As noted in the chapter, poverty and low educational attainment are the most important factors underlying health disparities.

Consider the following examples:

● *Overall health*. People living in poverty report worse health than people with higher incomes; within the latter group, however, more African Americans and Latinos rate their health as "bad" than do whites.

● *Infant mortality*. Rates of infant deaths go down as the education level of mothers goes up. Among mothers who are college graduates, however, African Americans have significantly higher rates of infant mortality than whites, Latinos, and Asian Americans. Overall, the rate of infant mortality among blacks is more than double that of whites, Asian Americans, or Hispanics.

Access to Appropriate Health Care

The health care reform bill passed by Congress in 2010 mandates insurance coverage for 32 million Americans without insurance. Major coverage expansion begins by 2014. The legislation should reduce the number of people without access to health care and without information about services and preventive care.

Although people with low incomes have tended to receive poorer quality health care, disparities among ethnic minorities persist even at higher income levels. For example, among nonpoor Americans, many more Latinos than whites or African Americans report no usual source of health care and no health care visits within the past year. Ongoing studies continually find that racial minorities have less access to better health care (such as complex surgery at high-volume hospitals) and receive lower quality care than whites.

Factors affecting such disparities may include the following:

● *Local differences in the availability of high-tech health care and specialists.* Minorities, regardless of income, may be more likely to live in medically underserved areas.

● *Problems with communication and trust.* People whose primary language is not English are more likely to be uninsured and to have trouble communicating with health care providers. They may also have problems interpreting health information from public health education campaigns. Language and cultural barriers may be compounded by an underrepresentation of minorities in the health professions.

● *Cultural preferences relating to health care.* Groups may vary in their assessment of when it is appropriate to seek medical care and what types of treatments are acceptable.

Culture and Lifestyle

As described in the chapter, ethnic groups may vary in health-related behaviors such as diet, tobacco and alcohol use, coping strategies, and health practices—and these behaviors can have important implications for wellness, both positive and negative. For example, African Americans are more likely to report consuming five or more servings of fruits and vegetables per day than people from other ethnic groups. American Indians report high rates of smoking and smoking-related health problems.

Cultural background can be an important protective factor. For example, poverty is strongly associated with increased rates of depression, but some groups, including Americans born in Mexico or Puerto Rico, have lower rates of mental disorders at a given level of income and appear to have coping strategies that provide special resilience.

Discrimination

Racism and discrimination are stressful events that can cause psychological distress and increase the risk of physical and psychological problems. Discrimination can contribute to lower socioeconomic status and its associated risks. Bias in medical care can directly affect treatment and health outcomes.

Conversely, research shows that better health care results when doctors ask patients detailed questions about their ethnicity. (Most medical questionnaires ask patients to put themselves in a vague racial or ethnic category, such as Asian or Caucasian.) Armed with more information on patients' backgrounds, medical professionals may find it easier to detect some genetic diseases or to overcome language or cultural barriers.

SOURCES: U.S. Department of Health and Human Services, Agency for Healthcare Research and Quality. 2010. *2009 National Healthcare Disparities Report.* Rockville, Md.: U.S. Department of Health and Human Services, Agency for Healthcare Research and Quality, AHRQ Pub. No. 10-0003; National Center for Health Statistics. 2010. *Health, United States, 2009: With Special Feature on Medical Technology.* Hyattsville, Md.: National Center for Health Statistics; National Center for Health Statistics. 2010. Deaths: Final Data for 2007. *National Vital Statistics Reports* 58(19).

In March 2010, President Barack Obama signed into law the new health care reform bill, officially titled the Health Care and Education Reconciliation Act of 2010. Many consider the legislation a landmark event, similar in importance to the creation in the 1960s of the Medicare and Medicaid programs, which provide health insurance to people over 65 and to people with low incomes and disabilities, respectively.

One of the new law's primary goals is to extend health insurance coverage to 32 million uninsured Americans by 2019. However, it will have far-reaching effects beyond that goal, touching the life of almost every American. One group affected by the bill is college students, who are allowed to stay on their parents' insurance policies until age 26 (instead of 24). This provision encourages older students to attend college and gives young graduates several years to establish careers before having to purchase their own insurance.

Other key provisions of the law include the following:

- **Individual Mandate** Starting in 2014, everyone must purchase health insurance or face a $695 annual fine. There are some exceptions for people with low incomes.

- **Employer Mandate** Employers with more than 50 employees must provide health insurance or pay a fine of $2000 per worker each year if any worker receives federal subsidies to purchase health insurance. Small businesses will receive tax credits to make employee insurance more affordable for them.

- **Health Insurance Exchanges** The uninsured and self-employed will be able to purchase insurance through state-based exchanges, with subsidies available to individuals and families with low incomes. Federal funding will be available to help states set up the exchanges.

- **Subsidies** Individuals and families with low incomes who want to purchase their own health insurance on an exchange are eligible for subsidies. They cannot be eligible for Medicare or Medicaid and cannot be covered by an employer. Eligible buyers will receive premium credits; there is a cap on how much they have to contribute to their premiums on a sliding scale.

- **Insurance Reforms**

  - Starting in September 2010, insurance companies can no longer deny coverage to children based on preexisting conditions. Starting in 2014, they cannot deny coverage to anyone with preexisting conditions.
  - Insurers will no longer be able to drop people from insurance plans when they get sick or place annual or lifetime limits on coverage.
  - Insurers will not be allowed to set up eligibility requirements that discriminate against lower-wage employees.
  - Insurers will have to spend 80–85% of premium dollars on medical services or else give rebates to policy holders.
  - Insurers will have to justify requested rate hikes.
  - Preventive services will be exempt from copayments and deductibles.

- **Abortion** The bill stipulates that no public funds can be used to pay for abortion, a provision backed up by an executive order signed by President Obama. Payments for abortion coverage will have to come from private insurance premium funds, not taxpayer funds. No health care plan will be required to offer abortion coverage, and states can pass legislation choosing to opt out of offering abortion coverage through the exchanges.

- **Immigration** Illegal immigrants will not be allowed to buy health insurance in the exchanges, even if they pay completely with their own money.

- **Medicare** The Medicare prescription drug program (Medicare Part D) will be amended to close a gap in coverage referred to as the "donut hole" and to give seniors a 50% discount on brand-name drugs. At the same time, the bill includes $500 billion in Medicare cuts over the next 10 years.

- **Medicaid** The bill expands Medicaid to cover more low-income families and adults without children.

- **Medical Services** The plan increases funding for community health centers and provides new funding to increase the number of primary care practitioners, including doctors, nurses, nurse practitioners, and physician assistants.

- **Consumer Protections** States will establish offices of health insurance consumer assistance, which will help people file complaints and appeals, and consumers will have access to independent appeals processes.

The plan is expected to cost $950 billion over 10 years and is expected to reduce the federal deficit by $143 billion in the first 10 years and by $1.2 trillion in the second 10 years. Costs of the plan will be paid by a Medicare payroll tax on investment income for families making more than $250,000 per year, by an excise tax on insurance companies for their so-called "Cadillac" high-end insurance plans, and by a 10% excise tax on indoor tanning services. The bill was subject to intense political debate (as evidenced by the provisions on abortion and immigration, for example), with proponents pointing out that the existing health care system was economically unsustainable and opponents charging that "big government" was not the solution. The debate will no doubt continue as the various parts of the bill go into effect between now and 2019.

SOURCE: U.S. Department of Health and Human Services. 2010. Health Care (http://www.healthcare.gov; retrieved October 21, 2010).

How often do you feel exuberant? Vital? Joyful? What makes you feel that way? Conversely, how often do you feel downhearted, de-energized, or depressed? What makes you feel that way? Have you ever thought about how you might increase experiences of vitality and decrease experiences of discouragement?

diverse community with varied health concerns. Their emotional wellness and personal safety are affected by factors relating to personal, family, and social acceptance of their sexual orientation. Gay, lesbian, bisexual, and transgender teens are more likely to engage in risky behaviors such as unsafe sex and drug use; they are also more likely to be depressed and to attempt suicide. HIV/AIDS is a major concern for gay men, and gay men and lesbians may have higher rates of substance abuse, depression, and suicide.

CHOOSING WELLNESS

Wellness is something everyone can have. Achieving it requires knowledge, self-awareness, motivation, and effort, but the benefits last a lifetime. Optimal health comes mostly from a healthy lifestyle—patterns of behavior that promote and support your health now and as you get older. In the pages that follow, you'll find current information and suggestions you can use to build a healthier lifestyle.

Factors That Influence Wellness

Our behavior, family health history, environment, and access to health care are all important influences on wellness. These factors, which vary for both individuals and groups, can interact in ways that produce either health or disease.

Health Habits Research continually reveals new connections between our habits and health. For example, heart disease is associated with smoking, stress, a hostile attitude, a poor diet, and being sedentary. Poor health habits take hold before many Americans reach adulthood.

TERMS

genome The complete set of genetic material in an individual's cells.

gene The basic unit of heredity; a section of genetic material containing chemical instructions for making a particular protein.

Other habits, however, are beneficial. Regular exercise can help prevent heart disease, high blood pressure, diabetes, osteoporosis, and depression and may reduce the risk of colon cancer, stroke, and back injury. A balanced and varied diet helps prevent many chronic diseases. As we learn more about how our actions affect our bodies and minds, we can make informed choices for a healthier life.

Heredity/Family History Your **genome** consists of the complete set of genetic material in your cells; it contains about 25,000 genes, half from each of your parents. **Genes** control the production of proteins that serve both as the structural material for your body and as the regulators of all your body's chemical reactions and metabolic processes. The human genome varies only slightly from person to person, and many of these differences do not affect health. However, some differences have important implications for health, and knowing your family health history can help you determine which conditions may be of special concern for you. Chapter 8 includes more information about creating a family health tree.

Errors in our genes are responsible for about 3500 clearly hereditary conditions, including sickle-cell disease and cystic fibrosis. Altered genes also play a part in heart disease, cancer, stroke, diabetes, and many other common conditions. However, in these more common and complex disorders, genetic alterations serve only to increase an individual's risk, and the disease itself results from the interaction of many genes with other factors. An example of the power of behavior and environment can be seen in the more than 60% increase in the incidence of diabetes that has occurred among Americans since 1990. This huge increase is not due to any sudden change in our genes; it is the result of increasing rates of obesity caused by poor dietary choices and lack of physical activity.

Environment Your environment includes substances and conditions in your home, workplace, and community. Are you frequently exposed to environmental tobacco smoke or the radiation in sunlight? Do you live in an area with high rates of crime and violence? Do you have access to nature? Today, environmental influences on wellness also include conditions in other countries and around the globe, particularly weather and climate changes occurring as a result of global warming (see the box "The Environmental Challenge").

Access to Health Care Adequate health care helps improve both quality and quantity of life through preventive care and the treatment of disease. For example, vaccinations prevent many dangerous infections, and screening tests help identify key risk factors and diseases in their early, treatable stages. As described earlier in the chapter, inadequate access to health care is tied to factors such as low income and lack of health insurance. Cost is one of many issues surrounding the development of advanced health-related technologies.

The effect of human activity on the environment has gradually become clear over several generations, and awareness has grown about environmental issues like air and water pollution, resource depletion, waste disposal, and overpopulation. Only in the last few years, however, has climate change attracted intensive attention worldwide. Most scientists agree that human activity—specifically, the burning of fossil fuels for energy and the release of greenhouse gases into the atmosphere—has caused changes that are raising the earth's temperature and threatening the health of the planet and its living systems. The evidence includes melting ice caps, shifting weather patterns, species extinctions, and a gradual increase in worldwide temperatures. Scientists are trying to determine how high the earth's temperature can climb before a tipping point is reached when damage becomes irreversible.

The complexity of the issues involved in global climate change was underscored by two recent events: the failure of the U.N. Climate Change Conference in December 2009 and the massive British Petroleum (BP) oil spill in the Gulf of Mexico in April 2010.

The goal of the Copenhagen Climate Change Conference was to reach agreement on a framework for climate change mitigation; the ultimate hope was for a legally binding treaty requiring countries worldwide to cut greenhouse gas and carbon emissions. Because of conflicting priorities between developed and developing nations, however, no agreement was reached. Developed countries, led by the United States, were willing to limit their emissions but wanted developing countries to do the same, since developing countries will be major contributors to global warming in the future. Developing countries, particularly China and India, argued that developed countries have caused most global warming and should bear the burden of reversing it. The top priority of developing countries, they said, is economic growth, which currently depends on energy production from fossil fuels. Because of the impasse, the only outcome of the conference was a vaguely worded, nonbinding agreement suggesting that individual countries take actions to limit global temperature increases.

Four months later, an explosion on the Deepwater Horizon offshore oil drilling platform operated by BP and the rupture of the underwater well sent millions of barrels of oil swirling into the waters of the Gulf of Mexico, causing untold damage to wildlife, ecosystems, and people's livelihoods. The public was shocked that BP had no workable emergency plan for containing the gushing oil a mile below the surface. The spill became the biggest environmental disaster in U.S. history.

Despite frustration, oil exploration continues. Since the 1950s, oil (petroleum) has been the world's most important energy source, powering all forms of transportation and driving industrial expansion. Oil is also a toxic pollutant—spilled on land and in water, it fouls the environment. When burned, it causes air pollution and produces carbon dioxide and other greenhouse gases. Although the damaging effects of oil extraction, refining, and consumption are well known, the world is hugely dependent on it—some say, addicted to it.

In the face of international stalemate and industrial ineptitude, is it possible for individuals to make a difference in climate change? Yes—in fact, some believe we have moved past the time when we can depend on experts to solve environmental problems. Instead, a broader understanding of environmental issues by the general public is needed, along with the willingness to make different choices in everyday life. Of course, government at every level is needed to lead the way, but there are hundreds of actions each of us can take

to reduce our impact on the environment. Here are just a few:

- Drive less; walk, bike, and take public transportation more.

- Use less energy. Use less heat, hot water, and air conditioning, and turn off lights and electronic devices, including power strips, when not in use.

- Buy energy-efficient products, from cars to appliances to compact fluorescent light bulbs.

- Eat responsibly. Buy locally grown foods to reduce the amount of fuel needed to transport food as well as air pollution and greenhouse gas emissions. Eating organically keeps petroleum-based pesticides and chemicals out of the food chain and water supply.

- Measure your personal carbon footprint with an online calculator, and learn what you can do to reduce it.

For a detailed discussion of environmental health—how the environment affects you and how you affect the environment—see Chapter 14.

Many more tips are provided throughout this text in On the Environment boxes, along with explorations of various aspects of environmental health and literacy, and environmental issues are described in detail in Chapter 19. Achieving a balance between global development and environmental protection is the great challenge facing the 21st century—and the next generation of world citizens.

Taking Personal Responsibility for Your Wellness In many cases, behavior can tip the balance toward good health, even when heredity or environment is a negative factor. For example, breast cancer can run in families, but it also may be associated with being overweight and inactive. A woman with a family history of breast cancer is less likely to develop the disease if she controls her weight, exercises regularly, and has regular mammograms to help detect the disease in its early, most treatable stage.

Similarly, a young man with a family history of obesity can maintain a normal weight by being careful to balance calorie intake against activities that burn calories. If your life is highly stressful, you can lessen the chances of heart disease and stroke by learning ways to manage and cope with stress. If you live in an area with severe air pollution, you can reduce the risk of lung disease by not smoking. You can also take an active role in improving your environment. Behaviors like these enable you to make a difference in how great an impact heredity and environment will have on your health.

REACHING WELLNESS THROUGH LIFESTYLE MANAGEMENT

As you consider the behaviors that contribute to wellness—being physically active, choosing a healthy diet, and so on—you may be doing a mental comparison with your own behaviors. If you are like most young adults, you probably have some healthy habits and some habits that place your health at risk. For example, you may be physically active and have a healthy diet but indulge in binge drinking on weekends. You may be careful to wear your safety belt in your car but smoke cigarettes or use chewing tobacco. Moving in the direction of wellness means cultivating healthy behaviors and working to overcome unhealthy ones. This approach to lifestyle management is called **behavior change.**

As you may already know from experience, changing an unhealthy habit can be harder than it sounds. When you embark on a behavior change plan, it may seem like too much work at first. But as you make progress, you will gain confidence in your ability to take charge of your life. You will also experience the benefits of wellness—more energy, greater vitality, deeper feelings of appreciation and curiosity, and a higher quality of life.

The rest of this chapter outlines a general process for changing unhealthy behaviors that is backed by research and that has worked for many people. The following sections offer many specific strategies and tips for change.

Getting Serious About Your Health

Before you can start changing a wellness-related behavior, you have to know that the behavior is problematic and that you *can* change it. To make good decisions, you need information about relevant topics and issues, including what resources are available to help you change.

Examine Your Current Health Habits Have you considered how your current lifestyle is affecting your health today and how it will affect your health in the future? Do you know which of your current habits enhance your health and which detract from it? Begin your journey toward wellness with self-assessment: Think about your own behavior, and talk with friends and family members about what they've noticed about your lifestyle and your health. Challenge any unrealistically optimistic attitudes or ideas you may hold—for example, "To protect my health, I don't need to worry about quitting smoking until I'm 40 years old," or "Being overweight won't put *me* at risk for diabetes." Health risks are very real, and health habits throughout life are important.

Many people start to consider changing a behavior when friends or family members express concern, when a landmark event occurs (such as turning 30), or when new information raises their awareness of risk. If you find yourself reevaluating some of your behaviors as you read this text, take advantage of the opportunity to make a change in a structured way.

Choose a Target Behavior Changing any behavior can be demanding. This is why it's a good idea to start small, by choosing one behavior you want to change—called a **target behavior**—and working on it until you succeed. Your chances of success will be greater if your first goal is simple, such as resisting the urge to snack between classes. As you change one behavior, make your next goal a little more significant, and build on your success.

Learn About Your Target Behavior Once you've chosen a target behavior, you need to learn its risks and benefits for you—both now and in the future. Ask these questions:

- How is your target behavior affecting your level of wellness today?
- What diseases or conditions does this behavior place you at risk for?
- What effect would changing your behavior have on your health?

As a starting point, use this text and the resources listed in the For More Information section at the end of each chapter; see the box "Evaluating Sources of Health Information" for additional guidelines.

Find Help Have you identified a particularly challenging target behavior or mood, something like alcohol addiction, binge eating, or depression, that interferes with your ability to function or places you at a serious health risk? Help may

> **8%** of Americans have diabetes, but about one-fourth of them don't know it.
>
> —American Diabetes Association, 2010

Evaluating Sources of Health Information

Believability of Health Information Sources

A 2007 survey conducted by the American College Health Association indicated that college students are smart about evaluating health information. They trust the health information they receive from health professionals and educators and are skeptical about popular information sources.

Rank	Source	Rank	Source
1	Health educators	8	Resident assistants/ advisers
2	Health center medical staff	9	Religious centers
3	Parents	10	Internet/World Wide Web
4	Faculty/coursework	11	Friends
5	Leaflets, pamphlets, flyers	12	Magazines
6	Campus newspaper articles	13	Television
7	Campus peer educators	14	Other sources

How good are you at evaluating health information? Here are some tips.

General Strategies

Whenever you encounter health-related information, take the following steps to make sure it is credible:

- **Go to the original source.** Media reports often simplify the results of medical research. Find out for yourself what a study really reported, and determine whether it was based on good science. What type of study was it? Was it published in a recognized medical journal? Was it an animal study or did it involve people? Did the study include a large number of people? What did the authors of the study actually report?

- **Watch for misleading language.** Reports that tout "breakthroughs" or "dramatic proof" are probably hype. A study may state that a behavior "contributes to" or is "associated with" an outcome; this does not prove a cause-and-effect relationship.

- **Distinguish between research reports and public health advice.** Do not change your behavior based on the results of a single report or study. If an agency such as the National Cancer Institute urges a behavior change, however, you should

be needed to change behaviors or conditions that are too deeply rooted or too serious for self-management. Don't be stopped by the seriousness of the problem; many resources are available to help you solve it. On campus, the student health center or campus counseling center can provide assistance. To locate community resources, consult the yellow pages, your physician, or the Internet.

Building Motivation to Change

Knowledge is necessary for behavior change, but it isn't usually enough to make people act. Millions of people

follow its advice. Large, publicly funded organizations issue such advice based on many studies, not a single report.

- **Remember that anecdotes are not facts.** A friend may tell you he lost weight on some new diet, but individual success stories do not mean the plan is truly safe or effective. Check with your doctor before making any serious lifestyle changes.

- **Be skeptical.** If a report seems too good to be true, it probably is. Be wary of information contained in advertisements. An ad's goal is to sell a product, even if there is no need for it.

- **Make choices that are right for you.** Friends and family members can be a great source of ideas and inspiration, but you need to make health-related choices that work best for you.

Internet Resources

Online sources pose special challenges; when reviewing a health-related Web site, ask these questions:

- **What is the source of the information?** Web sites maintained by government agencies, professional associations, or established academic or medical institutions are likely to present trustworthy information. Many other groups and individuals post accurate information, but it is important to look at the qualifications of the people who are behind the site. (Check the home page or click the "About Us" link.)

- **How often is the site updated?** Look for sites that are updated frequently. Check the "last modified" date of any Web page.

- **Is the site promotional?** Be wary of information from sites that sell specific products, use testimonials as evidence, appear to have a social or political agenda, or ask for money.

- **What do other sources say about a topic?** Be cautious of claims or information that appears at only one site or comes from a chat room, bulletin board, or blog.

- **Does the site conform to any set of guidelines or criteria for quality and accuracy?** Look for sites that identify themselves as conforming to some code or set of principles, such as those set forth by the Health on the Net Foundation or the American Medical Association. These codes include criteria such as use of information from respected sources and disclosure of the site's sponsors.

have sedentary lifestyles, for example, even though they know it's bad for their health. This is particularly true of young adults, who may not be motivated to change because they feel healthy in spite of their unhealthy behaviors. To succeed at behavior change, you need strong motivation.

Examine the Pros and Cons of Change Health behaviors have short-term and long-term benefits and costs. Consider the benefits and costs of an inactive lifestyle:

- Short-term, such a lifestyle allows you more time to watch TV and hang out with friends, but it leaves you less physically fit and less able to participate in recreational activities.

- Long-term, it increases the risk of heart disease, cancer, stroke, and premature death.

To successfully change your behavior, you must believe that the benefits of change outweigh the costs.

Carefully examine the pros and cons of continuing your current behavior and of changing to a healthier one. Focus on the effects that are most meaningful to you, including those that are tied to your personal identity and values. For example, if you see yourself as an active person who is a good role model for others, then adopting behaviors such as engaging in regular physical activity and getting adequate sleep will support your personal identity. If you value independence and control over your life, then quitting smoking will be consistent with your values and goals. To complete your analysis, ask friends and family members about the effects of your behavior on them. For example, a younger sister may say that your smoking habit influenced her decision to start smoking.

> To change a behavior, you need to recognize that you *are in control* of your actions.

The short-term benefits of behavior change can be an important motivating force. Although some people are motivated by long-term goals, such as avoiding a disease that may hit them in 30 years, most are more likely to be moved to action by shorter-term, more personal goals. Feeling better, doing better in school, improving at a sport, reducing stress, and increasing self-esteem are common short-term benefits of health behavior change.

Boost Self-Efficacy   When you start thinking about changing a health behavior, a big factor in your eventual success is whether you have confidence in yourself and in your ability to change. **Self-efficacy** refers to your belief in your ability to successfully take action and perform a specific task. Strategies for boosting self-efficacy include developing an internal locus of control, using visualization and self-talk, and getting encouragement from supportive people.

LOCUS OF CONTROL   Who do you believe is controlling your life? Is it your parents, friends, or school? Is it "fate"? Or is it you? **Locus of control** refers to the figurative "place" a person designates as the source of responsibility for the events in his or her life. People who believe they are in control of their own lives are said to have an *internal locus of control*. Those who believe that factors beyond their control determine the course of their lives are said to have an *external locus of control*.

For lifestyle management, an internal locus of control is an advantage because it reinforces motivation and commitment. An external locus of control can sabotage efforts to change behavior. For example, if you believe that you are destined to die of breast cancer because your mother died from the disease, you may view monthly breast self-exams and regular checkups as a waste of time. In contrast, if you believe that you can take action to reduce your risk of breast cancer in spite of hereditary factors, you will be motivated to follow guidelines for early detection of the disease.

If you find yourself attributing too much influence to outside forces, gather more information about your wellness-related behaviors. List all the ways that making lifestyle changes will improve your health. If you believe you'll succeed, and if you recognize that you are in charge of your life, you're on your way to wellness.

VISUALIZATION AND SELF-TALK   One of the best ways to boost your confidence and self-efficacy is to visualize yourself successfully engaging in a new, healthier behavior. Imagine yourself going for an afternoon run 3 days a week or no longer smoking cigarettes. Also visualize yourself enjoying all the short-term and long-term benefits that your lifestyle change will bring. Create a new self-image: What will you and your life be like when you become a regular exerciser or a nonsmoker?

You can also use *self-talk*, the internal dialogue you carry on with yourself, to increase your confidence in your ability to change. Counter any self-defeating patterns of thought with more positive or realistic thoughts: "I am a strong, capable person, and I can maintain my commitment to change." See Chapter 3 for more on self-talk.

ROLE MODELS AND SUPPORTIVE PEOPLE   Social support can make a big difference in your level of motivation and your chances of success. Perhaps you know people who have reached the goal you are striving for; they could be role models or mentors for you, providing information and support for your efforts. Gain strength from their experiences, and tell yourself, "If they can do it, so can I." Find a buddy who wants to make the same changes you do and who can take an active role in your behavior change program. For example, an exercise buddy can provide companionship and encouragement when you might be tempted to skip your workout.

IDENTIFY AND OVERCOME BARRIERS TO CHANGE   Don't let past failures at behavior change discourage you. They can be a great source of information you can use to boost your chances of future success. Make a list of the problems and challenges you faced in any previous behavior change attempts; to this, add the short-term costs of behavior change that you identified in your analysis of the pros and

TERMS

self-efficacy   The belief in one's ability to take action and perform a specific task.

locus of control   The figurative "place" a person designates as the source of responsibility for the events in his or her life.

cons of change. Once you've listed these key barriers to change, develop a practical plan for overcoming each one. For example, if you always smoke when you're with certain friends, decide in advance how you will turn down the next cigarette you are offered.

Enhancing Your Readiness to Change

The transtheoretical, or "stages of change," model has been shown to be an effective approach to lifestyle self-management. According to this model, you move through distinct stages as you work to change your target behavior. It is important to determine what stage you are in now so that you can choose appropriate strategies for progressing through the cycle of change. This approach can help you enhance your readiness and intention to change. Read the following sections to determine what stage you are in for your target behavior.

Precontemplation People at this stage do not think they have a problem and do not intend to change their behavior. They may be unaware of the risks associated with their behavior or may deny them. They may have tried unsuccessfully to change in the past and may now think the situation is hopeless. They may also blame other people or external factors for their problems. People in the precontemplation stage believe that there are more reasons or more important reasons not to change than there are reasons to change.

Contemplation People at this stage know they have a problem and intend to take action within 6 months. They acknowledge the benefits of behavior change but are also aware of the costs of changing. To be successful, people must believe that the benefits of change outweigh the costs. People in the contemplation stage wonder about possible courses of action but don't know how to proceed. There may also be specific barriers to change that appear too difficult to overcome.

Preparation People at this stage plan to take action within a month or may already have begun to make small changes in their behavior. They may be engaging in their new, healthier behavior but not yet regularly or consistently. They may have created a plan for change but may be worried about failing.

Action During the action stage, people outwardly modify their behavior and their environment. The action stage requires the greatest commitment of time and energy, and people in this stage are at risk for reverting to old, unhealthy patterns of behavior.

Maintenance People at this stage have maintained their new, healthier lifestyle for at least 6 months. Lapses may have occurred, but people in maintenance have been successful in quickly reestablishing the desired behavior. The maintenance stage can last months or years.

Termination For some behaviors, a person may reach the sixth and final stage of termination. People at this stage have exited the cycle of change and are no longer tempted to lapse back into their old behavior. They have a new self-image and total self-efficacy with regard to their target behavior.

Dealing with Relapse

People seldom progress through the stages of change in a straightforward, linear way; rather, they tend to move to a certain stage and then slip back to a previous stage before resuming their forward progress. Research suggests that most people make several attempts before they successfully change a behavior; 4 out of 5 people experience some degree of backsliding. For this reason, the stages of change are best conceptualized as a spiral, in which people cycle back through previous stages but are further along in the process each time they renew their commitment.

47 million living Americans have stopped smoking.
—CDC, 2010

QUICK STATS

If you experience a lapse (a single slip) or a relapse (a return to old habits) don't give up. Relapse can be demoralizing, but it is not the same as failure; failure means stopping before you reach your goal and never changing your target behavior. During the early stages of the change process, it's a good idea to plan for relapse so you can avoid guilt and self-blame and get back on track quickly.

If relapses keep occurring or you can't seem to control them, you may need to return to a previous stage of the behavior change process. If this is necessary, reevaluate your goals and strategy. A different or less stressful approach may help you avoid setbacks when you try again.

Developing Skills for Change: Creating a Personalized Plan

Once you are committed to making a change, it's time to put together a plan of action. Your key to success is a well-thought-out plan that sets goals, anticipates problems, and includes rewards.

1. Monitor Your Behavior and Gather Data Keep a record of your target behavior and the circumstances surrounding it. Record this information for at least a week or two. Keep your notes in a health journal or notebook or on your computer (see the sample journal entries in Figure 1.3). Record each occurrence of your behavior, noting the following:

- What the activity was
- When and where it happened
- What you were doing
- How you felt at that time

| Date | November 5 | | | | Day | M | TU | W | TH | F | SA | SU | | | |

Time of day	M/S	Food eaten	Cals.	H	Where did you eat?	What else were you doing?	How did someone else influence you?	What made you want to eat what you did?	Emotions and feelings?	Thoughts and concerns?
7:30	M	1 C Crispix cereal 1/2 C skim milk coffee, black 1 C orange juice	110 40 — 120	3	home	reading newspaper	alone	I always eat cereal in the morning	a little keyed up & worried	thinking about quiz in class today
10:30	S	1 apple	90	1	hall outside classroom	studying	alone	felt tired & wanted to wake up	tired	worried about next class
12:30	M	1 C chili 1 roll 1 pat butter 1 orange 2 oatmeal cookies 1 soda	290 120 35 60 120 150	2	campus food court	talking	eating w/ friends; we decided to eat at the food court	wanted to be part of group	excited and happy	interested in hearing everyone's plans for the weekend
	M/S = Meal or snack				H = Hunger rating (0–3)					

FIGURE 1.3 **Sample health journal entries.**

If your goal is to start an exercise program, track your activities to determine how to make time for workouts.

2. Analyze the Data and Identify Patterns After you have collected data on the behavior, analyze the data to identify patterns. When are you most likely to overeat? What events trigger your appetite? Perhaps you are especially hungry at midmorning or when you put off eating dinner until 9:00. Perhaps you overindulge in food and drink when you go to a particular restaurant or when you're with certain friends. Note the connections between your feelings and such external cues as time of day, location, situation, and the actions of others around you.

3. Be "SMART" About Setting Goals If your goals are too challenging, you will have trouble making steady progress and will be more likely to give up altogether. If, for example, you are in poor physical condition, it will not make sense to set a goal of being ready to run a marathon within 2 months. If you set goals you can live with, it will be easier to stick with your behavior change plan and be successful.

Experts suggest that your goals meet the "SMART" criteria; that is, your behavior change goals should be:

- *Specific.* Avoid vague goals like "eat more fruits and vegetables." Instead, state your objectives in specific terms, such as "eat 2 cups of fruit and 3 cups of vegetables every day."

- *Measurable.* Recognize that your progress will be easier to track if your goals are quantifiable, so give your goal a number. You might measure your goal in terms of time (such as "walk briskly for 20 minutes a day"), distance ("run 2 miles, 3 days per week"), or some other amount ("drink 8 glasses of water every day").

- *Attainable.* Set goals that are within your physical limits. For example, if you are a poor swimmer, it might not be possible for you to meet a short-term fitness goal by swimming laps. Walking or biking might be a better option.

- *Realistic.* Manage your expectations when you set goals. For example, it may not be possible for a long-time smoker to quit cold turkey. A more realistic approach might be to use nicotine-replacement patches or gum for several weeks while getting help from a support group.

- *Time frame–specific.* Give yourself a reasonable amount of time to reach your goal, state the time frame in your behavior change plan, and set your agenda to meet the goal within the given time frame.

Using these criteria, a sedentary person who wanted to improve his health and build fitness might set a goal of being able to run 3 miles in 30 minutes, to be achieved within a time frame of 6 months. To work toward that goal, he might set a number of smaller, intermediate goals that are easier to achieve. For example, his list of goals might look like this:

WEEK	FREQUENCY (DAYS/WEEK)	ACTIVITY	DURATION (MINUTES)
1	3	Walk < 1 mile	10–15
2	3	Walk 1 mile	15–20
3	4	Walk 1–2 miles	20–25
4	4	Walk 2–3 miles	25–30
5–7	3–4	Walk/run 1 mile	15–20
⋮			
21–24	4–5	Run 2–3 miles	25–30

4. Devise a Plan of Action   Develop a strategy that will support your efforts to change. Your plan of action should include the following steps:

  • *Get what you need.* Identify resources that can help you. For example, you can join a community walking club or sign up for a smoking cessation program. You may also need to buy some new running shoes or nicotine-replacement patches. Get the items you need right away; waiting can delay your progress.

  • *Modify your environment.* If there are cues in your environment that trigger your target behavior, try to control them. For example, if you normally have alcohol at home, getting rid of it can help prevent you from indulging. If you usually study with a group of friends in an environment that allows smoking, try moving to a non-smoking area. If you always buy a snack at a certain vending machine, change your route so you don't pass by it.

  • *Control related habits.* You may have habits that contribute to your target behavior; modifying these habits can help change the behavior. For example, if you usually plop down on the sofa while watching TV, try putting an exercise bike in front of the set so you can burn calories while watching your favorite programs.

  • *Reward yourself.* Giving yourself instant, real rewards for good behavior will reinforce your efforts. Plan your rewards; decide in advance what each one will be and how you will earn it. Tie rewards to achieving specific goals or subgoals. For example, you might treat yourself to a movie after a week of avoiding snacks. Make a list of items or events to use as rewards. They should be special to you and preferably unrelated to food or alcohol.

  • *Involve the people around you.* Tell family and friends about your plan, and ask them to help. To help them respond appropriately to your needs, create a specific list of dos and don'ts. For example, ask them to

support you when you set aside time to exercise or avoid second helpings at dinner.

  • *Plan for challenges.* Think about situations and people that might derail your program, and develop ways to cope with them. For example, if you think it will be hard to stick to your usual exercise program during exams, schedule short bouts of physical activity (such as a brisk walk) as stress-reducing study breaks.

5. Make a Personal Contract   A serious personal contract—one that commits you to your word—can result in a higher chance of follow-through than a casual, off-hand promise. Your contract can help prevent procrastination by specifying important dates and can also serve as a reminder of your personal commitment to change.

Your contract should include a statement of your goal and your commitment to reaching it. The contract should also include details, such as the following:

  • The date you will start
  • The steps you will take to measure your progress
  • The strategies you plan to use to promote change
  • The date you expect to reach your final goal

Have someone—preferably someone who will be actively helping you with your program—sign your contract as a witness.

Figure 1.4 shows a sample behavior change contract for someone who is committing to eating more fruit

Your environment contains powerful cues for both positive and negative lifestyle choices. Identifying and using the healthier options available to you throughout the day are a key part of a successful behavior change program.

Behavior Change Contract

1. I, __Tammy Lau__ , agree to __increase my consumption of fruit from__ __1 cup per week to 2 cups per day.__

2. I will begin on _____10/5_____ and plan to reach my goal of __2 cups__ __of fruit per day__ by __12/7__

3. To reach my final goal, I have devised the following schedule of mini-goals. For each step in my program, I will give myself the reward listed.

I will begin to have ½ cup of fruit with breakfast	10/5	see movie
I will begin to have ½ cup of fruit with lunch	10/26	new cd
I will begin to substitute fruit juice for soda 1 time per day	11/16	concert

   My overall reward for reaching my goal will be __trip to beach__

4. I have gathered and analyzed data on my target behavior and have identified the following strategies for changing my behavior: __Keep the__ __fridge stocked with easy-to-carry fruit. Pack fruit in my backpack__ __every day. Buy lunch at place that serves fruit.__

5. I will use the following tools to monitor my progress toward my final goal: __Chart on fridge door__ __Health journal__

   I sign this contract as an indication of my personal commitment to reach my goal: _____*Tammy Lau*_____ __9/28__

   I have recruited a helper who will witness my contract and __also increase__ __his consumption of fruit; eat lunch with me twice a week.__
   _____*Eric March*_____ __9/28__

FIGURE 1.4   A sample behavior change contract.

every day. You can apply the general behavior change planning framework presented in this chapter to any target behavior. Additional examples of behavior change plans appear in the Behavior Change Strategy sections at the end of many chapters in this text. In these sections, you will find specific plans for quitting smoking, starting an exercise program, and making other positive lifestyle changes.

Putting Your Plan into Action

When you're ready to put your plan into action, you need commitment, the resolve to stick with the plan no matter what temptations you encounter. Remember all the reasons you have to make the change—and remember that *you* are the boss. Use all your strategies to make your plan work. Make sure your environment is change-friendly, and get as much support and encouragement from others as possible. Keep track of your progress in your health journal, and give yourself regular rewards. And don't forget to give yourself a pat on the back—congratulate yourself, notice how much better you look or feel, and feel good about how far you've come and how you've gained control of your behavior.

BEING HEALTHY FOR LIFE

Your first few behavior change projects may never go beyond the planning stage. Those that do may not all succeed. But as you begin to see progress and changes, you'll start to experience new and surprising positive feelings about yourself. You'll probably find that you're less likely to buckle under stress. You may accomplish things you never thought possible—winning a race, climbing a mountain, quitting smoking. Being healthy takes extra effort, but the paybacks in energy and vitality are priceless.

Once you've started, don't stop. Remember that maintaining good health is an ongoing process. Tackle one area at a time, but make a careful inventory of your health strengths and weaknesses and lay out a long-range plan. Take on the easier problems first, and then use what you have learned to attack more difficult areas. Keep informed about the latest health news and trends; research is constantly providing new information that directly affects daily choices and habits.

You can't completely control every aspect of your health. At least three other factors—heredity, health care, and environment—play important roles in your well-being. After you quit smoking, for example, you may still be inhaling smoke from other people's cigarettes. Your resolve to eat better foods may suffer a setback when you can't find any healthy choices in vending machines.

But you can make a difference—you can help create an environment around you that supports wellness for everyone. You can help support nonsmoking areas in public places. You can speak up in favor of more nutritious foods and better physical fitness facilities. You can include non-alcoholic drinks at your parties.

You can also work on larger environmental challenges: air and water pollution, traffic congestion, overcrowding and overpopulation, global warming and climate change, toxic and nuclear waste, and many others. These difficult issues need the attention and energy of people who are informed and who care about good health. On every level, from personal to planetary, we can all take an active role in shaping our environment.

Ask Yourself

QUESTIONS FOR CRITICAL THINKING AND REFLECTION

Have you tried to change a behavior in the past, such as exercising more or quitting smoking? How successful were you? Do you feel the need to try again? If so, what would you do differently to improve your chances of success?

TIPS FOR TODAY AND THE FUTURE

You are in charge of your health. Many of the decisions you make every day have an impact on the quality of your life, both now and in the future. By making positive choices, large and small, you help ensure a lifetime of wellness.

RIGHT NOW YOU CAN

- Go for a 15-minute walk.
- Have a piece of fruit for a snack.
- Call a friend and arrange for a time to catch up with each other.
- Start thinking about whether you have a health behavior you'd like to change. If you do, consider the elements of a behavior change strategy. For example, begin a mental list of the pros and cons of the behavior, or talk to someone who can support you in your attempts to change.

IN THE FUTURE YOU CAN

- Stay current on health- and wellness-related news and issues.
- Participate in health awareness and promotion campaigns in your community—for example, support smoking restrictions in local venues.
- Be a role model for someone else who is working on a health behavior you have successfully changed.

SUMMARY

- Wellness is the ability to live life fully, with vitality and meaning. Wellness is dynamic and multidimensional; it incorporates physical, emotional, intellectual, spiritual, interpersonal and social, and environmental dimensions.

- As chronic diseases have become the leading cause of death in the United States, people have recognized that they have greater control over, and greater responsibility for, their health than ever before.

- The Healthy People initiative seeks to achieve a better quality of life for all Americans. The program's broad goals are to eliminate preventable disease, disability, injury, and premature death; achieve health equity for all groups; create social and physical environments that promote good health for all; and promote healthy development and healthy behaviors across every stage of life.

- Health-related differences among people that have implications for wellness can be described in the context of gender, ethnicity, income and education, disability, geographic location, and sexual orientation.

- Although heredity, environment, and health care all play roles in wellness and disease, behavior can mitigate their effects.

- To make lifestyle changes, you need information about yourself, your health habits, and resources available to help you change.

- You can increase your motivation for behavior change by examining the benefits and costs of change, boosting self-efficacy, and identifying and overcoming key barriers to change.

- The "stages of change" model describes six stages that people move through as they try to change their behavior: precontemplation, contemplation, preparation, action, maintenance, and termination.

- A specific plan for change can be developed by (1) monitoring behavior by keeping a journal; (2) analyzing the data; (3) setting specific goals; (4) devising strategies for modifying the environment, rewarding yourself, and involving others; and (5) making a personal contract.

- To start and maintain a behavior change program you need commitment, a well-developed plan, social support, and a system of rewards.

- Although we cannot control every aspect of our health, we can make a difference in helping create an environment that supports wellness for everyone.

FOR MORE INFORMATION

BOOKS

Claiborn, J., and C. Pedrick. 2001. *The Habit Change Workbook: How to Break Bad Habits and Form Good Ones.* Oakland, Ca.: New Harbinger Publications. *Provides step-by-step instructions for identifying and overcoming a variety of unhealthy behaviors, such as poor eating habits, reluctance to exercise, and addictive behavior.*

Komaroff, A. L., ed. 2005. *Harvard Medical School Family Health Guide.* New York: Free Press. *Provides consumer-oriented advice for the prevention and treatment of common health concerns.*

Litin, S. C., ed. 2009. *Mayo Clinic Family Health Book,* 4th ed. New York: HarperCollins Publishers. *A complete health reference for every stage of life, covering thousands of conditions, symptoms, and treatments.*

Murat, B., and G. Stewart. 2009. *Do I Need to See the Doctor? The Home-Treatment Encyclopedia—Written by Medical Doctors—That Lets You Decide,* 2nd ed. New York: John Wiley & Sons. *Fully illustrated, easy-to-read guide to hundreds of common symptoms and ailments, designed to help consumers determine whether they can treat themselves or should seek professional medical attention.*

Prochaska, J. O., J. C. Norcross, and C. C. DiClemente. 1994. *Changing for Good: The Revolutionary Program That Explains the Six Stages of Change and Teaches You How to Free Yourself from Bad Habits.* New York: Morrow. *Outlines the authors' model of behavior change and offers suggestions and advice for each stage of change.*

NEWSLETTERS

Consumer Reports on Health (800-274-7596; http://www.consumerreports.org/oh/index.htm)
Harvard Health Publications (877-649-9457; http://www.health.harvard.edu)
Harvard Men's Health Watch (877-649-9457)
Harvard Women's Health Watch (877-699-9457)
Mayo Clinic Health Letter (800-291-1128)
University of California, Berkeley, Wellness Letter (800-829-9170; http://www.wellnessletter.com)

ORGANIZATIONS, HOTLINES, AND WEB SITES

The Internet addresses (also called uniform resource locators, or URLs) listed here were accurate at the time of publication.

Centers for Disease Control and Prevention. Through phone, fax, and the Internet, the CDC provides a wide variety of health information.
http://www.cdc.gov

Federal Trade Commission: Consumer Protection — Health. Includes online brochures about a variety of consumer health topics, including fitness equipment, generic drugs, and fraudulent health claims.
http://www.ftc.gov/bcp/menus/consumer/health.shtm

FirstGov for Consumers: Health. Provides links to online brochures from a variety of government agencies.
http://consumer.gov/ncpw/category/health

Healthfinder. A gateway to online publications, Web sites, support and self-help groups, and agencies and organizations that produce reliable health information.
http://www.healthfinder.gov

Healthy Campus 2010. The American College Health Association's introduction to the Healthy Campus program.
http://www.acha.org/info_resources/hc2010.cfm

Healthy People 2010. Provides information on Healthy People objectives and priority areas.
http://www.healthypeople.gov

MedlinePlus. Provides links to news and reliable information about health from government agencies and professional associations; also includes a health encyclopedia and information on prescription and over-the-counter drugs.
http://www.medlineplus.gov

National Health Information Center (NHIC). Puts consumers in touch with the organizations that are best able to provide answers to health-related questions.
http://www.health.gov/nhic

National Institutes of Health. Provides information about all NIH activities as well as consumer publications, hotline information, and an A to Z listing of health issues with links to the appropriate NIH institute.
http://www.nih.gov

National Wellness Institute. Serves professionals and organizations that promote optimal health and wellness.
http://www.nationalwellness.org

National Women's Health Information Center. Provides information and answers to frequently asked questions.
http://www.womenshealth.gov

Office of Minority Health Resource Center. Promotes improved health among racial and ethnic minority populations.
http://minorityhealth.hhs.gov

Surgeon General. Includes information on activities of the Surgeon General and the text of many key reports on such topics as tobacco use, physical activity, and mental health.
http://www.surgeongeneral.gov

World Health Organization (WHO). Provides information about health topics and issues affecting people around the world.
http://www.who.int

The following are just a few of the many sites that provide consumer-oriented information on a variety of health issues:

CNN Health: http://www.cnn.com/health
FamilyDoctor.Org: http://familydoctor.org/online/famdocen/home.html
InteliHealth: http://www.intelihealth.com
MayoClinic.com: http://www.mayoclinic.com
MedlinePlus News: http://nlm.nih.gov/medlineplus/newsbydate.html
MedPage Today Medical News: http://www.medpagetoday.com
WebMD: http://www.webmd.com
Yahoo Health News: http://news.yahoo.com/health

SELECTED BIBLIOGRAPHY

American Cancer Society. 2010. *Cancer Facts and Figures—2010.* Atlanta: American Cancer Society.

American Heart Association. 2010. *Heart Disease and Stroke Statistics—2010 Update.* Dallas: American Heart Association.

Banks, J., et al. 2006. Disease and disadvantage in the United States and in England. *Journal of the American Medical Association* 295(17): 2037–2045.

Barr, D. A. 2008. *Health Disparities in the United States: Social Class, Race, Ethnicity, and Health.* Baltimore: The Johns Hopkins University Press.

Beckman, M. 2007. Help wanted: In the pursuit of a healthy lifestyle, sheer grit only takes you so far. *Stanford Medicine Magazine* 24(3).

Centers for Disease Control and Prevention. 2008. Racial/ethnic disparities in self-rated health status among adults with and without disabilities—United States, 2004–2006. *Morbidity and Mortality Weekly Report* 57(39): 1069–1073.

Centers for Disease Control and Prevention. 2010. *Racial and Ethnic Approaches to Community Health (REACH U.S.): Finding Solutions to Health Disparities, 2010* (http://www.cdc.gov/chronicdisease/resources/publications/AAG/reach.html; retrieved October 23, 2010).

Finkelstein, E. A., et al. 2008. Do obese persons comprehend their personal health risks? *American Journal of Health Behavior* 32(5): 508–516.

Flegal, K. M., et al. 2005. Excess deaths associated with underweight, overweight, and obesity. *Journal of the American Medical Association* 293 (15): 1861–1867.

Flegal, K. M., et al. 2007. Cause-specific excess deaths associated with underweight, overweight, and obesity. *Journal of the American Medical Association* 298(17): 2028–2037.

Flegal, K. M., et al. 2010. Prevalence and trends in obesity among U.S. adults, 1999–2008. *Journal of the American Medical Association* 3033: 235–241.

Gorman, B. K., and J. G. Read. 2006. Gender disparities in adult health: An examination of three measures of morbidity. *Journal of Health and Social Behavior* 47(2): 95–110.

Herd, P., et al. 2007. Socioeconomic position and health: The differential effects of education versus income on the onset versus progression of health problems. *Journal of Health and Social Behavior* 48(3): 223–238.

Horneffer-Ginter, K. 2008. Stages of change and possible selves: Two tools for promoting college health. *Journal of American College Health* 56(4): 351–358.

Martin, G., and J. Pear. 2007. *Behaviour Modification: What It Is and How to Do It,* 8th ed. Upper Saddle River, N.J.: Prentice-Hall.

Mokdad, A. H., et al. 2004. Actual causes of death in the United States, 2000. *Journal of the American Medical Association* 291(10): 1238–1245.

Mokdad, A. H., et al. 2005. Correction: Actual causes of death in the United States, 2000. *Journal of the American Medical Association* 293(3): 293–294.

National Center for Health Statistics. 2009. *Health, United States, 2009.* Hyattsville, Md.: National Center for Health Statistics.

National Center for Health Statistics. 2010. Deaths: Final data for 2007. *National Vital Statistics Report* 58(19).

National Center for Health Statistics. 2010. Health behaviors of adults: United States, 2005–07. *Vital and Health Statistics* 10(245).

Nothwehr, F., et al. 2008. Age group differences in diet and physical activity-related behaviors among rural men and women. *Journal of Nutrition, Health and Aging* 12(3): 169–174.

O'Loughlin, J., et al. 2007. Lifestyle risk factors for chronic disease across family origin among adults in multiethnic, low-income, urban neighborhoods. *Ethnicity and Disease* 17(4): 657–663.

Participants at the 6th Global Conference on Health Promotion. 2005. The Bangkok Charter for health promotion in a globalized world. Geneva, Switzerland: World Health Organization, Aug. 11. Accessed 2010.

Pinkhasov, R. M., et al. 2010. Are men shortchanged on health? Perspective on health care utilization and health risk behavior in men and women in the United States. *International Journal of Clinical Practice* 64(4): 475–487.

Song, J., et al. 2006. Gender differences across race/ethnicity in use of health care among Medicare-aged Americans. *Journal of Women's Health* 15(10): 1205–1213.

U.C. Berkeley. 2010 Update. *Evaluating Web Pages: Techniques to Apply and Questions to Ask* (http://www.lib.berkeley.edu/TeachingLib/Guides/Internet/Evaluate.html; retrieved May 10, 2010).

U.S. Census Bureau. 2005. *We the People: Women and Men in the United States.* Washington, D.C.: U.S. Census Bureau.

U.S. Census Bureau. 2009. *The 2008 American Community Survey: Hispanic or Latino Origin by Race.* Washington, D.C.: U.S. Census Bureau.

Walker, B., and C. P. Mouton. 2008. Environmental influences on cardiovascular health. *Journal of the National Medical Association* 100(1): 98–102.

Walsh, T., et al. 2006. Spectrum of mutations in BRCA1, BRCA2, CHEK2, and TP53 in families at high risk of breast cancer. *Journal of the American Medical Association* 295: 1379–1388.

World Health Organization. 2008. *Why Gender and Health?* (http://www.who.int/gender/genderandhealth/en; retrieved May 10, 2010).

World Health Organization. 2010 Update. *Gender Inequalities and HIV/AIDS* (http://www.who.int/gender/hiv_aids/en; retrieved May 10, 2010).

LOOKING AHEAD...

After reading this chapter, you should be able to:

- Explain what stress is and how people react to it—physically, emotionally, and behaviorally
- Describe the relationship between stress and disease
- List common sources of stress
- Describe techniques for preventing and managing stress
- Put together a plan for successfully managing the stress in your life

Stress: The Constant Challenge

2

L ike the term *wellness, stress* is a word many people use without really understanding its precise meaning. Stress is popularly viewed as an uncomfortable response to a negative event, which probably describes *nervous tension* more than the cluster of physical and psychological responses that actually constitute stress. In fact, stress is not limited to negative situations; it is also a response to pleasurable physical challenges and the achievement of personal goals. Whether stress is experienced as pleasant or unpleasant depends largely on the situation and the individual. Because learning effective responses to stress can enhance psychological health and help prevent a number of serious diseases, stress management can be an important part of daily life.

As a college student, you may be in one of the most stressful times of your life. This chapter explains the physiological and psychological reactions that make up the stress response and describes how these reactions can be risks to good health. The chapter also presents methods of managing stress.

WHAT IS STRESS?

In common usage, the term *stress* refers to two different things: situations that trigger physical and emotional reactions, *and* the reactions themselves. This text uses the more precise term **stressor** for a situation that triggers physical and emotional reactions and the term **stress response** for those reactions. A first date and a final exam are examples of stressors; sweaty palms and a pounding heart are symptoms of the stress response. We'll use the term **stress** to describe the general physical and emotional state that accompanies the stress response. So, a person taking a final exam experiences stress.

Each individual's experience of stress depends on many factors, including the nature of the stressor and how it is perceived. Stressors take many different forms. Some occur suddenly and don't last long or repeat, like a fire in the building you live in. Others, like air pollution or quarreling parents, can continue for a long time. The memory of a stressor can itself be a stressor years after the event, such as the memory of the loss of a loved one. Responses to stressors can include a wide variety of physical, emotional, and behavioral changes. A short-term response might be an upset stomach or insomnia, whereas a long-term response might be a change in your personality or social relations.

Physical Responses to Stressors

Imagine a near miss: As you step off the curb, a car careens toward you. With just a fraction of a second to spare, you leap safely out of harm's way. In that split second of danger and in the moments following it, you experience a predictable series of physical reactions. Your body goes from a relaxed state to one prepared for physical action to cope with a threat to your life.

Two systems in your body are responsible for your physical response to stressors: the nervous system and the endocrine system. Through rapid chemical reactions affecting almost every part of your body, you are primed to act quickly and appropriately in time of danger.

Actions of the Nervous System   The nervous system consists of the brain, spinal cord, and nerves. Part of the nervous system is under voluntary control, as when you tell your arm to reach for a chocolate. The part that is not under conscious supervision—for example, the part that controls the digestion of the chocolate—is the **autonomic nervous system.** In addition to digestion, it controls your heart rate, breathing, blood pressure, and hundreds of other involuntary functions.

The autonomic nervous system consists of two divisions:

- The **parasympathetic division** is in control when you are relaxed; it aids in digesting food, storing energy, and promoting growth.
- The **sympathetic division** is activated during times of arousal, including exercise, and when there is an emergency, such as severe pain, anger, or fear.

Sympathetic nerves use the neurotransmitter **norepinephrine** to exert their actions on nearly every organ, sweat gland, blood vessel, and muscle to enable your body to handle an emergency. In general, the sympathetic division commands your body to stop storing energy and to use it in response to a crisis.

Actions of the Endocrine System   During stress, the sympathetic nervous system triggers the **endocrine system.** This system of glands, tissues, and cells helps control body functions by releasing **hormones** and other chemical messengers into the bloodstream to influence metabolism and other body processes. These chemicals act on a variety of targets throughout the body. Along with the nervous system, the endocrine system prepares the body to respond to a stressor.

The Two Systems Together   How do both systems work together in an emergency? Let's go back to your near collision with a car. Both reflexes and higher cognitive

areas in your brain quickly make the decision that you are facing a threat—and your body prepares to meet the danger. Chemical messages and actions of sympathetic nerves cause the release of key hormones, including **cortisol** and **epinephrine.** These hormones trigger the physiological changes shown in Figure 2.1, including these:

- Heart and respiration rates accelerate to speed oxygen through the body.
- Hearing and vision become more acute.
- The liver releases extra sugar into the bloodstream to boost energy.
- Perspiration increases to cool the skin.
- The brain releases **endorphins**—chemicals that can inhibit or block sensations of pain—in case you are injured.

Taken together, these almost-instantaneous physical changes are called the **fight-or-flight reaction.** They give

Pupils dilate to admit extra light for more sensitive vision.

Mucous membranes of nose and throat shrink, while muscles force a wider opening of air passages to allow easier airflow.

Secretion of saliva and mucus decreases; digestive activities halt in an emergency.

Air passages dilate to allow more air into lungs.

Perspiration increases, especially in armpits, groin, hands, and feet, to flush out waste and cool the overheating body by evaporation.

Liver releases sugar into bloodstream to provide energy for muscles and brain.

Muscles of intestines stop contracting because digestion has halted.

Bladder relaxes. Emptying of bladder contents releases excess weight, making it easier to flee.

Blood vessels in skin and internal organs contract; those in skeletal muscles dilate. This increases blood pressure and delivery of blood to where it is most needed.

Endorphins are released to block any distracting pain.

Hearing becomes more acute.

Heart accelerates rate of beating, increases strength of contraction to allow more blood flow where it is needed.

Digestion, an unnecessary activity during an emergency, halts.

Spleen releases more red blood cells to meet an increased demand for oxygen and to replace any blood lost from injuries.

Adrenal glands stimulate secretion of epinephrine, increasing blood sugar, blood pressure, and heart rate; also spur increase in amount of fat in blood. These changes provide an energy boost.

Pancreas decreases secretions because digestion has halted.

Fat is removed from storage and broken down to supply extra energy.

Voluntary (skeletal) muscles contract throughout the body, readying them for action.

FIGURE 2.1   The fight-or-flight reaction. In response to a stressor, the autonomic nervous system and the endocrine system prepare the body to deal with an emergency.

you the heightened reflexes and strength you need to dodge the car or deal with other stressors. Although these physical changes may vary in intensity, the same basic set of physical reactions occurs in response to any type of stressor—positive or negative, physical or psychological.

The Return to Homeostasis   Once a stressful situation ends, the parasympathetic division of your autonomic nervous system takes command and halts the stress response. It restores **homeostasis,** a state in which blood pressure, heart rate, hormone levels, and other vital functions are maintained within a narrow range of normal. Your parasympathetic nervous system calms your body down, slowing a rapid heartbeat, drying sweaty palms, and returning breathing to normal. Gradually, your body resumes its normal "housekeeping" functions, such as digestion and temperature regulation. Damage that may have been sustained during the fight-or-flight reaction is repaired. The day after you narrowly dodge the car, you feel fine. In this way, your body can grow, repair itself, and acquire new reserves of energy. When the next crisis comes, you'll be ready to respond again, instantly.

The Fight-or-Flight Reaction in Modern Life   The fight-or-flight reaction is a part of our biological heritage, and it's a survival mechanism that has served humans well. In modern life, however, it is often absurdly inappropriate. Many stressors we face in everyday life do not

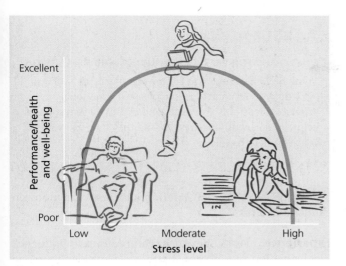

FIGURE 2.2   Stress level, performance, and well-being.
A moderate level of stress challenges individuals in a way that promotes optimal performance and well-being. Too little stress, and people are not challenged enough to improve; too much stress, and the challenges become stressors that can impair physical and emotional health.

require a physical response—for example, an exam, a mess left by a roommate, or a stop light. The fight-or-flight reaction prepares the body for physical action regardless of whether such action is a necessary or appropriate response to a particular stressor.

Emotional and Behavioral Responses to Stressors

We all experience a similar set of physical responses to stressors, which make up the fight-or-flight reaction. These responses, however, vary from person to person and from one situation to another. People's perceptions of potential stressors—and of their reactions to such stressors—also vary greatly. Remember, however, that not all stressors are negative. A certain amount of stress, if coped with appropriately, can help promote optimal performance (Figure 2.2).

Effective and Ineffective Responses   Common emotional responses to stressors include anxiety, depression, and fear. Although emotional responses are determined in part by inborn personality or temperament, we often can moderate or learn to control them. Coping techniques are discussed later in the chapter.

Behavioral responses to stressors—controlled by the **somatic nervous system,** which manages our conscious actions—are entirely under our control. Effective behavioral responses such as talking, laughing, exercising, meditating, learning time-management skills, and becoming more assertive can promote wellness and enable us to function at our best. Ineffective behavioral responses to stressors include overeating, expressing hostility, and using tobacco, alcohol, or other drugs.

Personality and Stress   Some people seem to be nervous, irritable, and easily upset by minor annoyances. Others are calm and composed even in difficult situations. Scientists remain unsure just why this is or how the brain's complex emotional mechanisms work. But **personality**—the sum of cognitive, behavioral, and emotional tendencies—clearly affects how people perceive and react to stressors. To investigate the links among personality, stress, and wellness, researchers examine different clusters of characteristics, or "personality types."

- **Type A.** People with Type A personality are described as ultracompetitive, controlling, impatient, aggressive, and even hostile. Type A people have a higher perceived stress level and more problems coping with stress. They react explosively to stressors and are upset by events that others would consider only annoyances. Studies indicate that certain characteristics of the Type A pattern—anger, cynicism, and hostility—increase the risk of heart disease.
- **Type B.** The Type B personality is relaxed and contemplative. Type B people are less frustrated by daily events and more tolerant of the behavior of others.
- **Type C.** The Type C personality is characterized by anger suppression, difficulty expressing emotions, feelings of hopelessness and despair, and an exaggerated response to minor stressors. This heightened response may impair immune functions.

Studies of Type A and C personalities suggest that expressing emotions is beneficial but habitually expressing exaggerated stress responses or hostility is unhealthy.

Researchers have also looked for personality traits that enable people to deal more successfully with stress. One such trait is *hardiness,* a particular form of optimism. People with a hardy personality view potential stressors as challenges and opportunities for growth and learning, rather than as burdens. They see fewer situations as stressful, and react less intensely to stress than nonhardy persons might. Hardy people are committed to their activities, have a sense of inner purpose and an inner locus of control, and feel at least partly in control of their lives.

QUICK STATS

85% of college students report feeling overwhelmed by their workload at least once in the last year.

—American College Health Association National College Health Assessment II, 2009

TERMS

somatic nervous system   The branch of the peripheral nervous system that governs motor functions and sensory information, largely under conscious control.

personality   The sum of behavioral, cognitive, and emotional tendencies.

The term *resilience* refers to personality traits associated with social and academic success in at-risk populations, such as people from low-income families and those with mental or physical disabilities. Resilient people tend to set goals and face adversity through individual effort. There are three basic types of resilience, and each one determines how a person responds to stress:

- *Nonreactive resilience,* in which a person does not react to a stressor
- *Homeostatic resilience,* in which a person may react strongly but returns to baseline functioning quickly
- *Positive growth resilience,* in which a person learns and grows from the stress experience

Resilience is associated with emotional intelligence and violence prevention.

You probably can't change your basic personality, but you can change your typical behaviors and patterns of thinking. You can also use positive stress-management techniques like those described later in the chapter.

Cultural Background   Young adults from around the world come to America for a higher education; most students finish college with a greater appreciation for other cultures and worldviews. The clashing of cultures, however, can be a big source of stress for many students—especially when it leads to disrespectful treatment, harassment, or violence. It is important to remember that everyone's reaction to stress is influenced by his or her family and cultural background. Learning to accept and appreciate the cultural backgrounds of other people is both a mind-opening experience and a way to avoid stress over cultural differences.

Gender   Our **gender role**—the activities, abilities, and behaviors our culture expects of us based on our sex—can affect our experience of stress. Some behavioral responses to stressors, such as crying or openly expressing anger, may be deemed more appropriate for one gender than the other.

Strict adherence to gender roles, however, can limit one's response to stress and can itself become a source of stress. Gender roles can also affect one's perception of a stressor. If a man derives most of his self-worth from his work, for example, retirement may be more stressful for him than for a woman whose self-image is based on several different roles.

See the box "Women, Men, and Stress" for more on gender and stress.

Experience   Past experiences can profoundly influence the evaluation of a potential stressor. Consider someone who has had a bad experience giving a speech in the past. He or she is much more likely to perceive an upcoming speech as stressful than someone who has had positive public speaking experiences.

STRESS AND HEALTH

According to the American Psychological Association, 43% of adult Americans suffer from stress-related health problems. The role of stress in health is complex, but evidence suggests that stress can increase vulnerability to many ailments. Several theories have been proposed to explain the relationship between stress and disease.

The General Adaptation Syndrome

Biologist Hans Selye was one of the first scientists to develop a comprehensive theory of stress and disease. Based on his work in the 1930s and 1940s, Selye coined the term **general adaptation syndrome (GAS)** to describe what he believed to be a universal and predictable response pattern to all stressors. As mentioned earlier, some stressors are pleasant (such as attending a party), and others are unpleasant (such as getting a bad grade). In the GAS theory, the stress triggered by a pleasant stressor is called **eustress;** stress brought on by an unpleasant stressor is called **distress.** The sequence of physical responses associated with GAS is the same for eustress and distress and occurs in three stages (Figure 2.3):

- *Alarm.* The alarm stage includes the complex sequence of events brought on by the fight-or-flight reaction. At this stage, the body is more susceptible to disease or injury because it is geared up to deal with a crisis. Someone in this stage may experience headaches, indigestion, anxiety, and disrupted eating or sleep patterns.
- *Resistance.* With continued stress, the body develops a new level of homeostasis in which it is more resistant to disease and injury than usual. In this stage, a person can cope with normal life and added stress.

Women, Men, and Stress

Men and women alike experience stress, but they experience it differently.

Women and Stress

Women are more likely than men to find themselves balancing multiple roles, such as those of student, spouse, and parent. Women who work outside the home still do most of the housework—although today's husbands are helping in greater numbers than previous generations did—and housework isn't limited to cleaning or doing laundry. For example, more than 60% of women make all decisions about their family's health care, including decisions about elderly parents. The combined pressures of home, workplace, and school can create very high stress levels.

Men and Stress

Men who fit a traditional male gender role may feel compelled to be in charge at all times. This may create tension in interpersonal situations and limit men's ability to build a support network. Such men may keenly feel the responsibility to support a family, which can compound existing pressures at home and work.

Perceptions of Stress

In late 2009, the American Psychological Association released the results of its annual "Stress in America" survey. The survey shows the different views American men and women have of their personal stress. Respondents said stress affects them in the following ways:

	Women	Men
Irritability or anger	51%	39%
Fatigue	49%	37%
Urge to cry	46%	16%
Lack of interest, motivation, energy	45%	35%
Headache	43%	24%
Feeling depressed or sad	42%	26%

The survey also shows that women are more likely than men to cope with stress through behaviors such as overeating or taking prescription medications.

Physiological Differences

Levels of testosterone (the primary male hormone, responsible for many masculine traits) increase from puberty onward, so men tend to have higher blood pressure than women of the same age. This factor contributes to greater wear on the male circulatory system, sometimes increasing a man's risk for cardiovascular disease. A part of the brain that regulates emotions, the amygdala, is sensitive to testosterone. This may be one reason that men are more likely than women to find certain situations (such as social interactions) to be stressful.

Conversely, women have higher levels of oxytocin (a hormone involved in social interaction and mood regulation) and are more likely to respond to stressors by seeking social support. This coping response may give women a longevity advantage over men by decreasing the risk of some stress-related disorders. It does not, however, free women from stress-related ailments, and women are more likely than men to suffer from stress-related hypertension, depression, and obesity.

connect
ACTIVITY

• *Exhaustion.* The first two stages of GAS require a great deal of energy. If a stressor persists, or if several stressors occur in succession, general exhaustion sets in. This is not the sort of exhaustion you feel after a long, busy day. Rather, it's a life-threatening type of physiological exhaustion.

Allostatic Load

Although the GAS model is still viewed as a key conceptual contribution to the understanding of stress, some aspects of it are outdated. For example, increased susceptibility to disease after repeated or prolonged stress is now thought to be due to the effects of the stress response itself rather than to a depletion of resources (exhaustion state). In particular, long-term overexposure to stress hormones such as cortisol has been linked with health problems. Further, although physical stress reactions promote homeostasis (resistance stage), they also have negative effects on the body.

Level of normal resistance to injury

| Alarm reaction | Stage of resistance | Stage of exhaustion |

FIGURE 2.3   The general adaptation syndrome. During the alarm phase, a lower resistance to injury is evident. With continued stress, resistance to injury is actually enhanced. With prolonged exposure to repeated stressors, exhaustion sets in, with a return of low resistance levels seen during acute stress.

The long-term wear and tear of the stress response is called the **allostatic load**. A person's allostatic load depends on many factors, including genetics, life experiences, and emotional and behavioral responses to stressors. A high allostatic load may be due to frequent stressors, poor adaptation to common stressors, an inability to shut down the stress response, or imbalances in the stress response of different body systems. High allostatic load is linked to heart disease, hypertension, obesity, and reduced brain and immune system functioning. In other words, when your allostatic load exceeds your ability to cope, you are more likely to get sick.

Psychoneuroimmunology

One of the most fruitful areas of current research into the relationship between stress and disease is **psychoneuroimmunology (PNI).** PNI is the study of the interactions among the nervous system, the endocrine system, and the immune system. The underlying premise of PNI is that stress, through the actions of the nervous and endocrine systems, impairs the immune system and thereby affects health.

A complex network of nerve and chemical connections exists among the nervous, endocrine, and immune systems. In general, increased levels of cortisol are linked to a decreased number of immune system cells, or lymphocytes (see Chapter 13 for more on the immune system). Epinephrine appears to promote the release of lymphocytes but at the same time reduces their efficiency. Scientists have identified hormone-like substances called *neuropeptides* that appear to translate stressful emotions into biochemical events, some of which impact the immune system, providing a physical link between emotions and immune function.

Different types of stress may affect immunity in different ways. For instance, during **acute stress** (typically lasting between 5 and 100 minutes), white blood cells move into the skin, where they enhance the immune response. During a stressful event sequence, such as a personal trauma and the events that follow, however, there are typically no overall significant immune changes. Chronic (ongoing) stressors such as unemployment have negative effects on almost all functional measures of immunity. **Chronic stress** may cause prolonged secretion of cortisol and may accelerate the course of diseases that involve inflammation, including multiple sclerosis, heart disease, and type 2 diabetes.

Ask yourself

QUESTIONS FOR CRITICAL THINKING AND REFLECTION

Have you ever been so stressed that you felt ill in some way? If so, what were your symptoms? How did you handle them? Did the experience affect the way you reacted to other stressful events?

Mood, personality, behavior, and immune functioning are intertwined. For example, people who are generally pessimistic may neglect the basics of health care, become passive when ill, and fail to engage in health-promoting behaviors. People who are depressed may reduce physical activity and social interaction, which may in turn affect the immune system and the cognitive appraisal of a stressor. Optimism, successful coping, and positive problem solving, on the other hand, may positively influence immunity.

Links Between Stress and Specific Conditions

Although much remains to be learned, it is clear that people who have unresolved chronic stress in their lives or who handle stressors poorly are at risk for a wide range of health problems. In the short term, the problem might be just a cold, a stiff neck, or a stomachache. Over the long term, the problems can be more severe—cardiovascular disease (CVD), high blood pressure, impaired immune function, or a host of other problems.

Cardiovascular Disease   During the stress response, heart rate increases and blood vessels constrict, causing blood pressure to rise. Chronic high blood pressure is a major cause of *atherosclerosis*, a disease in which blood vessels become damaged and caked with fatty deposits. These deposits can block arteries, causing heart attacks and strokes.

Certain types of emotional responses may increase a person's risk of CVD. As described earlier, people who tend to react to situations with anger and hostility are more likely to have heart attacks than are people with a less explosive, more trusting personality.

STATS

6.2% of American males and 8.3% of females age 18–21 suffer serious psychological distress.

—National Survey of Drug Use & Health, 2008

Psychological Problems   The hormones and other chemicals released during the stress response cause emotional as well as physical changes. Stress also activates the

Headaches: A Common Symptom of Stress

More than 45 million Americans suffer from chronic, recurrent headaches. Headaches come in various types but are often grouped into three major categories: tension headaches, migraines, and cluster headaches. Other types of headaches have underlying organic causes, such as sinus congestion or infection.

Tension Headaches

Approximately 90% of all headaches are *tension headaches*, characterized by a dull, steady pain, usually on both sides of the head. It may feel as though a band of pressure is tightening around the head, and the pain may extend to the neck and shoulders. Acute tension headaches may last from hours to days, while chronic tension headaches may occur almost every day for months or even years.

Psychological stress, poor posture, and immobility are the leading causes of tension headaches. There is no cure, but the pain can sometimes be relieved with over-the-counter painkillers and with therapies such as massage, acupuncture, relaxation, hot or cold showers, and rest.

If your headaches are frequent, keep a diary with details about the events surrounding each one. If you can identify the stressors that are consistently associated with your headaches, you can begin to gain more control over the situation. If you suffer persistent tension headaches, you should consult your physician.

Migraines

Migraines typically progress through a series of stages lasting from several minutes to several days. They may produce a variety of symptoms, including throbbing pain that starts on one side of the head and may spread; heightened sensitivity to light; visual disturbances such as flashing lights; nausea; and fatigue. About 70% of migraine sufferers are women, and migraine headaches may have a genetic component.

Research suggests that people who get migraines may have abnormally excitable nerve cells in their brains. When triggered, these nerve cells send a wave of electrical activity throughout the brain, which in turn causes migraine symptoms. Potential triggers include menstruation, stress, fatigue, atmospheric changes, specific sounds or odors, and certain foods. The frequency of attacks varies from a few in a lifetime to several per week.

Keeping a headache journal can help a migraine sufferer identify headache triggers—the first step to avoiding them. In addition, many new treatments can help reduce the frequency, severity, and duration of migraines.

Cluster Headaches

Cluster headaches are extremely severe headaches that cause intense pain in and around one eye. They usually occur in clusters of one to three headaches

each day over a period of weeks or months, alternating with periods of remission in which no headaches occur. About 90% of people with cluster headaches are male.

There is no known cause or cure for cluster headaches, but a number of treatments are available. During cluster periods, it is important to refrain from smoking cigarettes and drinking alcohol, because these activities can trigger attacks.

---

enzyme PKC, which influences the brain's prefrontal cortex. Excess PKC can negatively affect focus, judgment, and the ability to think clearly. Moreover, many stressors are inherently anxiety-producing, depressing, or both. Stress has been found to contribute to psychological problems such as depression, panic attacks, anxiety, eating disorders, and post-traumatic stress disorder (PTSD). PTSD, which afflicts war veterans, rape and child abuse survivors, and others who have suffered or witnessed severe trauma, is characterized by nightmares, flashbacks, and a diminished capacity to experience or express emotion.

Altered Functioning of the Immune System PNI research helps explain how stress affects the immune system. Some of the health problems linked to stress-related changes in immune function include vulnerability to

colds and other infections, asthma and allergy attacks, susceptibility to cancer, and flare-ups of chronic diseases such as genital herpes and HIV infection.

Other Health Problems Many other health problems may be caused or worsened by excessive stress, including the following:

- Digestive problems such as stomachaches, diarrhea, constipation, irritable bowel syndrome, and ulcers
- Tension headaches and migraines (see the box "Headaches: A Common Symptom of Stress")
- Insomnia and fatigue
- Injuries, including on-the-job injuries caused by repetitive strain
- Menstrual irregularities, impotence, and pregnancy complications

COMMON SOURCES OF STRESS

Recognizing potential sources of stress is an important step in successfully managing the stress in your life.

Major Life Changes

Any major change in your life that requires adjustment and accommodation can be a source of stress. Early adulthood and the college years are associated with many significant changes, such as moving out of the family home. Even changes typically thought of as positive—graduation, job promotion, marriage—can be stressful.

Clusters of life changes, particularly those that are perceived negatively, may be linked to health problems in some people. Personality and coping skills, however, are important moderating influences. People with a strong support network and a stress-resistant personality are less likely to become ill in response to life changes than people with fewer resources.

Daily Hassles

Although major life changes are stressful, they seldom occur regularly. Researchers have proposed that minor problems—life's daily hassles, such as losing your keys or wallet—can be an even greater source of stress because they occur much more often.

People who perceive hassles negatively are likely to experience a moderate stress response every time they are faced with one. Over time, this can take a significant toll on health. Studies indicate that for some people, daily hassles contribute to a general decrease in overall wellness.

College Stressors

College is a time of major changes and minor hassles. For many students, college means being away from home and family for the first time. Nearly all students share stresses like the following:

- *Academic stress.* Exams, grades, and an endless workload await every college student but can be especially troublesome for students just out of high school.
- *Interpersonal stress.* Most students are more than just students; they are also friends, children, employees, spouses, parents, and so on. Managing relationships while juggling the rigors of college life can be daunting, especially if some friends or family are less than supportive.
- *Time pressures.* Class schedules, assignments, and deadlines are an inescapable part of college life. But these time pressures can be drastically compounded for students who also have a job and/or family responsibilities.

- *Financial concerns.* The majority of college students need financial aid not just to cover the cost of tuition but to survive from day to day while in school. For many, college life isn't possible without a job, and the pressure to stay afloat financially competes with academic and other stressors.
- *Worries about the future.* As college life comes to an end, students face life after college. This means thinking about a career, choosing a place to live, and leaving the friends and routines of school behind.

As mentioned earlier, test anxiety is a source of stress for many students. To learn some proven techniques for overcoming test anxiety, see the Behavior Change Strategy at the end of this chapter.

Job-Related Stressors

Americans rate their jobs as a key source of stress in their lives. According to the 2009 Stress in America survey, about 41% of working Americans say they typically feel tense or stressed out while at work. Tight schedules and overtime leave little time to exercise, socialize, and engage in other stress-proofing activities. While daily work activities can be stressful enough on their own, stress can be even worse for people who are left out of important decisions relating to their jobs. When workers are given the opportunity to shape how their jobs are performed, job satisfaction goes up and stress levels go down.

If job-related (or college-related) stress is severe or chronic, the result can be **burnout,** a state of physical, mental, and emotional exhaustion. Burnout occurs most often in highly motivated and driven individuals who come to feel that their work is not recognized or that they are not accomplishing their goals. People in the helping professions—teachers, social workers, caregivers, police officers, and so on—are also prone to burnout. For some people who suffer from burnout, a vacation or leave of absence may be appropriate. For others, a reduced work schedule, better communication with superiors, or a change in job goals may be necessary. Improving time-management skills can also help.

Social Stressors

Social networks can be real or virtual. Both types can help improve your ability to deal with stress, but any social network can also become a stressor in itself.

Real Social Networks Although social support is a key buffer against stress, your interactions with others can themselves be a source of stress. The college years, in particular, can be a time of great change in interpersonal relationships. The larger community where you live can also act as a stressor.

Social stressors include prejudice and discrimination. You may feel stress as you try to relate to people of other ethnic or socioeconomic groups. If you are a member of a

TERMS

burnout A state of physical, mental, and emotional exhaustion.

Diverse Populations, Discrimination, and Stress

Stress is universal, but in diverse multiethnic and multicultural nations such as the United States, some groups face special stressors and have higher-than-average rates of stress-related physical and emotional problems. These groups include ethnic minorities, the poor, those with physical or mental disabilities, and those with atypical sexual orientations.

Discrimination occurs when people speak or act according to their prejudices—biased, negative beliefs or attitudes toward some group. Blatant examples are painting a swastika on a Jewish studies house or defacing a sculpture depicting a same-sex couple holding hands. More subtle examples are when an African American student notices that white shopkeepers in a mostly white college town tend to keep a close eye on him; a male-to-female transgender individual is treated with less respect by her professors and peers; a student using a wheelchair finds no accessible bathrooms; or an obese woman overhears remarks about eating and self-control.

Recent immigrants to the United States have to learn to live in a new society. This requires a balance between assimilating and changing to be like the majority, and maintaining a connection to their own culture, language, and religion. The process of acculturation is generally stressful, especially when the person's background is radically different from that of the people he or she is now living among. Parental expectations generate stress if they are too high or too low. If too high, the child may work too hard in an attempt to succeed at everything; if too low, the child may not work hard enough to succeed at anything.

Both immigrants and minorities that have lived for generations in the United States can face job- and school-related stressors because of stereotypes and discrimination. They may make less money in comparable jobs with comparable levels of education and may find it more difficult to achieve leadership positions.

However, on a positive note, many who experience hardship, disability, or

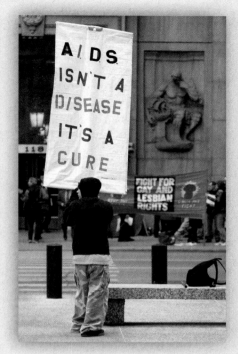

prejudice develop effective, goal-directed coping skills and are successful at overcoming obstacles and managing the stress they face.

---

minority ethnic group, you may feel pressure to assimilate into mainstream society, or to spend as much time as possible with others who share your ethnicity or background. If English is not your first language, you may face the added burden of conducting daily activities in a language with which you are not comfortable. All these pressures can become significant sources of stress. (See the box "Diverse Populations, Discrimination, and Stress.")

Virtual Social Networks Technology can help you save time, but it can also increase stress. Being electronically connected to work, family, and friends all the time can impinge on your personal space, waste time, and distract you from your current real situation. If you are "always on"—that is, always available by voice or text messaging—some friends or colleagues may think it's all right to contact you any time, even if you're in class or trying to work, and they may expect an immediate response. The convenience of staying electronically connected comes at a price.

Other Stressors

Have you tried to eat at a restaurant where the food was great, but the atmosphere was so noisy that it put you on edge? This is an example of an environmental stress—a

condition or event in the physical environment that causes stress.

Like the noisy atmosphere of some restaurants, many environmental stressors are mere inconveniences that are easy to avoid. Others, such as pollen or construction noise, may be an unavoidable daily source of stress. For those who live in poor or violent neighborhoods or in a war-torn country, environmental stressors can be major stressors (see the box "Coping After Violence on Campus").

Some stressors are found not in our environment but within ourselves. We pressure ourselves to reach goals and continuously evaluate our progress and performance. Striving to reach goals can enhance self-esteem if the goals are reasonable. Unrealistic expectations, however, can be

Ask Yourself

QUESTIONS FOR CRITICAL THINKING AND REFLECTION

What are the top two or three stressors in your life right now? Are they new to your life—as part of your college experience—or are they stressors you've experienced in the past? Do they include both positive and negative experiences (eustress and distress)?

Coping After Violence on Campus

Stories of violence on American campuses have become all too familiar:

- In May 2010, a University of Virginia student was beaten to death. Shortly afterward, her boyfriend was arrested and charged with murder.

- In December 2009, a disgruntled student opened fire in class at Northern Virginia Community College, apparently trying to shoot the teacher. No one was injured in the shooting.

- In March 2008, an Auburn University student died from gunshot wounds sustained during a robbery. A day later, a University of North Carolina student was killed while being robbed in Chapel Hill, N.C.

- On February 14, 2008, a former Northern Illinois University student walked into one of the school's lecture halls and fatally shot five students before killing himself. Gunfire injured at least 16 other people.

- On April 16, 2007, a student killed 28 students and 5 teachers and injured 29 others during two attacks at Virginia Polytechnic Institute and State University (Virginia Tech). The attacker was acting out fantasies of revenge in a drama that held the nation's attention for weeks.

School shootings are not uniquely American events. They also occur at schools in other countries, including countries where access to guns is much more tightly controlled than in the United States.

People react to news of school violence in different ways, depending on their proximity to the event and its recency. In the case of school massacres, people far from the site may suffer emotional reactions simply from watching endless coverage on television.

Responses to violence include disbelief, shock, fear, anger, resentment, anxiety, mood swings, irritability, sadness, depression, panic, guilt, apathy, feelings of isolation or powerlessness, and many of the symptoms of excess stress. Some people affected by such violence develop post-traumatic stress disorder (PTSD), a more serious condition.

In the case of the Virginia Tech shootings, the school and community mobilized quickly to respond to the expected surge in behavioral health needs generated by the attack. Hotline calls and emergency room visits increased dramatically, especially during the second and third weeks following the shootings. Information sources and support groups were established for people grieving the loss of friends, family, neighbors, or colleagues. Volunteers contacted each family that was directly affected by the shootings to offer help in making arrangements and other services.

If you are affected by a disastrous event such as a school shooting or terrorist attack, take these steps:

- Be sure that you have the best information about what happened, whether a continuing risk is present, and what you can do to avoid it. That information may be posted on Web sites or on local radio or TV stations.

- Don't expose yourself to so much media coverage that it overwhelms you.

- Take care of yourself. Use the stress-relief techniques discussed in this chapter.

- Share your feelings and concerns with others. Be a supportive listener.

- If you feel able, help others in any way you can, such as by volunteering to work with victims.

- If you feel emotionally distressed days or weeks after the event, consider asking for professional help.

---

a significant source of stress and can damage self-esteem. Other internal stressors are physical and emotional states such as illness and exhaustion; these can be both a cause and an effect of unmanaged stress.

MANAGING STRESS

You can control the stress in your life by taking the following steps:

- Shore up your support system.
- Improve your communication skills.
- Develop healthy exercise, eating, and sleeping habits.
- Learn to identify and moderate individual stressors.

The effort required is well worth the time. People who manage stress effectively not only are healthier but have more time to enjoy life and accomplish goals.

Social Support

Having the support of friends and family members seems to contribute to the well-being of body and mind. Social support can provide a critical counterbalance to the stress in our lives. Give yourself time to develop and maintain a network of people you can count on for emotional support, feedback, and nurturing. If you believe you don't have enough social support, consider becoming a volunteer to help build your network of friends and to enhance your spiritual wellness. (See the box "Altruism: Is Doing Good Good for Your Health?")

Altruism: Is Doing Good Good for Your Health?

Ethics and religion have long told us that it is more blessed to give than to receive. Now scientists from many disciplines are finding empirical support for the notion that altruism—unselfish love and giving—benefits the giver at least as much as the receiver. These benefits come in the form of better psychological health, better physical health, and longer life.

One study of more than 7000 older adults over the age of 70 found that volunteering was associated with delayed mortality—that is, the more frequently people volunteered, the longer they lived compared with people who didn't volunteer. Another study found that longer life was associated with more years of volunteering, suggesting that people who start giving early in life reap benefits over their lifetime. In surveys, people who volunteer report fewer colds and headaches, improved sleeping and eating patterns, and some relief from the discomfort of chronic diseases such as asthma and arthritis.

What is the chain of events leading from altruism to health benefits, from volunteering to improved well-being, better health, and longer life? Scientists have proposed several mechanisms:

- Better immune system functioning. Altruistic love may block or reduce the stress response, which is known to suppress the immune system. A healthier immune system is more effective at fighting off infection and illness.

- Better cardiovascular health. The stress response also affects the cardiovascular system, increasing heart rate and raising blood pressure. Altruistic love may protect the heart and blood vessels from the damaging effects of stress.

- Activation of the relaxation response. Altruistic love may activate the relaxation response, the opposite of the stress response, inducing feelings of warmth, calm, and happiness. This response may be mediated by the release of hormones and neurotransmitters.

- Pain relief. Altruistic love may reduce sensations of pain by inducing the release of endorphins, brain chemicals that block pain and produce feelings of euphoria. Endorphins may account for the experience known as "helper's high," similar to "runner's high," which makes people feel happier, stronger, and more energetic.

- Increase in the frequency and depth of positive emotions, such as happiness and calmness. Positive emotions may reduce the burden of psychological and physiological stress and thereby provide benefits for health-related physiological processes.

- Increased self-esteem and positive beliefs about self-efficacy and self-worth.

- Better overall mental health. The combination of positive feelings and increased self-esteem is conducive to improved mental health. Part of the effect may come from reducing self-absorption, taking an outer focus, and shifting attention away from one's own perceived problems.

- Better social integration, more social support. Volunteering provides people with meaningful social roles and a sense of purpose, as well as opportunities for social contact. For older adults, volunteering can enhance a shift toward developmentally appropriate goals, such as giving back and being generative, in contrast to an earlier focus on career.

- Improved spiritual health. Altruism provides an avenue for putting deeply felt values into practice.

Studies show that not all giving is the same—for example, donating money does not have the same beneficial health effects as volunteering that involves personal contact. A few simple guidelines can help you get the most out of giving:

- Choose a volunteer activity that puts you in contact with people.

- Make helping voluntary. Obligatory helping can actually increase stress levels.

- Volunteer with a group. Sharing your interests with other volunteers increases social support. Volunteering seems to have the most benefits for people who also have other close relationships and social interests.

- Know your limits. Helping that goes beyond what you can handle depletes your own resources and is detrimental to your health.

If you want to incorporate more giving and helping into your life, look for opportunities to volunteer on your campus or in your community. Many colleges have lists of volunteer opportunities, ranging from tutoring to assisting in community gardens. If your schedule doesn't allow volunteering at this time, you can still help others with small acts of kindness, empathy, and compassion, such as listening to a friend's problems or writing a note to an aging relative. Getting in the habit of helping now can set you on a lifetime course of health-promoting altruistic actions.

SOURCES: Harris, A. H. S., and C. E. Thoresen, 2005. Volunteering is associated with delayed mortality in older people: Analysis of the Longitudinal Study of Aging. *Journal of Health Psychology* 10(6), 739–752; Sternberg, E. M. 2001. *Approaches to Defining Mechanisms by Which Altruistic Love Affects Health.* Research Topic White Paper #3, Institute for Research on Unlimited Love, Altruism, Compassion, Service (http://www.altruists.org/f72; retrieved October 20, 2010); Pembroke, G. 2007. *Compassion Rx: The Many Health Benefits of Altruism* (http://epages.wordpress.com/2007/10/26/compassion-rx-the-many-health-benefits-of-altruism; retrieved October 20, 2010).

Communication

Communicating in an assertive way that respects the rights of others—while protecting your own rights—can prevent stressful situations from getting out of control. Better communication skills can help everyone form and maintain healthy relationships. If you typically suppress your feelings, you might want to take an assertiveness training course that can help you identify and change your patterns of communication. If you have trouble controlling your anger, you may benefit from learning anger management strategies.

Exercise

Exercise helps maintain a healthy body and mind and even stimulates the birth of new brain cells. Regular physical activity can also reduce many of the negative effects of stress. Consider the following examples:

- Taking a long walk can help decrease anxiety and blood pressure.
- A brisk 10-minute walk can leave you feeling more relaxed and energetic for up to 2 hours.
- People who exercise regularly react with milder physical stress responses before, during, and after exposure to stressors.
- In a study, people who took three brisk 45-minute walks each week for 3 months reported fewer daily hassles and an increased sense of wellness.

These findings should not be surprising, because the stress response mobilizes energy resources and readies the body for physical emergencies. If you experience stress and do not physically exert yourself, you are not completing the energy cycle. You may not be able to exercise while your daily stressors occur—during class, for example, or while sitting in a traffic jam—but you can be active at other times of the day. Physical activity allows you to expend the nervous energy you have built up and trains your body to more readily achieve homeostasis following stressful situations.

Most adults need 7–9 hours of sleep every night to stay healthy and perform their best.

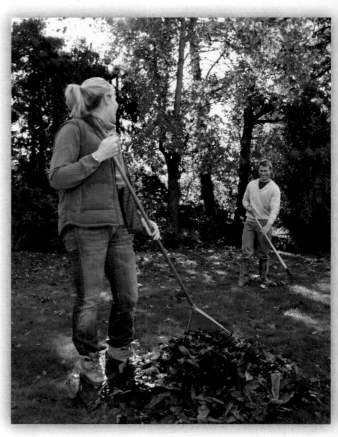

Exercise—even light activity—can be an effective antidote to stress.

Nutrition

A healthy diet gives you an energy bank to draw from whenever you experience stress. Eating wisely also can enhance your feelings of self-control and self-esteem. Learning the principles of sound nutrition is easy, and sensible eating habits rapidly become second nature when practiced regularly.

While your diet has an effect on the way your body handles stress, the reverse is also true. Excess stress can negatively affect the way you eat. Many people, for example, respond to stress by overeating; other people skip meals or stop eating altogether during stressful periods. Both responses are not only ineffective (they don't address the causes of stress), but potentially unhealthy.

Sleep

Most adults need 7–9 hours of sleep every night to stay healthy and perform their best. Getting enough sleep isn't just good for you physically. Adequate sleep also improves mood, fosters feelings of competence and self-worth, enhances mental functioning, and supports emotional functioning.

How Sleep Works Sleep occurs in two phases: **rapid eye movement (REM) sleep** and **non-rapid eye movement (NREM) sleep.** A sleeper goes through several cycles of NREM and REM sleep each night.

TERMS

rapid eye movement (REM) sleep The portion of the sleep cycle during which dreaming occurs.

non-rapid eye movement (NREM) sleep The portion of the sleep cycle that involves deep sleep; NREM sleep includes four states of successively deeper sleep.

NREM sleep actually includes four stages of successively deeper sleep. As you move through these stages of sleep, a variety of physiological changes occur, including the following:

- Blood pressure drops.
- Respiration and heart rates slow.
- Body temperature declines.
- Growth hormone is released.
- Brain wave patterns become slow and even.

During REM sleep, dreams occur. REM sleep is characterized by the rapid movement of the eyes under closed eyelids. Heart rate, blood pressure, and breathing rate rise, and brain activity increases to levels equal to or greater than those during waking hours. Muscles in the limbs relax completely, resulting in a temporary paralysis. (This total relaxation may prevent you from acting out your dreams while you're asleep.)

Sleep and Stress Stress hormone levels in the blood-stream vary throughout the day and are related to sleep patterns. Peak concentrations occur in the early morning, followed by a slow decline during the day and evening. Concentrations return to peak levels during the final stages of sleep and in the early morning hours. Stress hormone levels are low during NREM sleep and increase during REM sleep. With each successive sleep cycle during the night, REM sleep lasts a little longer. This increase in REM sleep duration with each sleep cycle may underlie the progressive increase in circulating stress hormones during the final stages of sleep.

Even though stress hormones are released during sleep, it is the *lack* of sleep that has the greatest impact on stress. In someone who is suffering from **sleep deprivation** (not getting enough sleep over time), mental and physical processes steadily deteriorate. A sleep-deprived person experiences headaches, feels irritable, is unable to concentrate, and is more prone to forgetfulness. Poor-quality sleep has long been associated with stress and depression. A small 2008 study of female college students further associated sleep deprivation with an increased risk of suicide.

Acute sleep deprivation slows the daytime decline in stress hormones, so evening levels are higher than normal. A decrease in total sleep time also causes an increase in the level of stress hormones. Together, these changes may cause an increase in stress hormone levels throughout the day and may contribute to physical and mental exhaustion. Extreme sleep deprivation can lead to hallucinations and other psychotic symptoms, as well as to a significant increase in heart attack risk.

Sleep Problems According to the National Sleep Foundation's 2009 Sleep in America Poll, 20% of American adults sleep an average of less than 6 hours per night. (Compare this to the recommended 7–9 hours per night.) Although many of us can attribute the lack of sleep to

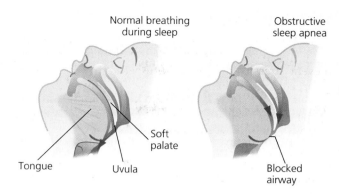

Normal breathing during sleep

Obstructive sleep apnea

Tongue

Soft palate

Uvula

Blocked airway

FIGURE 2.4 Sleep apnea. Sleep apnea occurs when soft tissues surrounding the airway relax, "collapsing" the airway and restricting airflow.

long work days and family responsibilities, as many as 70 million Americans suffer from chronic sleep disorders—medical conditions that prevent them from sleeping well.

According to National Sleep Foundation polls, more than 50% of adults report having trouble falling asleep or staying asleep—a condition called **insomnia.** The most common causes of insomnia are lifestyle factors, such as high caffeine or alcohol intake before bedtime; medical problems, such as a breathing disorder; and stress. About 75% of people who suffer from chronic insomnia report some stressful life event at the onset of their sleeping problems.

Another type of chronic sleep problem, called **sleep apnea,** occurs when a person stops breathing while asleep. Apnea can be caused by a number of factors, but it typically results when the soft tissue at the back of the mouth (such as the tongue or soft palate) "collapses" during sleep, blocking the airway (Figure 2.4). When breathing is interrupted, so is sleep, as the sleeper awakens repeatedly throughout the night to begin breathing again. In most cases, this occurs without the sleeper's even being aware of it. However, the disruption to sleep can be significant, and over time acute sleep deprivation can result from apnea. There are several treatments for apnea, including the use of medications, a special apparatus that helps keep the airway open during sleep, and surgery.

sleep deprivation A lack of sleep over a period of time.

insomnia A sleep problem involving the inability to fall or stay asleep.

sleep apnea The interruption of normal breathing during sleep.

TERMS

Time Management

Learning to manage your time can be crucial to coping with everyday stressors. Overcommitment, procrastination, and even boredom are significant stressors for many people. Along with gaining control of nutrition and exercise to maintain a healthy energy balance, time management is an important element in a wellness program. Try these strategies for improving your time-management skills:

- **Set priorities.** Divide your tasks into three groups: essential, important, and trivial. Focus on the first two, and ignore the third.
- **Schedule tasks for peak efficiency.** You've undoubtedly noticed you're most productive at certain times of the day (or night). Schedule as many of your tasks for those hours as you can, and stick to your schedule.
- **Set realistic goals and write them down.** Attainable goals spur you on. Impossible goals, by definition, cause frustration and failure. Fully commit yourself to achieving your goals by putting them in writing.
- **Budget enough time.** For each project you undertake, calculate how long it will take to complete. Then tack on another 10–15%, or even 25%, as a buffer.
- **Break up long-term goals into short-term ones.** Instead of waiting for large blocks of time, use short amounts of time to start a project or keep it moving.
- **Visualize the achievement of your goals.** By mentally rehearsing your performance of a task, you will be able to reach your goal more smoothly.
- **Keep track of the tasks you put off.** Analyze the reasons you procrastinate. If the task is difficult or unpleasant, look for ways to make it easier or more fun.
- **Consider doing your least-favorite tasks first.** Once you have the most unpleasant ones out of the way, you can work on the tasks you enjoy more.
- **Consolidate tasks when possible.** For example, try walking to the store so that you run your errands and exercise in the same block of time.
- **Identify quick transitional tasks.** Keep a list of 5- to 10-minute tasks you can do while waiting or between other tasks, such as watering your plants, doing the dishes, or checking a homework assignment.
- **Delegate responsibility.** Asking for help when you have too much to do is no cop-out; it's good time management. Just don't delegate the jobs you know you should do yourself.
- **Say no when necessary.** If the demands made on you don't seem reasonable, say no—tactfully, but without guilt or apology.
- **Give yourself a break.** Allow time for play—free, unstructured time when you can ignore the clock. Don't consider this a waste of time. Play renews you and enables you to work more efficiently.
- **Avoid your personal "time sinks."** You can probably identify your own time sinks—activities like watching television, surfing the Internet, or talking on the phone that consistently use up more time than you anticipate

and put you behind schedule. Some days, it may be best to avoid problematic activities altogether; for example, if you have a big paper due, don't sit down for a 5-minute TV break if it is likely to turn into a 2-hour break. Try a 5-minute walk if you need to clear your head.

- **Stop thinking or talking about what you're going to do, and just do it!** Sometimes the best solution for procrastination is to stop waiting for the right moment and just get started. You will probably find that things are not as bad as you feared, and your momentum will keep you going.

Striving for Spiritual Wellness

Spiritual wellness is associated with greater coping skills and higher levels of overall wellness. It is a very personal wellness component, and there are many ways to develop it. Researchers have linked spiritual wellness to longer life expectancy, reduced risk of disease, faster recovery, and improved emotional health.

Spirituality provides an ethical path to personal fulfillment that includes connectedness with self, others, and a higher power or larger reality. Spiritual wellness can make you more aware of your personal values and can help clarify them. Without an awareness of personal values, you might be driven by immediate desires and the passing demands of others. Living according to values means considering your options carefully before making a choice, choosing between options without succumbing to outside pressures that oppose your values, and making a choice and acting on it rather than doing nothing.

Confiding in Yourself Through Writing

Keeping a diary is analogous to confiding in others, except that you are confiding in yourself. This form of coping with severe stress may be especially helpful for those who are shy or introverted and find it difficult to open up to others. Although writing about traumatic and stressful events may have a short-term negative effect on mood, over the long term, stress is reduced and positive changes in health occur. A key to promoting health and well-being through journaling is to write about your emotional responses to stressful events. Set aside a special time each day or week to write down your feelings about stressful events in your life.

Problem-solving skills can improve your motivation, stress level, and grades.

Cognitive Techniques

Some stressors arise in our own minds. Ideas, beliefs, perceptions, and patterns of thinking can add to our stress level. Each of the following techniques can help you change unhealthy thought patterns to ones that will help you cope with stress. As with any skill, mastering these techniques takes practice and patience.

Think and Act Constructively Think back to the worries you had last week. How many of them were needless? Think about things you *can* control. Try to stand aside from the problem, consider the positive steps you can take to solve it, and then carry them out. Remember, if you can successfully predict that a stressor will occur, you can better control your response to it.

Take Control A situation often feels more stressful if you feel you're not in control of it. Time may seem to be slipping away before a big exam, for example. Unexpected obstacles may appear in your path, throwing you off course. When you feel your environment is controlling you instead of the other way around, take charge! Concentrate on what is possible to control, and set realistic goals. Be confident of your ability to succeed.

Problem-Solve Students with greater problem-solving abilities report easier adjustment to university life, higher motivation levels, lower stress levels, and higher grades. When you find yourself stewing over a problem, sit down with a piece of paper and do some problem solving. Try this approach:

1. Define the problem in one or two sentences.
2. Identify the causes of the problem.
3. Consider alternative solutions; don't just stop with the most obvious one.
4. Weigh positive and negative consequences for each alternative.
5. Make a decision—choose a solution.
6. Make a list of tasks you must perform to act on your decision.
7. Begin to carry out your list; if you're unable to do that, temporarily turn to other things.
8. Evaluate the outcome and revise your approach if necessary.

Modify Your Expectations Expectations are exhausting and restricting. The fewer expectations you have, the more you can live spontaneously and joyfully. The more you expect from others, the more often you will feel let down. And trying to meet the expectations others have of you is often futile.

Stay Positive If you beat up on yourself—"Late for class again! You can't even cope with college! How do you expect to ever hold down a professional job?"—change your inner dialogue. Talk to yourself as you would to a child you love: "You're a smart, capable person. You've solved other problems; you'll handle this one. Tomorrow you'll simply schedule things so you get to class with a few minutes to spare."

Practice Affirmations One way of cultivating the positive is to systematically repeat positive thoughts, or *affirmations,* to yourself. For example, if you react to stress with low self-esteem, you might repeat such sentences as "I approve and accept myself completely" and "It doesn't matter what others say, but what I believe." Saying affirmations to yourself every day may make them automatic and help you change the way you react.

Cultivate Your Sense of Humor When it comes to stress, laughter may be the best medicine. Even a fleeting smile produces changes in your autonomic nervous system that can lift your spirits. And a few minutes of belly laughing can be as invigorating as brisk exercise. Hearty laughter elevates your heart rate, aids digestion, eases pain, and triggers the release of endorphins and other pleasurable and stimulating chemicals in the brain. After a good laugh, your muscles go slack; your pulse and blood pressure dip below normal. You are relaxed. Cultivate the ability to laugh at yourself, and you'll have a handy and instantly effective stress reliever.

Focus on What's Important A major source of stress is trying to store too much data. Forget unimportant details (they will usually be self-evident) and organize important information. One technique you can try is to "chunk" the important material into categories. If your next exam covers three chapters from your textbook, consider each chapter a chunk of information. Then break down each chunk into its three or four most important features. Create a mental outline that allows you to trace your way from the most general category down to the most specific details. This technique can be applied to managing daily responsibilities as well.

Relaxation Techniques

The **relaxation response** is a physiological state characterized by a feeling of warmth and quiet mental alertness. This is the opposite of the fight-or-flight reaction. When the relaxation response is triggered by a relaxation technique, heart rate, breathing, and metabolism slow down. Blood pressure and oxygen consumption decrease. At the same time, blood flow to the brain and skin increases, and brain waves shift from an alert beta rhythm to a relaxed alpha rhythm. Practiced regularly, relaxation techniques can counteract the debilitating effects of stress. In addition, many people are familiar with the relaxing effects of nature; for more on this topic, see the box "The Green Way to Manage Stress."

relaxation response A physiological state characterized by a feeling of warmth and quiet mental alertness.

TERMS

The Green Way to Manage Stress

ON THE ENVIRONMENT

Need a way to beat your stress? Look no further than your own back yard, local park, or nearby hiking trail. Mounting evidence shows that people who get outdoors—or just get to look out a window once in a while—experience an almost instant, if short-term, reduction in stress. Scientists are investigating "natural stress reduction" as an easy and inexpensive boost to cognitive and behavioral approaches to stress management. High-tech replications of nature won't do, though—it has to be the real thing.

In a 2008 study at the University of Washington, participants were set up in two similar office environments with one difference. Some of the offices were equipped with plasma TV screens that displayed videos of a relaxing outdoor setting. The other offices were equipped with windows overlooking an actual outdoor setting. The volunteers were asked to perform a series of stress-inducing work tasks, and then their heart rates were measured. The volunteers with window views recovered from their stress significantly more quickly than the volunteers who viewed a natural scene on the TV. The study not only supported the idea that exposure to nature can reduce stress but also demonstrated that facsimiles of nature have little or no effect on stress.

Other studies have yielded similar results. For example, one study looked at hospital patients who were recovering from recent surgery. Patients whose rooms offered a window view of the outdoors needed fewer pain relievers than similar patients with no outdoor view.

Recent research on children with attention-deficit/hyperactivity disorder (ADHD) revealed that spending time in green play settings improved the children's ability to focus and concentrate, at least temporarily (see Chapter 3 for more on this topic).

Why do we benefit so much from communing with nature or even just seeing it through a window? Perhaps it's because we're born nature lovers. The term *biophilia* was coined to describe the innate affinity humans have for nature and living things. In his book, *Biophilia*, biologist Edward O. Wilson proposed that people feel a deep connection with the natural world and that this bond is rooted in our biology, perhaps because our species evolved in the context of living systems. According to this theory, we are attracted to plants and animals—we seek them out, surround ourselves with them, and get positive feelings from them—because they have always helped sustain life, including the life of our species.

Whether this hypothesis is true or not, many people are attracted to nature and experience relief from stress just being in natural settings. The next time you're struggling with a term paper or feeling frazzled by your electronic devices, try stepping outside and spending some time under the trees. You may find yourself feeling surprisingly soothed, relaxed, and refreshed.

For a detailed discussion of environmental health—how the environment affects you and how you affect the environment—see Chapter 14.

SOURCES: Grind, B., and G. G. Patil. 2009. Biophilia: Does visual contact with nature impact on health and well-being? *International Journal of Environmental Research and Public Health* 6(9): 2332–2343; Kahn, P. H., et al. 2008. A plasma display window? The shifting baseline problem in a technologically mediated natural world. *Journal of Environmental Psychology* 28(2008) 192–199; Faber Taylor, A., and W. C. Sullivan. 2001. Coping with ADD: The surprising connection to green play settings. *Environment and Behavior* 33(1): 54–77.

Progressive Relaxation Unlike most of the other methods of relaxation, progressive relaxation requires no imagination, willpower, or self-suggestion. You simply tense and relax the muscles in your body, group by group. The technique, also known as deep muscle relaxation, helps you become aware of the muscle tension that occurs when you're under stress. When you consciously relax those muscles, other systems of the body get the message and ease up on the stress response.

Start, for example, with your right fist. Inhale as you tense it. Exhale as you relax it. Repeat. Next, contract and relax your right upper arm. Repeat. Do the same with your left arm. Then, beginning at your forehead and ending at your feet, contract and relax your other muscle groups. Repeat each contraction at least once, breathing in as you tense, breathing out as you relax. To speed up the process, tense and relax more muscles at one time—both arms simultaneously, for instance. With practice, you'll be able to relax very quickly and effectively by clenching and releasing only your fists.

Visualization Also known as *imagery*, **visualization** lets you daydream without guilt. Next time you feel stressed, close your eyes. Imagine yourself floating on a cloud, sitting on a mountaintop, or lying in a meadow. Involve all your senses; imagine the sounds, the smells, and the other sensations that would be part of the scene. Your body will respond as if the imagery were real. An alternative: Close your eyes and imagine a deep purple light filling your body. Now change the color into a soothing gold. As the color lightens, so should your distress.

Visualization can also be used to rehearse for an upcoming event and enhance performance. By experiencing an event ahead of time in your mind, you can practice coping with any difficulties that may arise. Think positively, and you can "psych yourself up" for a successful experience.

Meditation The need to periodically stop our incessant mental chatter is so great that, from ancient times,

TERMS

visualization A technique for promoting relaxation or improving performance that involves creating or re-creating vivid mental pictures of a place or an experience; also called *imagery*.

Meditation and the Relaxation Response

Here is a simple technique for eliciting the relaxation response.

The Basic Technique

1. Pick a word, phrase, or object to focus on. If you like, you can choose a word or phrase that has a deep meaning for you, but any word or phrase will work. Some meditators prefer to focus on their breathing.

2. Take a comfortable position in a quiet environment, and close your eyes if you aren't focusing on an object.

3. Relax your muscles.

4. Breathe slowly and naturally. If you're using a focus word or phrase, silently repeat it each time you exhale. If you're using an object, focus on it as you breathe.

5. Keep a passive attitude. Disregard thoughts that drift in.

6. Continue for 10–20 minutes, once or twice a day.

7. When you're finished, sit quietly for a few minutes with your eyes first closed and then open. Then stand up.

Suggestions

● Allow relaxation to occur at its own pace; don't try to force it. Don't be surprised if you can't quiet your mind for more than a few seconds at a time; it's not a reason for anger or frustration. The more you ignore the intrusions, the easier doing so will become.

● If you want to time your session, peek at a watch or clock occasionally, but don't set a jarring alarm.

● The technique works best on an empty stomach, before a meal or about 2 hours after eating. Avoid times of day when you're tired—unless you want to fall asleep.

● Although you'll feel refreshed even after the first session, it may take a month or more to get noticeable results. Be patient. Eventually the relaxation response will become so natural that it will occur spontaneously, or on demand, when you sit quietly for a few moments.

---

hundreds of forms of **meditation** have developed in cultures all over the world. Meditation is a way of telling the mind to be quiet for a while, and it is potentially useful for reducing stress. According to a 2008 study, college students who learned how to use meditation for stress management were able to significantly reduce their daily stress levels. Further, those students found it easier to forgive others for perceived wrongdoings and spent less time focusing on negative thoughts.

Meditation helps you tune out the world temporarily, removing you from both internal and external sources of stress. The "thinker" takes time out to become the "observer"—calmly attentive, without analyzing, judging, comparing, or rationalizing. Regular practice of this quiet awareness will subtly carry over into your daily life, encouraging physical and emotional balance no matter what confronts you. For a step-by-step description of a basic meditation technique, see the box "Meditation and the Relaxation Response."

Another form of meditation, known as *mindfulness meditation,* involves paying attention to physical sensations, perceptions, thoughts, and imagery. Instead of focusing on a word or object to quiet the mind, you observe thoughts that occur without evaluating or judging them. Development of this ability requires regular practice but may eventually result in a more objective view of one's perceptions. It is believed that a greater understanding of one's moment-to-moment thought processes (mindful awareness) provides a richer and more vital sense of life and improves coping. Studies also suggest that people who rate high in mindfulness are less anxious and better able to deal with stress; among people with specific health problems, mindfulness can provide substantial benefits.

Deep Breathing Your breathing pattern is closely tied to your stress level. Deep, slow breathing is associated with relaxation. Rapid, shallow, often irregular breathing occurs during the stress response. With practice, you can learn to slow and quiet your breathing pattern, thereby also quieting your mind and relaxing your body. Breathing techniques can be used for on-the-spot tension relief as well as for long-term stress reduction.

The primary goal of many breathing exercises is to change your breathing pattern from chest breathing to diaphragmatic ("belly") breathing. To practice diaphragmatic breathing, lie on your back and place one hand on your chest and one hand on your abdomen to monitor your breathing. Take a slow, deep breath through your nose and into your belly. Your abdomen should rise significantly and your chest only slightly. Think of filling your belly with air. Exhale gently through your mouth. Once you become familiar with belly breathing, you can use it anywhere, any time, to dispel tension and stress.

Yoga Hatha yoga, the most common yoga style practiced in the United States, emphasizes physical balance and breath control. It

meditation A technique for quieting the mind by focusing on a particular word, object (such as a candle flame), or process (such as breathing).

TERMS

integrates components of flexibility, muscular strength and endurance, and muscle relaxation; it also sometimes serves as a preliminary to meditation. A session of yoga typically involves a series of postures, each held for a few seconds to several minutes, which involve stretching and balance and coordinated breathing. Yoga can induce the relaxation response and promote body awareness and flexibility. If you are interested in trying yoga, it's best to take a class from an experienced instructor.

Tai chi This martial art (in Chinese, *taijiquan*) is a system of self-defense that incorporates philosophical concepts from Taoism and Confucianism. In addition to self-defense, tai chi aims to bring the body into balance and harmony to promote health and spiritual growth. It teaches practitioners to remain calm and centered, to conserve and concentrate energy, and to manipulate force by becoming part of it—by "going with the flow." Tai chi is considered the gentlest of the martial arts. Instead of quick and powerful movements, tai chi consists of a series of slow, fluid, elegant movements, which reinforce the idea of moving *with* rather than *against* the stressors of everyday life. As with yoga, it's best to start tai chi with a class from an experienced instructor.

Listening to Music Listening to music is another method of inducing relaxation. It can influence pulse,

Listening to music is one of many techniques for inducing the relaxation response.

blood pressure, and the electrical activity of muscles. Exposure to soothing music leads to reduced levels of the stress hormone cortisol and causes changes in the electrical activity in the brain. To experience the stress-management benefits of music yourself, set aside a time to listen. Choose music that you enjoy and that makes you feel relaxed.

Other relaxation techniques include biofeedback, massage, hypnosis and self-hypnosis, and autogenic training. To learn more about these and other techniques for inducing the relaxation response, refer to For More Information at the end of the chapter.

Counterproductive Coping Strategies

College is a time when you'll learn to adapt to new and challenging situations and gain skills that will last a lifetime. It is also a time when many people develop counterproductive and unhealthy habits in response to stress. Such habits can last well beyond graduation.

Tobacco Use Cigarettes and other tobacco products contain nicotine, a chemical that enhances the actions of neurotransmitters. Nicotine can make you feel relaxed and even increase your ability to concentrate, but it is highly addictive. In fact, nicotine dependence itself is considered a psychological disorder. Cigarette smoke also contains substances that cause heart disease, stroke, lung cancer, and emphysema. These negative consequences far outweigh any beneficial effects, and tobacco use should be avoided. The easiest thing to do is to not start.

Use of Alcohol and Other Drugs Having a few drinks might make you feel temporarily at ease, and drinking until you're intoxicated may help you forget your current stressors. However, using alcohol to deal with stress places you at risk for all the short- and long-term problems associated with alcohol abuse. It also does nothing to address the actual causes of stress in your life. Although moderate alcohol consumption may have potential health benefits for some people, many college students have patterns of drinking that detract from wellness.

Using other psychoactive drugs to cope with stress is also usually counterproductive:

- Caffeine raises cortisol levels and blood pressure and can make you feel more stressed; caffeine also disrupts sleep. Other stimulants, such as amphetamine, can activate the stress response. They also affect the same areas of the brain that are involved in regulating the stress response.
- Marijuana use is relatively common among college students, who report that they smoke marijuana in an effort to induce relaxation and for "mind expansion." Use of marijuana causes a brief period of euphoria and

*The most important starting point for a successful stress-management plan is to **learn to listen to your body**.*

decreased short-term memory and attentional abilities. Physiological effects clearly show that marijuana use doesn't cause relaxation; in fact, some neurochemicals in marijuana act to enhance the stress response, and getting high on a regular basis can elicit panic attacks. To compound this, withdrawal from marijuana may also be associated with an increase in circulating stress hormones.

• Opioids such as morphine and heroin can mimic the effects of your body's natural painkillers and act to reduce anxiety. However, tolerance to opioids develops quickly, and many users become dependent.

Unhealthy Eating Habits Eating is psychologically rewarding. The feelings of satiation and sedation that follow eating produce a relaxed state. However, regular use of eating as a means of coping with stress may lead to unhealthy eating habits. In fact, a survey by the American Psychological Association revealed that about 25% of Americans use food as a means of coping with stress or anxiety. These "comfort eaters" are twice as likely to be obese as average Americans.

STRESS JOURNAL		DATE 9-18-09
TIME	STRESSOR	REACTION/COPING STRATEGY
7:45 AM	Tara wouldn't get out of the shower	Yelled at her, started an argument
8:35 AM	Late for class	Slouched in back of room; chewed my nails
11:55 AM	Dad called to discuss credit card debt	Cried, skipped lunch and went out to smoke with Greg
5:30 PM	Power outage at dorm, couldn't study	Took a walk with Tara, made up for arguing this morning, then went to library to study
7:45 PM	Ed called, asked to borrow money	Stayed calm, put down phone and counted to 10, then explained that he already owes me $50
8:30 PM	Ed called, angry, said he wanted to break up	Argued on phone, then went out with Tara for a drink

FIGURE 2.5   A sample stress journal. Tracking stressful events and reactions can help you understand how you normally cope with stress.

CREATING A PERSONAL PLAN FOR MANAGING STRESS

What are the most important sources of stress in your life? Are you coping successfully with these stressors? No single strategy or program for managing stress will work for everyone, but you can use the principles of behavior management described in Chapter 1 to tailor a plan specifically to your needs.

Identifying Stressors

Before you can learn to manage the stressors in your life, you have to identify them. Many experts recommend keeping a stress journal for a week or two (Figure 2.5). Each time you feel or express a stress response, record the time and the circumstances in your journal. Note what you were doing at the time, what you were thinking or feeling, and the outcome of your response.

After keeping your journal for a few weeks, you should be able to identify your key stressors and spot patterns in how you respond to them. Take note of the people, places, events, and patterns of thought and behavior that cause you the most stress. You may notice, for example, that mornings are usually the most stressful part of your day. Or you may discover that when you're angry at your roommate, you're apt to respond with behaviors that only make matters worse. Keeping a journal allows you to be analytical about what produces the most stress in your life and fills in where your conscious memory fails you.

Designing Your Plan

Once you've identified the key stressors in your life, choose the stress reduction techniques that will work best for you and create an action plan for change. Finding a buddy to work with you can make the process more fun and increase your chances of success. Some experts recommend drawing up a formal contract with yourself.

Whether or not you complete a contract, it's important to design rewards into your plan. You might treat yourself to a special breakfast in a favorite restaurant on the weekend (as long as you eat a nutritious breakfast every weekday morning). It's also important to evaluate your plan regularly and redesign it as your needs change. Under

Dealing with Test Anxiety

Do you have trouble performing well on tests? Does anxiety interfere with your ability to study effectively before a test and to think clearly in the test situation? If so, you may be experiencing test anxiety—an ineffective response to a stressful situation that can be replaced with more effective responses. If test anxiety is a problem for you, try some of the following strategies:

- Before the test, find out everything you can about it—its format, the material to be covered, the grading criteria. Ask the instructor for practice materials. Study in advance; don't just cram the night before. Avoid all-nighters.

- Devise a study plan. This might include forming a study group with one or more classmates or outlining what you will study, when, where, and for how long. Generate your own questions and answer them.

- In the actual test situation, sit away from possible distractions, listen carefully to instructions, and ask for clarification if you don't understand a direction.

- During the test, answer the easiest questions first. If you don't know an answer and there is no penalty for incorrect answers, guess. If there are several questions you have difficulty answering, review the ones you have already handled. Figure out approximately how much time you have to cover each question.

- For math problems, try to estimate the answer before doing the precise calculations.

- For true-false questions, look for qualifiers such as *always* and *never.* Such questions are likely to be false.

- For essay questions, look for key words in the question that indicate what the instructor is looking for in the answer. Develop a brief outline of your answer, sketching out what you will cover. Stick to your outline, and keep track of the time you're spending on your answer. Don't get caught with unanswered questions when time is up.

- Remain calm and focused throughout the test. Don't let negative thoughts rattle you. Avoid worrying about past performance, how others are doing, or the negative consequences of a poor test grade. If you start to become nervous, take some deep breaths and relax your muscles completely for a minute or so.

The best way to counter test anxiety is with successful test-taking experiences. The more times you succeed, the more your test anxiety will recede. If you find that these methods aren't sufficient to get your anxiety under control, you may want to seek professional help.

---

times of increased stress, for example, you might want to focus on good eating, exercise, and relaxation habits. Over time, your new stress-management skills will become almost automatic. You'll feel better, accomplish more, and reduce your risk of disease.

Getting Help

If the techniques discussed so far don't provide you with enough relief from the stress in your life, you might want to learn more about specific areas to work on. Excellent self-help guides can be found in bookstores or the library. Additional resources are listed in the For More Information section at the end of the chapter.

Your student health center or student affairs office can tell you whether your campus has a peer counseling program. Such programs are usually staffed by volunteer students with special training that emphasizes maintaining confidentiality. Peer counselors can guide you to other campus or community resources or can simply provide understanding. Support groups and short-term psychotherapy can also be tremendously helpful in dealing with stress-related problems.

TIPS FOR TODAY AND THE FUTURE

For the stress you can't avoid, develop a range of stress-management techniques and strategies.

RIGHT NOW YOU CAN

- Practice deep breathing for 5–10 minutes.
- Visualize a relaxing, peaceful place and imagine yourself experiencing it as vividly as possible. Stay there as long as you can.
- Do some stretching exercises.
- Get out your datebook and schedule what you'll be doing the rest of today and tomorrow. Pencil in a short walk and a conversation with a friend.

IN THE FUTURE YOU CAN

- Take a class or workshop that can help you overcome a source of stress, such as one in assertiveness training or time management.
- Find a way to build relaxing time into every day. Just 15 minutes of meditation, stretching, or massage can induce the relaxation response.

Connect to Your Choices

Have you ever thought about why you handle stress the way you do? Many factors can influence the choices we make about stress management, some not as obvious as others. Do you try to do too much and then take your frustration out on other people because that's how stress was handled in your family? Do you blow off steam with alcohol on weekends because that's what your friends are doing? Do you dismiss relaxation techniques like yoga, meditation, or deep breathing because you think they're only for a certain type of person?

What are the external factors that influence your choices about stress management? What are your inner motivations and core values, and how do they affect your choices? Based on what you learned in this chapter, will you make some different choices in the future? If so, what will they be?

Go online to Connect to complete this activity.
www.mcgraw-hillconnect.com

SUMMARY

• When confronted with a stressor, the body undergoes a set of physical changes known as the fight-or-flight reaction. The sympathetic nervous system and endocrine system act on many targets in the body to prepare it for action.

• Emotional and behavioral responses to stressors vary among individuals. Ineffective responses increase stress but can be moderated or changed.

• Factors that influence emotional and behavioral responses to stressors include personality, cultural background, gender, and past experiences.

• The general adaptation syndrome (GAS) has three stages: alarm, resistance, and exhaustion.

• A high allostatic load characterized by prolonged or repeated exposure to stress hormones can increase a person's risk of health problems.

• Psychoneuroimmunology (PNI) looks at how the physiological changes of the stress response affect the immune system and thereby increase the risk of illness.

• Health problems linked to stress include CVD, colds and other infections, asthma and allergies, cancer, flare-ups of chronic diseases, psychological problems, digestive problems, headaches, insomnia, and injuries.

• A cluster of major life events that require adjustment and accommodation can lead to increased stress and an increased risk of health problems. Minor daily hassles increase stress if they are perceived negatively.

• Sources of stress associated with college may be academic, interpersonal, time-related, or financial pressures.

• Job-related stress is common, particularly for employees who have little control over decisions relating to their jobs. If stress is severe or prolonged, burnout may occur.

• New and changing relationships, prejudice, and discrimination are examples of interpersonal and social stressors.

• Social support systems help buffer people against the effects of stress and make illness less likely. Good communication skills foster healthy relationships.

• Exercise, nutrition, sleep, and time management are wellness behaviors that reduce stress and increase energy.

• Cognitive techniques for managing stress involve developing new and healthy patterns of thinking, such as practicing problem solving, monitoring self-talk, and cultivating a sense of humor.

• The relaxation response is the opposite of the fight-or-flight reaction. Techniques that trigger it, including progressive relaxation, imagery, meditation, and deep breathing, counteract the effects of chronic stress. Counterproductive coping strategies include smoking, drinking, and unhealthy eating.

• A successful individualized plan for coping with stress begins with the use of a stress journal or log to identify and study stressors and inappropriate behavioral responses. Completing a contract and recruiting a buddy can help your stress-management plan succeed.

• Additional help in dealing with stress is available from self-help books, peer counseling, support groups, and psychotherapy.

FOR MORE INFORMATION

BOOKS

Blonna, R. 2012. *Coping with Stress in a Changing World,* 5th ed. New York: McGraw-Hill. *A comprehensive guide to stress management that includes separate chapters on college stressors and spirituality.*

Greenberg, J. 2010. *Comprehensive Stress Management,* 12th ed. New York: McGraw-Hill. *Provides a clear explanation of the physical, psychological, sociological, and spiritual aspects of stress and offers numerous stress-management techniques.*

Kabat-Zinn, J. 2006. *Coming to Our Senses: Healing Ourselves and the World Through Mindfulness.* New York: Hyperion. *Explores the connections among mindfulness, health, and physical and spiritual well-being.*

Pennebaker, J. W. 2004. *Writing to Heal: A Guided Journal for Recovering from Trauma and Emotional Upheaval.* Oakland, Calif.: New Harbinger Press. *Provides information about using journaling to cope with stress.*

Seaward, B. L. 2006. *Managing Stress: Principles and Strategies for Health and Well-Being,* 5th ed. Boston: Jones and Bartlett. *A comprehensive textbook for college students.*

ORGANIZATIONS AND WEB SITES

American Headache Society. Provides information for consumers and clinicians about different types of headaches, their causes, and their treatment.

> http://www.americanheadachesociety.org

American Psychiatric Association: Healthy Minds, Healthy Lives. Provides information on mental wellness developed especially for college students.

> http://www.healthyminds.org

American Psychological Association. Provides information on stress management and psychological disorders.

> http://www.apa.org
> http://apa.org/helpcenter

Association for Applied Psychophysiology and Biofeedback. Provides information about biofeedback and referrals to certified biofeedback practitioners.

> http://www.aapb.org

Benson-Henry Institute for Mind Body Medicine. Provides information about stress-management and relaxation techniques.

> http://www.massgeneral.org/bhi/

National Institute of Mental Health (NIMH). Publishes informative brochures about stress and stress management as well as other aspects of mental health.

> http://www.nimh.nih.gov

National Sleep Foundation. Provides information about sleep and how to overcome sleep problems such as insomnia and jet lag.

> http://www.sleepfoundation.org

The American Institute of Stress. A resource of in-depth information on stress, its causes, and its treatments.

> http://www.stress.org

SELECTED BIBLIOGRAPHY

American College Health Association. 2009. *American College Health Association-National College Health Assessment II Reference Group Executive Summary, Fall 2009.* Linthicum, Md.: American College Health Association.

American Psychological Association. 2009. *Stress in America 2009.* Washington, D.C.: American Psychological Association.

American Psychological Association. 2010. *How Does Stress Affect Us?* (http://www.apa.org/helpcenter/stress-effects.aspx; retrieved October 20, 2010).

American Psychological Association. 2010. *Learning to Deal with Stress* (http://www.apa.org/helpcenter/stress-learning.aspx; retrieved October 20, 2010).

American Psychological Association. 2010. *Mind/Body Health: Stress.* (http://www.apa.org/helpcenter/stress.aspx; retrieved October 20, 2010).

Caldwell, K., et al. 2010. Developing mindfulness in college students through movement-based courses: Effects on self-regulatory self-efficacy, mood, stress, and sleep quality. *Journal of American College Health* 58(5): 433–442.

Centers for Disease Control. 2010. *Coping with a Disaster or Traumatic Event: Information for Individuals and Families* (http://emergency.cdc.gov/mentalhealth/general.asp; retrieved October 20, 2010).

Cohen, S., W. J. Doyle, and A. Baum. 2006. Socioeconomic status is associated with stress hormones. *Psychosomatic Medicine* 68(3): 414–420.

Hefner, J., and D. Eisenberg. 2009. Social support and mental health among college students. *American Journal of Orthopsychiatry* 79(4): 491–499.

Flugel Colle, K. F., et al. 2010. Measurement of quality of life and participant experience with the mindfulness-based stress reduction program. *Complementary Therapies in Clinical Practice* 16(1): 36–40.

Freedman, N. 2010. Treatment of obstructive sleep apnea syndrome. *Clinics in Chest Medicine* 31(2): 187–201.

Frequent headaches, hidden dangers. 2006. *Consumer Reports on Health,* June.

Headaches. 2006. *Journal of the American Medical Association* 295(19): 2320.

Hook, J. N., et al. 2010. Empirically supported religious and spiritual therapies. *Journal of Clinical Psychology* 66(1): 46–72.

How stress can make you forgetful, age faster. 2005. *Tufts University Health & Nutrition Letter,* February, 1.

Institute of Medicine Committee on Sleep Medicine and Research. 2006. *Sleep Disorders and Sleep Deprivation: An Unmet Public Health Problem,* ed. H. R. Colton and B. M. Altevogt. Washington, D.C.: National Academies Press.

Lauderdale, D. S., et al. 2006. Objectively measured sleep characteristics among early-middle-aged adults: The CARDIA study. *American Journal of Epidemiology* 164(1): 17–18.

Mayo Foundation for Medical Education and Research. 2008. *Stress: Win Control over the Stress in Your Life* (http://www.mayoclinic.com/health/stress/SR00001; retrieved October 20, 2010).

National Health Information Center. 2010. *Manage Stress* (http://healthfinder.gov/prevention/PrintTopic.aspx?topicID=45; retrieved October 20, 2010).

National Sleep Foundation. 2010. *2010 Sleep in America Poll.* Washington, D.C.: National Sleep Foundation.

Nordboe, D. J., et al. 2007. Immediate behavioral health response to the Virginia Tech shootings. *Disaster Medicine and Public Health Preparedness* 1 (Suppl. 1): S31–S32.

Roddenberry, A., and K. Renk. 2010. Locus of control and self-efficacy: Potential mediators of stress, illness, and utilization of health services in college students. *Child Psychiatry and Human Development* 41(4): 353–370.

Sax, L. J., et al. 2006. *The American Freshman: National Norms for Fall 2005.* Los Angeles: UCLA Higher Education Research Institute.

Telles, S., et al. 2009. Effect of a yoga practice session and a yoga theory session on state anxiety. *Perceptual and Motor Skills* 109(3): 924–930.

The New York Times. 2010 Update. *Times Topics: School Shootings* (http://topics.nytimes.com/top/reference/timestopics/subjects/s/school_shootings/index.html; retrieved October 20, 2010).

Torpy, J. M. 2008. Chronic stress and the heart. *Journal of the American Medical Association* 298(14): 1722.

U.S. Department of Health and Human Services, National Institutes of Health. 2009. *Stress* (http://www.nlm.nih.gov/medlineplus/stress.html; retrieved October 20, 2010).

Wittstein, I. S., et al. 2005. Neurohumoral features of myocardial stunning due to sudden emotional stress. *New England Journal of Medicine* 352(6): 539–548.

Yaggi, H. K., and K. P. Strohl. 2010. Adult obstructive sleep apnea/hypopnea syndrome: Definitions, risk factors, and pathogenesis. *Clinics in Chest Medicine* 31(2): 179–186.

Psychological Health

3

Psychological health contributes to every dimension of wellness. It can be very difficult to maintain emotional, social, or even physical wellness if you are not psychologically healthy.

Psychological health, however, is a broad concept—one that is as difficult to define as it is important to understand. That is why the first section of this chapter is devoted to explaining what psychological health is and is not. The rest of the chapter discusses a number of common psychological problems, their symptoms, and their treatments.

DEFINING PSYCHOLOGICAL HEALTH

Psychological health (*or mental health*) can be defined either negatively as the absence of sickness or positively as the presence of wellness. The narrow, negative definition has two advantages: It concentrates attention on the worst problems and on the people most in need, and it avoids value judgments about the best way to lead our lives. If we think of everyone who is not severely mentally disturbed as being mentally healthy, however, we end up ignoring common problems that can be addressed. Finally, freedom from disorders is only one factor in psychological wellness.

Positive Psychology

A positive definition—psychological health as the presence of wellness—is a more ambitious goal.

During the 1960s, Abraham Maslow adopted a perspective that he called positive psychology in his book *Toward a Psychology of Being.* Maslow defined a *hierarchy of needs* (Figure 3.1) listed here in order of decreasing importance:

- Physiological needs
- Safety
- Being loved
- Maintaining self-esteem
- Self-actualization

When urgent (life-sustaining) needs—such as the need for food and water—are satisfied, less basic needs take priority. Maslow's conclusions were based on his study of

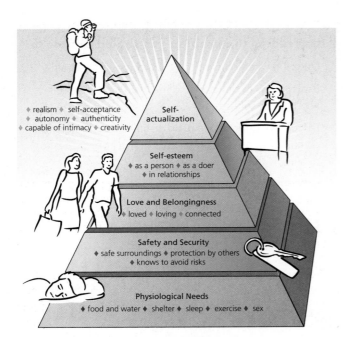

FIGURE 3.1 Maslow's hierarchy of needs.

SOURCE: Maslow, A. 1970. *Motivation and Personality,* 2nd ed. New York: Harper & Row.

Ask Yourself

QUESTIONS FOR CRITICAL THINKING AND REFLECTION

Have you ever had a reason to feel concerned about your own psychological health? If so, what was the reason? Did your concern lead you to talk to someone about the issue, or to seek professional help? If you did, what was the outcome, and how do you feel about it now?

a group of visibly successful people who seemed to have lived, or be living, at their fullest. He said that these people had achieved **self-actualization;** they had fulfilled a good measure of their human potential. Maslow suggested that self-actualized people all share certain qualities:

- *Realism.* Self-actualized people know the difference between what is real and what they want. As a result, they can cope with the world as it exists without demanding that it be different; they know what they can and cannot change. Just as important, realistic people accept evidence that contradicts what they want to believe.
- *Acceptance.* Psychologically healthy people have a **self-concept,** or *self-image;* that is positive but realistic. Such a person typically feels satisfaction and confidence in him- or herself, and so is said to have healthy **self-esteem.** Self-acceptance also means being tolerant of one's own imperfections, an ability that makes it easier to accept the imperfections of others.

- *Autonomy.* Psychologically healthy people are *autonomous,* meaning they can direct themselves, acting independently of their social environment. **Autonomy** is more than physical independence; it is social, emotional, and intellectual independence as well.
- *Authenticity.* Autonomous people are not afraid to be themselves; sometimes their capacity for being "real" may give them a certain childlike quality. They respond in a genuine, or authentic, spontaneous way to whatever happens, without pretense or self-consciousness.
- *Capacity for intimacy.* Healthy people can share their feelings and thoughts without fear of rejection. A psychologically healthy person is open to the pleasure of physical contact and the satisfaction of being close to others—but without being afraid of the risks involved in intimacy, such as the risk of having one's feelings hurt. (Chapters 4 and 5 discuss intimacy in more detail.)
- *Creativity.* Psychologically healthy people continually look at the world with renewed appreciation. Such appreciation can inform one's creativity, which helps explain why so many mentally healthy people are creative.

Self-actualization is an ideal to strive for. Rather than dwelling on the past, we need to concentrate on meeting current challenges in ways that lead to long-term mental wellness. We must not consider ourselves failures if we do not achieve our full potential in every way or at every moment.

Positive psychology more recently has focused on clearly defining positive goals and on concrete, measurable ways of achieving them. According to psychologist Martin Seligman, happiness can be achieved by travelling three quite different but equally valid roads:

- *The Pleasant Life.* This life is dedicated to maximizing

TERMS

psychological health   Mental health, defined negatively as the absence of illness or positively as the presence of wellness.

self-actualization   The highest level of growth in Maslow's hierarchy of needs.

self-concept   The ideas, feelings, and perceptions one has about oneself; also called *self-image.*

self-esteem   Satisfaction and confidence in oneself; the valuing of oneself as a person.

autonomy   Independence; the sense of being self-directed.

positive **emotions** about the past, present, and future and to minimizing pain and negative emotions. Your feelings about the past should be of contentment, satisfaction, and serenity; those about the present should include both immediate bodily pleasure and learned pleasures, such as the enjoyment of music. About the future, you should cultivate optimism and hopefulness.

- **The Engaged Life.** This life involves cultivating a strong character and exercising your talents. Most cultures admire personality traits such as courage, leadership, kindness, integrity, and originality along with the capacity to love someone and be loved. In this life, you become engaged and absorbed in what you do. You experience "flow" with complete immersion in what you do. Time stops, you are concentrated, you feel completely at home.

Emotional intelligence is a positive personality trait and a key to being engaged and successful in life. An emotionally intelligent person can identify and manage his or her own emotions and the emotions of others. People with higher emotional intelligence can perceive their own emotions and also can harness them to reach their intended goals. They can read and understand the emotions of others and use that understanding to get along with people. Psychologists and educators believe that emotional intelligence is less fixed than abstract intelligence and can be taught.

> *Emotional intelligence is not only a positive personality trait but a key to being engaged and successful in life.*

- **The Meaningful Life.** Another road to happiness is to belong to and serve institutions that enable the best in human nature. Examples are institutions that educate and that cultivate strong families, democracy, or a free press. Many people find meaning in a connection to families, friends, religious institutions, and their work. Ultimately, meaning derives from belonging to and serving something larger than oneself. It is strongest when meaning comes from more than one source.

Seligman and his colleagues are developing methods of assessing these three ways of life and of teaching people how to become happier by adopting one or more of them. They need not be mutually exclusive.

Not everyone accepts the ideas of positive psychology—or even the concept of psychological health—because they involve value judgments that are inconsistent with psychology's claim to be a science. Defining psychological health requires making assumptions and value judgments about what human goals are desirable, and some think these are matters for religion or philosophy.

Positive psychology has also been criticized as promoting a short-sighted denial of reality and unwarranted optimism. In particular, therapists informed by existential philosophy believe that psychological health comes from acknowledging and accepting the painful realities of life.

What Psychological Health Is Not

Psychological health is not the same as psychological normality. Being mentally normal simply means being close to average. We can define normal body temperature because a few degrees above or below this temperature means physical sickness. But your ideas and attitudes can vary tremendously without your losing efficiency or feeling emotional distress. In fact, psychological diversity—with its wide range of ideas, lifestyles, and attitudes—is a valuable asset to society.

Never seeking help for personal problems does not prove you are psychologically healthy, any more than seeking help proves you are mentally ill. Unhappy people may avoid seeking help for many reasons, and severely disturbed people may not even realize they need help.

Further, we can't say people are "mentally ill" or "mentally healthy" based solely on the presence or absence of symptoms. Consider the symptom of anxiety, for example. Anxiety can help you face a problem and solve it before it becomes too big. Someone who shows no anxiety may be refusing to recognize problems or to do anything about them. A person who is anxious for good reason is likely to be judged more psychologically healthy in the long run than someone who is inappropriately calm.

Finally, we cannot judge psychological health from the way people look. All too often, a person who seems to be OK and even happy suddenly takes his or her own life. Usually, such people lack close friends who might have known their desperation. At an early age, we learn to conceal our feelings and even to lie about them. We may believe that our complaints put unfair demands on others. While suffering in silence may sometimes be a virtue, it can also prevent one from getting help.

75% of all people who intend to commit suicide warn a family member or friend of their intention.

QUICK STATS

—**American Foundation for Suicide Prevention, 2008**

---

emotion A feeling state involving some combination of thoughts, physiological changes, and an outward expression or behavior.

emotional intelligence The capacity to identify and manage your own emotions and the emotions of others.

TERMS

MEETING LIFE'S CHALLENGES

Life is full of challenges—large and small. Everyone, regardless of heredity and family influences, must learn to cope successfully with new situations and new people.

Growing Up Psychologically

Our responses to life's challenges influence the development of our personality and identity.

Developing an Adult Identity A primary task beginning in adolescence is the development of an adult identity: a unified sense of self, characterized by attitudes, beliefs, and ways of acting that are genuinely one's own. People with adult identities know who they are, what they are capable of, what roles they play, and their place among their peers. They have a sense of their own uniqueness but also appreciate what they have in common with others. They view themselves realistically and can assess their strengths and weaknesses without relying on the opinions of others. Achieving an identity also means that one can form intimate relationships with others while maintaining a strong sense of self.

Our identities evolve as we interact with the world and make choices about what we'd like to do and whom we'd like to model ourselves after. Developing an adult identity is particularly challenging in a heterogeneous, secular, and relatively affluent society like ours, in which many roles are possible, many choices are tolerated, and ample time is allowed for experimenting and making up one's mind.

Early identities are often modeled after parents—or the opposite of parents, in rebellion against what they represent. Over time, peers, rock stars, sports heroes, and religious figures are added to the list of possible models. In high school and college, people often join cliques that assert a certain identity, such as the "jocks," the "brains," or the "slackers." Although much of an identity is internal—a way of viewing oneself and the world—certain aspects of it can be external, such as styles of talking and dressing, ornaments like earrings, and hairstyles.

Early identities are rarely permanent. A student who works for good grades and approval one year can turn into a dropout devoted to hard rock and wild parties a year later. At some point, however, most of us adopt a more stable, individual identity that ties together the experiences of childhood and the expectations and aspirations of adulthood. However, we don't suddenly assume our final identity and never change after that. Life is more interesting for people who continue evolving into more distinct individuals, rather than being rigidly controlled by their pasts. Identity reflects a lifelong process, and it changes as a person develops new relationships and roles.

Developing an adult identity is an important part of psychological wellness. Without a personal identity, we begin to feel confused about who we are; this situation is called an **identity crisis.** Until we have "found ourselves," we cannot have much self-esteem, because a self is not firmly in place.

Developing Intimacy Learning to live intimately with others and finding a productive role for yourself in society are other tasks of adulthood—to be able to love and work. People with established identities can form intimate relationships and sexual unions characterized by sharing, open communication, long-term commitment, and love. Those who lack a firm sense of self may have difficulty establishing relationships because they feel overwhelmed by closeness and the needs of another person. As a result, they experience only short-term, superficial relationships with others and may remain isolated.

Developing Values and Purpose in Your Life Values are criteria for judging what is good and bad; they underlie our moral decisions and behavior. The first morality of the young child is to consider "good" to mean what brings immediate and tangible rewards, and "bad," whatever results in punishment. An older child will explain right and wrong in terms of authority figures and rules. But the final stage of moral development, one that not everyone attains, is being able to conceive of right and wrong in more abstract terms such as justice and virtue.

As adults we need to assess how far we have evolved morally and what values we actually have adopted. Without an awareness of our personal values, our lives may be hurriedly driven forward by immediate desires and the passing demands of others. Living according to values means doing the following:

- Considering your options carefully before making a choice
- Choosing between options without succumbing to outside pressures that oppose your values
- Making a choice and acting on it rather than doing nothing

Your actions and how you justify them proclaim to others what you stand for.

TERMS

identity crisis Internal confusion about who one is.

values Criteria for judging what is good and bad, which underlie one's moral decisions and behavior.

Achieving Healthy Self-Esteem

Having a healthy level of self-esteem means regarding your self, which includes all aspects of your identity, as good, competent, and worthy of love. It is a critical component of wellness.

Developing a Positive Self-Concept   Ideally, a positive self-concept begins in childhood, based on experiences both within the family and outside it. Children need to develop a sense of being loved and being able to give love and to accomplish their goals. If they feel rejected or neglected by their parents, they may fail to develop feelings of self-worth. They may grow to have a negative concept of themselves.

Another component of self-concept is *integration*. An integrated self-concept is one that you have made for yourself—not someone else's image of you or a mask that doesn't quite fit. Important building blocks of self-concept are the personality characteristics and mannerisms of parents, which children may adopt without realizing it. Later, they may be surprised to find themselves acting like one of their parents. Eventually, such building blocks should be reshaped and integrated into a new, individual personality.

A further aspect of self-concept is *stability*. Stability depends on the integration of the self and its freedom from contradictions. People who have gotten mixed messages about themselves from parents and friends may have contradictory self-images, which defy integration and make them vulnerable to shifting levels of self-esteem. At times they regard themselves as entirely good, capable, and lovable—an ideal self—and at other times they see themselves as entirely bad, incompetent, and unworthy of love. Neither of these extreme self-concepts allows people to see themselves or others realistically, and their relationships with other people are filled with misunderstandings and ultimately with conflict.

> *Healthy self-esteem means regarding your self as **good, competent, and worthy of love**.*

Meeting Challenges to Self-Esteem   As an adult, you sometimes run into situations that challenge your self-concept. People you care about may tell you they don't love you or feel loved by you, for example, or your attempts to accomplish a goal may end in failure.

You can react to such challenges in several ways. The best approach is to acknowledge that something has gone wrong and try again, adjusting your goals to your abilities without radically revising your self-concept. Less productive responses are denying that anything went wrong and blaming someone else. These attitudes may preserve your self-concept temporarily, but in the long run they keep you from meeting the challenge.

The worst reaction is to develop a lasting negative self-concept in which you feel bad, unloved, and ineffective—in other words, to become demoralized. Instead of coping, the demoralized person gives up, reinforcing the negative self-concept and setting in motion a cycle of bad self-concept and failure. In people who are genetically predisposed to depression, demoralization can progress to additional symptoms, which are discussed later in the chapter.

One method for fighting demoralization is to recognize and test the negative thoughts and assumptions you may have about yourself and others. Try to note exactly when an unpleasant emotion—feeling worthless, wanting to give up, feeling depressed—occurs or gets worse, to identify the events or daydreams that trigger that emotion, and to observe whatever thoughts come into your head just before or during the emotional experience. It is helpful to keep a daily journal about such events.

People who are demoralized tend to use all-or-nothing thinking. They overgeneralize from negative events. They overlook the positive and jump to negative conclusions, minimizing their own successes and magnifying the successes of others. They take responsibility for unfortunate

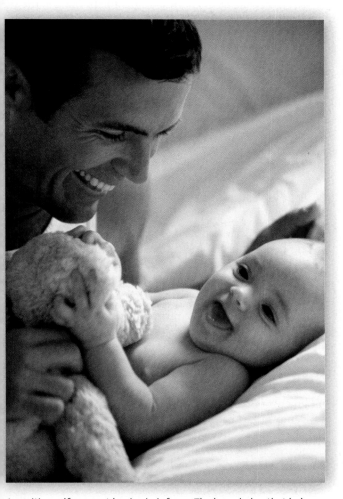

A positive self-concept begins in infancy. The knowledge that he's loved and valued by his parents gives this baby a solid basis for lifelong psychological health.

Realistic Self-Talk

Do your patterns of thinking make events seem worse than they truly are? Do negative beliefs about yourself become self-fulfilling prophecies? Substituting realistic self-talk for negative self-talk can help you build and maintain self-esteem and cope better with the challenges in your life. Here are some examples of common types of distorted, negative self-talk, along with suggestions for more accurate and rational responses.

Cognitive Distortion	Negative Self-Talk	Realistic Self-Talk
Focusing on negatives	School is so discouraging—nothing but one hassle after another.	School is pretty challenging and has its difficulties, but there certainly are rewards. It's really a mixture of good and bad.
Expecting the worst	Why would my boss want to meet with me this afternoon except to fire me?	I wonder why my boss wants to meet with me. I guess I'll just have to wait and see.
Overgeneralizing	(After getting a poor grade on a paper) Just as I thought—I'm incompetent at everything.	I'll start working on the next paper earlier. That way, if I have problems, I'll have time to talk to the TA.
Minimizing	I won the speech contest, but none of the other speakers was very good. I wouldn't have done as well against stiffer competition.	It may not have been the best speech I'll ever give, but it was good enough to win the contest. I'm really improving as a speaker.
Blaming others	I wouldn't have eaten so much last night if my friends hadn't insisted on going to that restaurant.	I overdid it last night. Next time I'll make different choices.
Expecting perfection	I should have scored 100% on this test. I can't believe I missed that one problem through a careless mistake.	Too bad I missed one problem through carelessness, but overall I did very well on this test. Next time I'll be more careful.
Believing you're the cause of everything	Sarah seems so depressed today. I wish I hadn't had that argument with her yesterday; it must have really upset her.	I wish I had handled the argument better, and in the future I'll try to. But I don't know if Sarah's behavior is related to what I said or even if she's depressed. In any case, I'm not responsible for how Sarah feels or acts; only she can take responsibility for that.
Thinking in black and white	I've got to score 10 points in the game today. Otherwise, I don't belong on the team.	I'm a good player or else I wouldn't be on the team. I'll play my best—that's all I can do.
Magnifying events	They went to a movie without me. I thought we were friends, but I guess I was wrong.	I'm disappointed they didn't ask me to the movie, but it doesn't mean our friendship is over. It's not that big a deal.

SOURCE: Adapted from Schafer, W. *Stress Management for Wellness*, 4th ed. Copyright © 2000 Wadsworth, a part of Cengage Learning, Inc. Reproduced by permission. www.cengage.com/permissions.

situations that are not their fault, then jump to more negative conclusions and more unfounded overgeneralizations. Patterns of thinking that make events seem worse than they are in reality are called **cognitive distortions.**

When you react to a situation, an important piece of that reaction is your **self-talk**—the statements you make to yourself inside your own mind. Rational thinking and self-talk will not only help get you through the situation without feeling upset, but also help you avoid damaging your own self-concept.

In your own fight against demoralization, it may be hard to think of a rational response until hours or days after the event that upset you. Responding rationally can be especially hard when you are having an argument with someone else, which is why people often say things they don't mean in the heat of the moment or develop hurt feelings even when the other person had no intention of hurting them.

Once you get used to noticing the way your mind works, however, you may be able to catch yourself thinking negatively and change the process before it goes too far. This approach to controlling your reactions is not the same as positive thinking—which means substituting a positive thought for a negative one. Instead, you simply try to make your thoughts as logical and accurate as possible, based on the facts of the situation as you know them, and not on snap judgments or conclusions that may turn out to be false.

Demoralized people can be tenacious about their negative beliefs—so tenacious that they make their beliefs come true in a self-fulfilling prophesy. For example, if you conclude that you are so boring that no one will like you anyway, you may decide not to bother socializing. This behavior could make the negative belief become a reality.

For additional tips on changing distorted, negative ways of thinking, see the box "Realistic Self-Talk."

cognitive distortion A pattern of negative thinking that makes events seem worse than they are.

self-talk The statements a person makes to himself or herself.

Table 3.1 — Defense and Coping Mechanisms

MECHANISM	DESCRIPTION	EXAMPLE
Projection	Reacting to unacceptable inner impulses as if they were from outside the self	A student who dislikes his roommate feels that the roommate dislikes him.
Repression	Expelling from awareness an unpleasant feeling, idea, or memory	The child of an alcoholic, neglectful father remembers only when his father showed consideration and love.
Denial	Refusing to acknowledge to yourself what you really know to be true	A person believes that smoking cigarettes won't harm her because she's young and healthy.
Displacement	Shifting your feelings about a person to another person	A student who is angry with one of his professors returns home and yells at one of his housemates.
Dissociation	Falling into a state of altered consciousness to avoid emotional distress	A woman who was raped experiences frightening images and confusion when something reminds her of the event.
Rationalization	Giving a false, acceptable reason when the real reason is unacceptable	A shy young man decides not to attend a dorm party, telling himself he'd be bored.
Reaction formation	Concealing emotions or impulses by exaggerating the opposite ones	A student struggling with homosexual impulses engages in gay-bashing.
Substitution	Replacing an unacceptable or unobtainable goal with an acceptable one	In love with an unavailable partner, a man throws himself into training for a marathon.
Passive-aggressive behavior	Expressing hostility toward someone by being covertly uncooperative or passive	A person tells a coworker, with whom she competes for assignments, that she'll help him with a report but then never follows through.
Humor	Finding something funny in unpleasant situations	A student whose bicycle has been stolen thinks how surprised the thief will be when he or she starts downhill and discovers the brakes don't work.

Being Less Defensive

Sometimes our wishes come into conflict with people around us or with our conscience, and we become frustrated and anxious. If we cannot resolve the conflict by changing the external situation, we try to resolve the conflict internally by rearranging our thoughts and feelings. Some standard **defense mechanisms** are listed in Table 3.1. The drawback of many of these coping mechanisms is that they succeed temporarily, but make finding ultimate solutions much harder.

*Defense mechanisms may work right now, but they can **keep you from finding long-term solutions to conflicts.***

Recognizing your own defense mechanisms can be difficult, because they've probably become habits, occurring unconsciously. But we each have some inkling about how our mind operates. By remembering the details of conflict situations you have been in, you may be able to figure out which defense mechanisms you used in successful or unsuccessful attempts to cope. Try to look at yourself as an objective, outside observer would and analyze your thoughts and behavior in a psychologically stressful situation from the past. Having insight into what strategies you typically use can lead to new, less defensive and more effective ways of coping in the future.

Being Optimistic

Most of us have a tendency toward optimism or pessimism. **Pessimism** is a tendency to focus on the negative and expect an unfavorable outcome; **optimism** is a tendency to dwell on the hopeful and expect a favorable outcome. Pessimists not only expect repeated failure and rejection but also accept it as deserved. They do not see themselves as capable of success and irrationally dismiss any evidence of their own accomplishments. This negative point of view is learned, typically at a young age from parents and other authority figures. Optimists, on the other hand, consider bad events to be more temporary than permanent, consider failure to be limited to the area of life in which it occurred rather than pervasive, hope that the causes of negative events are temporary, and ascribe negative events to other causes instead of blaming themselves.

You can learn to be optimistic by recording adverse events in a diary along with the reactions and beliefs with which you met those events. By doing so, you learn to recognize and dispute the false, negative predictions you generate about yourself, like "The problem is going to last forever and ruin everything, and it's all my fault." Refuting such negative self-talk frees energy for realistic coping.

defense mechanism A mental mechanism for coping with conflict or anxiety.

pessimism The tendency to expect an unfavorable outcome.

optimism The tendency to expect a favorable outcome.

TERMS

Maintaining Honest Communication

Another important area of psychological functioning is communicating honestly with others. It can be very frustrating for us and for people around us if we cannot express what we want and feel. Others can hardly respond to our needs if they don't know what those needs are. We must recognize what we want to communicate and then express it clearly.

Some people know what they want others to do but don't state it clearly because they fear denial of the request, which they interpret as personal rejection. Such people might benefit from **assertiveness** training: learning to insist on their rights and to bargain for what they want. Assertiveness includes being able to say no or yes depending on the situation.

Dealing with Loneliness

It can be hard to strike the right balance between being alone and being with others. Some people are motivated to socialize by a fear of being alone—not the best reason to spend time with others. If you discover how to be happy by yourself, you'll be better able to cope with periods when you're forced to be alone—for example, when you've just broken off a romantic relationship or when your usual friends are away on vacation.

Unhappiness with being alone may come from interpreting it as a sign of rejection—that others are not interested in spending time with you. Before you reach such a conclusion, be sure that you give others a real chance to get to know you. Examine your patterns of thinking: You may harbor unrealistic expectations about other people—for example, that everyone you meet must like you and, if they don't, you must be terribly flawed.

If you decide that you're not spending enough time with people, take action to change the situation. College life provides many opportunities to meet people. If you're shy, you may have to push yourself to join a group. Look for something you've enjoyed in the past or in which you have a genuine interest.

Dealing with Anger

Common wisdom holds that expressing anger is beneficial for psychological and physical health. However, recent studies have questioned this idea by showing that overtly hostile people seem to be at higher risk for heart attacks. Angry words or actions don't contribute to psychological wellness if they damage relationships or produce feelings of guilt or loss of control. Perhaps the best way to resolve this

College offers many antidotes to loneliness, in the forms of clubs, organized activities, sports, and just hanging out with friends.

contradiction is to distinguish between a gratuitous expression of anger and a reasonable level of self-assertiveness.

At one extreme are people who never express anger or any opinion that might offend others, even when their own rights and needs are being jeopardized. If you have trouble expressing your anger, consider training in assertiveness and appropriate expressions of anger to help you learn to express yourself constructively.

At the other extreme are people whose anger is explosive or misdirected—a condition called *intermittent explosive disorder (IED)*. IED is often accompanied by depression or another disorder. Explosive anger or rage, like a child's tantrum, renders one temporarily unable to think straight or to act in his or her own best interest. During an IED episode, a person may lash out uncontrollably, hurting someone else or destroying property. Anyone who expresses anger this way should seek professional help.

Managing Your Own Anger   If you feel explosive anger coming on, consider the following two strategies to head it off.

First, try to *reframe* what you're thinking at that moment. You'll be less angry at another person if there is a possibility that his or her behavior was not intentionally directed against you. Imagine that another driver suddenly cuts in front of you. You would certainly be angry if you knew the other driver did it on purpose, but you probably would be less angry if you knew he simply did not see you. If you're angry because you've just been criticized, avoid mentally replaying scenes from the past when you received other unjust criticisms. Think about what is happening now, and try to act differently than in the past—less defensively and more analytically.

Second, until you're able to change your thinking, try to *distract* yourself. Use the old trick of counting to 10 before you respond, or start concentrating on your breathing. If necessary, cool off by leaving the situation until your anger has subsided. This does not mean that you should permanently avoid the issues and people who make you angry. Return to the matter after you've had a chance to think clearly about it.

Dealing with Anger in Other People   Anger can be infectious, and it disrupts cooperation and communication. If someone you're with becomes very angry, respond "asymmetrically" by reacting not with anger but with calm. Try to validate the other person by acknowledging that he or

she has some reason to be angry. This does not mean apologizing if you don't think you're to blame, or accepting verbal abuse, which is always inappropriate. Try to focus on solving the problem by allowing the person to explain why he or she is so angry and what can be done to alleviate the situation. Finally, if the person cannot be calmed, it may be best to disengage, at least temporarily. After a time-out, you may have better luck trying to solve the problem rationally.

PSYCHOLOGICAL DISORDERS

All of us feel anxious at times. In dealing with anxiety, we may avoid doing something that we want to do or should do. Most of us have periods of feeling down when we become pessimistic, less energetic, and less able to enjoy life. Many of us are bothered at times by irrational thoughts or odd feelings. Such feelings and thoughts can be normal responses to the ordinary challenges of life, but when emotions or irrational thoughts start to interfere with daily activities and rob us of our peace of mind, they can be considered symptoms of a psychological disorder. (Table 3.2 shows the likelihood of these disorders occurring during one's lifetime and during the past year.)

Psychological disorders are generally the result of many factors. Genetic differences, which underlie differences in how the brain processes information and experiences, are known to play an important role, especially in certain

VITAL STATISTICS

| Table 3.2 | Prevalence of Selected Psychological Disorders Among Americans |

DISORDER	MEN		WOMEN	
	LIFETIME PREVALENCE (%)	PAST YEAR PREVALENCE (%)	LIFETIME PREVALENCE (%)	PAST YEAR PREVALENCE (%)
Anxiety disorders				
Simple phobia	6.7	4.4	15.7	13.2
Social phobia	11.1	6.6	15.5	9.1
Panic disorder	2.0	1.3	5.0	3.2
Generalized anxiety disorder	3.6	2.0	6.6	4.3
Obsessive-compulsive disorder	1.7	0.5	2.8	0.8
Post-traumatic stress disorder	5.0	1.5	10.4	3.5
Mood disorders				
Major depressive episode	12.0	5.5	20.4	7.7
Manic episode	1.6	1.4	1.7	1.3
Schizophrenia and related disorders	1.0	0.8	0.5	0.4
Dementia	Depends on life expectancy	6.4 (age >=65)	Depends on life expectancy	5.7 (age >=65)

NOTE: Rates of the prevalence of dementia are highly dependent on how much impairment is considered dementia and on the age range of the population.

SOURCES: Kessler, R. C., et al. 2003. The epidemiology of major depressive disorder: Results from the National Comorbidity Survey Replication (NCS-R). *Journal of the American Medical Association* 289(23): 3095–3105; U.S. Department of Health and Human Services. 1999. *Mental Health: A Report of the Surgeon General.* Rockville, Md.: DHHS; Kessler, R. C., et al. 1995. Posttraumatic stress disorder in the National Comorbidity Survey. *Archives of General Psychiatry* 52(12): 1048–1060; Kessler, R. C., et al. 1994. Lifetime and 12-month prevalence of DSM-III-R psychiatric disorders in the United States. *Archives of General Psychiatry* 51(1): 8–19; Ferri, C. P., et al. 2005. Global prevalence of dementia: A Delphi consensus. *Lancet* 366: 2112–2117; Kukull, W. A., et al. 2002. Dementia and Alzheimer disease incidence. *Archives of Neurology* 59(Nov.): 1737–1776.

57.7 million adult Americans suffer from a diagnosable psychological disorder.

—National Institute of Mental Health, 2009

disorders. However, exactly which genes are involved, and how they alter the structure and chemistry of the brain, are still under study. Learning and life events are important, too: Identical twins often don't have the same psychological disorders in spite of having identical genes. Some people have been exposed to more traumatic events than others, leading either to greater vulnerability to future traumas or, conversely, to the development of better coping skills. Further, what your parents, peers, and others have taught you strongly influences your level of self-esteem and how you deal with frightening or depressing life events (see the box "Ethnicity, Culture, and Psychological Disorders").

Anxiety Disorders

Fear is a basic and useful emotion. Its value for our ancestors' survival cannot be overestimated. For modern humans, it provides motivation for self-protection and for learning to cope with new or potentially dangerous situations. We consider fear to be a problem only when it is out of proportion to real danger. **Anxiety** is another word for fear, especially a feeling of fear that is not in response to any definite threat. Anxiety is a disorder only when it occurs almost daily or in life situations that recur and cannot be avoided.

---

anxiety A feeling of fear that is not directed toward any definite threat.

simple (specific) phobia A persistent and excessive fear of a specific object, activity, or situation.

social phobia An excessive fear of being observed in public; speaking in public is the most common example.

panic disorder A syndrome of severe anxiety attacks accompanied by physical symptoms.

agoraphobia An anxiety disorder characterized by fear of being alone away from help and avoidance of many different places and situations; in extreme cases, a fear of leaving home.

generalized anxiety disorder (GAD) An anxiety disorder characterized by excessive, uncontrollable worry about all kinds of things and anxiety in many situations.

obsessive-compulsive disorder (OCD) An anxiety disorder characterized by uncontrollable, recurring thoughts and the performing of senseless rituals.

obsession A recurrent, irrational, unwanted thought or impulse.

Simple Phobia The most common and understandable anxiety disorder, called **simple (specific) phobia**, is a fear of something definite like lightning, a particular type of animal, or a place. Snakes, spiders, and dogs are commonly feared animals; frightening locations are often high places or enclosed spaces. Sometimes, but not always, these fears originate in bad experiences, such as being bitten by a snake.

Social Phobia The 15 million Americans with **social phobia** fear humiliation or embarrassment while being observed by others. Fear of speaking in public is perhaps the most common phobia of this kind. Extremely shy people can have social fears that extend to almost all social situations.

Panic Disorder People with **panic disorder** experience sudden unexpected surges in anxiety, accompanied by symptoms such as rapid and strong heartbeat, shortness of breath, loss of physical equilibrium, and a feeling of losing mental control. Such attacks usually begin in one's early twenties and can lead to a fear of being in crowds or closed places or of driving or flying. Sufferers fear that a panic attack will occur in a situation from which escape is difficult (such as while in an elevator), where the attack could be incapacitating and result in a dangerous or embarrassing loss of control (such as while driving a car or shopping), or where no medical help would be available if needed (such as when a person is alone away from home). Fears such as these lead to avoidance of situations that might cause trouble. The fears and avoidance may spread to a large variety of situations until a person is virtually housebound, a condition called **agoraphobia**.

Generalized Anxiety Disorder A basic reaction to future threats is to worry about them. **Generalized anxiety disorder (GAD)** is a diagnosis given to people whose worries have taken on a life of their own, pushing out other thoughts and refusing banishment by any effort of will. For someone with GAD, ordinary concerns can become sources of overwhelming worries.

The GAD sufferer's worrying is not completely unjustified—after all, thinking about problems can result in solving them. But this kind of thinking seems to just go around in circles, and the more you try to stop it, the more you feel at its mercy. The end result is a persistent feeling of nervousness, often accompanied by depression.

Obsessive-Compulsive Disorder Someone diagnosed with **obsessive-compulsive disorder (OCD)** contends with obsessions, compulsions, or both.

• **Obsessions** are recurrent, unwanted thoughts or impulses. Unlike the worries of GAD, they are not ordinary concerns but improbable fears such as of suddenly committing an antisocial act or of having been contaminated by germs.

Ethnicity, Culture, and Psychological Disorders

Psychological disorders differ in incidence and symptoms across cultures and ethnic groups around the world. This variability is usually attributable to cultural differences—factors such as how symptoms are interpreted and communicated, whether treatment is sought, and whether a social stigma is attached to a particular symptom or disorder.

Expression of Symptoms

People from different cultures or groups may manifest or describe symptoms differently. Consider the following examples:

- In Japan, people with social phobia may be more distressed about the imagined harm their social clumsiness causes to others than about their own embarrassment.

- Older African Americans may express depression in atypical ways—for example, denying depression by taking on a multitude of extra tasks.

- Somatization, the indirect reporting of psychological distress through nonspecific physical symptoms, is more prevalent among African Americans, Puerto Ricans, and Chinese Americans.

- Schizophrenia may manifest with different delusions depending on the local culture.

Differing Attitudes

It is relatively easy for Americans of northern European descent to regard an emotional problem as psychological in nature and to therefore accept a psychological treatment. For other groups, symptoms of psychological distress may be viewed as a spiritual problem, best dealt with by religious figures.

People from some groups may have little hesitation about communicating intimate, personal problems to professional care providers. However, for others, particularly men and members of certain ethnic groups, loss of emotional control may be seen as a weakness.

In addition, the use of mental health services is viewed negatively in many cultures; this stigma may partly account for the fact that African Americans and Asian American/ Pacific Islanders are only about half as likely as whites to use any type of mental health service.

Assimilation

One of the largest immigrant groups in the United States is from Mexico. Surprisingly, surveys show that these immigrants are psychologically healthier than their own children born in the United States. Mexican, Cuban, and Puerto Rican Hispanics in this country come from a culture where family bonds are valued and divorce is rare. As they assimilate and begin using English exclusively, however, these family bonds tend to weaken, but less so for Cubans than for Puerto Ricans or Mexicans. With assimilation, the incidence of anxiety, depression, and substance abuse increases.

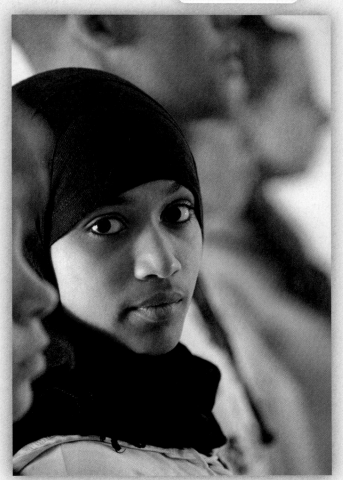

Biological Risk Factors

Biology can also play a role in the differences seen among patients of different ethnic groups. For example, psychotropic drugs are broken down in the body by a specific enzyme known as CYP2C19. Reduction of the activity of this enzyme is caused by two mutations, one of which appears to be found only in Asian populations. These "poor metabolizers" are very sensitive to medications that are broken down by this enzyme. The percentage of poor metabolizers among Asians is about 20%; among Latinos, about 5%; and among whites, 3%. Asian patients thus tend to have more adverse reactions to the doses of drugs standardized principally on white patients in the United States.

SOURCES: Alegria, M., et al. 2007. Understanding differences in past year psychiatric disorders for Latinos living in the US. *Social Science & Medicine* 65(2): 214–230; Kleinman, A. 2004. Culture and depression. *New England Journal of Medicine* 351(10): 951–953; Kirmayer, L. J. 2001. Cultural variations in the clinical presentation of depression and anxiety: Implications for diagnosis and treatment. *Journal of Clinical Psychiatry* 62 (Suppl. 13): 22–28; Lin, K. M. 2001. Biological differences in depression and anxiety across races and ethnic groups. *Journal of Clinical Psychiatry* 62 (Suppl. 13): 13–19.

- **Compulsions** are repetitive, difficult-to-resist actions usually associated with obsessions. A common compulsion is hand washing, associated with an obsessive fear of contamination by dirt. Other compulsions are counting and repeatedly checking whether something has been done—for example, whether a door has been locked or a stove turned off.

People with OCD feel anxious, out of control, and embarrassed. Their rituals can occupy much of their time and make them inefficient at work and difficult to live with.

Post-Traumatic Stress Disorder   People who suffer from **post-traumatic stress disorder (PTSD)** are reacting to severely traumatic events (events that produce a sense of terror and helplessness) such as physical violence to oneself or loved ones. Trauma occurs in personal assaults (rape, military combat), natural disasters (floods, hurricanes), and tragedies like fires and airplane or car crashes.

Symptoms include reexperiencing the trauma in dreams and in intrusive memories, trying to avoid anything associated with the trauma, and numbing of feelings. Hyperarousal, sleep disturbances, and other symptoms of anxiety and depression also commonly occur. Such symptoms can last months or even years.

7.7 million adult Americans suffer from PTSD.

—**National Institute of Mental Health, 2010**

The terrorist attacks on September 11, 2001, brought PTSD into the public spotlight. Among those affected were survivors, rescue workers, passersby, residents of Manhattan in general, and to some extent, television viewers around the world who saw countless repeated images of the devastation. An estimated 150,000 New Yorkers suffered PTSD following the attacks; some were still experiencing symptoms 5 years later. Hurricane Katrina had a similarly devastating effect; in one survey, 19% of police officers and 22% of firefighters in the Gulf Coast states reported symptoms of PTSD. Soldiers wounded in combat are also at risk for PTSD; among soldiers wounded in Iraq or Afghanistan, rates of PTSD

increased during the first year after the injury, suggesting that the emotional impact deepens with time. When symptoms persist and daily functioning is disrupted, professional help is needed.

Treating Anxiety Disorders   Therapies for anxiety disorders range from medication to psychological interventions concentrating on a person's thoughts and behavior. Both drug treatments and cognitive-behavioral therapies are effective in panic disorder, OCD, and GAD. Simple phobias are best treated without drugs. (For a more natural approach, see the box "Does Exercise Improve Mental Health?")

Mood Disorders

Daily, temporary mood changes typically don't affect our overall emotional state or level of wellness. A person with a **mood disorder,** however, experiences emotional disturbances that are intense and persistent enough to affect normal functioning. The two most common mood disorders are depression and bipolar disorder.

Depression   The National Institutes of Health estimates that **depression** strikes nearly 10% of Americans annually, making it the most common mood disorder. Depression affects the young as well as adults; nearly 50% of college students report depression severe enough to hinder their daily functioning. Depression tends to be more severe and persistent in blacks than in people of other races. Despite this, less than 50% of blacks affected by depression are treated for it.

Depression takes different forms but usually involves demoralization and can include the following:

- A feeling of sadness and hopelessness
- Loss of pleasure in doing usual activities
- Poor appetite and weight loss
- Insomnia or disturbed sleep
- Restlessness or, alternatively, fatigue
- Thoughts of worthlessness and guilt
- Trouble concentrating or making decisions
- Thoughts of death or suicide

A person experiencing depression may not have all of these symptoms. Sometimes instead of poor appetite and insomnia, the opposite occurs—eating too much and sleeping too long. (Depression may contribute to weight gain in young women.) People can have multiple symptoms of depression without feeling depressed, although they usually experience a loss of interest or pleasure.

In major depression, symptoms are often severe; a diagnosis of *dysthymic disorder* may be applied to people who experience persistent symptoms of mild or moderate depression for 2 years or longer. In some cases, depression is a clear-cut reaction to specific events, such as the

compulsion   An irrational, repetitive, forced action, usually associated with an obsession.

post-traumatic stress disorder (PTSD)   An anxiety disorder characterized by reliving traumatic events through dreams, flashbacks, and hallucinations.

mood disorder   An emotional disturbance that is intense and persistent enough to affect normal function; two common mood disorders are depression and bipolar disorder.

depression   A mood disorder characterized by loss of interest, sadness, hopelessness, loss of appetite, disturbed sleep, and other physical symptoms.

Does Exercise Improve Mental Health?

Since 1995, more than 30 major population-based studies (involving 175,000 Americans) have been published on the association between physical activity and mental health. The overall conclusion is that exercise—even modest activity such as taking a daily walk—can help combat a variety of mental health problems. For example, studies found that regular physical activity protects against depression and the onset of major depressive disorder; it can also reduce symptoms of depression in otherwise healthy people. Other studies found that physical activity protects against anxiety and the onset of anxiety disorders (such as specific phobia, social phobia, generalized anxiety, and panic disorder); it also helps reduce symptoms in people affected with an anxiety disorder.

Physical activity can enhance feelings of well-being in some people, which may provide some protection against psychological distress. Overall, physically active people are about 25–30% less likely to feel distressed than inactive people. Regardless of the number, age, or health status of the people being studied, those who were active managed stress better than their inactive counterparts.

Researchers have also looked at specific aspects of the activity/stress association. For example, one study found that taking a long walk can be effective at reducing anxiety and blood pressure. Another showed that a brisk walk of as little as 10 minutes' duration can leave people feeling more relaxed and energetic for up to 2 hours. People who took three brisk 45-minute walks a week for 3 months reported that they perceived fewer daily hassles and had a greater sense of general wellness.

Physical activity also helps you sleep better, and consistently sound sleep is critical to stress management and mental health. According to the National Sleep Foundation, about two-thirds of Americans have trouble sleeping at least a few nights a week, and 41% say they have difficulty sleeping virtually every night. There are about 70 known sleep disorders, and disordered sleep is associated with a variety of physical and neurological problems, including health problems relating to stress. Although only a few small-scale studies have been done on the relationship between physical activity and sleep, most experts have concluded that regular activity promotes better sleep and provides some protection against sleep interruptions such as insomnia and sleep apnea. Consistent, restful sleep is now regarded as a protective factor in disorders such as depression, anxiety, obesity, and heart disease.

SOURCES: Physical Activity Guidelines Advisory Committee. 2008. *Physical Activity Guidelines Advisory Committee Report, 2008*. Washington, D.C.: U.S. Department of Health and Human Services; National Sleep Foundation. 2009. *2009 Sleep in America Poll: Summary of Findings*. Washington, D.C.: National Sleep Foundation.

---

loss of a loved one or failing in school or work, whereas in other cases no trigger event is obvious.

One of the principal dangers of severe depression is suicide, which is discussed later in this chapter.

TREATING DEPRESSION Although treatments are highly effective, only about 35% of people who suffer from depression currently seek treatment. Treatment for depression depends on its severity and on whether the depressed person is suicidal. The best initial treatment for moderate to severe depression is probably a combination of drug therapy and psychotherapy. Newer prescription antidepressants work well, although they may need several weeks to take effect, and patients may need to try multiple medications before finding one that works well. Therefore, when suicidal impulses are strong, hospitalization may be necessary.

Antidepressants work by affecting key neurotransmitters in the brain, including serotonin. The herbal supplement St. John's wort may also affect serotonin levels and may be effective in helping with mild to moderate symptoms of depression. However, it is not subject to the same testing and regulation as prescription medications, and it may interact with certain medications, reducing their effectiveness. These include oral contraceptives and some medications for heart disease, depression, HIV infection, and seizures. The safety of St. John's wort in pregnancy has not been established. Anyone who may be suffering from depression should seek a medical evaluation rather than self-treating with supplements.

Electroconvulsive therapy (ECT) is effective for severe depression when other approaches have failed, including medications and other electronic therapies such as magnetic stimulation. In ECT, an epileptic-like seizure is induced by an electrical impulse transmitted through electrodes placed on the head. Patients are given an anesthetic and a muscle relaxant to reduce anxiety and prevent injuries associated with seizures. ECT usually includes 3 treatments per week for 2 to 4 weeks.

One type of depression is treated by having sufferers sit with eyes open in front of a bright light source every morning. These patients have **seasonal affective disorder (SAD)**; their depression worsens during winter months as daylight hours diminish, then improves in the spring and summer. The American Psychiatric Association estimates that 10–20% of Americans suffer symptoms that may be linked to SAD. SAD is more common among people who live at higher latitudes, where there

electroconvulsive therapy (ECT) The use of electric shock to induce brief, generalized seizures; used in the treatment of selected psychological disorders.

seasonal affective disorder (SAD) A mood disorder characterized by seasonal depression, usually occurring in winter, when there is less daylight.

Antidepressant Use in Young People

In 2004, a Food and Drug Administration (FDA) advisory committee recommended a warning label for antidepressant drugs based on evidence that their use increases the risk of suicidal thinking and behavior in children and adolescents.

Effectiveness

Drug treatment for depression is part of a success story in which people take seriously symptoms of depression and hints of suicidal thinking in children and teens. Over the past decade, the suicide rate among adolescents has fallen. Many factors have contributed to the decline, including stricter gun laws that make it harder for young people to get guns. Drug treatment has also been considered a key factor in the decline in suicide rates.

A 2005 review of reported childhood depression cases showed that between 1995 and 2002 the number of pediatric psychotherapy sessions declined significantly while prescriptions for antidepressants rose. Most of those prescriptions were for drugs that had not been approved for use in children. To date, only one drug—fluoxetine (Prozac)—has been approved for use specifically in children and teens. Studies have found that fluoxetine causes a greater improvement than a placebo, but the combination of drug therapy and cognitive-behavioral therapy is more beneficial than either treatment alone. The placebo effect, in which people improve while taking pills containing inactive compounds, is significant in studies of depression and can exceed 30%—meaning almost a third of people receiving a placebo experience an improvement in their symptoms.

Many antidepressants other than fluoxetine, especially other SSRIs, are also prescribed to young people, but these other drugs haven't been shown to be effective for that age group. Unpublished research data indicate that some SSRIs are *not* effective in children and teens or are only slightly more effective than a placebo.

Safety

SSRIs may increase the risk of suicide in some young people. The risk is especially high immediately after starting the medication. When study results were pooled, researchers found that in the short term, about 2–3% of users have an increased risk of suicidal thoughts and actions beyond the risk inherent from depression itself.

Researchers aren't exactly sure what causes this effect. One theory is that SSRIs reverse the lethargy associated with depression more quickly than they relieve the depression itself, giving users the energy to contemplate suicide in the interim. Antidepressants may work differently on the brains of young people than on the brains of adults, so there may be as yet unidentified effects.

In October 2004, the FDA published a public health advisory about using antidepressants in children and teens. It emphasizes that young people who take antidepressants should be monitored closely, especially when starting a new medication or changing the dosage of a drug. The FDA told manufacturers to add a boxed warning and expanded warning statements to product labels.

Depression is a serious illness that can increase the risk of suicide, and mental health professionals and patients must balance the risks of doing nothing against the potential risks and benefits of different types of treatments. These points were emphasized by the American Academy of Child and Adolescent Psychiatry in response to the FDA advisory.

Results of the Warning

Following the FDA advisory, the number of SSRI prescriptions for this age group fell by more than 20%. At the same time, however, the group's suicide rate rose by 15%. A similar advisory was issued in the Netherlands at about the same time, with the same result. These statistics do not prove a cause-effect relationship but certainly are a reason for concern. In

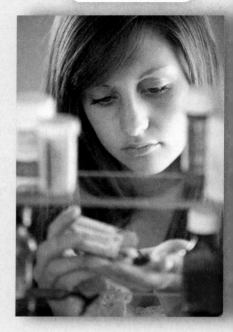

some cases, psychological treatment for depression may not have been a practical alternative to medication because it was not available or not accepted.

The FDA has limited persuasive power. Although it had recommended that young SSRI users be monitored through frequent face-to-face contacts in the first months of treatment, insurance claim statistics show that this did not happen.

SOURCES: Busch, S. H., et al. 2010. Antidepressants and suicide risk: How did specific information in FDA safety warnings affect treatment patterns? *Psychiatric Services* 61(1): 11–16; Gibbons, R. D. 2007. Early evidence on the effects of regulators' suicidality warnings on SSRI prescriptions and suicide in children and adolescents. *American Journal of Psychiatry* 164(9): 1356–1363; Newman, T. B. 2004. Treating depression in children: A black-box warning for antidepressants in children? *New England Journal of Medicine* 351(16): 1595–1598; Treatment for Adolescents with Depression Study (TADS) Team. 2004. Fluoxetine, cognitive-behavioral therapy, and their combination for adolescents with depression. *Journal of the American Medical Association* 292(7): 807–820; Stafford, R. S., et al. 2005. Depression treatment during outpatient visits by U.S. children and adolescents. *Journal of Adolescent Health* 37(6): 434–442.

are fewer hours of light in winter. Light therapy may work by extending the perceived length of the day and thus convincing the brain that it is summertime even during the winter months.

Mania and Bipolar Disorder People who experience **mania,** a less common feature of mood disorders, are restless, have a lot of energy, need little sleep, and often talk nonstop. They may devote themselves to fantastic projects and spend more money than they can afford. Many manic people swing between manic and depressive states, a syndrome called **bipolar disorder** because of the two opposite poles of mood. Bipolar disorder affects men and women equally. Tranquilizers are used to treat individual manic episodes, while special drugs such as the salt lithium carbonate taken daily can prevent future mood swings. Anticonvulsants (used to prevent epileptic seizures) are also prescribed to stabilize moods; examples are Tegretol (carbamazepine) and Lamictal (lamotrigene).

Schizophrenia

Schizophrenia is a disorder that affects one's thinking and perceptions of reality. The disease can be severe and debilitating or so mild that it's hardly noticeable. Although people are capable of diagnosing their own depression, they usually don't diagnose their own schizophrenia because they often can't see that anything is wrong. This disorder is not rare; in fact, 1 in every 100 people has a schizophrenic episode sometime in his or her lifetime, most commonly starting in adolescence.

> *1 in 100 Americans has a schizophrenic episode at least once in his or her lifetime.*

Scientists are uncertain about the exact causes of schizophrenia. Researchers have identified possible chemical and structural differences in the brains of people with the disorder as well as several genes that appear to increase risk. Schizophrenia is likely caused by a combination of genes and environmental factors that occur during pregnancy and development. For example, children born to older fathers have higher rates of schizophrenia, as do children with prenatal exposure to certain infections or medications.

Some general characteristics of schizophrenia include the following:

- *Disorganized thoughts.* Thoughts may be expressed in a vague or confusing way.
- *Inappropriate emotions.* Emotions may be either absent or strong but inappropriate.
- *Delusions.* People with delusions—firmly held false beliefs—may think that their minds are controlled by outside forces, that people can read their minds, that they are great personages like Jesus Christ or the president of the United States, or that they are being persecuted by a group such as the CIA.
- *Auditory hallucinations.* Schizophrenic people may hear voices when no one is present.
- *Deteriorating social and work functioning.* Social withdrawal and increasingly poor performance at school or work may be so gradual that they are hardly noticed at first.

None of these characteristics is invariably present. Some schizophrenic people are quite logical except on the subject of their delusions. Others show disorganized thoughts but no delusions or hallucinations.

A schizophrenic person needs help from a mental health professional. Suicide is a risk in schizophrenia, and expert treatment can reduce that risk and minimize the social consequences of the illness by shortening the period when symptoms are active. The key element in treatment is regular medication. At times medication is like insulin for diabetes—it makes the difference between being able to function or not. Sometimes hospitalization is temporarily required to relieve family and friends.

SUICIDE

In the United States, suicide is the third leading cause of death for young people ages 15–24 and the 11th leading cause for all ages. About 15 attempts are made for every death. In this country, men have much higher suicide rates than women; white men over age 65 have the highest suicide rate (Figure 3.2). Whites and Native Americans have higher rates than most other groups, but rates

Ask Yourself

QUESTIONS FOR CRITICAL THINKING AND REFLECTION

Have you ever wondered if you were depressed? Try to recall your situation at the time. How did you feel, and what do you think brought about those feelings? What, if anything, did you do to bring about change and to feel better?

mania A mood disorder characterized by excessive elation, irritability, talkativeness, inflated self-esteem, and expansiveness.

bipolar disorder A mental illness characterized by alternating periods of depression and mania.

schizophrenia A psychological disorder that involves a disturbance in thinking and in perceiving reality.

TERMS

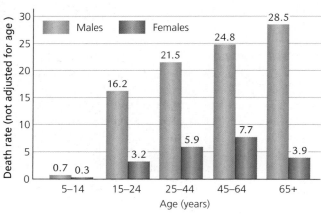

(a) Suicide rate by age and gender

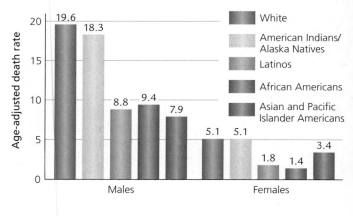

(b) Suicide rate by ethnicity and gender (all ages)

FIGURE 3.2   Rates of suicide per 100,000 people in the United States. The rate of suicide varies by gender, age, and ethnicity. Rates are higher among men than women at all ages and are higher among whites compared to other groups. White men over age 65 have the highest rates of suicide. The age-adjusted national suicide rate is 10.9 per 100,000 people. These statistics are from 2006.

SOURCE: National Center for Health Statistics. 2009. *Health, United States, 2009.* Hyattsville, Md.: National Center for Health Statistics.

among blacks have been rising. Women attempt three times as many suicides as men, yet men succeed at more than three times the rate of women (see the box "Depression, Anxiety, and Gender"). Suicide rates among adolescents and young adults and among adults over 65 have been falling for the last two decades.

Self-inflicted injuries—including cutting, burning, hitting, and other self-injury—are sometimes mistaken for suicide attempts. The prevalence of self-injury is estimated at 3–4% in the general population but is higher in adolescents, especially females. In a 2007 study, 25% of college-age females surveyed said they had injured themselves intentionally. A maladaptive coping strategy, self-injury is believed to provide relief from unbearable psychological distress or pain, perhaps through the release of endorphins. A variety of psychotherapeutic interventions can help people who injure themselves. Whatever the reason behind it, however, self-harm should be taken very seriously because it may signal an increased risk for suicide. According to a 2007 British study, young persons who purposefully hurt themselves were much more likely to commit suicide than the general population.

Suicide rarely occurs without warning signs. About 60% of people who commit suicide are depressed. The more symptoms of depression a person has, the greater the risk. Other warning signs include the following:

- Expressing the wish to be dead or revealing contemplated methods
- Increasing social withdrawal and isolation
- A sudden, inexplicable lightening of mood (which can mean the person has decided to commit suicide)

Certain risk factors increase the likelihood of suicide:

- A history of previous attempts
- A suicide by a family member or friend
- Readily available means, such as guns or pills
- A history of substance abuse or eating disorders
- Serious medical problems

If you are severely depressed or know someone who is, expert help from a mental health professional is essential. Don't be afraid to discuss the possibility of suicide with someone you fear is suicidal. You won't give them an idea they haven't already thought of. Asking direct questions is the best way to determine whether someone seriously intends to commit suicide. Encourage your friend to talk and to take positive steps to improve his or her situation.

Most communities have emergency help available, often in the form of a hotline telephone counseling service run by a suicide prevention agency. If you feel there is an immediate danger of suicide, do not leave the person alone. Call for help or take him or her to an emergency room.

Firearms are used in more suicides than homicides. 83% of gun-related deaths in the home are the result of suicide, often by someone other than the gun owner. If you learn someone at high risk for suicide has access to a gun, try to convince him or her to put it in safekeeping.

52% of American suicides are committed with guns.

—National Center for Health Statistics, 2009

STATS

Depression, Anxiety, and Gender

The common belief that females are more emotional than males has both a positive and a negative side. On the one hand, women are thought to express positive emotions more clearly than men, especially those related to sympathy and caring. On the other hand, women are more prone to negative emotions such as depression and worry.

One of the defining characteristics of a psychiatric disorder is that it interferes with daily activities and the ability to live a happy life. Thus, the higher incidence of anxiety and mood disorders in women is convincing evidence that they are more likely to suffer from emotional distress than are men.

Anxiety Disorders

Panic disorder is more than twice as common in women as in men, whereas obsessive-compulsive disorder occurs in men and women at about the same rate. In population surveys, social anxiety disorder is more common in women than in men, but men are more likely to seek treatment for it—perhaps because men are more likely to find it a barrier to success in white-collar jobs. In some surveys, PTSD is more common in women, but the incidence of PTSD depends on the incidence of traumatic events, which varies in different environments. Men are more often exposed to military combat, and women to rape. Trauma from motor vehicle crashes is a fairly common cause of PTSD in both sexes.

Depression and Suicide

Over their lifetimes, about 20% of women and 12% of men have serious depression. When women are depressed, they are more likely than men to experience guilt, anxiety, increased appetite and weight gain, and increased sleep. When women take antidepressants, they may need a lower dose than men;

at the same dosage, blood levels of medication tend to be higher in women. An issue for women who may become pregnant is whether antidepressants can harm a fetus or newborn. The best evidence indicates that the most frequently prescribed types of antidepressants do not cause birth defects, although some studies have reported withdrawal symptoms in some newborns whose mothers used certain antidepressants.

Although suicidal behavior is strongly associated with depression, and depression is more prevalent in women, many more men than women commit suicide. Overall, about three times as many women as men attempt suicide, but women's attempts are less likely to be lethal.

Underlying Factors

Why women have more anxiety and depression than men is a matter of debate. Some experts think much of the difference is due to reporting bias: Women are more willing to admit to experiencing negative emotions, being stressed, or having difficulty coping. Women may also be more likely to seek treatment.

Other experts point to biologically based sex differences, particularly in the level and action of hormones. Greater anxiety and depression in women compared with men are most pronounced between puberty and menopause, when female hormones are most active. However, this period of life is also the time in which women's social roles and expectations may be the most different from those of men. Women may put more emphasis on relationships in determining self-esteem, so the deterioration of a relationship is a cause of depression that can hit women harder than men. In addition, culturally determined gender roles are more likely to place women in situations where they have less control

over key life decisions, and lack of autonomy is associated with depression.

The higher suicide rate among young men may relate to gender norms and expectations that men assert independence and physical prowess—sometimes expressed in risky, dangerous, and potentially self-destructive behavior. Such behavior, often involving drugs and alcohol and resulting in motor vehicle crashes, occurs more often in young people who later commit suicide. Even when suicidal intention is never expressed, suicidal impulses are often suspected of contributing to sudden deaths in this age group.

SOURCES: Gentile, S. 2010. On categorizing gestational, birth, and neonatal complications following late pregnancy exposure to antidepressants: The prenatal antidepressant exposure syndrome. *CNS Spectrums* 15(3): 167–185: Kessler, R. C. 2003. Epidemiology of women and depression. *Journal of Affective Disorders* 74: 5–13: World Health Organization. 2002. *Gender and Mental Health*. Geneva: World Health Organization.

GETTING HELP

Knowing when self-help or professional help is required for mental health problems is usually not as difficult as knowing how to start or which professional to choose.

Self-Help

If you have a personal problem to solve, a smart way to begin is by finding out what you can do on your own. Some problems are specifically addressed in this book. Behavioral and some cognitive approaches are especially

ADHD and Exposure to Nature

Attention-deficit/hyperactivity disorder (ADHD)—characterized by impulsivity, hyperactivity, and/or an inability to stay focused—is the most commonly diagnosed mental disorder among American children and adolescents. Children with ADHD can struggle with conflict and aggression, peer rejection, and academic problems. Up to 7% of American children are affected by some form of ADHD, and about 4% of adults develop symptoms in any given year.

ADHD is commonly treated with the drug methylphenidate (Ritalin), a psychostimulant that has the seemingly paradoxical effect in people with ADHD of improving attention and decreasing distractibility. Although Ritalin is approved by the FDA for the treatment of ADHD, the long-term effects are not known.

In recent years, interest has grown in supplementing drug and behavioral therapy for children with ADHD by exposing them to natural environments. Researchers have found that when children spend time outdoors in natural settings, ADHD symptoms diminish. In one study, children with ADHD took 20-minute walks in a park, a residential neighborhood, and an urban downtown area, and their concentration was measured after each walk. After the nature walk, concentration improved significantly, comparable to the effects of medication. No one suggests that nature exposure replaces medication, and some believe that the positive effects are overstated, but researchers suggest that "doses of nature" may serve as safe, inexpensive complements to other ADHD treatments.

Some experts worry that all American children are missing out on nature these days, largely as a result of increased time spent on video games, computers, and TV. The term *nature deficit disorder* has been coined to describe this lack of exposure to the outside world, with associated childhood obesity and mental health problems like depression and anxiety. A grassroots movement called the No Child Left Inside Coalition has sprung up to get children outside and to teach them environmental responsibility. Many school districts participate in the program, incorporating environmental literacy into their curricula, beginning in elementary school. The U.S. government is also getting involved. In 2009, the No Child Left Inside Act was introduced in Congress, extending funding for environmental education programs in public schools. As part of the U.S. Department of Education's budget for fiscal year 2011, $1 billion was included specifically for environmental literacy programs.

Advocates say that, in addition to helping with ADHD, there are other good reasons for encouraging children to spend time outdoors. Today's children, they contend, may be losing their fundamental connection to nature, possibly resulting in an entire generation of Americans who feel less connected to—and less sympathy for—the environment. Given the urgency of global warming, pollution, and other environmental issues, experts say, future generations must be environmentally literate and understand their role in protecting the planet—or risk causing more harm for themselves and their own children.

For a detailed discussion of environmental health—how it affects you and how you affect it—see Chapter 19.

SOURCES: Bennett, L. 2009. *Greening a K-12 Curriculum.* (http://www.ecoliteracy.org/essays/greening-k-12-curriculum; retrieved June 2, 2010); Education.com. 2010. *Nature Deficit Disorder* (http://www.education.com/topic/nature-deficit-disorder/; retrieved June 2, 2010); Faber, T. A., and F. E. Kuo. 2009. Children with attention deficits concentrate better after walk in the park. *Journal of Attention Disorders* 12(5): 402–409; Luov, R. 2008. *Last Child in the Woods.* Chapel Hill, N.C.: Algonquin.

useful for helping yourself. They all involve becoming more aware of self-defeating actions and ideas and combating them in some way: by being more assertive; by communicating honestly; by raising your self-esteem by counteracting negative thoughts, people, and actions that undermine it; and by confronting, rather than avoiding, the things you fear. You can get more information from books in the psychology and self-help sections of libraries and bookstores, but be selective. Watch out for self-help books making fantastic claims that deviate from mainstream approaches.

Some people find it helpful to express their feelings in a journal. Grappling with a painful experience in this way provides an emotional release and can help you develop more constructive ways of dealing with similar situations in the future. Research indicates that using a journal this way can improve physical as well as emotional wellness.

For some people, religious belief and practice may promote psychological health. Religious organizations provide a social network and a supportive community, and religious practices, such as prayer and meditation, offer a path for personal change and transformation. Spending time in nature can have psychological benefits as well (see the box "ADHD and Exposure to Nature").

Peer Counseling and Support Groups

Sharing your concerns with others is another helpful way of dealing with psychological health challenges. Just being able to share what's troubling you with an accepting, empathetic person can bring relief. Comparing notes with people who have problems similar to yours can give you new ideas about coping.

Many colleges offer peer counseling through a health center or through the psychology or education department. Peer counseling is usually done by volunteer students who have special training that emphasizes confidentiality. Peer counselors may steer you toward an appropriate campus or community resource or simply offer a sympathetic ear.

Many self-help groups work on the principle of bringing together people with similar problems to share their experiences and support one another. Support groups are typically organized around a specific problem, such as eating disorders or substance abuse. Self-help groups may be listed in the phone book or the campus newspaper.

Professional Help

Sometimes self-help or talking to nonprofessionals is not enough. More objective, more expert, or more discreet help is needed. Many people have trouble accepting the need for professional help, and often those who most need help are the most unwilling to get it. You may someday find yourself having to overcome your own reluctance, or that of a friend, about seeking help.

Determining the Need for Professional Help In some cases, professional help is optional. Some people are interested in improving their psychological health in a general way by going into individual or group therapy to learn more about themselves and how to interact with others. Seeking professional help for these reasons is a matter of individual choice. In some situations, such as friction among family members or between partners, professional help can mean the difference between a painful divorce and a satisfying relationship.

Professional help is appropriate in any of the following situations:

- Depression, anxiety, or other emotional problems interfere seriously with school or work performance or in getting along with others.
- Suicide is attempted or is seriously considered. (See the warning signs listed earlier in the chapter.)
- Symptoms such as hallucinations, delusions, incoherent speech, or loss of memory occur.
- Alcohol or drugs are used to the extent that they impair normal functioning during much of the week, finding or taking drugs occupies much of the week, or reducing their dosage leads to psychological or physiological withdrawal symptoms.

Types of Psychotherapy There are several approaches to treating psychological disorders:

- *Pharmacological therapy* is based on the premise that the mind's activity depends on an organic structure, the brain, whose composition is genetically determined. Pharmacological therapy relies on a wide variety of prescription medications to treat psychological disorders, but often in combination with one or more other therapies.
- *Behavioral therapy* focuses on current behavior patterns. The goal is to help the patient replace unhealthy, maladaptive behaviors with more positive ones. Shaping one's environment is a key part

of this therapy. Behavioral therapy is often used to treat phobias and other anxiety disorders. For example, a person might be exposed to a feared object or situation in gradual stages in order to overcome an irrational fear of it.

- *Cognitive therapy* emphasizes the effect of ideas on behavior and feeling. People in cognitive therapy are taught to notice their unrealistic thoughts and to substitute more realistic ones. Cognitive and behavioral therapies are frequently combined. For example, treatment of social anxiety might include gradual exposure to a feared situation like a party along with practice in identifying and changing unrealistic, negative self-talk.
- *Psychodynamic therapy* emphasizes the role of the past and of unconscious thoughts and impulses in shaping present behavior. Uncovering feelings and building self-awareness are common therapy goals.

Although these types of therapies may be described as distinctive orientations, most therapists offer a variety of approaches. Multiple therapies may be combined in various ways to meet the needs of a given patient's disorder or needs.

TIPS FOR TODAY AND THE FUTURE

Most of life's psychological challenges can be met with self-help and everyday skills. You can take many steps to maintain your mental health.

RIGHT NOW YOU CAN

- Take a serious look at how you've been feeling recently. If you have any feelings that are especially hard to handle, consider how you can get help with them.
- Think of the way in which you are most creative (an important part of self-actualization), whether it's in music, art, or whatever you enjoy. Try to focus at least an hour each week on this activity.
- Review the list of defense mechanisms in Table 3.1. Have you used any of them recently or consistently over time? Think of a situation in which you used one of those mechanisms, and determine how you could have coped with it differently.

IN THE FUTURE YOU CAN

- Write 100 positive adjectives that describe you. This exercise may take several days to complete. Post your list in a place where you will see it often.
- Record your reactions to upsetting events in your life. Are your reactions and self-talk typically negative or neutral? Decide whether you are satisfied with your reactions and if they are healthy.

Choosing and Evaluating Mental Health Professionals

College students are usually in a good position to find convenient, affordable mental health care. Larger schools typically have both health services that employ psychiatrists and psychologists and counseling centers staffed by professionals and student peer counselors. Resources in the community may include a school of medicine, a hospital, and a variety of professionals who work independently. Although independent practitioners are listed in the telephone book, it's a good idea to get recommendations from physicians, clergy, friends who have been in therapy, or community agencies rather than pick a name at random.

Financial considerations are also important. Find out how much different services will cost and what your health insurance will cover. If you're not adequately covered by a health plan, don't let that stop you from getting help; investigate low-cost alternatives. City, county, and state governments often support mental health clinics for those who can afford to pay little or nothing for treatment. Some on-campus services may be free or offered at very low cost.

The cost of treatment is linked to how many therapy sessions will be needed, which in turn depends on the type of therapy and the nature of the problem. Psychological therapies focusing on specific problems may require eight or ten sessions at weekly intervals. Therapies aiming for psychological awareness and personality change can last months or years.

Deciding whether a therapist is right for you will require meeting the therapist in person. Before or during your first meeting, find out about the therapist's background and training:

- Does she or he have a degree from an appropriate professional school and a state license to practice?

- Has she or he had experience treating people with problems similar to yours?

- How much will therapy cost?

You have a right to know the answers to these questions and should not hesitate to ask them. After your initial meeting, evaluate your impressions:

- Does the therapist seem like a warm, intelligent person who would be able to help you and interested in doing so?

- Are you comfortable with the personality, values, and beliefs of the therapist?

- Is he or she willing to talk about the techniques in use? Do these techniques make sense to you?

If you answer yes to these questions, this therapist may be satisfactory for you. If you feel uncomfortable—and you're not in need of emergency care—it's worthwhile to set up one-time consultations with one or two others before you make up your mind. Take the time to find someone who feels right for you.

Later in your treatment, evaluate your progress:

- Are you being helped by the treatment?

- If you are displeased, is it because you aren't making progress, or because therapy is raising difficult, painful issues you don't want to deal with?

- Can you express dissatisfaction to your therapist? Such feedback can improve your treatment.

If you're convinced your therapy isn't working or is harmful, thank your therapist for her or his efforts, and find another.

Connect to your Choices

Have you ever thought about why you approach emotional and psychological problems the way you do? Many factors can influence the choices we make about psychological health, some not as obvious as others. Do you hold in your feelings and hide them from others because that's what was modeled in your family? Do you drink or use drugs when you feel depressed or anxious because you aren't aware of any other options? Do you think getting professional help for a psychological problem is a sign that you're weak or crazy?

What are the external factors that influence your choices about psychological health? What are your inner motivations and core values, and how do they affect your choices? Based on what you learned in this chapter, will you make some different choices in the future? If so, what will they be?

Go online to Connect to complete this activity.
www.mcgraw-hillconnect.com

Choosing a Mental Health Professional Mental health workers belong to several different professions and have different roles. Psychiatrists are medical doctors. They are experts in deciding whether a medical disease lies behind psychological symptoms, and they are usually involved in treatment if medication or hospitalization is required. Clinical psychologists typically hold a Ph.D. degree; they are often experts in behavioral and cognitive therapies. Other mental health workers include social workers, licensed counselors, and clergy with special training in pastoral counseling. In hospitals and clinics, various mental health professionals may join together in treatment teams.

For more on finding appropriate help, see the box "Choosing and Evaluating Mental Health Professionals."

SUMMARY

- Psychological health encompasses more than a single particular state of normality. Psychological diversity is valuable among groups of people.

Dealing with Social Anxiety

Shyness is often the result of both high anxiety levels and lack of key social skills. To help overcome shyness, you need to learn to manage your fear of social situations and to develop social skills such as making appropriate eye contact, initiating topics in conversations, and maintaining the flow of conversations by asking questions and making appropriate responses.

To reduce your anxiety in social situations, try some of the following strategies:

- Refocus your attention away from the stress reaction you're experiencing and toward the social task at hand. Your nervousness is much less visible than you think.

- Allow a warm-up period for new situations. Realize that you will feel more nervous at first, and take steps to relax and become more comfortable. Refer to the suggestions for deep breathing and other relaxation techniques in Chapter 2.

- If possible, take breaks during anxiety-producing situations. For example, if you're at a party, take a moment to visit the restroom or step outside. Alternate between speaking with good friends and striking up conversations with new acquaintances.

- Practice realistic self-talk. Replace your self-critical thoughts with more supportive ones: "No one else is perfect, and I don't have to be either." "It would have been good if I had a funny story to tell, but the conversation was interesting anyway."

Starting and maintaining conversations can be difficult for shy people, who may feel overwhelmed by their physical stress reaction. If small talk is a problem for you, try the following strategies:

- Introduce yourself early in the conversation. If you tend to forget names, repeat your new acquaintance's name to help fix it in your mind ("Nice to meet you, Amelia").

- Ask questions and look for shared topics of interest. Simple, open-ended questions like "How's your presentation coming along?" or "How do you know our host?" encourage others to carry the conversation for a while and help bring up a variety of subjects.

- Take turns talking, and elaborate on your answers. Simple yes and no answers don't move the conversation along. Try to relate something in your life—a course you're taking or a hobby you have—to something in the other person's life. Match self-disclosure with self-disclosure.

- Have something to say. Expand your mind and become knowledgeable about current events and local or campus news. If you have specialized knowledge about a topic, practice discussing it in ways that both beginners and experts can understand and appreciate.

- If you get stuck for something to say, try giving a compliment ("Great presentation!" or "I love your earrings.") or performing a social grace (pass the chips or get someone a drink).

- Be an active listener. Reward the other person with your full attention and with regular responses. Make frequent eye contact and maintain a relaxed but alert posture.

At first, your new behaviors will likely make you anxious. Don't give up—things *will* get easier. Create lots of opportunities to practice your new behaviors; your goal is to make them routine activities.

Eventually, you'll be able to sustain social interactions with comfort and enjoyment. If you find that social anxiety is a major problem for you and self-help techniques don't seem to work, consider looking into a shyness clinic or treatment program on your campus.

SOURCES: University of Texas at Dallas, Student Counseling Center. 2008 Update. *Self-Help: Overcoming Social Anxiety* (http://www.utdallas.edu/counseling/selfhelp/social-anxiety.html; retrieved June 2, 2010); Carducci, B. J. 2000. *Shyness: A Bold New Approach.* New York: Harper Paperbacks.

- Defining psychological health as the presence of wellness means that to be healthy you must strive to fulfill your potential.

- Self-actualized people have high self-esteem and are realistic, inner-directed, authentic, capable of emotional intimacy, and creative.

- Crucial parts of psychological wellness include developing an adult identity, establishing intimate relationships, and developing values and purpose in life.

- A pessimistic outlook can be damaging; it can be overcome by developing more realistic self-talk.

- Honest communication requires recognizing what needs to be said and saying it clearly. Assertiveness enables people to insist on their rights and to participate in the give-and-take of good communication.

- People may be lonely if they haven't developed ways to be happy on their own or if they interpret being alone as a sign of rejection. Lonely people can take action to expand their social contacts.

- Dealing successfully with anger involves distinguishing between a reasonable level of assertiveness and gratuitous expressions of anger, heading off rage by reframing thoughts and distracting oneself, and responding to the anger of others with an asymmetrical, problem-solving orientation.

- People with psychological disorders have symptoms severe enough to interfere with daily living.

- Anxiety is a fear that is not directed toward any definite threat. Anxiety disorders include simple phobias, social phobias, panic disorder, generalized anxiety disorder, obsessive-compulsive disorder, and post-traumatic stress disorder.

- Depression is a common mood disorder; loss of interest or pleasure in things seems to be its most universal symptom. Severe depression carries a high risk of suicide, and suicidally depressed people need professional help.

- Symptoms of mania include exalted moods with unrealistically high self-esteem, little need for sleep, and rapid speech. Mood swings between mania and depression characterize bipolar disorder.

- Schizophrenia is characterized by disorganized thoughts, inappropriate emotions, delusions, auditory hallucinations, and deteriorating social and work performance.

- Help is available in a variety of forms, including self-help, peer counseling, support groups, and therapy with a mental health professional. For serious problems, professional help may be the most appropriate.

FOR MORE INFORMATION

BOOKS

Antony, M. M. 2008. *The Shyness & Social Anxiety Workbook: Proven, Step-by-Step Strategies for Overcoming Your Fear,* 2nd ed. Oakland, Calif.: New Harbinger. *Practical suggestions for fears of interacting with people you don't know.*

Grieco, R. 2009. *The Other Depression: Bipolar Disorder.* New York: Routledge. *Provides a complete introduction to bipolar disorder, its symptoms, and its current treatments.*

Jenkins, J., D. Keltner, and K. Oatley. 2006. *Understanding Emotions,* 2nd ed. Oxford: Blackwell. *A comprehensive guide to emotions, including current research on the neuroscience of emotions, evolutionary and cultural approaches to emotion, and the expression and communication of emotions.*

Nathan, P. E., and J. M. Gorman. 2007. *A Guide to Treatments That Work,* 3rd ed. New York: Oxford University Press. *A balanced and comprehensive report on various treatments for psychological disorders.*

Seligman, M. E. 2006. *Learned Optimism: How to Change Your Mind and Your Life* (Vintage Reprint Edition). New York: Vintage. *Introduces methods for overcoming feelings of helplessness and building a positive self-image that can contribute to emotional well-being.*

Thase, M. E., and S. S. Lang. 2006. *Beating the Blues: New Approaches to Overcoming Dysthymia and Chronic Mild Depression.* New York: Oxford University Press. *Describes strategies for changing negative thinking patterns that lead to discouragement and pessimism; also discusses newer medications and alternative therapies.*

ORGANIZATIONS, HOTLINES, AND WEB SITES

American Association of Suicidology. Provides information about suicide and resources for people in crisis.
http://www.suicidology.org

Anxiety Disorders Association of America (ADAA). Provides information and resources related to anxiety disorders.
http://www.adaa.org

Cope, Care, Deal. Offers information on mental health issues specifically for teens.
http://www.copecaredeal.org

Depression and Bipolar Support Alliance (DBSA). Provides educational materials and information about support groups.
http://www.dbsalliance.org

Mental Health America. Provides consumer information on a variety of issues, including how to find help.
http://www.nmha.org

NAMI (National Alliance on Mental Illness). Provides information and support for people affected by mental illness.
800-950-NAMI (Help Line)
http://www.nami.org

National Hopeline Network. 24-hour hotline for people who are thinking about suicide or know someone who is; calls are routed to local crisis centers.
800-SUICIDE
http://www.hopeline.com

National Institute of Mental Health (NIMH). Provides helpful information about anxiety, depression, eating disorders, and other challenges to psychological health.
http://www.nimh.nih.gov

National Mental Health Information Center. A one-stop source for information and resources relating to mental health.
http://mentalhealth.samhsa.gov

SELECTED BIBLIOGRAPHY

American Psychiatric Association. 2000. *Diagnostic and Statistical Manual of Mental Disorders,* 4th ed., Text Revision *(DSM-IV-TR).* Washington, D.C.: American Psychiatric Association Press.

Antidepressants for children and adolescents: An update. 2006. *Harvard Mental Health Letter* 22(12): 4–5.

Avagianou, P. A., and M. Zafiropoulou. 2008. Parental bonding and depression: Personality as a mediating factor. *International Journal of Adolescent Medicine & Health* 20(3): 261–269.

Beard, C., et al. 2010. Health-related quality of life across the anxiety disorders: Findings from a sample of primary care patients. *Journal of Anxiety Disorders* 24(6): 559–564.

Brenes, G. A. 2006. Age differences in the presentation of anxiety. *Aging and Mental Health* 10(3): 298–302.

Centers for Disease Control and Prevention. 2010. Attitudes toward mental illness—35 states, District of Columbia, and Puerto Rico, 2007. *Morbidity and Mortality Weekly Report* 59(20): 619–625.

Coryell, W. H. 2006. Clinical assessment of suicide risk in depressive disorder. *CNS Spectrums* 11(6): 455–461.

Eranti, S., et al. 2007. A randomized, controlled trial with 6-month follow-up of repetitive transcranial magnetic stimulation and electroconvulsive therapy for severe depression. *American Journal of Psychiatry* 164(1): 73–81.

Favaro, A., et al. 2007. Self-injurious behavior in a community sample of young women: Relationship with childhood abuse and other types of self-damaging behaviors. *Journal of Clinical Psychiatry* 68(1): 122–131.

Fazel, S., and M. Grann. 2006. The population impact of severe mental illness on violent crime. *American Journal of Psychiatry* 163(8): 1397–1403.

Ferrier-Auerback, A. G., et al. 2010. Predictors of emotional distress reported by soldiers in the combat zone. *Journal of Psychiatric Research* 44(7): 470–476.

Forty, L., et al. 2009. Polarity at illness onset in bipolar I disorder and clinical course of illness. *Bipolar Disorders* 11(1): 82–88.

Hamilton, B. E., et al. 2007. Annual summary of vital statistics: 2005. *Pediatrics* 119(2): 345–360.

Healy, D. 2006. Did regulators fail over selective serotonin reuptake inhibitors? *British Medical Journal* 333: 92–95.

Hettema, J. M., et al. 2006. A population-based twin study of the relationship between neuroticism and internalizing disorders. *American Journal of Psychiatry* 163(5): 857–864.

Jones, S. H., and G. Burrell-Hodgson. 2008. Cognitive-behavioral treatment of first diagnosis bipolar disorder. *Clinical Psychology & Psychotherapy* 15(6): 367–377.

Kasper, S., et al. 2006. Superior efficacy of St. John's wort extract WS(R) 5570 compared to placebo in patients with major depression: A randomized, double-blind, placebo-controlled, multi-center trial. *BMC Medicine* 4(1): 14.

Kendler, K. S., J. Myers, and C. A. Prescott. 2005. Sex differences in the relationship between social support and risk for major depression: A longitudinal study of opposite-sex twin pairs. *American Journal of Psychiatry* 162(2): 250–256.

Licinio, J., and M. L. Wong. 2005. Opinion: Depression, antidepressants and suicidality: A critical appraisal. *Nature Reviews: Drug Discovery* 4(2): 165–171.

Lin, Y. R., et al. 2008. Evaluation of assertiveness training for psychiatric patients. *Journal of Clinical Nursing* 17(21): 2875–2883.

McGirr, A., et al. 2006. An examination of DSM-IV depressive symptoms and risk for suicide completion in major depressive disorder: A psychological autopsy study. *Journal of Affective Disorders,* 17 July.

Nemeroff, C. B. 2007. The burden of severe depression: A review of diagnostic challenges and treatment alternatives. *Journal of Psychiatric Research* 41(3–4): 189–206.

Ozer, D. J., and V. Benet-Martinez. 2006. Personality and prediction of consequential outcomes. *Annual Review of Psychology* 57: 401–421.

Rothwell, J. D. 2009. *In the Company of Others: An Introduction to Communication,* 3rd ed. New York: McGraw-Hill.

Saewyc, E. M., and R. Tonkin. 2008. Surveying adolescents: Focusing on positive development. *Pediatrics & Child Health* 13(1): 43–47.

Schatzberg, A. F., J. O. Cole, and C. DeBattista. 2007. *Manual of Clinical Psychopharmacology,* 6th ed. Washington, D.C.: American Psychiatric Publishing.

Seligman, M. E. P. 2008. Positive health. *Applied Psychology: An International Review* 57, 3–18.

Simon, G. E., and J. Savarino. 2007. Suicide attempts among patients starting depression treatment with medications or psychotherapy. *American Journal of Psychiatry* 164(7): 1029–1034.

Simon, G. 2009. Collaborative care for mood disorders. *Current Opinion in Psychiatry* 22(1): 37–41.

Singh, N. N., et al. 2007. Individuals with mental illness can control their aggressive behavior through mindfulness training. *Behavior Modification* 31(3): 313–328.

Verhaak, P. F., et al. 2009. Receiving treatment for common mental disorders. *General Hospital Psychiatry* 31(1): 46–55.

Williams, D., et al. 2007. Prevalence and distribution of major depressive disorder in African Americans, Caribbean blacks, and non-Hispanic whites. *Archives of General Psychiatry* 64: 305–315.

Zarit, S. H., and J. M. Zarit. 2006. *Mental Disorders in Older Adults: Fundamentals of Assessment and Treatment,* 2nd ed. New York: Guilford Press.

LOOKING AHEAD...

After reading this chapter, you should be able to:

- Explain the qualities that help people develop intimate relationships
- Describe different types of love relationships and the stages they often go through
- Identify common challenges of forming and maintaining intimate relationships
- Explain some elements of healthy and productive communication
- List some characteristics of successful families and some potential problems families face

Intimate Relationships and Communication

4

Human beings need social relationships; we cannot thrive as solitary creatures. Nor could the human species survive if adults didn't cherish and support each other, if we didn't form strong mutual attachments with our infants, and if we didn't create families in which to raise children. Simply put, people need people.

Although people are held together in relationships by a variety of factors, the foundation of many relationships is the ability to both give and receive love. Love in its many forms—romantic, passionate, platonic, parental—is the wellspring from which much of life's meaning and delight flows. In our culture, it binds us together as partners, parents, children, and friends.

Just as important, we also need to develop a healthy relationship to ourselves, which includes the ability to self-soothe, to regulate our emotions, and to be alone with ourselves at times.

DEVELOPING INTIMATE RELATIONSHIPS

People who develop successful intimate relationships believe in themselves and in the people around them. They are willing to give of themselves—to share their ideas, feelings, time, needs—and to accept what others want to give them.

Self-Concept and Self-Esteem

The principal element that we all bring to our relationships is our *selves*. To have successful relationships, we must first accept and feel good about ourselves. A positive self-concept and a healthy level of self-esteem help us love and respect others.

As discussed in Chapter 3, the roots of our identity and sense of self can be found in childhood, in the relationships we had with our parents and other family members. As adults, we probably have a sense that we're basically lovable, worthwhile people and that we can trust others if, as babies and children, we experienced the following:

- We felt loved, valued, and respected.
- Adults responded to our needs in a reasonably appropriate way.
- They gave us the freedom to explore and develop a sense of being separate individuals.

Gender Role Another thing we learn in early childhood is *gender role*—the activities, abilities, and characteristics our culture deems appropriate for us based on our sex. In our society, men have traditionally been expected to provide for their families; to be aggressive, competitive, and power-oriented; and to use logic to solve problems. Women have been expected to take care of home and children; to be cooperative, supportive, and nurturing; and to approach life emotionally and intuitively. More egalitarian gender roles have emerged in our society, but the stereotypes we absorb in childhood can be deeply ingrained.

Attachment Our ways of relating to others are also rooted in childhood. Some researchers have suggested that our adult styles of loving may be based on the style of **attachment** we established in infancy with our mother, father, siblings, or other primary caregiver. According to this view, people who are secure in their intimate relationships probably had a secure, trusting, mutually satisfying attachment to their mother, father, or other parenting figure. As adults, they find it relatively easy to get close to others. They don't worry about being abandoned or having someone get too close to them. They feel that other people like them and are generally well-intentioned.

People who are clinging and dependent in their relationships may have had an "anxious/ambivalent" attachment. Their parents' inconsistent responses made them unsure that their needs would be met. As adults, they worry whether their partners really love them and will stay with them. They tend to feel that others don't want to get as close as they do. They want to merge completely with another person, which can scare others away.

People who seem to run from relationships may have had an "anxious/avoidant" attachment, in which a parent's inappropriate responses made them want to escape from his or her sphere of influence. As adults, they feel uncomfortable being close to others. They're distrustful and fearful of becoming dependent. Their partners usually want more intimacy than they do.

Even if people's earliest experiences and relationships were less than ideal, however, they can still establish satisfying relationships in adulthood. In fact, relationships in adolescence and adulthood give us a golden opportunity to work on and through unresolved issues and conflicts from the past.

The type and strength of our attachment to our parents can affect other relationships throughout our lives.

People can be resilient and flexible. They have the capacity to change their ideas, beliefs, and behavior. They can learn ways to raise their self-esteem; they can become more trusting, accepting, and appreciative of others; and they can acquire the communication and conflict-resolution skills required for maintaining successful relationships. Although it helps to have a good start in life, it may be even more important to begin again, right from where you are. Most important is to be accepting and kind to ourselves as we are in the present and do our best to grow and develop emotionally.

Friendship

The first relationships we form outside the family are friendships. The friendships we form in childhood are important in our development; through them we learn about tolerance, sharing, and trust. Friendships usually include most or all of the following characteristics:

- *Companionship.* Friends are usually relaxed and happy when they're together. They typically have common values and interests and plan to spend time together.

attachment The emotional tie between an infant and his or her caregiver or between two people in an intimate relationship.

- *Respect.* Friends have a basic respect for each other's humanity and individuality. Good friends respect each other's feelings and opinions and work to resolve their differences without demeaning or insulting each other. They also show their respect by being honest.
- *Acceptance.* Friends feel free to be themselves and express their feelings without fear of ridicule or criticism.
- *Help.* Sharing time, energy, and even material goods is important to friendship. Friends know they can rely on each other in times of need.
- *Trust.* Friends are secure in the knowledge that they will not intentionally hurt each other.
- *Loyalty.* Friends can count on one another. They stand up for each other in both word and deed.
- *Mutuality.* Friends retain their individual identities, but close friendships are characterized by a sense of mutuality—"what affects you affects me." Friends share the ups and downs in each other's lives.
- *Reciprocity.* Friendships are reciprocal. There is give-and-take between friends and the feeling that both share joys and burdens more or less equally over time.

As important as friendships are, however, the average American's social circle is shrinking. In 2006, sociologists from Duke University and the University of Arizona released details of a study on this issue. According to the study, Americans have fewer close friends than ever before. Most have only two friends they consider close enough to discuss problems with.

A study released in 2009 by the Pew Internet and American Life Project verified this decline in the size of many American's core networks, but it differed from the 2006 study in one important respect. That is, the Pew study refuted the assumption that our social circles are shrinking because of our increasing use of technology. Many relationship experts contend that the rising use of the Internet and cell phones has resulted in less person-to-person interaction and that this is a primary reason for the falling number of confidants. The Pew study shows, however, that among demographically similar people, those who use technology to communicate do not have fewer close friends than those who don't use the Internet or a cell phone. On the contrary, the study found that technology users had larger and more diverse core discussion networks and were just as involved in their communities as people who do not communicate via the Internet or a cell phone.

Love, Sex, and Intimacy

Love is one of the most basic and profound human emotions. It is a powerful force in all our intimate relationships. Love encompasses opposites: affection and anger, excitement and boredom, stability and change, bonds and freedom. Love does not give us perfect happiness, but it does give our lives meaning.

For most people, love, sex, and commitment are closely linked ideals in intimate relationships. Love reflects the positive factors that draw people together and sustain them in a relationship. It includes trust, caring, respect, loyalty, interest in the other, and concern for the other's well-being. Sex brings excitement and passion to the relationship. It intensifies the relationship and adds fascination and pleasure.

6% of Americans feel that they have no one "especially significant" in their life.

—Pew Internet & American Life Project, 2009

Commitment, the determination to continue, reflects the stable factors that help maintain the relationship. Responsibility, reliability, and faithfulness are characteristics of commitment. Although love, sex, and commitment are related, they are not necessarily connected. One can exist without the others. Despite the various "faces" of love, sex, and commitment, most of us long for a special relationship that contains them all.

Other elements can be identified as features of love, such as euphoria, preoccupation with the loved one, idealization or devaluation of the loved one, and so on, but these tend to be temporary. These characteristics may include **infatuation,** which will fade or deepen into something more substantial. As relationships progress, the central aspects of love and commitment take on more importance.

Men and women tend to have different views of the relationship between love (or intimacy) and sex (or passion). Numerous studies have found that men can separate love from sex rather easily, although many men find that their most erotic sexual experiences occur in the context of a love relationship. Women generally view sex from the point of view of a relationship. Some people believe you can have satisfying sex without love—with friends, acquaintances, or strangers. Although sex with love is an important norm in our culture, it is frequently disregarded in practice, as the high incidence of extrarelational affairs attests.

The Pleasure and Pain of Love The experience of intense love has confused and tormented lovers throughout history. They live in a tumultuous state of excitement, subject to wildly fluctuating feelings of joy and despair. They lose their appetite, can't sleep, and can think of nothing but the loved one. Is this happiness? Misery? Both?

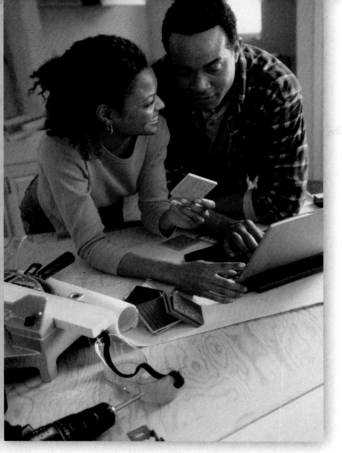

Although passion and physical intimacy often decline with time, other aspects of a relationship—such as commitment—tend to grow as the relationship matures.

The contradictory nature of passionate love can be understood by recognizing that human emotions have two components: physiological arousal and an emotional explanation for the arousal. Love is just one of many emotions accompanied by physiological arousal. Many unpleasant emotions can also generate arousal, such as fear, rejection, frustration, and challenge. Although experiences like attraction and sexual desire are pleasant, extreme excitement is similar to fear and is unpleasant. For this reason, passionate love may be too intense for some people to enjoy. Over time, the physical intensity and excitement tend to diminish. When this happens, pleasure may actually increase.

The Transformation of Love   All human relationships change over time, and love relationships are no exception. At first, love is likely to be characterized by high levels of passion and rapidly increasing intimacy. After a while, passion decreases as we become habituated to it and to the person. The diminishing of romance or passionate love is often experienced as a crisis in a relationship. If a more lasting love fails to emerge, the relationship will likely break up.

Unlike passion, however, commitment does not necessarily diminish over time. When intensity diminishes, partners often discover a more enduring love. They can now move from absorption in each other to a relationship that includes external goals and projects, friends, and family. In this kind of intimate, more secure love, satisfaction comes not just from the relationship itself but also from achieving other creative goals, such as work or child rearing. The key to successful relationships is in transforming passion into an intimate love, based on closeness, caring, and the promise of a shared future.

Challenges in Relationships

Many people believe that love naturally makes an intimate relationship easy to begin and maintain, but in fact, obstacles arise and challenges occur. Even in the best of circumstances, a loving relationship will be tested. Partners enter a relationship with diverse needs and wants, some of which emerge only at times of change or stress.

Honesty and Openness   It's usually best to be yourself from the start to give both you and your potential partner a chance to find out if you are comfortable with each other's beliefs, interests, and lifestyles. Getting close to another person by sharing thoughts and feelings is emotionally risky, but it is necessary for a relationship to deepen. Take your time, and self-disclose at a slow but steady rate—one that doesn't make you feel too vulnerable or your partner too uncomfortable. Over time, you and your partner will learn more about each other and feel more comfortable sharing.

9.8% of college students say that relationship problems affect their academic performance.

—American College Health Association, 2009

Unequal or Premature Commitment   Sometimes one person in an intimate partnership becomes more serious about the relationship than the other partner. In this situation, it can be difficult to maintain a friendship without hurting the other person. Sometimes a couple makes a premature commitment, and then one of the partners has second thoughts and wants to break off the relationship. Sometimes both partners begin to realize that something is wrong, but each is afraid to tell the other. Such problems usually can be resolved only by honest and sensitive communication.

Unrealistic Expectations   Each partner brings hopes and expectations to a relationship, some of which may be unrealistic, unfair, and, ultimately, damaging to the relationship. For example, if you believe that love will eliminate all of your problems, you may start to blame your

Strategies for Enhancing Support in Relationships

- *Be aware of the importance of support.* Time and energy spent on support will help both you and your partner deal with stress and create a positive atmosphere that will help when differences or conflicts do occur.

- *Learn to ask for help from your partner.* Try different ways of asking for help and support from your partner and make note of which approaches work best for your relationship.

- *Help your partner the way she or he would like to be helped.* Some people prefer empathy and emotional support, whereas others like more practical help with problems.

- *Avoid negativity, especially when being asked for help.* Asking for help puts a person in a vulnerable position. If your partner asks for your aid, be gracious and supportive; don't use phrases like "I told you so" or "You should have just. . . ." Otherwise, your partner may learn not to ask for your help or support at all.

- *Make positive attributions.* If you're unsure about the reasons for your partner's behavior, give her or him the benefit of the doubt. For example, if your partner arrives for a date 30 minutes late and in a bad mood, assume it's because she or he had a bad day rather than attributing it to a character flaw or relationship problem. Offer appropriate support.

- *Help yourself.* Develop coping strategies for times your partner won't be available. These might include things you can do for yourself, such as going for a walk, or other people you can turn to for support.

- *Keep relationship problems separate.* Avoid bringing up relationship problems when you are offering or asking for help.

- *Avoid giving advice.* Immediately offering advice when asked for help implies that you are smarter or more capable than your partner at solving your partner's difficulty. Begin by providing emotional support and validating your partner's feelings. Then, if asked, help brainstorm solutions.

SOURCE: Plante, T., and K. Sullivan. 2000. *Getting Together and Staying Together: The Stanford Course on Intimate Relationships.* Bloomington, Ind.: 1st Books Library. Reprinted with permission.

---

partner for anything that goes wrong in your life. Other unrealistic expectations include the following:

- Expecting your partner to change
- Assuming that your partner has all the same opinions, priorities, interests, and goals as you
- Believing that a relationship will fulfill all of your personal, financial, intellectual, and social needs

Competitiveness If one partner always feels the strong need to compete and win, it can detract from the sense of connectedness, interdependence, equality, and mutuality between partners. The same can be said for a perfectionistic need to be right in every instance—to "win" every argument.

If competitiveness is a problem for you, ask yourself if your need to win is more important than your partner's feelings or the future of your relationship. Try noncompetitive activities or an activity where you are a beginner and your partner excels. Accept that your partner's views may be just as valid and important to your partner as your own views are to you.

Balancing Time Spent Together and Apart You may enjoy time together with your partner, but you may also want to spend time alone or with other friends. If you or your partner interprets time apart as rejection or lack of commitment, it can damage the relationship. Talk with your partner about what time apart means, and share your feelings about what you expect from the relationship in terms of time together. Consider your partner's feelings carefully, and try to reach a compromise that satisfies both of you.

Differences in expectations about time spent together can mirror differences in ideas about emotional closeness. Any romantic relationship involves giving up some degree of autonomy in order to develop an identity as a couple. But remember that every person is unique and has different needs for distance and closeness in a relationship.

Jealousy Jealousy is the angry, painful response to a partner's real, imagined, or likely involvement with a third person. Some people think that the existence of jealousy proves the existence of love, but jealousy is actually a sign of insecurity or possessiveness. In its irrational and extreme forms, jealousy can destroy a relationship by its insistent demands and attempts at control. Jealousy is a factor in precipitating violence in dating relationships among both high school and college students, and abusive spouses often use jealousy to justify their violence.

People with a healthy level of self-esteem are less likely to feel jealous. When jealousy occurs in a relationship, it's important for the partners to communicate clearly with each other about their feelings.

Supportiveness Another key to successful relationships is the ability to ask for and give support. Partners need to know that they can count on each other during difficult times. If you are having trouble getting or giving the support that you or your partner needs, try some of the suggestions in the box "Strategies for Enhancing Support in Relationships."

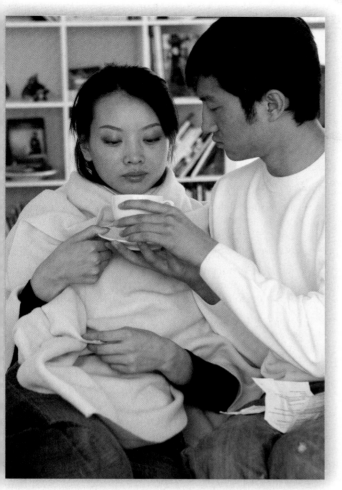

Supportiveness is a sign of commitment and compassion and is an important part of any healthy relationship.

Unhealthy Relationships

Everyone should be able to recognize when a relationship is unhealthy. Relatively extreme examples of unhealthy relationships are those that are physically or emotionally abusive or that involve codependency; strategies for addressing these problems are presented in Chapters 7 and 16, respectively. Even relationships that are not abusive or codependent can still be unhealthy. If your relationship lacks love and respect and places little value on the time you and your partner have spent together, it may be time to get professional help or to end the partnership. Further, if your relationship is characterized by communication styles that include criticism, contempt, defensiveness, and withdrawal—despite real efforts to repair these destructive patterns—the relationship may not be salvageable. Spiritual leaders suggest that relationships are unhealthy when you feel that your sense of spontaneity, your potential for inner growth and joy, and your connection to your spiritual life is deadened. There are negative physical and mental consequences of being in an unhappy relationship; although breaking up is painful and difficult, it is ultimately better than living in a toxic relationship.

Ask Yourself

QUESTIONS FOR CRITICAL THINKING AND REFLECTION

Have you ever ended an intimate relationship? If so, how did you handle it? How did you feel after the breakup? How did the breakup affect your former partner? Did the experience help you in other relationships?

Ending a Relationship

Even when a couple starts out with the best of intentions, an intimate relationship may not last. Some breakups occur quickly following direct action by one or both partners, but many others occur over an extended period as the couple goes through a cycle of separating and reconciling.

Ending an intimate relationship is usually difficult and painful. Both partners may feel attacked and abandoned, but feelings of distress are likely to be more acute for the rejected partner. If you are involved in a breakup, the following suggestions may help make the ending easier:

- Give the relationship a fair chance before breaking up.
- Be fair and honest.
- Be tactful and compassionate.
- If you are the rejected person, give yourself time to resolve your anger and pain.
- Recognize the value in the experience.

Use the recovery period following a breakup for self-renewal. Redirect more of your attention to yourself, and reconnect with people and areas of your life that may have been neglected as a result of the relationship. Time will help heal the pain of the loss of the relationship.

COMMUNICATION

The key to developing and maintaining any type of intimate relationship is good communication.

Nonverbal Communication

Even when we're silent, we're communicating. We send messages when we look at someone or look away, lean forward or sit back, smile or frown. Especially important forms of nonverbal communication are touch, eye contact, and proximity. If someone we're talking to touches our hand or arm, looks into our eyes, and leans toward us when we talk, we get the message that the person is interested in us and cares about what we're saying. If a person keeps looking around the room while we're talking or takes a step backward, we get the impression the person is uninterested or wants to end the conversation.

The ability to interpret nonverbal messages correctly is important to the success of relationships. It's also

Guidelines for Effective Communication

Getting Started

- When you want to have a serious discussion with your partner, choose a private place and time when you won't be interrupted or rushed.

- Face your partner and maintain eye contact. Use nonverbal feedback to show that you are interested and involved in the communication process.

Being an Effective Speaker

- State your concern or issue as clearly as you can.

- Use "I" statements rather than statements beginning with "You." When you use "I" statements, you take responsibility for your feelings. "You" statements are often blaming or accusatory and will probably get a defensive or resentful response. The statement "I feel unloved," for example, sends a clearer, less blaming message than the statement "You don't love me."

- Focus on a behavior, not the whole person. Be specific about the behavior you like or don't like. Avoid generalizations beginning with "You always" or "You never." Such statements make people feel defensive.

- Make constructive requests. Opening your request with "I would like" keeps the focus on your needs rather than your partner's supposed deficiencies.

- Avoid blaming, accusing, and belittling. Even if you are right, you have little to gain by putting your partner down. Studies have shown that when people feel criticized or attacked, they are less able to think rationally or solve problems constructively.

- Ask for action ahead of time, not after the fact. Tell your partner what you would like to have happen in the future; don't wait for him or her to blow it and then express anger or disappointment.

Being an Effective Listener

- Provide appropriate nonverbal feedback (nodding, smiling, making eye contact, and so on).

- Don't interrupt.

- Listen reflectively. Don't judge, evaluate, analyze, or offer solutions (unless asked to do so). Your partner may just need to sort out his or her feelings. By jumping in to "fix" the problem, you may cut off communication.

- Don't give unsolicited advice. Giving advice implies that you know more about what a person needs to do than he or she does; therefore, it often evokes anger or resentment.

- Clarify your understanding of what your partner is saying by restating it in your own words and asking if your understanding is correct. "I think you're saying that you would feel uncomfortable having dinner with my parents and that you'd prefer to meet them in a more casual setting. Is that right?" This type of specific feedback prevents misunderstandings and helps validate the speaker's feelings and message.

- Be sure you are really listening, not off somewhere in your mind rehearsing your reply. Try to tune in to your partner's feelings as well as the words.

- Let your partner know that you value what he or she is saying and want to understand. Respect for the other person is the cornerstone of effective communication.

---

important, when sending messages, to make sure our body language agrees with our words. When our verbal and nonverbal messages don't correspond, we send a mixed message.

Communication Skills

Three keys to good communication in relationships are self-disclosure, listening, and feedback.

- *Self-disclosure* involves revealing personal information that we ordinarily wouldn't reveal because of the risk involved. It usually increases feelings of closeness and moves the relationship to a deeper level of intimacy. Friends often disclose the most to each other, sharing feelings, experiences, hopes, and disappointments. Married couples may share less because they think they already know everything about each other.

- *Listening* requires that we spend more time and energy trying to fully understand another person's "story" and less time judging, evaluating, blaming, advising, analyzing, or trying to control. Empathy, warmth, respect, and genuineness are qualities of skillful listeners. Attentive listening encourages friends or partners to share more and, in turn, to be attentive listeners.

- *Feedback*, a constructive response to another's self-disclosure, is the third key to good communication. Giving positive feedback means acknowledging that the friend's or partner's feelings are valid—no matter how upsetting or troubling—and offering self-disclosure in response. Self-disclosure and feedback can open the door to change, whereas other responses block communication and change. (For tips on improving your skills, see the box "Guidelines for Effective Communication.")

Gender and Communication

Some of the difficulties people encounter in relationships can be traced to common gender differences in communication. Men and women generally approach conversation and communication differently. Men tend to use conversation in a *competitive* way, perhaps hoping to establish dominance in relationships. When male conversations are over, men often find themselves in a one-up or a one-down position. Women tend to use conversation in a more

Gender and Communication

From an early age, girls and boys receive different messages regarding emotion from parents, teachers, and society. Boys learn to suppress their feelings, especially fear and other emotions that make them feel vulnerable. Girls are encouraged to express their feelings.

These differences are reinforced by peer groups. Gender segregation is apparent in preschool and increases throughout middle childhood for most children. Boys and girls spend most of their time with same-sex peers, and their communication styles are different. For example, when conflict arises, girls care

more about preserving their relationships, and boys care more about maintaining the game they were playing.

Research also shows that men have a more intense physiological response to certain emotions. In discussions around conflict, a man's blood pressure and heart rate rise and remain elevated longer. When one is physiologically or emotionally overwhelmed, productive communication is impossible.

A common pattern that arises between men and women is called "confront-withdraw." A woman approaches her male partner because she is upset and wants to talk about it. The man tries to calm her down, provides solutions he sees as rational, and/or withdraws. This response may make his partner even more upset and demanding, which causes the man to further shut down. Given what we know about gender differences, we might understand the man's response as one of self-protection, because he is in a situation that is both emotionally and physically unpleasant.

To enhance intimacy, couples must try to understand each other and develop compatible communication styles.

Advice for Men

- When your partner raises an emotional topic, be aware of uncomfortable feelings and the desire to retreat.

- Do not run away, physically or emotionally. Telling her to "calm down" will likely create the opposite response.

- Stay connected. This is the best way to prevent the conflict from escalating.

- Empathize. Listen to what she is saying. Even if you disagree, tell her you understand how she is feeling and where she is coming from. Often, a person needs only to feel genuinely heard.

- Try not to think of her comments as attacks; instead, continue to empathize.

- Calm yourself. Take long deep breaths, tell yourself that your partner needs to air her feelings, and remember that she also wants the conflict to end.

- Take a short break so you can soothe yourself; don't replay upsetting thoughts.

Advice for Women

- Try to be calm when approaching conflict. Practice relaxation techniques like those described in "Advice for Men."

- Try to speak in ways that will not provoke defensiveness. Don't criticize. Be specific. Use "I" statements.

- Don't be critical of your partner's responses or attempts to communicate.

- Be aware if he is withdrawing, and, if appropriate, help him relax by using methods discussed previously.

SOURCE: Gottman, J. 1994. *Why Marriages Succeed or Fail . . . and How You Can Make Yours Last.* New York: Simon & Schuster.

---

affiliative way, perhaps hoping to establish friendships. They negotiate various degrees of closeness, seeking to give and receive support. Men tend to talk more—though without disclosing more—and listen less. Women tend to use good listening skills such as eye contact, frequent nodding, focused attention, and asking relevant questions. Even when a man and a woman are talking about the same subject, their unconscious goals may be very different.

The woman may be looking for understanding and closeness, while the man may be trying to demonstrate his competence by giving advice and solving problems. Both styles are valid; the problem comes when differences in style result in poor communication and misunderstanding. See the box "Gender and Communication" for more information.

Sometimes communication is not the problem in a relationship—the partners understand each other all too well. The problem is that they're unable or unwilling to change or compromise. Although good communication can't salvage a bad relationship, it does enable couples to see their differences and make more informed decisions.

Conflict and Conflict Resolution

Conflict is natural in intimate relationships. No matter how close two people become, they still remain separate individuals with their own needs, desires, past experiences, and ways of seeing the world. In fact, the closer the relationship, the more differences and the more opportunities for conflict there will be.

Conflict itself isn't dangerous to a relationship. In fact, it may indicate that the relationship is growing. But if it isn't handled constructively, conflict can damage—and ultimately destroy—the relationship.

Conflict is often accompanied by anger—a natural emotion, but one that can be difficult to handle. If we express anger aggressively, we risk creating distrust, fear, and distance; if we act it out without thinking things through, we can cause the conflict to escalate; if we suppress anger, it turns into resentment and hostility. The best way to handle anger in a relationship is to recognize it as a symptom of something that requires attention and needs to be changed. When angry, partners should exercise restraint so as not to become abusive. It is important to express anger skillfully and not in a way that is out of proportion to the issue at hand.

The sources of conflict for couples change over time but primarily revolve around the basic tasks of living together: dividing the housework, handling money, spending time together, and so on. Sexual interaction is also a source of disagreement for many couples.

The following strategies can be helpful when negotiating with a partner:

1. *Clarify the issue.* Take responsibility for thinking through your feelings and discovering what's really bothering you. Agree that one partner will speak first and have the chance to speak fully while the other listens. Then reverse the roles. Try to understand your partner's position fully by repeating what you've heard and asking questions to clarify or elicit more information. Agree to talk only about the topic at hand and not get distracted by other issues. Sum up what your partner has said.

2. *Find out what each person wants.* Ask your partner to express his or her desires. Don't assume you know what your partner wants and don't speak for him or her.

3. *Determine how you both can get what you want.* Brainstorm to come up with a variety of options.

4. *Decide how to negotiate.* Work out a plan for change. For example, one partner will do one task and the other will do another task. Be willing to compromise, and avoid trying to "win."

5. *Solidify the agreements.* Go over the plan and write it down, if necessary, to ensure that you both understand and agree to it.

6. *Review and renegotiate.* Decide on a time frame for trying out your plan, and set a time to discuss how it's working. Make adjustments as needed.

To resolve conflicts, partners have to feel safe in voicing disagreements. They have to trust that the discussion won't get out of control, that they won't be abandoned by the other, and that the partner won't take advantage of their vulnerability. Partners should follow some basic ground rules when they argue, such as avoiding ultimatums, resisting the urge to give the silent treatment, refusing to "hit below the belt," and not using sex to smooth over disagreements. When you argue, maintain a spirit of goodwill and avoid being harshly critical or contemptuous. If you and your partner find that you argue again and again over the same issue, it may be better to stop trying to resolve that problem and instead come to accept the differences between you.

PAIRING AND SINGLEHOOD

Although most people eventually marry or commit to a partner, everyone spends some time as a single person, and nearly all make some attempt, consciously or unconsciously, to find a partner. Intimate relationships are as important for singles as for couples.

Choosing a Partner

Most men and women select partners for long-term relationships through a fairly predictable process, although they may not be consciously aware of it. First attraction is

For many college students today, group activities have replaced dating as a way to meet and get to know potential partners.

Interfaith and Intrafaith Partnerships

Interfaith marriage is common among Americans; for example, about 50% of Jews and 25% of Roman Catholics marry a partner of a different faith. There are many types of interfaith partnerships, including partners from two completely different religions, two religions with similar roots, two divisions of the same religion, and two denominations from the same religious division. The latter two are often called intrafaith partnerships.

Marrying someone of a different faith can broaden the partners' worldview and enrich their lives, but it can also be a stressor and challenge the relationship. The impact of being an interfaith couple depends on how religious the partners are. There isn't one right way to address religious diversity in a partnership, but the following are potential approaches.

Withdrawal: In some cases, both partners withdraw from their respective religions. Religious differences may be minimized, but the withdrawal may not last. If a partner was observant prior to the relationship, he or she may want to become actively involved again. This may occur with a significant event such as the birth of a child or death of a parent.

Conversion: One partner might choose to convert to the other's religion. Religious differences are decreased, but problems can arise if the converted partner becomes resentful, has difficulties with her or his family, misses the old religion, or feels guilty or betrayed.

Compromise: Some couples convert together to a new religion, possibly to a religion or denomination at a "midpoint" between their two religions. The couple may find a happy medium that is satisfying to both. However, both may have the problems associated with conversion.

Multifaith: Some couples join both religions—formally or informally. They may alternate places of worship weekly or make other creative arrangements. The advantage of this pattern is that both partners maintain their religions and learn more about each other. Problems may arise if the religions have conflicting values or practices.

Ecumenical: Partners can also merge their religions. They may combine the "best" of each or observe only the areas where the religions intersect. They may get the best of both worlds and/or discover that their religions have more in common than they thought. In some cases, however, the original religious institutions may condemn compromise.

Diversity: In some couples, each partner chooses to follow his or her own religion. If both partners are very religious, they do not then have to give up an important part of their lives. However, some partners consider this approach undesirable because it means more time apart.

Do Nothing: Some couples find no need to address religious differences because neither partner is observant or committed to a religion to an extent that it is a relationship challenge. They address specific issues if and when they arise.

Couples often handle their religious differences without a problem until they marry or have children. Planning an interfaith wedding can be fraught with unique stressors, such as differing ritu-

als and the expectations of guests from different faiths. When children arrive, decisions may need to be made about issues such as baptism, circumcision, religious upbringing, and others.

To maintain a successful partnership, couples should communicate about religious issues before getting married and having children, discuss the importance of their religions and religious needs, and consider ways to honor each other's religious traditions.

SOURCES: Robinson, B. A. 2007. *Inter-Faith Marriages* (http://www.religioustolerance.org/ ifm_menu.htm; retrieved October 26, 2010); Robinson, B. A. 1999. *How Inter-Faith and Intra-Faith Couples Handle Religious Differences* (http://www.religioustolerance.org/ifm_diff. htm; retrieved October 26, 2010).

---

based on easily observable characteristics: looks, dress, social status, and reciprocated interest. Most people pair with someone who:

- Lives in the same geographic area
- Is from a similar ethnic and socioeconomic background
- Has similar educational attainment
- Lives a similar lifestyle
- Is like them in terms of physical attractiveness

Once the euphoria of romantic love winds down, personality traits and behaviors become more significant factors in how the partners view each other. The emphasis shifts to basic values and future aspirations regarding career, family, and children. At some point, they decide whether the relationship feels viable and is worthy of their continued commitment.

Perhaps the most important question for potential mates to ask is, "How much do we have in common?" Although differences add interest to a relationship, similarities increase the chances of a relationship's success. Differences can affect a relationship in the areas of values, religion, ethnicity, attitudes toward sexuality and gender roles, socioeconomic status, familiarity with each other's culture, and interactions with the extended family (see the box "Interfaith and Intrafaith Partnerships").

Online Relationships

Online dating sites like Match.com, eHarmony, and OkCupid have become incredibly popular in recent years, especially among young adults seeking an intimate partner or new friends.

Connecting with people online has its advantages and its drawbacks. It allows people to communicate in a relaxed way, to try out different personas, and to share things they might not share with family or friends face-to-face. It's easier to put yourself out there without too much investment; you can get to know someone from the comfort of your own home, set your own pace, and start and end relationships at any time. With millions of singles using dating sites that let them describe exactly what they are seeking, the Internet can increase a person's chance of finding a good match.

There are drawbacks, however, to meeting people online. Too often, participants misrepresent themselves, pretending to be very different—older or younger or even of a different sex—than they really are. Investing time and emotional resources in such relationships can be painful. In rare cases, online romances become dangerous or even deadly (see Chapter 16 for information on cyberstalking).

Because people have greater freedom to reveal only what they want to, users should also be aware of a greater tendency to idealize online partners—setting themselves up for later disappointment. If your online friend seems perfect, take that as a warning sign. Conversely, looking for partners online can be like shopping—all the choices may increase your tendency to search for perfection or find fault quickly, and prevent you from giving people a chance. Keep your expectations realistic.

Relationship sites also remove an important and powerful source of information from the process: chemistry and in-person intuition. Much of our communication is transmitted through body language and tone, which aren't obvious in text messages and can't be fully captured even by Web cams and microphones. Trust your feelings about the process of the relationship. Are you revealing more than the other person? Is there a balance in the amount of time spent talking by each of you? Is the other person respecting your boundaries? Just as in real-life dating, online relationships require you to use common sense and to trust your instincts.

If you pursue an online relationship, the following strategies can help you have a positive experience and stay safe:

- To improve your chances of meeting people interested in you as a person, avoid sexually oriented Web sites. Some sites that seem like dating sites are actually used for "hooking up"—that is, arranging meetings for casual sex—rather than for building relationships. Inspect each site thoroughly before registering or providing any information about yourself. If you aren't comfortable with a site's content or purpose, close your Web browser and clear out its cache and its store of cookies. (If you don't know how to do this, check your browser's help system for instructions.)

- Know what you are looking for as well as what you have to offer someone else. If you are looking for a relationship, make that fact clear. Find out the other person's intentions.

- Dating sites let users upload photos, but your photo can be downloaded by anyone, distributed to other individuals or sites, and even altered. Don't post photos unless you are completely comfortable with the potential consequences.

- Don't give out personal information, including your real full name, school, or place of employment, until you feel sure that you are giving the information to someone who is trustworthy. Do not give out your contact information over the Internet.

- Set up a second e-mail account for sending and receiving dating-related e-mails. Don't use your primary e-mail account for dealing with relationship Web sites.

- If someone does not respond to a message, don't take it personally. There are many reasons why a person may not pursue the connection. Don't send messages to an unresponsive person; doing so could lead to an accusation of stalking. If someone stops responding, drop the interaction completely.

- Before deciding whether to meet an online friend in person, arrange to talk over the phone a few times.

- Don't agree to meet someone face-to-face unless you feel completely comfortable about it. Always meet initially in a very public place—a museum, a coffee shop, or a restaurant—not in private, and especially not at your home. Bring along a friend to increase your safety, and let others know where you will be.

If you pursue online relationships, don't let them interfere with your other personal relationships and social activities. Online dating can become addictive. To protect your emotional and personal wellness, use the Internet to widen your circle of friends, not shrink it.

Acceptance and communication skills go a long way toward making a relationship work, no matter how different the partners.

Dating

Many people find romantic partners through some form of dating. Typically, casual dating might evolve into steady or exclusive dating, then engagement, and finally marriage. Although the American cultural norm is personal choice in courtship and mate selection, the popularity of dating services and online matchmaking suggests that many people want help finding a suitable partner (see the box "Online Relationships").

In recent years, traditional dating has given way to a more casual form of getting together in groups. Two people may begin to spend more time together, but often in the group context. If sexual involvement develops, it is more likely to be based on friendship, respect, and common interests than on expectations related to gender roles. In this model, mate selection may progress from getting together to living together to marriage.

Hooking Up

A current tend among teenagers and young adults is hooking up—having casual sexual encounters with acquaintances or strangers with no commitment or investment in a relationship. The sexual activity can be anything from kissing to intercourse, but the key element is the lack of emotional intimacy. Although casual sex is not new, the difference today is that hooking up seems to be the main form of sexual activity for many people, as opposed to sexual activity within a relationship. Some data indicate that more than 80% of college students have had at least one hook-up experience. If dating occurs at all, it happens after people have had sex and become a couple.

Hooking up most likely has its roots in the changing social and sexual patterns of the 1960s. Since then, changes in college policies have contributed to the shift, such as the move away from colleges acting "in loco parentis" (in the place of parents), the trend toward co-ed dorms, and the increase in the percentage of women in student populations and the decreased availability of men.

Because hooking up is often fueled by alcohol, it is associated with sexual risk taking and negative health effects, including the risk of acquiring a sexually transmitted disease. In 2007, for example, young adults age 15 to 24 had rates of chlamydia that were 4 to 5.5 times the overall incidence for the general population, according to the CDC. Hooking up can also have emotional and mental health consequences, including sexual regret, negative emotional reactions, psychological distress, depression, and anxiety. Women are more likely to suffer these reactions after hooking up, but men experience them too. Biological anthropologists suggest that having sex—even casual sex—sets off hormones that cause feelings of bonding and attachment, which are inevitably thwarted in the hook-up.

On some campuses, a backlash against hooking up has taken place. In some cases, individuals are deciding they don't want to be part of the hook-up culture. In other cases, groups and organizations have formed to call for a return to traditional dating or at least some middle ground between dating and hooking up that doesn't have the potential to cause physical and emotional harm. The existence of alternative social and sexual norms can help students think twice when it comes to choices about their sexual activities.

SOURCES: Downing-Matibag, T. M., and B. Geisenger. 2009. Hooking up and sexual risk taking among college students: A health belief model perspective. *Qualitative Health Research* 19(9): 1196–1209; Bachtel, M. Is dating really dead? Emerging evidence on the college hookup culture and health issues. *Action Newsletter, American College Health Association* 49(2): 16–18; Chen, S. 2010. *No Hooking Up, No Sex for Some Coeds* (http://www.cnn.com/2010/LIVING/04/19/college.anti.hookup.culture/index.html?hpt=Sbin; retrieved October 26, 2010).

Among some teenagers and young adults, dating has been all but supplanted by hooking up—casual sexual activity without any relationship commitment. For more on this trend, see the box "Hooking Up."

Living Together

According to the U.S. Census Bureau's American Community Survey for 2006–2008, 5.4 million opposite-sex couples and 700,000 same-sex couples were living together during that period. The Human Rights Campaign, however, estimates that the number of same-sex couples in the United States is closer to 1.6 million. Living together, or **cohabitation,** is one of the most rapid and dramatic social changes that has ever occurred in our society. It seems to be gaining acceptance as part of the normal mate-selection process. By age 30, about half of all men and women will have cohabited.

Cohabitation provides many of the benefits of marriage: companionship; a setting for an enjoyable and meaningful relationship; a chance to develop greater intimacy through learning, compromising, and sharing; a satisfying sex life; and a way to save on living costs.

Living together has certain advantages over marriage. For one thing, it can give the partners a greater sense of autonomy. Not bound by the social rules and expectations that are part of the institution of marriage, partners may find it easier to keep their identity and more of their independence. Cohabitation doesn't incur the same obligations as marriage. If things don't work out, the partners may find it easier to leave a relationship that hasn't been legally sanctioned.

But living together has some drawbacks, too. In most cases, the legal protections of marriage are absent, such as health insurance benefits and property and inheritance rights. These considerations can be particularly serious if the couple has children. Couples may feel social or family pressure to marry or otherwise change their living arrangements, especially if they have young children. The general trend, however, is toward legitimizing nonmarital partnerships; for example, some employers, communities, and states now extend benefits to unmarried domestic partners.

Although many people choose cohabitation as a kind of trial marriage, unmarried partnerships tend to be less stable than marriages. A 2010 survey conducted by the

> **QUICK STATS**
>
> **Roughly 50%** of cohabitating couples get married.
>
> —National Institute of Child Health and Human Development, 2002

> **TERMS**
>
> **cohabitation** Living together in a sexual relationship without being married.

National Center for Health Statistics revealed that cohabitation is much less likely than marriage to survive the 1-, 3-, and 5-year milestones. There is little evidence that cohabitation before marriage leads to happier or longer-lasting marriages. In fact, some studies have found slightly less marital satisfaction and slightly higher divorce rates among couples who had previously cohabited.

Same-Sex Partnerships

Regardless of **sexual orientation,** most people look for love in a committed relationship. A person whose sexual orientation is lesbian, gay, or bisexual (LGB) may be involved in a same-sex (**homosexual**) relationship. Same-sex couples have many similarities with **heterosexual** couples (those who seek members of the opposite sex). According to one study, most gay men and lesbians have experienced at least one long-term relationship with a single partner. Like any intimate relationship, same-sex partnerships provide intimacy, passion, and security.

Same-sex partnerships tend to be more egalitarian (equal) and less organized around traditional gender roles. Same-sex couples put greater emphasis on partnership than on role assignment. Domestic tasks are shared or split, and both partners usually support themselves financially.

Another difference between heterosexual and homosexual relationships is that same-sex partners often have to deal with societal hostility or ambivalence toward their relationship, in contrast to the societal approval and rights given to heterosexual couples (see the box "Same-Sex Marriage and Civil Unions"). *Homophobia,* fear or hatred of homosexuals, can be obvious, as in the case of violence or discrimination, or subtle, such as how same-sex couples are portrayed in the media. Because of societal disapproval, community resources and support may be more important for same-sex couples than for heterosexuals as a source of identity and social support.

People with diverse sexual orientations and gender identities are often grouped together in the category "LGBT," "LGBTQ," or LGBTQI," where T is for transgender, Q is for questioning or queer, and I is for intersex. Transgender individuals—people whose biological sex doesn't match their gender identity—and intersex individuals—people born with ambiguous genitals—may

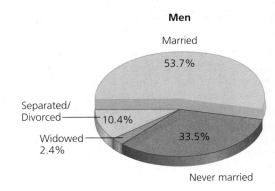

Men

Married
53.7%

Separated/Divorced — 10.4%

Widowed
2.4%

33.5%

Never married

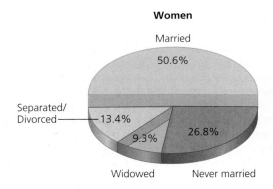

Women

Married
50.6%

Separated/Divorced — 13.4%

9.3%

26.8%

Widowed   Never married

VITAL STATISTICS

FIGURE 4.1   Marital status of the U.S. population age 15 years and older, 2009

SOURCE: U.S. Census Bureau. 2009. *America's Families and Living Arrangements, 2009* (http://www.census.gov/population/www/socdemo/hh-fam.html; retrieved October 26, 2010).

be heterosexual, homosexual, or bisexual, or they may feel that current definitions of sexual orientation and gender are too narrow to apply to them.

Singlehood

Despite the prevalence and popularity of marriage, a significant and growing number of adults in our society are unmarried—nearly 115 million single individuals. The largest group of unmarried adults have never been married (Figure 4.1).

Several factors contribute to the growing number of single people. One is the changing view of singlehood, which is increasingly being viewed as a legitimate alternative to marriage. Education and career are delaying the age at which young people are marrying. The median age for marriage is now 27.7 years for men and 26.1 years for women. More young people are living with their parents as they complete their education, seek jobs, or strive for financial independence. Many other single people live together without being married. Gay people who would marry their partners if they were legally permitted to do so are counted among the single population. High divorce rates mean more singles, and people who have experienced divorce

Same-Sex Marriage and Civil Unions

Marriage is an institution defined by the state and federal statutes that confer legal and economic rights and responsibilities to every married couple. The U.S. General Accountability Office reports that more than 1000 federal laws make distinctions based on marriage. Marital status affects many aspects of life, such as Social Security benefits, federal tax status, inheritance, and medical decision making.

The push for legal recognition of same-sex partnerships has gone on for decades. Supporters of same-sex marriage rights, however, have met opposition at the local, state, and federal levels, in both the public and private sectors.

The majority of states and the federal government have passed laws and amendments that effectively ban same-sex marriage. The federal Defense of Marriage Act (DOMA), enacted in 1996, defines marriage as the legal union between one man and one woman and refuses federal recognition of same-sex marriages. It also allows states to refuse to recognize same-sex marriages and civil unions performed in other states or countries. (Such action might otherwise be in violation of the Constitution's provision that each state give "full faith and credit" to the laws of other states.)

In 2009, the Respect for Marriage Act was introduced in the U.S. House of Representatives. If enacted, the legislation would overturn the Defense of Marriage Act and entitle legally married same-sex couples to the benefits of marriage under federal law. The act would also ensure same-sex couples that their federal rights would follow them if they moved to another state that does not approve same-sex marriages. The act would not force states to recognize or license same-sex marriages or to change any existing state laws on the issue.

Another proposed piece of federal legislation, called the Domestic Partnership Benefits and Obligations Act, would extend the same benefits to domestic partners of federal civilian employees as those offered to employees' spouses. These benefits would include participation in retirement programs, compensation for work-related injuries, and life and health insurance benefits. Such benefits would be available to both same- and opposite-sex domestic partners of federal employees.

As of early 2010, the status of same-sex marriage and civil union laws was as follows in the United States:

- Most states had enacted their own DOMAs and/or passed state constitutional amendments that ban same-sex marriages and/or civil unions. Most of these states further refuse to recognize same-sex marriages from other states.

- The District of Columbia, Connecticut, Iowa, Massachusetts, New Hampshire, and Vermont issue marriage licenses to same-sex couples.

- New York recognizes marriages of same-sex couples who are legally wed in another state. New York does not issue marriage licenses to same-sex couples.

- Several states now provide some or all state-level spousal rights to same-sex couples. The type of union and scope of rights vary from state to state.

- A growing number of municipalities and private corporations now extend health insurance coverage and other benefits to the same-sex spouses and domestic partners of their gay and lesbian employees.

Opponents of civil unions and same-sex marriage offer several arguments against such unions. For example, opponents claim that the purpose of marriage is to procreate, that the Bible forbids same-sex unions, that homosexuals are seeking special rights, that same-sex unions are bad for children and families, and that most Americans oppose such unions. (Many recent polls show that most Americans oppose legalizing same-sex marriage, but a growing number support civil unions.) The growing argument, however, is that same-sex marriage undermines the sanctity and validity of marriage as it is traditionally understood and thus un-

dermines society. Rules and restrictions on who can marry preserve the value of the institution of marriage, according to this view. The underlying assumption of this position is that homosexual behavior is a choice and that people can change their orientation, though the process may be difficult.

Proponents of civil unions and same-sex marriage believe that sexual orientation is outside the control of the individual and results from genetic and environmental factors that create an unchangeable orientation. The issue of same-sex union is then seen as one of basic civil rights, in which a group is being denied rights—to publicly express their commitment to one another, to provide security for their children, and to receive the legal and economic benefits afforded to married heterosexual couples—on the basis of something as unalterable as skin color.

Opponents and proponents of same-sex marriage agree that marriage is healthy for both men and women and is the main social institution promoting family values; both sides see this assertion as supportive of their position. What remains to be seen is how society in general is going to view same-sex marriage in the future—as a furthering of American values or as an attack on them.

MIND/BODY/SPIRIT

Findings suggest that there are intrinsic benefits to marriage. Married people, on average, live longer than unmarried people—whether single, divorced, or widowed—and they score higher on measures of mental health. They have a lower prevalence of headaches, low-back pain, inactivity, and psychological distress. Married people consistently report being happier than unmarried people.

The benefits of intimate relationships have been demonstrated for a range of conditions: People with strong social support are less likely to catch colds. They recover better from heart attacks, live longer with heart disease, and have higher survival rates for certain cancers. Married men with prostate cancer live significantly longer than those who are single, divorced, or widowed. Women in satisfying marriages are less likely to develop risk factors associated with cardiovascular diseases

than unmarried or unhappily married women. People who never marry have a higher chance of dying prematurely than people who have been divorced, separated, or widowed.

What is it about marriage that supports wellness? Some studies suggest that partners may encourage and reinforce healthy habits, such as exercising, eating right, and seeing a physician when needed. In times of illness, a loving partner can give practical help and emotional support. Feeling loved, esteemed, and valued brings comfort in times of vulnerability, reduces anxiety, and mitigates the damaging effects of stress and social isolation.

Although good relationships may help people stay well, bad relationships may have the opposite effect. The impact of relationship quality on health may be partly explained by its effects on the immune system: A study of married couples

who engaged in fighting, criticism, and name calling found that they had weaker immune responses than couples who were more civil. Hostile couples need more time for injuries to heal; their systems tend to contain higher levels of inflammatory agents, which have been linked to long-term illness. High marital stress is linked with risky lifestyle choices and non-adherence to medical regimens. Unhappy marriages are associated with risk factors for heart disease, such as depression, hostility, and anger.

Marriage, of course, isn't the only support system available. If you have supportive people in your life, you are likely to enjoy better physical and emotional health than if you feel isolated and alone. So when you start planning lifestyle changes to improve your health and well-being, don't forget to nurture your relationships with family and friends. Strong relationships are powerful medicine.

---

may have more negative attitudes about marriage and more positive attitudes about singlehood.

Being single doesn't mean not having close relationships, however. Single people date, enjoy active and fulfilling social lives, and have a variety of sexual experiences and relationships. Other advantages of being single include more opportunities for personal and career development without concern for family obligations and more freedom and control in making life choices. Disadvantages include loneliness and a lack of companionship, as well as economic hardships (mainly for single women). Single men and women alike experience some discrimination and often are pressured to get married.

Nearly everyone has at least one episode of being single in adult life, whether prior to marriage, between marriages, following divorce or the death of a spouse, or for his or her entire life. How enjoyable and valuable this single time is depends on several factors, including how deliberately the person has chosen it; how satisfied the person is with his or her social relationships, standard of living, and job; how comfortable the person feels when alone; and how resourceful and energetic the person is about creating an interesting and fulfilling life.

MARRIAGE

The majority of Americans marry at some time in their life. Marriage continues to remain popular because it satisfies several basic needs. There are many important social, moral, economic, and political aspects of marriage, all of

which have changed over the years. In the past, people married mainly for practical reasons, such as raising children or forming an economic unit. Today, people marry more for personal, emotional reasons.

> **Nearly 2.2** million marriages took place in the U.S. in 2008.
> —**National Center for Health Statistics, 2009**

Benefits of Marriage

The primary functions and benefits of marriage are those of any intimate relationship: affection, personal affirmation, companionship, sexual fulfillment, and emotional growth. Marriage also provides a setting in which to raise children, although an increasing number of couples choose to remain childless, and people can also choose to raise children without being married. Marriage is also important for providing for the future. By committing themselves to the relationship, people establish themselves with lifelong companions as well as some insurance for their later years.

Research shows that good marriages have myriad positive effects on individuals' health (see the box "Are Intimate Relationships Good for Your Health?").

Issues in Marriage

Although we might like to believe otherwise, love is not enough to make a successful marriage. Couples have to be strong and successful in their relationship before getting married, because relationship problems will be magnified rather than solved by marriage. The following relationship characteristics appear to be the best predictors of a happy marriage:

- The partners have realistic expectations about their relationship.
- Each feels good about the personality of the other.
- They communicate well.
- They have effective ways of resolving conflicts.
- They agree on religious/ethical values.
- They have an egalitarian role relationship.
- They have a good balance of individual versus joint interests and leisure activities.

Once married, couples must provide each other with emotional support, negotiate and establish marital roles, establish domestic and career priorities, handle their finances, make sexual adjustments, manage boundaries and relationships with their extended family, and participate in the larger community.

Marital roles and responsibilities have undergone profound changes over time. Many couples no longer accept traditional role assumptions, such as that the husband is solely responsible for supporting the family and the wife is solely responsible for domestic work. Many husbands share domestic tasks, and many wives work outside the home. In fact, over 50% of married women are in the labor force, including women with babies under 1 year of age. Although women still take most of the responsibility for home and children even when they work and although men still suffer more job-related stress and health problems than women do, the trend is toward an equalization of responsibilities in the home.

The Role of Commitment

Coping with all these challenges requires that couples be committed to remaining in the relationship through its inevitable ups and downs. They need to be tolerant of each other's imperfections and keep their perspective and sense of humor. Commitment is based on conscious choice rather than on feelings, which, by their very nature, are transitory. Commitment is a promise of a shared future, a promise to be together, come what may. Commitment has become an important concept in recent years. To many people, commitment is a more important goal than living together or marriage.

Separation and Divorce

People marrying today have a 50–55% chance of divorcing. The high rate of divorce in the United States reflects our extremely high expectations for emotional fulfillment and satisfaction in marriage (Figure 4.2). It also indicates that we no longer believe in the permanence of marriage.

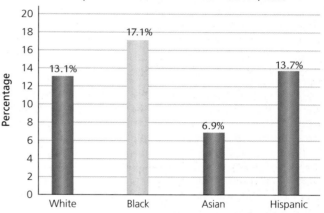

FIGURE 4.2 Percentage of separated and divorced Americans, 2009.

SOURCE: U.S. Census Bureau. 2009. *America's Families and Living Arrangements, 2009* (http://www.census.gov/population/www/socdemo/hh-fam-html; retrieved October 26, 2010).

The process of divorce usually begins with an emotional separation. Often one partner is unhappy and looks beyond the relationship for other forms of validation. Dissatisfaction increases until the unhappy partner decides he or she can no longer stay. Physical separation follows, although it may take some time for the relationship to be over emotionally.

Except for the death of a spouse or family member, divorce is the greatest stress-producing event in life. Research shows that divorced women are more likely to develop heart disease than married, remarried, or widowed women. Both men and women experience turmoil, depression, and lowered self-esteem during and after divorce. People experience separation distress and loneliness for about a year and then begin a recovery period of 1–3 years. During this time they gradually construct a postdivorce identity, along with a new pattern of life. Most people are surprised by how long it takes to recover from divorce.

Children are especially vulnerable to the trauma of divorce, and sometimes counseling is appropriate to help them adjust to the changes in their lives. However, recent research has found that children who spend substantial time with both parents are usually better adjusted than those in sole custody arrangements and as well adjusted as their peers from intact families.

FAMILY LIFE

American families are very different today than they were even a few decades ago. Currently, nearly 75% of families with children under the age of 18 are headed by a married couple, while 14% are headed by a single parent. The remaining 11% of families involve some other arrangement, such as households being headed by an unmarried couple (of the same or opposite gender), by grandparents, or by other relatives or friends.

Becoming a Parent

Few new parents have any preparation for the job of parenting, yet they have to assume that role literally overnight. They have to learn quickly how to hold and feed a baby, how to change diapers, and how to differentiate a cry of hunger from the cry caused by pain or fear. No wonder the birth of the first child is one of the most stressful transitions for any couple.

Even couples with an egalitarian relationship before their first child is born find that their marital roles become more traditional with the arrival of the new baby. The father becomes the primary provider and protector, and the mother becomes the primary nurturer. Most research indicates that mothers have to make greater changes in their lives than fathers do. Although men today spend more time caring for their infants than ever before, women still take the ultimate responsibility for the baby. Women are usually the ones who make job changes, either quitting work or reducing work hours in order to stay home with the baby for several months or more. Many mothers juggle the multiple roles of mother, homemaker, and employer/employee and feel guilty that they never have enough time to do justice to any of these roles.

Parenting

Sometimes being a parent is a source of unparalleled pleasure and pride—the first smile (at you), the first word, the

first home run. But at other times parenting can seem like an overwhelming responsibility.

Most parents worry about their ability to raise a healthy, responsible, and well-adjusted child. Parents may wonder about the long-term impact of each decision they make on their child's well-being and personality. According to parenting experts, no one action or decision (within limits) will determine a child's personality or development. Instead, *parenting style,* or overall approach to parenting, is most important. Parenting styles vary according to the levels of two characteristics of the parent:

- *Demandingness* encompasses the use of discipline and supervision, the expectation that children act responsibly and maturely, and the direct reaction to disobedience.

- *Responsiveness* refers to a parent's warmth and intent to facilitate independence and self-confidence in a child by being supportive, connected, and understanding of the child's needs.

Several parenting styles have been identified, and each style emerges according to the parents' balance of demandingness and responsiveness. For example:

- *Authoritarian* parents are high in demandingness and low in responsiveness. They give orders and expect obedience, giving very little warmth or consideration to their children's special needs.

- *Authoritative* parents are high in both demandingness and responsiveness. They set clear boundaries and expectations, but they are also loving, supportive, and attuned to their children's needs.

- *Permissive* parents are high in responsiveness and low in demandingness. They do not expect their children to act maturely but instead allow them to follow their own impulses. They are very warm, patient, and accepting, and they are focused on not stifling their child's innate creativity.

- *Uninvolved* parents are low in both demandingness and responsiveness. They require little from their children and respond with little attention, frequency, or effort. In extreme cases, this style of parenting might reach the level of child neglect.

Parenting and the Family Life Cycle Parenting that is responsive and demanding is the most beneficial for children. Providing a balance of firm limits and clear structure along with plenty of warmth, nurturing, and respect for the child's own special needs and temperament as well as her or his growing independence is the best predictor for raising a healthy child.

At each stage of the family life cycle, the relationship between parents and children changes. And with those changes come new challenges. The parents' primary responsibility to a small, helpless baby is to ensure its physical well-being around the clock. As babies grow into

? Ask Yourself

QUESTIONS FOR CRITICAL THINKING AND REFLECTION
How do you define "commitment" in a relationship? Is it simply a matter of staying faithful to a partner, or is there more? In your own relationships, what signs of commitment do you look for from your partner? What signs of commitment does your partner see in you?

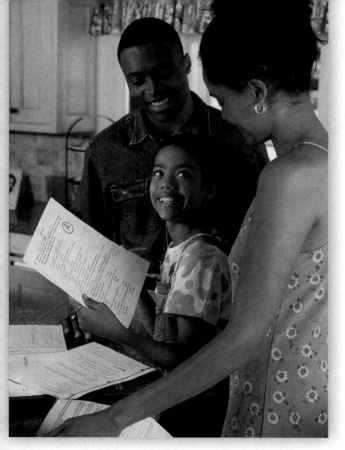

Setting clear boundaries, holding children to high expectations, and responding with warmth to children's needs are all positive parenting strategies.

toddlers and begin to walk and talk, they begin to be able to take care of some of their own physical needs. For parents, the challenge at this stage is to strike a balance between giving children the freedom to explore and setting limits that will keep the children safe and secure. As children grow toward adolescence, parents need to give them increasing independence and gradually be willing to let them risk success or failure on their own.

Marital satisfaction for most couples tends to decline while the children are in school. Reasons include the financial and emotional pressures of a growing family and the increased job and community responsibilities of parents in their thirties, forties, and fifties. Once the last child has left home, marital satisfaction usually increases because the couple has time to enjoy each other once more.

Single Parents

According to the U.S. Census Bureau, about 26% of all children under 18 live with only one parent. In some single-parent families, the traditional family life cycle is reversed and the baby comes before the marriage. In these families, the single parent is usually a teenage mother; she may very well be black or Hispanic, and she may never get married or may not marry for several years. In 2009, about 59% of all black children were living with single parents, as were 27% of Hispanic children.

Economic difficulties are the primary problem for single mothers, especially for unmarried mothers who have not finished high school and have difficulty finding work. Divorced mothers usually experience a sharp drop in income the first few years on their own, but if they have job skills or education they usually can eventually support themselves and their children adequately. Other problems for single mothers are the often-conflicting demands of playing both father and mother and the difficulty of satisfying their own needs for adult companionship and affection.

Financial pressures are also a complaint of single fathers, but they do not experience them to the extent that single mothers do. Because they are likely to have less practice than mothers in juggling parental and professional roles, they may worry that they do not spend enough time with their children. Because single fatherhood is not as common as single motherhood, however, the men who choose it are likely to be stable, established, and strongly motivated to be with their children.

Research about the effect on children of growing up in a single-parent family is inconclusive. Evidence seems to indicate that these children tend to have less success in school and in their careers than children from two-parent families, but these effects may be associated more strongly with low educational attainment of the single parent than with the absence of the second parent. Two-parent families are not necessarily better if one of the parents spends little time relating to the children or is physically or emotionally abusive.

Stepfamilies

Single parenthood is usually a transitional stage: About three out of four divorced women and about four out of five divorced men will ultimately remarry. Rates are lower for widowed men and women, but overall, almost half the marriages in the United States are remarriages for the husband, the wife, or both. If either partner brings children from a previous marriage into the new family unit, a stepfamily (or "blended family") is formed.

Stepfamilies are significantly different from primary families and should not be expected to duplicate the emotions and relationships of a primary family. Research has shown that healthy stepfamilies are less cohesive and more adaptable than healthy primary families; they have a greater capacity to allow for individual differences and accept that biologically related family members will have emotionally closer relationships. Stepfamilies gradually gain more of a sense of being a family as they build a history of shared daily experiences and major life events.

Successful Families

Family life can be extremely challenging. A strong family is not a family without problems; it's a family that copes successfully with stress and crisis. Successful families are intentionally connected—members share experiences and meanings.

An excellent way to build strong family ties is to develop family rituals and routines—organized, repeated activities that have meaning for family members. Families with regular routines and rituals have healthier children, more satisfying marriages, and stronger family relationships. Some of the most common routines identified in research studies are dinner time, a regular bedtime, and household chores; common rituals include birthdays, holidays, and weekend activities. Family routines may even serve as protective factors, balancing out potential risk factors associated with single-parent families and families with divorce and remarriage. Incorporating a regular family mealtime into a family's routine allows parents and children to develop closer relationships and leads to better parenting, healthier children, and better school performance.

Although there is tremendous variation in American families, researchers have proposed that six major qualities or themes appear in strong families:

1. *Commitment.* The family is very important to its members. Sexual fidelity between partners is included in commitment.
2. *Appreciation.* Family members care about one another and express their appreciation. The home is a positive place for family members.
3. *Communication.* Family members spend time listening to one another and enjoying one another's company. They talk about disagreements and attempt to solve problems.
4. *Time together.* Family members do things together, often simple activities that don't cost money.
5. *Spiritual wellness.* The family promotes sharing, love, and compassion for other human beings.
6. *Coping with stress and crisis.* When faced with illness, death, marital conflict, or other crises, family members pull together, seek help, and use other coping strategies to meet the challenge.

It may surprise some people that members of strong families are often seen at counseling centers. They know that the smartest thing to do in some situations is to get help.

Connect to Your Choices

Have you ever thought about why you handle your relationships the way you do? Many factors can influence the relationship choices we make, some not as obvious as others. Do you avoid intimate relationships because you don't want to replicate the patterns you saw in your parents' relationship? Are you frequently disappointed with your relationships because they aren't as blissful—or as exciting—as the relationships you see in movies or on TV? Do you go along with your partner's ideas because you're not sure what you want?

What are the external factors that influence your choices about relationships? What are your inner motivations and core values, and how do they affect your choices? Based on what you learned in this chapter, will you make some different choices in the future? If so, what will they be?

Go online to Connect to complete this activity. www.mcgraw-hillconnect.com

TIPS FOR TODAY AND THE FUTURE

A balanced life includes ample time for nourishing relationships with friends, family, and intimate partners.

RIGHT NOW YOU CAN

- Seek out an acquaintance or a new friend and arrange a coffee date to get to know the person better.
- Call someone you love and tell him or her how important the relationship is to you. Don't wait for a crisis.

IN THE FUTURE YOU CAN

- Think about the conflicts you have had in the past with your close friends or loved ones and consider how you handled them. Decide whether your conflict-management methods were helpful. Using the suggestions in this chapter and Chapter 3, determine how you could better handle similar conflicts in the future.
- Think about your prospects as a parent. What kind of example have your parents set? How do you feel about having children in the future (if you don't have children already)? What can you do to prepare yourself to be a good parent?

SUMMARY

- Successful relationships begin with a positive sense of self and reasonably high self-esteem. Personal identity, gender roles, and attachment styles are all rooted in childhood experiences.

- Characteristics of friendship include companionship, respect, acceptance, help, trust, loyalty, and reciprocity.

- Love, sex, and commitment are closely linked ideals in intimate relationships. Love includes trust, caring, respect, and loyalty. Sex brings excitement, fascination, and passion to the relationship.

- Common challenges in relationships relate to issues of self-disclosure, commitment, expectations, competitiveness, balancing time together and apart, and jealousy.

- Partners in successful relationships have strong communication skills and support each other in difficult times.

- The keys to good communication in relationships are self-disclosure, listening, and feedback.

- Conflict is inevitable in intimate relationships; partners need to have constructive ways to negotiate their differences.

- People usually choose partners like themselves. If partners are very different, acceptance and good communication skills are necessary to maintain the relationship.

- Most Americans find partners through dating or getting together in groups. Cohabitation is a growing social pattern that allows partners to get to know each other intimately without being married.

- Gay and lesbian partnerships are similar to heterosexual partnerships, with some differences. Partners often don't conform to traditional gender roles, and they may experience hostility or ambivalence rather than approval of their partnership from society.

- Singlehood is a growing option in our society. Advantages include greater variety in sex partners and more freedom in making life decisions; disadvantages include loneliness and possible economic hardship, especially for single women.

- Marriage fulfills many functions for individuals and society. It can provide people with affection, affirmation, and sexual fulfillment; a context for child rearing; and the promise of life-long companionship.

- Love isn't enough to ensure a successful marriage. Partners must be realistic, feel good about each other, have communication and conflict-resolution skills, share values, and balance their individual and joint interests.

- When problems can't be worked out, people often separate and divorce. Divorce is traumatic for all involved, especially children, but the negative effects are usually balanced in time by positive ones.

- At each stage of the family life cycle, relationships change. Marital satisfaction may be lower during the child-rearing years and higher later.

- Many families today are single-parent families. Problems for single parents include economic difficulties, conflicting demands, and time pressures.

- Stepfamilies are formed when single, divorced, or widowed people remarry and create new family units. Stepfamilies gradually gain more of a sense of being a family as they build a history of shared experiences.

- Important qualities of successful families include commitment to the family, appreciation of family members, communication, time spent together, spiritual wellness, and effective methods of dealing with stress.

FOR MORE INFORMATION

For resources in your area, check your campus directory for a counseling center or peer counseling program, or check the agencies listed in the Mental Health section of the phone book.

BOOKS

Brooks, J. B. 2010. *The Process of Parenting,* 8th ed. New York: McGraw-Hill. *Demonstrates how parents and caregivers can translate their love and concern for children into effective parenting behavior.*

DeGenova, M. K., and F. P. Rice. 2010. *Intimate Relationships, Marriages, and Families,* 8th ed. New York: McGraw-Hill. *A comprehensive introduction to relationships.*

McKay, M., P. Fanning, and K. Paleg. 2007. *Couple Skills: Making Your Relationship Work,* 2nd rev. ed. New York: New Harbinger. *A comprehensive guide to improving communication, resolving conflict, and developing greater intimacy and commitment in relationships.*

Miller, R., D. Perlman, and S. S. Brehm. 2008. *Intimate Relationships,* 5th ed. New York: McGraw-Hill. *A balanced presentation of both the positive and the problematic aspects of intimate relationships.*

Olson, D., and J. DeFrain. 2007. *Marriages and Families: Intimacy, Diversity, and Strengths,* 6th ed. New York: McGraw-Hill. *A comprehensive introduction to relationships and families.*

ORGANIZATIONS AND WEB SITES

American Association for Marriage and Family Therapy. Provides information on a variety of relationship issues and referrals to therapists.
  http://www.aamft.org
Association for Couples in Marriage Enrichment (ACME). An organization that promotes activities to strengthen marriage; a resource for books, tapes, and other materials.
  http://www.bettermarriages.org
Conflict Resolution Information Source. Provides links to a broad range of Internet resources on conflict resolution. Information covers interpersonal, marriage, family, and other types of conflicts.
  http://www.crinfo.org/
Family Education Network. Provides information about education, safety, health, and other family-related issues.
  http://www.familyeducation.com
Gottman Institute. Includes tips and suggestions for relationships and parenting, including an online relationships quiz.
  http://www.gottman.com
Parents Without Partners (PWP). Provides educational programs, literature, and support groups for single parents and their children. Search the online directory for a referral to a local chapter.
  http://www.parentswithoutpartners.org
United States Census Bureau. Provides current statistics on births, marriages, and living arrangements.
  http://www.census.gov

Yahoo! Directory: Lesbian, Gay, Bisexual and Transgender. A directory of links to information and support for lesbians, gays, bisexuals, and transgendered persons.

http://dir.yahoo.com/society_and_culture/cultures_and_groups/lesbian_gay_bisexual_and_transgendered/transgendered/

See also the listings for Chapters 3 and 8.

SELECTED BIBLIOGRAPHY

American College Health Association. 2009. *American College Health Association-National College Health Assessment II: Reference Group Executive Summary Fall 2009.* Linthicum, Md.: American College Health Association.

Centers for Disease Control and Prevention. 2004. Marital status and health: United States, 1999–2002. *Advance Data from Vital and Health Statistics,* No. 351.

Centers for Disease Control and Prevention, National Center for Health Statistics. 2010. *Early Release of Selected Estimates Based on Data from the January–September 2009 National Health Interview Survey.* Hyattsville, Md.: National Center for Health Statistics.

Centers for Disease Control and Prevention, National Center for Health Statistics. 2010. Marriage and cohabitation in the United States: A statistical portrait based on Cycle 6 (2002) of the National Survey of Family Growth. *Vital and Health Statistics* 23(28): 1–46.

Chistakis, N. A., et al. 2006. Mortality after hospitalization of a spouse. *New England Journal of Medicine* 354(7): 719–730.

Federal Interagency Forum on Child and Family Statistics. 2009. *America's Children: Key National Indicators of Well-Being, 2009.* Washington, D.C.: U.S. Government Printing Office.

Gallup, Inc. 2010. *Marriage* (http://www.gallup.com/poll/117328/Marriage.aspx#1; retrieved March 29, 2010).

Godoy, M. 2009. *NPR: Gay Marriage Laws Interactive Map* (http://www.npr.org/news/specials/gaymarriage/map; retrieved March 31, 2010).

Hampton, K., et al. 2009. *Social Isolation and New Technology: How the Internet and Mobile Phones Impact Americans' Social Networks* (http://www.pewinternet.org/Reports/2009/18–Social-Isolation-and-New-Technology.aspx; retrieved March 29, 2010).

Human Rights Campaign. 2010. *Marriage Equality and Other Relationship Recognition Laws* (http://www.hrc.org/state_laws; retrieved March 31, 2010).

Human Rights Campaign. 2010. *Relationship Recognition in the United States* (http://www.hrc.org/issues/marriage.asp; retrieved March 31, 2010).

McPherson, M., L. Smith-Lovin, and M. Brashears. 2006. Social isolation in America: Changes in core discussion networks over two decades. *American Sociological Review* 71: 353–375.

National Conference of State Legislatures. 2010. *Same Sex Marriage, Civil Unions and Domestic Partnerships* (http://www.ncsl.org/IssuesResearch/HumanServices/SameSexMarriage/tabid/16430/Default.aspx; retrieved March 31, 2010).

Pleis, J. R., and M. Lethbridge-Cejku. 2007. Summary health statistics for U.S. adults: National Health Interview Survey, 2006. *Vital and Health Statistics* 10(235): 1–153.

Roisman, G. I., et al. 2008. Adult romantic relationships as contexts of human development: A multimethod comparison of same-sex couples with opposite-sex dating, engaged, and married dyads. *Developmental Psychology* 44(1): 91–101.

Schoen, R., et al. 2007. Family transitions in young adulthood. *Demography* 44(4): 807–820.

Strong, B., et al. 2009. *Human Sexuality: Diversity in Contemporary America,* 7th ed. New York: McGraw-Hill.

U.S. Census Bureau. 2009. *2006–2008 American Community Survey 3-Year Estimates: Table B11009–Unmarried-Partner Households by Sex of Partner.* Washington, D.C.: U.S. Census Bureau.

U.S. Census Bureau. 2009. *2006–2008 American Community Survey 3-Year Estimates: Table B12007–Median Age at First Marriage.* Washington, D.C.: U.S. Census Bureau.

U.S. Census Bureau. 2010. *2009 Community Population Survey Reports: Families, 2009* (http://www.census.gov/population/www/socdemo/hh-fam.html; retrieved April 1, 2010).

Sexuality, Pregnancy, and Childbirth

5

Humans are sexual beings. Sexual activity is the source of our most intense physical pleasures, a central ingredient in many of our intimate emotional relationships, and the key to reproduction.

Sexuality is more than just sexual behavior. It is a complex, interacting group of biological characteristics and acquired behaviors people learn over the course of growing up in a particular family, community, and society. Sexuality includes biological sex (being biologically male or female), gender (masculine and feminine behaviors), sexual anatomy and physiology, sexual functioning and practices, and social and sexual interactions with others. Our individual sense of identity is powerfully influenced by our sexuality. We think of ourselves in fundamental ways as male or female; as heterosexual or homosexual; as single, attached, married, or divorced.

Basic information about the body, sexual functioning, and sexual behavior is vital to healthy adult life. Once we understand the facts, we have a better basis for making informed, responsible choices about our sexual activities.

SEXUAL ANATOMY

In spite of their different appearances, the sex organs of men and women arise from the same structures and fulfill similar functions. Each person has a pair of **gonads:** ovaries in females and testes in males. The gonads produce **germ cells** and sex hormones. The germ cells are **ova** (eggs) in females and **sperm** in males. Ova and sperm are the basic units of reproduction; their union results in the creation of a new life.

Female Sex Organs

The external sex organs, or genitals, of the female are called the **vulva** (Figure 5.1). The *mons pubis,* a rounded mass of fatty tissue over the pubic bone, becomes covered with hair during puberty (biological maturation). Below it are two paired folds of skin called the labia majora (major lips) and the labia minora (minor lips). Enclosed within these folds are the clitoris, the opening of the urethra, and the opening of the vagina.

FIGURE 5.1   The female sex organs.

Fallopian tube
Ovary
Uterus
Bladder
Pubic bone
Mons pubis
Urethra
Clitoris
Urethral opening
Labia majora

Cervix
Rectum
Vagina
Anus
Perineum
Vaginal opening
Labia minora

TERMS

sexuality   A dimension of personality shaped by biological, psychosocial, and cultural forces and concerning all aspects of sexual behavior.

gonads   The primary reproductive organs that produce germ cells and sex hormones; the ovaries and testes.

germ cells   Sperm and ova (eggs).

ovum   A germ cell produced by a female, which combines with a male germ cell (sperm) to create a fetus; plural, *ova*. Also called an *egg*.

sperm   A germ cell produced by a male, which combines with a female germ cell (ovum) to create a fetus.

vulva   The external female genitals, or sex organs.

clitoris   The highly sensitive female genital structure.

prepuce   The foreskin of the clitoris or penis.

urethra   The duct that carries urine from the bladder to the outside of the body.

vagina   The passage leading from the female genitals to the internal reproductive organs; the birth canal.

hymen   A fold of mucous membrane that surrounds or partially covers the external vaginal opening. It forms part of the vulva, or external genitalia.

cervix   The end of the uterus opening toward the vagina.

uterus   The hollow, thick-walled, muscular organ in which the fertilized egg develops; the womb.

fetus   The developmental stage of a human from the 9th week after conception to the moment of birth.

fallopian tube   A duct that guides a mature ovum from the ovary to the uterus. Also called an *oviduct*.

ovaries   The paired female reproductive glands that produce ova (eggs) and sex hormones; ovaries are the female gonads.

penis   The male genital structure consisting of spongy tissue that becomes engorged with blood during sexual excitement.

scrotum   The loose sac of skin and muscle fibers that contains the testes.

testis   One of two male gonads, the site of sperm production; plural, *testes*. Also called *testicle*.

The **clitoris** is highly sensitive to touch and plays an important role in female sexual arousal and orgasm. The clitoris consists of a shaft, glans, and spongy tissue that fills with blood during sexual excitement. The glans is the most sensitive part of the clitoris and is covered by the clitoral hood, or **prepuce**, which is formed from the upper portion of the labia minora.

The female **urethra** is a duct that leads directly from the urinary bladder to its opening between the clitoris and the opening of the vagina. The urethra conducts urine from the bladder to the outside of the body. The female urethra is not part of the reproductive tract.

The **vagina** is the passage that leads to the internal reproductive organs. It is the female structure for heterosexual sexual intercourse and serves as the birth canal. The vaginal opening is partially covered by a membrane called the **hymen.** This membrane can be stretched or torn during athletic activity or when a woman has sexual intercourse for the first time. In some virgins, the hymen covers much of the vaginal opening, but it is also common for the hymenal membrane to be minimal or entirely lacking in women who have never had vaginal intercourse. Thus, the idea that an intact hymen is a sign of virginity is a myth.

Projecting into the upper part of the vagina is the **cervix,** which is the opening of the **uterus**—or *womb*—where a fertilized egg is implanted and grows into a **fetus.** A pair of **fallopian tubes** (or *oviducts*) extends from the top of the uterus. The end of each oviduct surrounds an **ovary** and guides the mature ovum down into the uterus after the egg exits the ovary.

Male Sex Organs

A man's external sex organs, or genitals, are the penis and the scrotum (Figure 5.2).

The **penis** consists of spongy tissue that becomes engorged with blood during sexual excitement, causing the organ to enlarge and become erect.

FIGURE 5.2 The male sex organs.

Bladder
Pubic bone
Vas deferens
Corpus spongiosum
Penis
Urethra
Glans
Opening of urethra

Seminal vesicle
Rectum
Prostate
Cowper's gland
Anus
Epididymis
Testis
Scrotum

The **scrotum** is a pouch that contains a pair of sperm-producing male gonads, called **testes.** The scrotum maintains the testes at a temperature approximately 5°F below that of the rest of the body. The process of sperm production is extremely heat-sensitive. In hot temperatures the muscles in the scrotum relax, and the testes move away from the heat of the body.

The male urethra is a tube that runs through the entire length of the penis. The urethra carries both urine and *semen* (sperm-carrying fluid) to the opening at the tip of the penis. Although urine and semen share a common passage, they are prevented from mixing together by muscles that control their entry into the urethra. During its brief lifetime, a sperm takes the following route:

1. Sperm are produced inside a maze of tiny, tightly packed tubules within the testes. As they mature, sperm flow into a tube called the **epididymis,** which lies on the surface of each testis.

2. Sperm move from each epididymis into another tube—called the **vas deferens**—which carries them upward into the abdominal cavity and through an organ called the **prostate gland.** This gland produces some of the fluid in semen, which helps transport and nourish the sperm.

3. The two *vasa deferentia* eventually merge into a pair of **seminal vesicles,** whose secretions provide nutrients for the semen.

4. On the final stage of their journey, sperm flow into the **ejaculatory ducts,** which join the urethra.

The **Cowper's glands** are two small structures flanking the urethra. During sexual arousal, these glands secrete a clear, preejaculatory fluid that appears at the tip of the penis. Preejaculatory fluid may contain sperm, so withdrawal of the penis before ejaculation is not a reliable form of contraception.

The smooth, rounded tip of the penis is the highly sensitive **glans,** an important component in sexual arousal. The glans is partially covered by the foreskin, or prepuce, a retractable fold of skin that is removed by **circumcision** in about 55% of newborn males in the United States. Circumcision is performed for cultural, religious, and hygienic reasons, and rates of circumcision vary widely among different groups (see the box "Genital Alteration").

20 million or more sperm per milliliter of semen is considered a normal sperm count.

—Mayo Clinic
(www.mayoclinic.com), 2008

QUICK STATS

epididymis A storage duct for maturing sperm, located on the surface of each testis.

vas deferens A tube that carries sperm from the epididymis through the prostate gland to the seminal vesicles; plural, *vasa deferentia.*

prostate gland A male reproductive organ; produces some of the fluid in semen, which helps transport and nourish sperm.

seminal vesicle A tube leading from the vas deferens to the ejaculatory duct; secretes nutrients for the semen.

ejaculatory duct A tube that carries mature sperm to the urethra so they can exit the body upon ejaculation.

Cowper's gland In the male reproductive system, a small organ that produces preejaculatory fluid.

glans The rounded head of the penis or the clitoris.

circumcision Surgical removal of the foreskin of the penis.

TERMS

Many societies have a tradition of altering the appearance and function of their children's genitalia, either shortly after birth or as part of a puberty rite. Such cultural customs can seem strange, and sometimes even barbaric, to those who are not part of that particular culture. Male circumcision and female genital cutting are both examples of genital alteration, and both are subjects of considerable controversy.

The most common form of genital alteration worldwide is male circumcision, the removal of the foreskin of the penis. Circumcision is a relatively minor surgical procedure that is performed for a variety of cultural, religious, aesthetic, and medical reasons. Worldwide, an estimated one-third of males are circumcised, making it the world's most common surgery. Circumcision rates vary widely from country to country and even within countries. In parts of Africa, the Middle East, South Korea, and the Philippines, more than 80% of males are circumcised. In Europe, Russia, China, Japan, and Central and South America, circumcision is relatively rare, with rates of circumcision generally running less than 10%. In the United States, circumcision rates differ dramatically among religious, ethnic, and racial groups and from region to region. Most Jews and Muslims circumcise boys in accordance with religious custom. Whites and blacks have much higher rates of circumcision than Latinos and Asian Americans. In the Midwest, about three-fourths of male infants are circumcised, compared to about one-third in the West. Nationwide, the rate today is about 55%, down dramatically from the 1960s, when nearly 90% of males were circumcised.

Currently, major medical groups in the United States recommend the routine circumcision of male infants. The procedure, even though minor, carries some medical risks including bleeding, infection, and damage to the penis. Circumcision causes pain to the infant, although most pain can be alleviated with appropriate use of local anesthetic. Circumcision may change the sensitivity of the penis, and some critics claim that it can diminish a man's sexual pleasure. Opponents of circumcision point to the fact that most of the world's men are uncircumcised; why perform surgery, they ask, when there is no clear need for it?

On the other side of the debate, there are a number of health benefits of circumcision. Citing research findings, proponents argue that it promotes cleanliness and reduces the risk of urinary tract infections in newborns and the risk of sexually transmitted diseases, including HIV, later in life, as well as the risk of penile cancer. Studies conducted in developing countries have shown that circumcision can reduce a man's risk of acquiring HIV through heterosexual contact by as much as 60%. However, STD education and the practice of abstinence or low-risk sexual behaviors have a far greater impact on the transmission of STDs than does circumcision. For many parents, the decision about circumcision comes down to questions of aesthetics and appearance.

Far more controversial is the practice of female genital cutting (FGC), also called female genital mutilation. There are no medical or health reasons to perform these procedures, which range from removal of the external genitalia (including the clitoris and labia) to narrowing of the vaginal opening with a surgically created seal to less drastic forms of harm to the genitalia. These practices were probably originally developed to control a woman's sexuality and ensure that she remained a virgin before marriage. Where FGC is cultural convention, the practice is preserved by social pressure to conform and by notions of how a girl should be raised properly and prepared for adulthood and marriage.

Each year, about 3 million female children undergo FGC, usually between infancy and age 15, and about 140 million women worldwide are estimated to have had some form of genital cutting. The practice is most common in parts of Africa, in some countries in Asia and the Middle East, and in some immigrant groups in Europe and North America. FGC is often performed under unsterile conditions and without adequate anesthesia. Serious complications are common and include severe pain, infection, bleeding, and death. Common long-term health issues include infertility, difficulties with childbirth, and problems with urinary and sexual function.

The World Health Organization has come out strongly against FGC, declaring it a violation of the human rights of girls and women. The WHO reports that when a practicing community decides to abandon FGC, the practice can be eliminated very rapidly. FGC is now illegal in many countries, but is still performed on large numbers of girls where the cultural tradition persists.

SOURCES: Circumcision Reference Library. 2008. *United States Circumcision Incidence* (http://www.cirp.org/library/statistics/USA/; retrieved October 26, 2010); World Health Organization. 2010. *Female Genital Mutilation* (http://www.who.int/topics/female_genital_mutilation/en/; retrieved October 26, 2010); World Health Organization. 2010. *Male Circumcision for HIV Prevention* (http://www.who.int/hiv/topics/malecircumcision/en/; retrieved October 26, 2010).

HORMONES AND THE REPRODUCTIVE LIFE CYCLE

The sex hormones produced by the ovaries or testes have a major influence on the development and function of the reproductive system throughout life. In addition to their effects on the reproductive organs, sex hormones influence many other organs in the body, including the brain.

The sex hormones made by the testes are called **androgens,** the most important of which is *testosterone.* The female sex hormones, produced by the ovaries, belong to two groups: **estrogens** and **progestagens,** the most important of which is *progesterone.* The ovaries also produce a small amount of testosterone. The **adrenal glands** also produce androgens in both males and females.

Sex hormones are regulated by the hormones of the **pituitary gland,** located at the base of the brain. This gland in turn is controlled by hormones produced by the **hypothalamus** in the brain. Substances that act like hormones are also found in the environment; see the box "Environmental Hazards and Reproductive Health."

Differentiation of the Embryo

The biological sex of an individual is determined by the fertilizing sperm at the time of conception. All human cells normally contain 23 pairs of chromosomes. In 22 of the pairs, the two partner chromosomes match. But in the twenty-third pair, the **sex chromosomes,** two configurations are possible. Individuals with two matching X chromosomes are female, and individuals with one X and one Y chromosome are male. Thus, at the time of conception, the genetic sex is established: Females are XX and males are XY.

Abnormalities sometimes occur in the sex chromosomes; the two most common disorders of sex chromosomes are Klinefelter's syndrome and Turner's syndrome. Klinefelter's syndrome, a condition where a male carries two or more X chromosomes in addition to the Y chromosome, occurs in about 1 in 1000 males and causes infertility and small genitalia. Turner's syndrome occurs in about 1 in 2500 females. Women with Turner's have only a single complete X chromosome. These women are usually not able to have children and can sometimes have other medical problems.

Genetic sex dictates whether the undifferentiated gonads become ovaries or testes. If a Y chromosome is present, the gonads become testes and produce the male hormone **testosterone.** Testosterone circulates throughout the body and causes the undifferentiated reproductive structures to develop into male sex organs (penis, scrotum, and so on). If a Y chromosome is not present, there is no testosterone and the gonads become ovaries and the reproductive structures develop into female sex organs (clitoris, labia, and so on).

Female Sexual Maturation

Although humans are fully sexually differentiated at birth, the differences between males and females are accentuated at **puberty,** the period during which the reproductive system matures, secondary sex characteristics develop, and the bodies of males and females become more distinctive. The changes of puberty are induced by testosterone in males and estrogen and **progesterone** in females.

Physical Changes   The first sign of puberty in girls is breast development, followed by a rounding of the hips and buttocks. As the breasts develop, hair appears in the pubic region and later in the underarms. Shortly after the onset of breast development, girls show an increase in growth rate. Breast development usually begins between ages 8 and 13, and the time of rapid body growth occurs between ages 9 and 15.

The Menstrual Cycle   A major landmark of puberty for young women is the onset of the **menstrual cycle,** the

---

TERMS

androgens   Sex hormones; produced by the testes in males, the ovaries in females, and the adrenal glands in both sexes.

estrogens   A class of female sex hormones, produced by the ovaries, that bring about sexual maturation at puberty and maintain reproductive functions.

progestagens   A class of female sex hormones, produced by the ovaries, that sustain reproductive functions.

adrenal glands   Endocrine glands, located over the kidneys, that produce sex hormones.

pituitary gland   An endocrine gland at the base of the brain that produces follicle-stimulating hormone (FSH) and luteinizing hormone (LH), among others.

hypothalamus   A region of the brain above the pituitary gland whose hormones control the secretions of the pituitary; also involved in the control of many bodily functions, including hunger, thirst, temperature regulation, and sexual functions.

sex chromosomes   The X and Y chromosomes, which determine an individual's biological sex.

testosterone   The most important male sex hormone; stimulates an embryo to develop into a male and induces the development of male secondary sex characteristics during puberty.

puberty   The period of biological maturation during adolescence.

progesterone   The most important female sex hormone; regulates the menstrual cycle and sustains pregnancy.

menstrual cycle   The monthly ovarian cycle, regulated by hormones; in the absence of pregnancy, menstruation occurs.

Ask Yourself

QUESTIONS FOR CRITICAL THINKING AND REFLECTION

What are your personal views on circumcision? Who or what has influenced those opinions? Are the bases of your views primarily cultural, moral, or medical?

Environmental Hazards and Reproductive Health

ON THE ENVIRONMENT

For many years, scientists have known that certain chemicals in the environment can have a significant impact on the reproductive health of animals. One of the best known examples is DDT, a pesticide that nearly caused the extinction of the bald eagle and many other species before its use was banned in the United States in 1972. Another well-known example is DES (diethylstilbestrol), a drug given to women between about 1940 and 1970 to prevent miscarriage. DES was subsequently found to cause reproductive cancers and other adverse effects in the women's daughters, sons, and possibly even grandchildren.

DDT and DES are examples of *endocrine-disrupting chemicals (EDCs)*, substances that act like hormones and disrupt normal hormone activity, particularly activity related to reproduction and development. The most studied EDCs are environmental estrogens, which mimic the female sex hormone estrogen and can duplicate or exaggerate its effects. Other EDCs can block estrogen, mimic or block androgens (male sex hormones), or otherwise alter hormonal responses in the body.

The effects of EDCs on normal sexual and reproductive development were first observed in wildlife species, including birds, frogs, alligators, polar bears, and dozens of others. The effects of EDCs on humans are less clear. At high doses, as in the case of DES, they clearly affect reproductive development and physiology, but at low doses, like those found in the environment, no adverse health effects have been definitively documented. However, according to a 2009 Endocrine Society Scientific Statement, the evidence for adverse reproductive outcomes in humans, including infertility and anatomical malformations, is strong.

The widespread use of EDCs began in the late 1930s and 1940s, when the chemical and plastics industries were taking off. They include industrial solvents and lubricants, plastics, pesticides, flame retardants, and pharmaceuticals. These chemicals are so ubiquitous in our environment and food supply today that their residues have been found as part of the "body burden" of virtually every animal or human who is tested. Many common chemicals used both indoors and outdoors are EDCs, and exposure occurs through the food and water we ingest, the air we breathe, and the products we use in our everyday lives. Although some EDCs rapidly deteriorate in the environment, others are persistent organic pollutants that remain in the environment long after they are no longer produced and bioaccumulate in the food chain. EDCs also occur naturally as

phytoestrogens in plants such as soybeans.

The effects of EDCs include the following:

- DDT, a pesticide still used as an antimalaria insecticide in Africa and Southeast Asia, inhibits development of female reproductive organs, causes decreased female fertility, and may increase the risk of childhood obesity.

- PCBs (polychlorinated biphenyls), used as industrial coolants and lubricants, are toxic to the liver and thyroid, increase the risk of childhood obesity, and may increase the risk of diabetes. Persistent organic pollutants that accumulate in marine sediments, they were banned worldwide in 1977.

monthly ovarian cycle that leads to menstruation (loss of blood and tissue lining the uterus) in the absence of pregnancy. The timing of **menarche** (the first *menstrual period*) varies with several factors, including ethnicity, genetics, and nutritional status. The current average age of menarche in the United States is around 12 and a half years, but it may also normally start several years earlier or later.

The day of the onset of bleeding is considered to be day 1 of the menstrual cycle. For the purposes of our discussion, a cycle of 28 days will be used; however, normal cycles vary in length from 21 to 35 days. The menstrual cycle consists of the following four phases.

1. Menses. During **menses**, characterized by the menstrual flow, blood levels of hormones from the ovaries and the pituitary gland are relatively low. This phase of the cycle usually lasts from day 1 to about day 5.

2. Estrogenic Phase. The estrogenic phase begins when the menstrual flow ceases and the pituitary gland begins to produce increasing amounts of follicle-stimulating hormone (FSH) and luteinizing hormone (LH). Under the influence of FSH, an egg-containing ovarian **follicle** begins to mature, producing increasingly higher amounts of estrogen. Stimulated by estrogen, the **endometrium**, the uterine lining, thickens with large numbers of blood vessels and uterine glands.

3. Ovulation. A surge of a potent estrogen called estradiol from the follicle causes the pituitary to release a large burst of LH and a smaller amount of FSH. The high

---

TERMS

menarche The first menstrual period, experienced by most young women at some point during adolescence.

menses The portion of the menstrual cycle characterized by menstrual flow.

follicle A saclike structure within the ovary, in which eggs (ova) mature.

endometrium The lining of the uterus.

- BPA (bisphenol A), found in some plastic water bottles and in baby bottles, plastic and metal food containers, and dental materials, has been implicated in reproductive problems in lab animals, as well as obesity, mammary and prostate cancers, diabetes, and neurological problems. Nalgene and other manufacturers removed BPA from their products as of 2008, and some politicians have proposed bans on BPA.

- PBDEs (polybrominated diphenyl ethers), a flame-retardant additive used in the plastic cases of TVs and computers, carpets, bedding, clothing, car components, and textiles, may disrupt thyroid hormone balance and contribute to neurological and developmental deficits, including low intelligence, learning disabilities, and behavior problems. Many PBDEs were banned in Europe in 2006.

- Phthalates (pronounced *tha-lates*), used mainly as plasticizers (chemicals that soften plastics and make them more durable), are known to disrupt the endocrine system in animals, and some research has implicated them in the rise of birth defects involving the male reproductive system in humans. In 2002 the FDA cautioned against exposing male babies to a particular phthalate, citing concerns about its effects on the male reproductive system, the production of normal sperm, and masculine neurological development. Phthalates are found in hundreds of common products, including children's toys, personal care items, cleaning products, home products, pharmaceuticals, medical devices, and pesticides. California and some European countries have banned the use of phthalates in children's toys.

Besides birth defects, prenatal and early childhood exposure to EDCs may have long-term effects. A concept known as the developmental origins of health and disease suggests that early exposure can cause problems that show up only later in life, including early onset of puberty in females, decreased quantity and quality of sperm, infertility, and breast and testicular cancer. Women exposed to DES prenatally, for example, have a higher incidence of breast cancer once they reach the age of breast cancer prevalence. Researchers are also looking at other complex conditions and diseases for possible connections to EDCs, including obesity, metabolic syndrome, diabetes, cardiovascular disease, ADHD, autism, and gender dysphoria and transgenderism.

Given the ubiquity of EDCs in our environment, it is difficult or impossible for individuals to avoid exposure, although consumers might opt not to buy water in plastic bottles or to buy more organic foods. Instead, more scientific research is needed to determine the effects of these chemicals on human development and health, and government action is needed to phase out their production as their effects are documented. One concrete step that could be taken is labeling foods with high levels of EDCs. The biggest challenge is eliminating EDCs from the environment. Some cleanup projects are under way, such as the dredging of PCB-contaminated sediment from the Hudson River by General Electric with oversight by the Environmental Protection Agency, which began in 2009. As more evidence becomes available, similar programs will need to be undertaken to reduce the health effects of these chemicals on future generations.

For a detailed discussion of environmental health—how the environment affects you and how you affect the environment—see Chapter 19.

SOURCES: Diamanti-Kandarakis, E., et al. 2009. Endocrine-disrupting chemicals: An Endocrine Society Scientific Statement. *Endocrine Reviews* 30(4): 293–342; National Institute of Environmental Health Sciences, National Institutes of Health. 2009. *Environmental Agents: Endocrine Disruptors* (http://www.niehs.nih.gov/health/topics/agents/endocrine/index.cfm; retrieved October 26, 2010); Hood, E. 2009. Are EDCs blurring issues of gender? *Environmental Health Perspectives* 113: A670–A677.

---

concentration of LH stimulates the developing follicle to release its ovum. This event is known as **ovulation.** After ovulation, the follicle is transformed into the **corpus luteum,** which produces progesterone and estrogen.

Ovulation theoretically occurs about 14 days prior to the onset of menstrual flow, with the window of greatest fertility occurring from a few days before ovulation to about one day after. This information has been used to attempt to predict the most fertile time during the menstrual cycle for fertility treatments and natural family planning methods. However, a recent study showed that even women with regular menstrual cycles often have unpredictable ovulation and can actually be fertile on any day of the month, including during menstruation. The "window of fertility" is especially unpredictable in teenagers and women who are approaching menopause.

4. Progestational Phase. During the progestational phase of the cycle, the amount of progesterone secreted from the corpus luteum increases and remains high until the onset of the next menses. Under the influence of estrogen and progesterone, the endometrium continues to develop, readying itself to receive and nourish a fertilized ovum. When pregnancy occurs, the fertilized egg produces the hormone human chorionic gonadotropin (HCG), which maintains the corpus luteum. Thus, levels of ovarian hormones remain high and the uterine lining is preserved, preventing menses.

If pregnancy does not occur, the corpus luteum degenerates, and estrogen and progesterone levels gradually fall. Below certain hormonal levels, the endometrium can no longer be maintained, and it begins to slough off, initiating menses. As the levels of ovarian hormones fall, a slight rise in the amounts of LH and FSH occurs, and a new menstrual cycle begins.

---

ovulation   The release of a mature egg (ovum) from an ovary.

corpus luteum   The part of the ovarian follicle left after ovulation, which secretes estrogen and progesterone during the second half of the menstrual cycle.

TERMS

MENSTRUAL PROBLEMS Menstruation is a normal biological process, but physical and/or emotional symptoms associated with the menstrual cycle are very common. Many women experience menstrual cramps, the severity of which tends to vary from cycle to cycle. **Dysmenorrhea,** discomfort associated with menstruation, can include any combination of the following symptoms: lower abdominal cramps, backache, vomiting, nausea, bloating, diarrhea, headache, and fatigue. Many of these symptoms can be attributed to uterine muscular contractions caused by chemicals called *prostaglandins.* Non-steroidal anti-inflammatory drugs (NSAIDs) such as ibuprofen (Motrin, Advil) block the effects of prostaglandins and are often effective in relieving dysmenorrhea. Oral contraceptives are also effective in reducing dysmenorrheal symptoms in most women.

Many women experience transient emotional symptoms prior to the onset of their menstrual flow. Depending on their severity, these symptoms may be categorized along a continuum: **premenstrual tension, premenstrual syndrome (PMS),** and **premenstrual dysphoric disorder (PMDD).** Premenstrual tension symptoms are mild and may include negative mood changes and physical symptoms such as abdominal cramping and backache. More severe symptoms are classified as PMS; very severe symptoms that impair normal daily and social functioning are classified as PMDD. All three conditions share a definite pattern. Symptoms appear prior to the onset of menses and disappear within a few days after the start of menstruation. Premenstrual tension is quite common, PMS affects about 1 in 5 women, and PMDD affects less than 1 in 10 women.

Symptoms associated with PMS and PMDD can include breast tenderness, water retention (bloating), headache, fatigue, insomnia or excessive sleep, appetite changes, food cravings, irritability, anger, increased interpersonal conflict, depression, anxiety, tearfulness, inability to concentrate, social withdrawal, and the sense of being out of control or overwhelmed.

Despite many research studies, the causes of PMS and PMDD are still unknown, and it is unclear why some women are more vulnerable than others. Most researchers feel that PMS is probably caused by a combination of hormonal, neurological, genetic, dietary, and psychological factors.

The following strategies provide relief for many women with premenstrual symptoms, and all of them can contribute to a healthy lifestyle at any time:

- *Limit salt intake.* Salt promotes water retention and bloating.
- *Exercise.* Women who exercise experience many fewer symptoms before and after menstrual periods.
- *Don't use alcohol or tobacco.* Alcohol and tobacco may aggravate certain symptoms of PMS and PMDD.
- *Eat a nutritious diet.* Choose a low-fat diet rich in complex carbohydrates from vegetables, fruits, and whole-grain breads, cereals, and pasta. Get enough calcium from calcium-rich foods and, if needed, supplements. Minimize your intake of sugar and caffeine, and avoid chocolate, which is rich in both.
- *Relax.* Stress reduction is always beneficial, and stressful events can trigger PMS symptoms. Try relaxation techniques during the premenstrual time.

If you're a female with persistent premenstrual symptoms, keep a daily diary to track the symptoms, their severity, and how they correlate with your menstrual cycle. See your physician for an evaluation and to learn about treatments that are available only by prescription.

Selective serotonin reuptake inhibitors (SSRIs), such as Prozac and Zoloft, are often used to treat PMS and PMDD. Until recently, women using SSRIs took the medication throughout the entire menstrual cycle, but taking the medication during just the progestational phase of the cycle is effective in some women.

Other drug treatments for PMS and PMDD include certain oral contraceptives, diuretics to minimize water retention, and NSAIDs such as ibuprofen. A number of vitamins, minerals, and other dietary supplements have also been studied for PMS relief. Only one supplement, calcium, has been shown to provide relief in rigorous clinical studies; several others show promise, but more research is needed.

Male Sexual Maturation

Reproductive maturation of boys occurs about 2 years later than that of girls; it usually begins at about age 10 or 11. Testicular growth is usually the first obvious sign of sexual maturity in boys. The penis also grows at this time, reaching adult size by about age 18. Pubic hair starts to develop after the genitals begin increasing in size, with underarm and facial hair gradually appearing. Hair on the

QUICK STATS

75% of women experience premenstrual symptoms during their childbearing years.

—National Institutes of Health, 2010

TERMS

dysmenorrhea Painful or problematic menstruation.

premenstrual tension Mild physical and emotional changes associated with the time before the onset of menses.

premenstrual syndrome (PMS) A disorder characterized by physical discomfort, psychological distress, and behavioral changes that begin after ovulation and cease when menstruation begins.

premenstrual dysphoric disorder (PMDD) A severe form of PMS, characterized by symptoms serious enough to interfere with daily activities and relationships.

chest, back, and abdomen increases later in development. Facial hair often continues to get thicker and darker for several years after puberty. The voice deepens as a result of the lengthening and thickening of the vocal chords.

Boys grow taller for about 6 years after the first signs of puberty, with a very rapid period of growth about 2 years after puberty starts. Largely because of the influence of testosterone, muscle development and bone density are much greater in males than females. By adulthood, men on average have one and a half times the lean body mass of women, and nearly half the body fat.

Aging and Human Sexuality

Hormone production and sexual functioning change as we age. Sexual "performance" may diminish, but sexuality and sensuality can continue to be a source of great pleasure and satisfaction. A study of sexuality in older Americans found that three-fourths of 57–64-year-olds were sexually active (defined as having at least one sexual partner in the last year). Half of those age 65–74 and about one-fourth of people age 75–85 remained sexually active. People who remain healthy and active are much more likely to continue to be sexually active in their older years.

Menopause   As a woman approaches age 50, her ovaries gradually cease to function and she enters **menopause,** the cessation of menstruation. For some women, the associated drop in hormone production causes troublesome symptoms. The most common physical symptom of menopause is the hot flash, a sensation of warmth rising to the face from the upper chest, with or without perspiration and chills. During a hot flash, skin temperature can rise by more than 10 degrees. Other menopausal symptoms can include night sweats, insomnia, vaginal dryness, thinning of head hair, and mood changes. Osteoporosis—decreasing bone density—can develop, making older women more vulnerable to fractures.

As a result of decreased estrogen production during menopause, the vaginal walls become thin and lubrication in response to sexual arousal diminishes. Sexual intercourse may become painful. Hormonal treatment or the use of lubricants during intercourse can minimize these problems.

For many decades it was common for postmenopausal women to be prescribed estrogen for relief from hot flashes, vaginal dryness, bone loss, and a host of other symptoms. However, doctors discovered that giving estrogen alone to postmenopausal women resulted in higher rates of endometrial cancer. To alleviate this problem, it became customary to prescribe estrogen with a progestagen (called *hormone therapy,* or *HT*), since this combination reduced the risk for uterine cancer but still reduced menopausal symptoms. The medical community was taken by surprise when a large study in 2002 showed that women taking a common form of estrogen/progestagen therapy

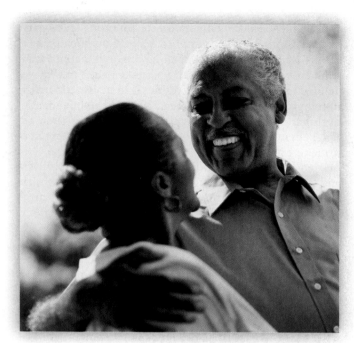

Although sexual physiology changes as people get older, many men and women readily adjust to these alterations.

had higher rates of cardiovascular disease, blood clots, and breast cancer than postmenopausal women not taking hormones. Prescriptions for hormone therapy plummeted after this news. Breast cancer rates dropped over the next few years, but experts are not sure if the fall in breast cancer rates was due to the decrease in hormone therapy or if other factors were responsible.

In the last several years, re-analysis of the data and information from newer studies has resulted in a more individualized approach to hormone therapy. It appears that younger women who have just become menopausal are more likely to benefit from hormone therapy and less likely to have serious side effects than older women. Current forms of hormone therapy include low-dose estrogen, sometimes in the form of a patch, cream, or vaginal ring, designed to treat specific symptoms of menopause, with less risk of side effects.

Aging Male Syndrome   Between the ages of 35 and 65, men experience a gradual decline in testosterone production resulting in the aging male syndrome, sometimes referred to as *male menopause* or *andropause*. Symptoms can include loss of muscle mass, increased fat mass, decreased sex drive, erectile problems, depressed mood, irritability, difficulties with concentration, increased urination, loss of bone mineral density, and sleep difficulties. In some cases, testosterone replacement therapy can help. Although taking testosterone can be harmful in young

menopause   The cessation of menstruation, occurring gradually around age 50.

healthy men, older men with low testosterone levels may benefit from carefully prescribed testosterone treatment.

As men get older, they depend more on direct physical stimulation for sexual arousal. They take longer to achieve an erection and find it more difficult to maintain; orgasmic contractions are less intense. Older men with erectile dysfunction are often prescribed medications such as Viagra that increase blood flow to the penis, resulting in a firmer erection.

Men continue to produce sperm throughout their lives and can sometimes father children well into their eighties and even nineties. Starting at about age 30, however, men become gradually less fertile. Regardless of the age of their female partners, couples in which the male is over age 35 have a 50% lower pregnancy rate than couples in which the man is 30 years old or younger. Men over age 40 are more likely to produce children with health problems such as autism, schizophrenia, and Down syndrome.

SEXUAL FUNCTIONING

Sexual activity is based on stimulus and response. Erotic stimulation leads to sexual arousal (excitement), which may culminate in the intensely pleasurable experience of orgasm. But sexual activity should not be thought of only in terms of the sex organs. Responses to sexual stimulation involve not just the genitals but the entire body and mind.

Sexual Stimulation

Sexual excitement can come from many sources, both physical and psychological. Although physical stimuli have an obvious and direct effect, some people believe psychological stimuli—thoughts, fantasies, desires, perceptions—are even more powerfully erotic.

Physical Stimulation Physical stimulation comes through the senses: We are aroused by things we see, hear, taste, smell, and feel. The most obvious and effective physical stimulation is touching. Even though culturally defined practices vary and individual people have different preferences, most sexual encounters eventually involve some form of touching with hands, lips, and body surfaces. Kissing, caressing, fondling, and hugging are as much a part of sexual encounters as they are of expressing affection.

The most intense form of stimulation by touching involves the genitals. The clitoris and the glans of the penis are particularly sensitive to such stimulation. Other highly responsive areas include the vaginal opening, the nipples, the breasts, the insides of the thighs, the buttocks, the anal region, the scrotum, the lips, and the earlobes. Such sexually sensitive areas, or **erogenous zones,** are especially susceptible to sexual arousal for most people, most of the time. Often, though, what determines the response is not *what* is touched but how, for how long, and by whom. Under the right circumstances, touching any part of the body can cause sexual arousal.

Psychological Stimulation Sexual arousal also has an important psychological component, regardless of the nature of the physical stimulation. Fantasies, ideas, memories of past experiences, and mood can all generate sexual excitement.

Arousal is also powerfully influenced by emotions. How you feel about a person and how the person feels about you matter tremendously in how sexually responsive you are likely to be. Even the most direct forms of physical stimulation carry emotional overtones. Kissing, caressing, and fondling express affection and caring. The emotional charge they give to a sexual interaction is at least as significant to sexual arousal as the purely physical stimulation achieved by touching.

The Sexual Response Cycle

Men and women respond physiologically with a predictable set of reactions, regardless of the nature of the stimulation.

Two physiological mechanisms explain most genital and bodily reactions during sexual arousal and orgasm. These mechanisms are vasocongestion and muscular tension. **Vasocongestion** is the engorgement of tissues that results when more blood flows into an organ than is flowing out. Increased muscular tension culminates in rhythmical muscular contractions during orgasm.

Four phases characterize the sexual response cycle:

1. In the *excitement phase,* the penis becomes erect as its tissues become engorged with blood. The testes expand and are pulled upward within the scrotum. In women, the clitoris, labia, and vaginal walls are similarly engorged with blood and the vaginal walls become moist with lubricating fluid.

2. The *plateau phase* is an extension of the excitement phase. Reactions become more marked. In men, the penis becomes harder, and the testes become larger.

TERMS

erogenous zone   Any region of the body highly responsive to sexual stimulation.

vasocongestion   The accumulation of blood in tissues and organs.

Ask Yourself

QUESTIONS FOR CRITICAL THINKING AND REFLECTION
Think about your own experience as you matured sexually during puberty and adolescence. In what ways did these changes affect your life? How did they contribute to the person you are today?

In women, the lower part of the vagina swells, as its upper end expands and vaginal lubrication increases.

3. In the *orgasmic phase,* or **orgasm,** rhythmic contractions occur along the man's penis, urethra, prostate gland, seminal vesicles, and muscles in the pelvic and anal regions. These involuntary muscular contractions lead to the ejaculation of **semen,** which consists of sperm cells from the testes and secretions from the prostate gland and seminal vesicles. In women, contractions occur in the lower part of the vagina and in the uterus, as well as in the pelvic region and the anus.

4. In the *resolution phase,* all the changes initiated during the excitement phase are reversed. Excess blood drains from tissues, the muscles in the region relax, and the genital structures return to their unstimulated state.

More general physical reactions accompany the genital changes in both men and women. Beginning with the excitement phase, nipples become erect, the woman's breasts begin to swell, and in both sexes the skin of the chest becomes flushed; these changes are more marked in women. The heart rate doubles by the plateau phase, and respiration becomes faster. During orgasm, breathing becomes irregular and the person may moan or cry out. A feeling of warmth leads to increased sweating during the resolution phase. Deep relaxation and a sense of well-being pervade the body and the mind.

Male orgasm is marked by the ejaculation of semen. After ejaculation, men enter a *refractory period,* during which they cannot be restimulated to orgasm. Women do not have a refractory period, and immediate restimulation to orgasm is possible for some women.

Sexual Problems

Both physical and psychological factors can interfere with sexual functioning. Many diseases specifically affect the sex organs. Any illness that affects your general health is likely to have some affect on your ability to function sexually. Disturbances in sexual desire, performance, or satisfaction are referred to as **sexual dysfunctions.** These problems may be due to psychological issues, physical problems, or both.

Common Sexual Health Problems   Medical conditions that affect women's sexual organs include the following:

• *Vaginitis* (inflammation of the vagina) is a common problem that can be caused by a variety of organisms: *Candida* (yeast infection), *Trichomonas* (trichomoniasis), and the overgrowth of a variety of bacteria (bacterial vaginosis). Symptoms include vaginal discharge, vaginal irritation, and pain during intercourse. Vaginitis is treated with a variety of topical and oral medications.

• *Endometriosis* is the growth of endometrial tissue outside the uterus. Endometriosis can cause serious problems if left untreated because endometrial tissue can scar and partially or completely block the oviducts, causing infertility (difficulty conceiving) or sterility (the inability to conceive).

• *Pelvic inflammatory disease* (PID) is an infection of the uterus, oviducts, or ovaries caused when microorganisms spread to these areas from the vagina. Approximately 50–75% of PID cases are caused by sexually transmitted organisms associated with diseases such as gonorrhea and chlamydia. PID can cause scarring of the oviducts, resulting in infertility or sterility.

Sexual health problems affecting men include the following:

• *Prostatitis* is an inflammation or infection of the prostate gland.

• *Testicular cancer* occurs most commonly in men in their twenties and thirties. A rare cancer, it has a very high cure rate if detected early. Every man should perform testicular self-exams regularly (see Chapter 12).

• *Epididymitis* is an inflammation of the epididymis (the coiled tube located on the top and back of each testicle). The most common cause of epididymitis is infection, often sexually transmitted. Symptoms include tenderness over the testicle, swelling, fever, and pain with ejaculation. The treatment is antibiotics.

• *Testicular torsion* occurs when the spermatic cord, which supplies blood to the testicle, becomes twisted. Decreased blood flow to the testicle causes severe, sudden pain, and if not treated quickly, it can cause permanent damage to the testicle. Testicular pain should be evaluated by a medical professional promptly; sudden, severe pain is a medical emergency.

Systematic diseases—illnesses that affect organs throughout the body—affect both men and women and often affect sexual function. A common example is diabetes, which often results in sexual dysfunction because of poor

orgasm   The discharge of accumulated sexual tension with characteristic genital and bodily manifestations and a subjective sensation of intense pleasure.

semen   Seminal fluid, consisting of sperm cells and secretions from the prostate gland and seminal vesicles.

sexual dysfunction   A disturbance in sexual desire, performance, or satisfaction.

TERMS

blood flow to the sexual organs, along with impaired sensation and nerve function. Smoking, alcoholism, and obesity are also major causes of sexual dysfunctions. Sexual difficulties are frequently the first sign of serious health problems because any disease that affects the cardiovascular, nervous, or endocrine system is likely to have an impact on sexual function.

Sexual Dysfunctions   The term *sexual dysfunction* encompasses disturbances in sexual desire, performance, or satisfaction. Many physical conditions and drugs can interfere with sexual functioning. Psychological causes and relationship problems can be important factors as well. Sexual satisfaction is highly individual, so no one should feel that it is necessary to live up to a particular standard of sexual performance or "normalcy." Only you can determine if some aspect of your sexuality is creating a problem for you or your partner.

COMMON SEXUAL DYSFUNCTIONS   Three of the most common sexual difficulties in men are erectile dysfunction, premature ejaculation, and retarded ejaculation. **Erectile dysfunction** (previously called *impotence*) is the inability to achieve or maintain an erection sufficient for sexual intercourse. Erectile dysfunction occurs in men of all ages, but becomes much more common as men age. **Premature ejaculation** (ejaculation before or just after penetration of the vagina or anus) is also common, especially among younger men. If the problem is persistent and bothersome to the man and his partner, there are numerous treatments. **Retarded ejaculation** is the inability to ejaculate once an erection is achieved. Many men experience occasional difficulty achieving an erection or ejaculating because of excessive alcohol consumption, fatigue, or stress.

Female sexual problems generally involve a lack of desire to have sex, the failure to become physically aroused even when sex is desired, the failure to have an orgasm **(orgasmic dysfunction),** or pain during sexual contact. All of these problems can have physical and psychological components. Many medical problems can influence a woman's desire and ability to respond sexually. Hormonal factors, especially menopause, also have a major influence. Psychological and social issues such as relationship difficulties, family stresses, depression, and past sexual trauma are all frequent causes of sexual dysfunction.

TERMS

erectile dysfunction   The inability to achieve or maintain an erection sufficient for sexual intercourse.

premature ejaculation   Involuntary orgasm before or shortly after the penis enters the vagina or anus; ejaculation that takes place sooner than desired.

retarded ejaculation   The inability to ejaculate when one wishes to during intercourse.

orgasmic dysfunction   The inability to experience orgasm.

Many women experience orgasm but not during intercourse, or they experience orgasm during intercourse only if the clitoris is directly stimulated at the same time. In general, the inability to experience orgasm under certain circumstances is a problem only if the woman considers it so.

Dyspareunia (painful intercourse) is a common symptom in women with many possible causes. Infection, lack of lubrication, endometriosis, past sexual trauma, and scarring due to childbirth are a few common reasons for pain during intercourse. In a small percentage of women, *vaginismus* (the involuntary contraction of pubic muscles) makes sexual penetration impossible.

TREATING SEXUAL DYSFUNCTION   Most forms of sexual dysfunction are treatable. The first step is to have a physical examination to find a possible medical cause. Heart disease, diabetes, smoking, the use of alcohol or recreational drugs, and certain over-the-counter and prescription medications can all inhibit sexual response. Obesity is also a common cause of erectile dysfunction. Being overweight makes a man more vulnerable to cardiovascular problems, and it also can affect his hormonal balance.

Many treatments are available for erectile dysfunction. Viagra (sildenafil citrate), Cialis (tadalafil), and Levitra (vardenafil) work by enhancing the effects of nitric oxide, a chemical that relaxes smooth muscles in the penis. This increases blood flow and allows a natural erection to occur in response to sexual stimulation. The medications are generally safe for healthy men, but they should not be used by men who have a high risk of heart attack or stroke. They are effective in about 70% of users, but there are potential side effects, including headaches, indigestion, facial flushing, back pain, visual and hearing disturbances, and changes in blood pressure. Viagra, Cialis, and Levitra should never be taken by anyone who takes nitrate medication (usually prescribed for heart problems), and the recreational drugs amyl nitrate or nitrite (sometimes called "poppers") should never be combined with drugs for erectile dysfunction. The combination of nitrates and Viagra-like drugs can cause a sudden potentially lethal drop in blood pressure.

Viagra use by men between the ages of 18 and 45 has risen dramatically—possibly due to use of the drug for recreational purposes. The drug may cut the refractory period in men who do not have erectile dysfunction; younger men may also be using it to cope with performance anxiety or the effects of other drugs, such as antidepressants.

Although Viagra is not approved by the FDA for use by women, a growing number of women are trying the drug. Research findings are mixed as to whether

> *Any disease affecting the cardiovascular, nervous, or endocrine system may also affect sexual function.*

Viagra can increase sex drive and satisfaction levels in women. Recent studies have shown, however, that the drug can sometimes help women with sexual dysfunction caused by the use of antidepressant drugs. Meanwhile, pharmaceutical companies around the world are trying to develop a "Viagra for women," and it may not be long before the FDA begins considering such drugs for approval.

Many people with no obvious physical disorder have sexual problems because of psychological and social issues. Too often, sexual difficulties are treated with drugs when nondrug strategies may be more appropriate. Psychosocial causes of dysfunction include troubled relationships, a lack of sexual skills, irrational attitudes and beliefs, anxiety, and psychosexual trauma, such as sexual abuse or rape. Many of these problems can be addressed by sex therapy.

Premature ejaculation is an example of a common sexual problem that often responds well to nondrug therapy. On average, men typically ejaculate between 2 and 10 minutes after intercourse begins, but most men periodically ejaculate more quickly. There are several nondrug techniques that are frequently helpful for men who habitually ejaculate sooner than they would like. Kegel exercises, which strengthen and improve control of the pelvic muscles, are often helpful, as are other techniques that, with practice, increase control of ejaculation. Certain antidepressants delay ejaculation and are sometimes prescribed for this purpose.

Women who seek treatment for orgasmic dysfunction often have not learned what types of stimulation will excite them and bring them to orgasm. Most sex therapists treat this problem with **masturbation** (genital self-stimulation). Women are taught about their own anatomy and sexual responses and then are encouraged to experiment with masturbation until they experience orgasm.

Substances being tested for the treatment of female sexual dysfunction include prostaglandin creams and testosterone patches. A prostaglandin cream that improves blood flow to the clitoris is currently being developed and may be available to treat female sexual arousal disorder in the future. Another option is a device that creates suction over the clitoris to increase blood flow and sensitivity.

Dyspareunia and vaginismus are treated by first diagnosing and treating any underlying physical cause of the problem. The use of generous amounts of lubricant during sexual activity is important. Sexual therapy for vaginismus often involves gradual desensitization techniques. Recently, Botox (a chemical that paralyzes muscles) injections have been used successfully in relaxing the pubic muscles in some women with vaginismus.

SEXUAL BEHAVIOR

Many behaviors stem from sexual impulses, and sexual expression takes a variety of forms. Probably the most basic aspect of sexuality is reproduction. But sexual excitement and satisfaction are aspects of sexual behavior separate from reproduction. The intensely pleasurable sensations of arousal and orgasm are probably the strongest motivators for human sexual behavior. People are infinitely varied in the ways they seek to experience erotic pleasure.

Sexual Orientation

Sexual orientation is a consistent pattern of emotional, romantic, and sexual attraction to men, women, or both sexes. It exists along a continuum that ranges from exclusive heterosexuality (attraction to people of the other sex) through bisexuality (attraction to people of both sexes) to exclusive homosexuality (attraction to people of one's own sex). The terms *straight* and *gay* are often used to refer to heterosexuals and homosexuals, respectively, and female homosexuals are also referred to as *lesbians*. In recent years, the term *queer* has been reclaimed as a self-identifier by some elements of the gay community.

Sexual orientation involves feelings and self-concept, and individuals may or may not express their sexual orientation in their behavior. In national surveys, about 2–6% of men identify themselves as homosexuals and about 2% of women identify themselves as lesbians. Many theories try to account for the development of sexual orientation. At this time, most experts agree that sexual orientation results from multiple genetic, biological, cultural, social, and psychological factors. In addition, a person's expressed sexual identity may be quite different from his or her actual sexual practices. For example, some people who identify as heterosexual have sex primarily with members of their own sex.

So far, most studies on the origin of sexual orientation have focused on males. The factors that determine sexual orientation in women may be even more complex. Perhaps the most important message is that sexual orientation is most likely the result of the complex interaction of biological, psychological, and social factors, possibly different in the case of each individual.

Varieties of Human Sexual Behavior

Some sexual behaviors are aimed at self-stimulation only, whereas other practices involve interaction with a partner. Some people choose not to express their sexuality at all.

Celibacy   Continuous abstention from sexual activities, termed **celibacy,** can be a conscious and deliberate choice, or it can be necessitated by circumstances. Health considerations and religious and moral beliefs may lead

---

masturbation   Self-stimulation for the purpose of sexual arousal and orgasm.

celibacy   Continuous abstention from sexual activity.

TERMS

some people to celibacy, particularly until marriage or until an acceptable partner appears. Many people use the related term *abstinence* to refer to avoidance of just one sexual activity—intercourse.

Autoeroticism and Masturbation   The most common form of **autoeroticism** is **erotic fantasy,** creating imaginary experiences that range from fleeting thoughts to elaborate scenarios. Masturbation involves manually stimulating the genitals, rubbing them against objects, or using stimulating devices such as vibrators. It may be used as a substitute for sexual intercourse or as part of sexual activity with a partner.

Touching and Foreplay   Touching is integral to sexual experiences, whether in the form of massage, kissing, fondling, or holding. Our entire body surface is a sensory organ, and touching almost anywhere can enhance intimacy and sexual arousal. Touching can convey a variety of messages, including affection, comfort, and a desire for further sexual contact.

   During arousal, many men and women manually and orally stimulate each other by touching, stroking, and caressing their partner's genitals. Men and women vary greatly in their preferences for the type, pacing, and vigor of such **foreplay.** Working out the details to accommodate each other's pleasure is a key to enjoying these activities. Direct communication about preferences can enhance sexual pleasure and protect both partners from physical and psychological discomfort.

Oral-Genital Stimulation   **Cunnilingus** (the stimulation of the female genitals with the lips and tongue) and **fellatio** (the stimulation of the penis with the mouth) are common practices. Oral sex may be practiced either as part of foreplay or as a sex act culminating in orgasm. Although prevalence varies in different populations, 90% of men, 88% of women, and more than 50% of teens report that they have engaged in oral sex. Like all acts of sexual expression between two people, oral sex requires the cooperation and consent of both partners.

Anal Intercourse   About 10% of heterosexuals and 50% of homosexual males regularly practice anal stimulation and penetration by the penis or a finger. Because the

This couple's physical experiences together will be powerfully affected by their emotions, ideas, and values and by the quality of their relationship.

anus is composed of delicate tissues that tear easily under such pressure, anal intercourse is one of the riskiest of sexual behaviors associated with the transmission of HIV and all other sexually transmitted infections. Anal intercourse is also associated with increased risk of anal cancer, hemorrhoids, anal fissures, prolapsed rectum, and fecal incontinence. The use of condoms is highly recommended for anyone engaging in anal sex.

Sexual Intercourse   For most adults, most of the time, **sexual intercourse** (*coitus*) is the ultimate sexual experience. The most common heterosexual practice is the man inserting his erect penis into the woman's dilated and lubricated vagina after sufficient arousal. Men and women engage in vaginal intercourse to fulfill both sexual and psychological needs. In

One of the commonly stated reasons for having sex is to express emotional attachment to one's partner.

TERMS

autoeroticism   Behavior aimed at sexual self-stimulation.

erotic fantasy   Sexually arousing thoughts and daydreams.

foreplay   Kissing, touching, and any form of oral or genital contact that stimulates people toward intercourse.

cunnilingus   Oral stimulation of the female genitals.

fellatio   Oral stimulation of the penis.

sexual intercourse   Sexual relations involving genital union; also called *coitus,* and also known as making love.

---

a 2006 study by the National Center for Health Statistics, 87% of men age 15–44 and 98% of women in the same age group reported having had vaginal intercourse.

Atypical and Problematic Sexual Behaviors

In American culture, many kinds of sexual behavior are accepted. However, some types of sexual expression are considered harmful; they may be illegal, classified as mental disorders, or both. Because sexual behavior occurs on a continuum, it is sometimes difficult to differentiate a behavior that is simply atypical from one that is harmful. When attempting to evaluate an unusual sexual behavior, experts consider the issues of consent between partners and whether physical or psychological harm is done to the individual or to others.

The use of force and coercion in sexual relationships is one of the most serious problems in human interactions. The most extreme manifestation of **sexual coercion**—forcing a person to submit to another's sexual desires—is rape, but sexual coercion occurs in many subtler forms, such as sexual harassment.

Commercial Sex

Conflicting feelings about sexuality are apparent in the attitudes of Americans toward commercial sex: prostitution and sexually oriented materials in a variety of formats. Our society supposedly disapproves of prostitution, but it also provides their customers. Pornography is readily available and widely viewed in our society, although many people are concerned about its ubiquitous nature and the blurring of pornography with popular culture.

Pornography   Derived from the Greek word meaning "the writing of prostitutes," **pornography** (*porn*) is now often defined as obscene literature, art, or movies. A major problem in identifying pornographic material is that different people and communities have different opinions about what is obscene. Differing definitions of obscenity have led to many legal battles over potentially pornographic materials. Currently, the sale and rental of pornographic materials are restricted so that only adults can legally obtain them; materials depicting children in sexual contexts are illegal in any format or setting.

Much of the debate about pornography focuses on whether it is harmful. Some people argue that adults who want to view pornographic materials in the privacy of their own homes should be allowed to do so. Others feel that the exposure to explicit sexual material can lead to delinquent or criminal behavior, such as rape or the sexual abuse of children. Currently, there is no reliable evidence that pornography by itself leads to violence or harmful sexual behavior, and debate is likely to continue.

Online Porn and Cybersex   The appearance of thousands of sexually oriented Web sites has expanded the number of people with access to pornography and has made it more difficult for authorities to enforce laws regarding porn. Of special concern is the increased availability of child pornography, which previously could be acquired only with great difficulty and at great legal risk. Online porn is now a multibillion-dollar industry.

Hundreds of thousands of people also use the Internet to engage in **cybersex,** or *virtual sex*. Cybersex is erotic interaction between people who are communicating over the Internet. People who become addicted to cybersex or viewing online porn may become isolated and perform poorly at work or school. Their addiction may also have a negative impact on their interpersonal relationships. For more on this topic, see the box "Sex Addiction."

"Sexting," sending provocative photos from cell phone to cell phone, has become popular among teens, sometimes with serious consequences. Images can end up traveling from person to person by cell phone and from there onto social networking Web sites like Facebook. These images can haunt individuals years later when they are viewed by potential employers or partners. Teens have found themselves charged with child pornography and have even faced jail time as a result of forwarding a sexually explicit photo of an underage person to a friend.

Prostitution   The exchange of sexual services for money is **prostitution.** Prostitutes may be men, women, or children, and the buyer of a prostitute's services is nearly always a man. Except in parts of Nevada, prostitution is illegal in the United States. Most customers are white, middle-class, middle-aged, and married. Although they come from a wide variety of backgrounds, prostitutes are usually motivated to join the profession because of money.

AIDS and other STDs are major concerns for prostitutes and their customers. Many prostitutes are injection drug users or are involved with men who are. The rate of HIV infection among prostitutes varies widely, but in some parts of the country it is as high as 25–50%. Unfortunately, many prostitutes are children. The majority of prostitutes, both female and male, began working as prostitutes before they were 16 years of age. A majority of prostitutes report that they were sexually abused as children. Many

---

sexual coercion   The use of physical or psychological force or intimidation to make a person submit to sexual demands.

pornography   The explicit or obscene depiction of sexual activities in pictures, writing, or other material.

cybersex   Erotic interaction between people who are not in physical contact, conducted over a network such as the Internet; also called *virtual sex*.

prostitution   The exchange of sexual services for money.

TERMS

Sex Addiction

"It's hard to admit that I need help, but I do." With these words, spoken in February 2010, pro golfer Tiger Woods acknowledged that he was receiving treatment for what the media referred to as his "sex addiction." Woods joined a long line of public figures and celebrities, including movie stars, athletes, politicians, and even a U.S. president, who have suffered negative consequences as a result of their sexual activities. With 24/7 access to sexual material on the Internet available to all, some experts worry that an increasing number of individuals in our society are at risk for sex addiction.

Sex addiction is generally defined as compulsive, out-of-control sexual behavior that has severe negative consequences. Although it is not considered a diagnosable disorder by the American Psychiatric Association, many psychiatric experts compare it to obsessive-compulsive and impulse-control disorders. Sex addiction has more in common with compulsive gambling and substance dependence than with typical forms of sexual expression.

The sex addict may be preoccupied or obsessed with the next sexual encounter, may try to have sex several times a day with as many partners as possible, may masturbate compulsively, and may put him- or herself in danger to fulfill sexual cravings. The cybersex addict may spend hours every day watching porn, interacting with anonymous strangers in chat rooms, pursuing online hookups, and

surfing the Internet for sexual material. Sex addicts risk their personal lives, relationships, jobs, health, and legal status to pursue sexual gratification.

Many sex addicts suffer from depression, low self-esteem, and concurrent addictions, such as alcoholism and eating disorders. They often have problems with emotional intimacy and use sex to block out feelings of emptiness, loneliness, and lack of connection. Many sex addicts have a history of childhood trauma or abuse. Since sexual acting out does not meet underlying emotional needs, it serves as a distraction rather than a solution.

If you worry that you might be at risk for sex addiction, consider these five questions:

● Do you often feel driven to engage in sexual behaviors or activities even though you know they are not good for you?

● Have you tried to spend less time or stop engaging in these sexual behaviors and been unable to do so?

● Do you fantasize or think about sex so often that it interferes with other areas of your life, such as school, work, or socializing?

● Are your relationships with a partner, family, or friends suffering because of your sexual habits?

● Do you place yourself in sexual situations that are risky to your health or that could result in your getting arrested or otherwise experiencing legal problems?

If you answered yes to any of these questions, you may be at risk for sex addiction. Don't wait until you experience negative consequences—talk to a mental health professional on your campus. Treatment for sex addiction focuses on stopping the problematic behavior, understanding its underlying causes, and learning skills to prevent relapse. Social support, 12-step work, partner and family involvement, and psychoeducation are also part of a successful treatment program.

SOURCES: Sexual Recovery Institute. *About Sexual Addiction* (http://www.sexualrecovery.com; retrieved October 26, 2010); Bancroft, J., and Z. Vukadinivic. 2004. Sexual addiction, sexual compulsivity, sexual impulsivity, or what? Toward a theoretical model. *Journal of Sex Research* 41(3): 225–234.

prostitutes start out as child runaways, escaping abusive homes and turning to prostitution as a way to survive.

Responsible Sexual Behavior

Healthy sexuality is an important part of adult life. It can be a source of pleasurable experiences and emotions and an important part of intimate partnerships. But sexual behavior also carries many responsibilities, as well as potential consequences such as pregnancy, STDs, and emotional changes in the relationship.

Open, Honest Communication Each partner needs to clearly indicate what sexual involvement means to him or her. Does it mean love, fun, a permanent commitment, or something else? The intentions of both partners should

be clear. For strategies on talking about sexual issues with your partner, see the box "Communicating about Sexuality."

Agreed-On Sexual Activities No one should pressure or coerce a partner. Sexual behaviors should be consistent with the sexual values, preferences, and comfort level of both partners. Everyone has the right to refuse sexual activity at any time.

Sexual Privacy Intimate relationships involving sexual activity are based on trust, and that trust can be violated if partners reveal private information about the relationship to others. Sexual privacy also involves respecting other people—not engaging in activities in the presence of others that would make them uncomfortable.

Communicating about Sexuality

To talk with your partner about sexuality, follow the general suggestions for effective communication in Chapter 4. Getting started may be the most difficult part. Some people feel more comfortable if they begin by talking about talking—that is, initiating a discussion about why people are so uncomfortable talking about sexuality. Talking about sexual histories—how partners first learned about sex or how family and cultural background influenced sexual values and attitudes—is another way to get started. Reading about sex can also be a good beginning: Partners can read an article or book and then discuss their reactions.

Be honest about what you feel and what you want from your partner. Cultural and personal obstacles to discussing sexual subjects can be difficult to overcome, but self-disclosure is important for successful relationships. Research indicates that when one partner openly discusses attitudes and feelings, the other partner is more likely to do the same. If your partner seems hesitant to open up, try asking open-ended or either/or questions: "Where do you like to be touched?" or "Would you like to talk about this now or wait until later?"

If something is bothering you about your sexual relationship, choose a good time to initiate a discussion with your partner. Be specific and direct but also tactful. Focus on what you actually observe, rather than on what you think the behavior means. Try focusing on a specific behavior that concerns you rather than on the person as a whole—your partner can change behaviors but not his or her entire personality. For example, you could say "I'd like you to take a few minutes away from studying to kiss me" instead of "You're so caught up in your work, you never have time for me."

If you are going to make a statement that your partner may interpret as criticism, try mixing it with something positive: "I love being with you, but I feel annoyed when you . . . ." Similarly, if your partner says something that upsets you, don't lash back. An aggressive response may make you feel better in the short run, but it will not help the communication process or the quality of the relationship.

If you want to say no to some sexual activity, say no unequivocally. Don't send mixed messages. If you are afraid of hurting your partner's feelings, offer an alternative if it's appropriate: "I am uncomfortable with that. How about . . . ?"

If you're in love, you may think that the sexual aspects of a relationship will work out magically without discussion. However, partners who never talk about sex deny themselves the opportunity to increase their closeness and improve their relationship.

Using Contraception If pregnancy is not desired, contraception should be used during sexual intercourse. Both partners need to take responsibility for protecting against unwanted pregnancy. Partners should discuss contraception before sexual involvement begins.

Safer Sex Both partners should be aware of and practice safer sex to guard against STDs. Many sexual behaviors carry the risk of STDs, including HIV infection. Partners should be honest about their health and any medical conditions and work out a plan for protection.

Sober Sex The use of alcohol or drugs in sexual situations increases the risk of unplanned, unprotected sexual activity. This is particularly true of young adults, many of whom binge-drink during social events. Alcohol and drugs impair judgment and should not be used in association with sexual activity. Be honest with yourself; if you need to drink in order to engage in sexual activities, maybe it's time to rethink your social life and relationships.

UNDERSTANDING FERTILITY

Conceiving a child is a highly complex process. Although many couples conceive readily, others can testify to the difficulties that can be encountered.

Conception

The process of conception involves the **fertilization** of a woman's ovum (egg) by a man's sperm. Every month during a woman's fertile years, her body prepares itself for conception and pregnancy. In one of her ovaries, an egg matures and is released from its follicle. The egg, about the size of a pinpoint, travels through an oviduct, or fallopian tube, to the uterus in 3–4 days. The endometrium, or lining of the uterus, has already thickened for the implantation of a **fertilized egg,** or *zygote*. If the egg is not fertilized, it lasts about 24 hours and then disintegrates.

> **fertilization** The initiation of biological reproduction: the union of the nucleus of an egg cell with the nucleus of a sperm cell.
>
> **fertilized egg** The egg after penetration by a sperm; a *zygote*.

TERMS

The woman's body expels the egg's remains and the uterine lining during menstruation.

Fertilization   Sperm cells are produced in the man's testes and ejaculated from his penis into the woman's vagina during sexual intercourse. Sperm cells are much smaller than eggs. The typical ejaculate contains millions of sperm, but only a few complete the journey through the uterus and up the fallopian tube to the egg.

Of those that reach the egg, only one will penetrate its hard outer layer. As sperm approach the egg, they release enzymes that soften this outer layer. Enzymes from hundreds of sperm must be released in order for the egg's outer layer to soften enough to allow one sperm cell to penetrate. The first sperm cell that bumps into a spot that is soft enough can swim into the egg cell. It then merges with the nucleus of the egg, and fertilization occurs. The sperm's tail, its means of locomotion, gets stuck in the egg's outer membrane and drops off, leaving the sperm's head inside the egg. The egg then releases a chemical that makes it impenetrable by other sperm.

The ovum carries the hereditary characteristics of the mother and her ancestors; sperm cells carry the hereditary characteristics of the father and his ancestors. Each parent cell—egg or sperm—contains 23 chromosomes, each of which contains **genes**, packages of chemical instructions for the developing baby. Genes provide the blueprint for a unique individual based on the functional and health characteristics of his or her ancestors.

Twins

In the usual course of events, one egg and one sperm unite to produce one fertilized egg and one baby. But if the ovaries release two or more eggs during ovulation and if both eggs are fertilized, twins develop. (The development of two or more fetuses in the same pregnancy is called *multiple gestation* and leads to a *multiple birth*.) These twins will be no more alike than siblings from different pregnancies, because each will have come from a different fertilized egg. Twins who develop this way are referred to as **fraternal twins**; they may be the same sex or different sexes. About 70% of twins are fraternal. Twins can also develop from the division of a single fertilized egg into two cells that develop separately. Because these babies share all genetic material, they will be **identical twins.**

The most serious complication of multiple births is preterm delivery (delivery before the fetus is adequately mature). The more fetuses a woman carries simultaneously, the shorter the gestational period will be.

Infertility

About 2 million American couples have difficulty conceiving. **Infertility** is defined as the inability to conceive after trying for a year or more. It affects about 15% of the reproductive-age population of the United States.

Female Infertility   Female infertility usually results from one of two key causes—tubal blockage (40%) or failure to ovulate (40%). An additional 10% of cases of infertility are due to anatomical abnormalities, benign growths in the uterus, thyroid disease, and other uncommon conditions; the remaining 10% of cases are unexplained.

Blocked fallopian tubes are most commonly the result of pelvic inflammatory disease (PID), a serious complication of several sexually transmitted diseases. Each year, PID renders more than 100,000 American women infertile. More than 1 million cases of PID are treated each year, but physicians estimate that just as many may go untreated because of an absence of symptoms. Tubal blockages can also be caused by prior surgery or by endometriosis, which is typically treated with hormonal therapy and surgery.

Age impacts fertility; beginning at around age 30, a woman's fertility naturally begins to decline. Age is probably the main factor in ovulation failure. Exposure to toxic chemicals or radiation also appears to reduce fertility, as does cigarette smoking.

Male Infertility   Male factor infertility accounts for about 20% of infertile couples. The leading causes of male infertility can be divided into four main categories: hypothalamic pituitary disease or congenital disorders, testicular disease, disorders of sperm transport, and unexplained. Some acquired disorders of the testes can lead to infertility, such as damage from drug use, smoking, infection, or environmental toxins.

The sons of mothers who took DES may have increased sperm abnormalities and fertility problems. Studies have identified a link between infertility and overweight and obesity in men, although the mechanism responsible for the relationship was not clear.

Treating Infertility   The cause of infertility can be determined for about 85% of infertile couples. Most cases of infertility are treated with conventional medical therapies. Surgery

142,435 ART procedures were performed in the United States in 2007, resulting in more than 57,569 babies.

—CDC, 2009

Home Pregnancy Tests

connect
ACTIVITY

Women have access to a variety of over-the-counter home pregnancy tests today, but all of them work in basically the same way—by detecting the presence of the hormone human chorionic gonadotropin (HCG) in the pregnant woman's urine. HCG is released by the implanted fertilized egg and can be detected within about 2 weeks after ovulation. Home pregnancy tests vary in such minor details as how the woman uses the test strips and how the strips display results.

Home pregnancy tests have become extremely accurate, typically providing accurate results 99% of the time. However, there is variation among women in how long it takes for a fertilized egg to implant in the uterus and begin releasing HCG. Implantation occurs between 6 and 12 days after ovulation, usually by 10 days. The earliest you can get a positive result is 7 days after ovulation, but it makes sense to wait until 10 to 12 days after ovulation to take a test. Even then, a significant percentage of women who are pregnant will show a negative result. HCG levels double every 2 to 3 days, and many women won't have a positive test result until the first day of a missed period or even a few days later.

A clinical pregnancy test can also be done, measuring HCG levels in the woman's blood. Blood tests are more accurate—measuring the exact number of units of HCG in the blood—but not necessarily more sensitive than a home pregnancy test. That is, they cannot detect pregnancy sooner than urine tests.

If you use a home pregnancy test kit, be aware of the limitations. If you elect to take the test as early as the day after you've missed your period, a negative result isn't 100% certain. If you're comfortable waiting, a sensitive test taken a week after your period is due will almost certainly give you accurate results. Remember that a positive result may mean either a viable pregnancy or a pregnancy destined to end shortly after it began. With either of those results, you should plan on testing again a week later, just to be sure. For that reason, it's a good idea to buy tests in pairs; 15 of the 18 commercially available home testing products come in multiple-test kits.

---

can repair oviducts, clear up endometriosis, and correct anatomical problems in men and women. Fertility drugs can help women ovulate, but may cause multiple births. If these conventional treatments don't work, couples can turn to **assisted reproductive technology (ART)** techniques, as described in the following sections. According to 2010 estimates from the CDC, about 1% of births in the United States are the result of ART treatments.

INTRAUTERINE INSEMINATION Male infertility can sometimes be overcome by collecting and concentrating the man's sperm and introducing it by syringe into a woman's vagina or uterus, a procedure known as **artificial (intrauterine) insemination.** To increase the probability of success, the woman is often given fertility drugs to induce ovulation prior to the insemination procedure. The success rate is about 60–70%.

IVF, GIFT, AND ZIFT Three related techniques involve removing mature eggs from a woman's ovary.

- In **in vitro fertilization (IVF),** the harvested eggs are mixed with sperm in a laboratory dish. If eggs are successfully fertilized, one or more of the resulting embryos are inserted into the woman's uterus. IVF is often used by women with blocked oviducts.

- In **gamete intrafallopian transfer (GIFT),** eggs and sperm are surgically placed into the fallopian tubes prior to fertilization.

- In **zygote intrafallopian transfer (ZIFT),** eggs are fertilized outside the woman's body and surgically introduced into the oviducts after they begin to divide.

GIFT and ZIFT can be used by women who have at least one open fallopian tube.

SURROGATE MOTHERHOOD Surrogate motherhood involves a contract between an infertile couple and a fertile woman who agrees to carry a fetus. The surrogate mother agrees to be artificially inseminated by the father's sperm or to undergo IVF with the couple's embryo, to carry the baby to term, and to give it to the couple at birth. In return, the couple pays her for her services (typically around $50,000). There are thought to be several hundred births to surrogate mothers each year in the United States.

PREGNANCY

Pregnancy is usually discussed in terms of **trimesters**—3 periods of about 3 months (or 13 weeks) each. During the first trimester, the mother experiences a few physical changes and some fairly common symptoms (see the box "Home Pregnancy Tests"). During the second trimester, often the most peaceful time of pregnancy, the

TERMS

assisted reproductive technology (ART) Advanced medical techniques used to treat infertility.

artificial (intrauterine) insemination The introduction of semen into the vagina by artificial means.

in vitro fertilization (IVF) Combining egg and sperm outside of the body and inserting the fertilized egg into the uterus.

gamete intrafallopian transfer (GIFT) Surgically placing eggs and sperm in the fallopian tube prior to fertilization.

zygote intrafallopian transfer (ZIFT) Surgically placing a fertilized egg into the fallopian tube.

trimester One of the three 3-month periods of pregnancy.

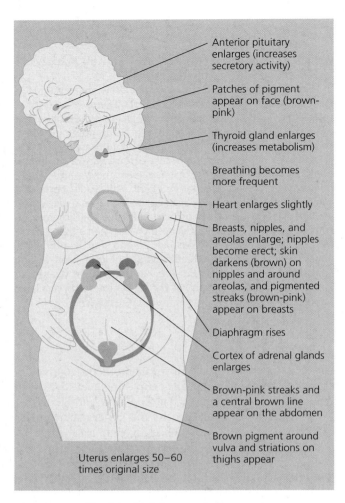

Anterior pituitary enlarges (increases secretory activity)

Patches of pigment appear on face (brown-pink)

Thyroid gland enlarges (increases metabolism)

Breathing becomes more frequent

Heart enlarges slightly

Breasts, nipples, and areolas enlarge; nipples become erect; skin darkens (brown) on nipples and around areolas, and pigmented streaks (brown-pink) appear on breasts

Diaphragm rises

Cortex of adrenal glands enlarges

Brown-pink streaks and a central brown line appear on the abdomen

Brown pigment around vulva and striations on thighs appear

Uterus enlarges 50–60 times original size

FIGURE 5.3 Physiological changes during pregnancy.

mother gains weight, looks noticeably pregnant, and may experience a general sense of well-being if she is happy about having a child. The third trimester is the hardest for the mother because she must breathe, digest, excrete, and circulate blood for herself and the growing fetus.

Changes in the Woman's Body

Hormonal changes begin as soon as the egg is fertilized, and for the next 9 months the woman's body nourishes the fetus and adjusts to its growth (Figure 5.3).

Early Signs and Symptoms Early recognition of pregnancy is important, especially for women with physical problems and nutritional deficiencies. The following symptoms are not absolute indications of pregnancy, but they are reasons to visit a gynecologist:

- *A missed menstrual period.* When a fertilized egg implants in the uterine wall, the endometrium is retained to nourish the embryo.

- *Slight bleeding.* Slight bleeding follows implantation of the fertilized egg in about 14% of pregnant women. Because this happens about the time a period is expected, the bleeding is sometimes mistaken for menstrual flow. It usually lasts only a few days.

- *Nausea.* About two-thirds of pregnant women feel nauseated, probably as a reaction to increased levels of progesterone and other hormones. Although this nausea is often called *morning sickness,* some women have it all day long. It frequently begins during the 6th week and disappears by the 12th week. In some cases, it lasts throughout the pregnancy.

- *Breast tenderness.* Some women experience breast tenderness, swelling, and tingling, usually described as different from the tenderness experienced before menstruation.

- *Increased urination.* Increased frequency of urination can occur soon after the missed period.

- *Sleepiness, fatigue, and emotional upset.* These symptoms result from hormonal changes.

The first reliable physical signs of pregnancy can be distinguished about 4 weeks after a woman misses her menstrual period. A softening of the uterus just above the cervix, called *Hegar's sign,* and other changes in the cervix and pelvis are apparent during a pelvic examination. The labia minora and the cervix may take on a purple color rather than their usual pink hue.

Continuing Changes in the Woman's Body During the first 3 months, the uterus enlarges to about three times its nonpregnant size, but it still cannot be felt in the abdomen. By the 4th month, it is large enough to make the abdomen protrude. By the 7th or 8th month, the uterus pushes up into the rib cage, which makes breathing slightly more difficult. The breasts enlarge and are sensitive; by week 8, they may tingle or throb. The pigmented area around the nipple, called the *areola,* darkens and broadens.

Early in pregnancy, the muscles and ligaments attached to bones begin to soften and stretch. The joints between the pelvic bones loosen and spread, making it easier to have a baby but harder to walk. The circulatory system becomes more efficient to accommodate the blood volume, which increases by 50%, and the heart pumps it more rapidly. The mother's lungs also become more efficient, and her rib cage widens to permit her to inhale up to 40% more air.

The average weight gain during a healthy pregnancy is 27.5 pounds, although actual weight change varies with the individual. About 60% of the weight gain is directly related to the baby (such as the fetus and placenta); the rest accumulates over the woman's body as fluid and fat.

Changes During the Later Stages of Pregnancy By the end of the 6th month, the increased needs of the fetus place a burden on the mother's lungs, heart, and kidneys.

Her back may ache from the pressure of the baby's weight and from having to throw her shoulders back to keep her balance while standing. Her body retains more water, perhaps up to 3 extra quarts of fluid. Her legs, hands, ankles, or feet may swell, and she may be bothered by leg cramps, heartburn, or constipation. Despite discomfort, both her digestion and her metabolism are working at top efficiency.

The uterus prepares for childbirth with preliminary contractions, called *Braxton Hicks contractions.* Unlike true labor contractions, these are usually short, irregular, and painless. The mother may only be aware that at times her abdomen is hard to the touch. These contractions become more frequent and intense as the delivery date approaches.

In the 9th month, the baby settles into the pelvic bones, usually head down, fitting snugly. This process, called **lightening,** allows the uterus to sink down about 2 inches, producing a visible change in the mother's profile. Pelvic pressure increases, and pressure on the diaphragm lightens. Breathing becomes easier; urination becomes more frequent. Sometimes, after a first pregnancy, the baby doesn't settle down into the pelvis until labor begins.

The third trimester is the time of greatest physical stress during the pregnancy. A woman may find that her physical abilities are limited by her size. Because some women feel physically awkward and sexually unattractive, they may experience periods of depression. But many also feel a great deal of happy excitement and anticipation. The fetus may already be looked on as a member of the family, and both parents may begin talking to the fetus and interacting with it by patting the mother's belly. The upcoming birth will probably be a focus for both the woman and her partner (see the box "Pregnancy Tasks for Fathers").

Fetal Development

Now that we've seen what happens to the mother's body during pregnancy, let's consider the development of the fetus (Figure 5.4).

The First Trimester   About 30 hours after an egg is fertilized, the cell divides, and this process of cell division repeats many times. As the cluster of cells drifts along the oviduct, several different kinds of cells emerge. The entire set of genetic instructions is passed to every cell, but each

---

lightening   A process in which the uterus sinks down because the baby's head settles into the mother's pelvic area.

FIGURE 5.4   A chronology of milestones in prenatal development.

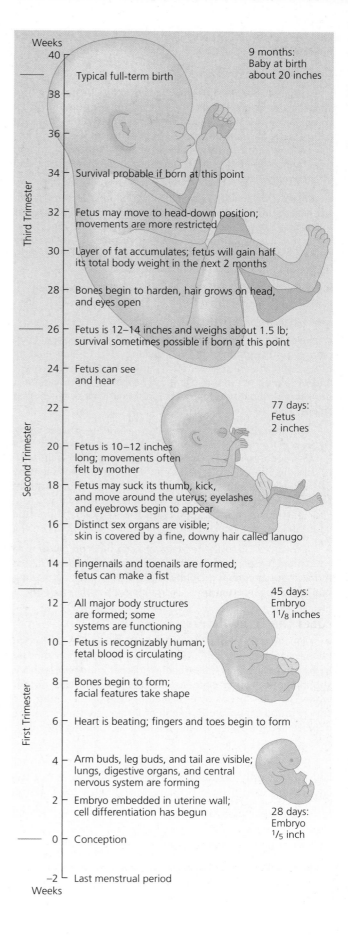

Weeks
- 40 — Typical full-term birth
- 9 months: Baby at birth about 20 inches
- Third Trimester
- 38
- 36
- 34 — Survival probable if born at this point
- 32 — Fetus may move to head-down position; movements are more restricted
- 30 — Layer of fat accumulates; fetus will gain half its total body weight in the next 2 months
- 28 — Bones begin to harden, hair grows on head, and eyes open
- 26 — Fetus is 12–14 inches and weighs about 1.5 lb; survival sometimes possible if born at this point
- 24 — Fetus can see and hear
- Second Trimester
- 22 — 77 days: Fetus 2 inches
- 20 — Fetus is 10–12 inches long; movements often felt by mother
- 18 — Fetus may suck its thumb, kick, and move around the uterus; eyelashes and eyebrows begin to appear
- 16 — Distinct sex organs are visible; skin is covered by a fine, downy hair called lanugo
- 14 — Fingernails and toenails are formed; fetus can make a fist
- 45 days: Embryo 1 1/8 inches
- 12 — All major body structures are formed; some systems are functioning
- 10 — Fetus is recognizably human; fetal blood is circulating
- First Trimester
- 8 — Bones begin to form; facial features take shape
- 6 — Heart is beating; fingers and toes begin to form
- 4 — Arm buds, leg buds, and tail are visible; lungs, digestive organs, and central nervous system are forming
- 2 — Embryo embedded in uterine wall; cell differentiation has begun
- 28 days: Embryo 1/5 inch
- 0 — Conception
- −2 — Last menstrual period
- Weeks

Pregnancy Tasks for Fathers

GENDER MATTERS

Before the Pregnancy

● *Consider your lifestyle and health habits.* A healthy lifestyle can help boost fertility and improve pregnancy outcome. Being too thin or too heavy may lower a man's sperm count, as may marijuana use. Men who smoke and drink have a lower concentration of sperm and a lower percentage of active sperm. Exposure to chemicals on the job may also affect pregnancy.

● *Check your budget, financial situation, and insurance status.* Make sure your finances are in order, and that you have as much life, health, and disability insurance as you can afford. See a financial planner for advice. Try putting away extra money every month now—both to practice living on a tighter budget and to actually save up for the baby.

● *Get any necessary health checks and genetic counseling.*

During the Pregnancy

● *Help your partner stay healthy during the pregnancy.* If you smoke, quit; secondhand smoke is dangerous to a developing fetus. Support your partner by making other lifestyle changes and/or joining her in any changes she's making; for example, drink nonalcoholic beverages, take walks with her, and get extra sleep.

● *Help around the home and with planning for the baby.* Help shop for necessities, and help get your home ready for a baby. Pregnancy is hard work, so providing extra help with household chores and errands can be an important element of support. (Due to the risk of infection by toxoplasmosis, pregnant women should avoid handling cat litter; if you and your partner have a cat, emptying the litter box should be your job.)

● *Be involved.* Go to all the prenatal visits, birth preparation or education classes, hospital and nursery tours, and so on. Learn more about pregnancy, childbirth, and parenting by reading books, visiting Internet sites, and talking with other parents.

After the Baby Arrives

● *Help meet your baby's needs.* If your job allows, take parental leave to help with the new baby. Support the new mother by helping with baby care (feeding, diaper changes), laundry, shopping, and other chores. Take turns or join the mother when the baby needs care or feeding during the night; one survey found that more than half of fathers continue to sleep or pretend to be asleep when their babies cry during the night.

● *Support your partner, and reach out to others for help.* It is normal for a new mother to be tired and to experience mood changes, and new fathers often experience anxiety about their changing role. Good communication between partners and help from supportive relatives and friends can help new parents adjust.

● *Give mom some time off.* A new mother needs time to recover from childbirth, even after she leaves the hospital or birthing center. This is especially true if the delivery was difficult, if a cesarean section was performed, or if an episiotomy was required. Aside from pitching in with daily chores, the father can aid the mother's recuperation by taking the baby for a few hours at a time. If the baby is being bottlefed, the dad may be able to take charge for a morning, an afternoon, or even the entire day.

---

cell follows only certain instructions; if this were not the case, there would be no different organs or body parts. For example, all cells carry genes for hair color and eye color, but only the cells of the hair follicles and irises (of the eye) respond to that information.

On about the 4th day after fertilization, the cluster, now about 32–128 cells and hollow, arrives in the uterus; this is a **blastocyst.** On about the sixth or seventh day, the blastocyst attaches to the uterine wall, usually along the upper curve. Over the next few days, it becomes firmly implanted and begins to draw nourishment from the endometrium, the uterine lining.

TERMS

blastocyst   A stage of development, days 4–14, before the cell cluster becomes the embryo and placenta.

The blastocyst becomes an **embryo** by about the end of the 2nd week after fertilization. The inner cells of the blastocyst separate into three layers. One layer becomes inner body parts, the digestive and respiratory systems; the middle layer becomes muscle, bone, blood, kidneys, and sex glands; and the third layer becomes the skin, hair, and nervous tissue.

The outermost shell of cells becomes the **placenta, umbilical cord,** and **amniotic sac.** A network of blood vessels called *chorionic villi* eventually forms the placenta. The human placenta allows a two-way exchange of nutrients and waste materials between the mother and the fetus. The placenta brings oxygen and nutrients to the fetus and transports waste products out. The placenta does not provide a perfect barrier between the fetal circulation and the maternal circulation, however. Some blood cells are exchanged and certain substances, such as alcohol, pass freely from the maternal circulation through the placenta to the fetus.

The period between weeks 2 and 9 is a time of rapid differentiation and change. All the major body structures are formed during this time, including the heart, brain, liver, lungs, and sex organs. The eyes, nose, ears, arms, and legs also appear. Some organs begin to function as well; the heart begins to beat, and the liver starts producing blood cells. Because body structures are forming, the developing organism is vulnerable to damage from environmental influences such as drugs and infections.

By the end of the 2nd month, the brain sends out impulses that coordinate the functioning of other organs. The embryo is now a fetus, and most further changes will be in the size and refinement of working body parts. In the 3rd month, the fetus becomes active. By the end of the first trimester, the fetus is about an inch long and weighs less than 1 ounce.

The Second Trimester To grow during the second trimester, to about 14 inches and 1.5 pounds, the fetus must have large amounts of food, oxygen, and water, which come from the mother through the placenta. All body systems are operating, and the fetal heartbeat can be heard with a stethoscope. The mother can detect fetal movements beginning in the 4th or 5th month. Against great odds, a fetus born prematurely at the end of the second trimester might survive.

Against great odds, a fetus born at the end of the second trimester might survive.

Ultrasonography provides information about the position, size, and physical condition of a fetus in the uterus.

The Third Trimester The fetus gains most of its birth weight during the last 3 months. Some of the weight is fat under the skin that insulates the fetus and supplies food. About 85% of the calcium and iron the mother consumes goes into the fetal bloodstream.

The fetus may live if it is born during the 7th month, but it needs the fat layer acquired in the 8th month and time for organs—especially the respiratory and digestive organs—to develop. It also needs the immunity supplied by the antibodies in the mother's blood during the final

embryo The stage of development between blastocyst and fetus; about weeks 2–8.

placenta The organ through which the fetus receives nourishment and empties waste via the mother's circulatory system; after birth, the placenta is expelled from the uterus.

umbilical cord The cord connecting the placenta and fetus, through which nutrients pass.

amniotic sac A membranous pouch enclosing and protecting the fetus; also holds amniotic fluid.

DIMENSIONS OF DIVERSITY

Genes carry the chemical instructions that determine the development of hundreds of individual traits, including disease risks, in every human being. Many traits and conditions involve multiple genes and environmental influences. Some diseases, however, can be traced to a mutation in a single gene.

Children inherit one set of genes from each parent. If only one copy of an abnormal gene is necessary to produce a disease, then it is called a *dominant* gene. Diseases caused by dominant genes seldom skip a generation; anyone who carries the gene will probably get the disease.

If two copies of an abnormal gene (one from each parent) are necessary for a disease to occur, then the gene is called *recessive*. Many diseases caused by recessive genes occur disproportionately in certain ethnic groups. Prospective parents who come from the same ethnic group can be tested for any recessive diseases that are known to occur in that group. If both parents are carriers, each of their children will have about a 25% chance of developing the disease.

The following list describes a few common conditions with proven genetic links in certain ethnic populations. If there is a history of any of these conditions in your family and you plan to have children, genetic tests and counseling can help assess the risk to your prospective children.

- *Sickle-cell disease* occurs in about 1 out of every 500 African American births and in 1 out of every 36,000 Hispanic American births, according to the CDC. In this disease, red blood cells, which carry oxygen to the body's tissues, change shape; the normally disc-shaped cells become sickle-shaped. The altered cells carry less oxygen and can block small blood vessels. People who inherit one gene for sickle-cell disease (about 1 in 12 African Americans) experience only mild symptoms; those with two genes become severely, often fatally, ill.

If you are at risk for sickle-cell disease, you should take care to reduce stress and respond to minor infections, because red blood cells become sickle-shaped when the body is under stress. You should also have regular checkups and appropriate treatment, if required.

- *Hemochromatosis* ("iron overload") affects about 1 in 200 people. At highest risk are people of Northern European (especially Irish), Mediterranean, and Hispanic descent. In hemochromatosis, the body absorbs and stores up to ten times the normal amount of iron. Iron deposits form in the joints, liver, heart, and pancreas. If untreated, the disease can cause organ failure and death.

Early symptoms are often vague and include weakness, lethargy, darkening of the skin, and joint pain. Early detection and treatment are necessary to prevent damage. Treatment involves reducing iron stores by removing blood from the body (a process known as phlebotomy or "bloodletting").

- *Tay-Sachs disease,* another recessive disorder, occurs in about 1 in 3000 Jews of Eastern European ancestry. People with Tay-Sachs disease cannot properly metabolize fat. As a result, the brain and other nerve tissues deteriorate. Affected children show weakness in their movements and eventually develop blindness (by age 12–18 months) and seizures. This disease is fatal, and death usually occurs by age 6. No effective treatment is currently available.

- *Cystic fibrosis* affects 1 in 2500–3000 Caucasians; about 1 in 29 carries one copy of the cystic fibrosis gene. In cystic fibrosis, essential enzymes are deficient so the body cannot properly absorb nutrients. Thick mucus impairs functioning in the lungs and intestinal tracts of people with this disease. Cystic fibrosis is often fatal in early childhood, but treatments are increasingly effective in reducing symptoms and prolonging life. In some cases, symptoms do not appear until early adulthood.

- *Lactose intolerance,* or intolerance to lactose-containing foods (primarily dairy products), often has a genetic component. In the United States, the prevalence is 80–95% in Native Americans, 65–75% among Africans and African Americans, 50% in Hispanics, and 20% in Caucasians. The prevalence exceeds 90% in some populations in eastern Asia.

Clinical symptoms of lactose intolerance include diarrhea, abdominal pain, and flatulence after ingestion of milk or milk-containing products. These symptoms result from low intestinal levels of the enzyme lactase-phlorizin hydrolase.

If you suspect lactose intolerance, see your doctor for a lactose absorption test. Lactose malabsorption is treated by reducing lactose intake, finding alternatives to foods containing lactose, taking an enzyme substitute, and maintaining calcium and vitamin D intake.

Other health problems that have a hereditary component and that disproportionately affect certain ethnic groups include thalassemia, diabetes, osteoporosis, high blood pressure, alcoholism, and certain cancers. Later chapters discuss many of these links.

---

3 months. The antibodies protect the fetus against many of the diseases to which she has acquired immunity.

TERMS

ultrasonography The use of high-frequency sound waves to view the fetus in the uterus; also known as *ultrasound*.

sonogram The visual image of the fetus produced by ultrasonography.

Diagnosing Fetal Abnormalities About 3% of babies are born with a major birth defect. Information about the health and sex of a fetus can be obtained prior to birth through prenatal testing.

Ultrasonography (also called *ultrasound*) uses high-frequency sound waves to create a **sonogram,** or visual image, of the fetus in the uterus. Sonograms show the fetus' position, size, gestational age, and the presence of certain anatomical problems. Sonograms can sometimes be used to determine the sex of the fetus. Sonograms are considered safe for a pregnant woman and the fetus, but the FDA advises against "keepsake" sonograms performed for no medical purpose.

Amniocentesis involves the removal of fluid from the uterus with a long, thin needle inserted through the abdominal wall. It is usually performed between 15 and 18 weeks into the pregnancy, although earlier amniocentesis is available. A genetic analysis of the fetal cells in the fluid can reveal the presence of chromosomal disorders, such as Down syndrome, and some genetic diseases, including Tay-Sachs disease (see the box "Ethnicity and Genetic Diseases"). The sex of the fetus can also be determined.

Another prenatal test is **chorionic villus sampling (CVS),** which can be performed earlier in pregnancy than amniocentesis, between weeks 10 and 12. This procedure involves removal through the cervix (by catheter) or abdomen (by needle) of a tiny section of chorionic villi, which contain fetal cells that then can be analyzed.

The **quadruple marker screen (QMS)** is a maternal blood test that can be used to help identify fetuses with neural tube defects, Down syndrome, and other anomalies. Blood is taken from the mother at 16–19 weeks of pregnancy and analyzed for four hormone levels—human chorionic gonadotropin (HCG), unconjugated estriol, alpha-fetoprotein (AFP), and inhibin-A. The hormone levels are compared to appropriate standards, and the results are used to estimate the probability that the fetus has particular anomalies. QMS is a screening test rather than a diagnostic test; in the case of abnormal QMS results, parents may choose further testing such as ultrasonography or amniocentesis.

A new first-trimester screening test for Down syndrome combines ultrasound evaluation of nuchal translucency (the thickness of the back of the fetus's neck) with maternal blood testing. This test can be done between the 10th and 14th week of pregnancy. If results indicate an increased risk of abnormality, further diagnostic studies such as amniocentesis can be done for confirmation.

Fetal Programming   Amniocentesis, CVS, and QMS look for chromosomal, genetic, and other anomalies that typically cause immediate problems. A new area of study known as *fetal programming theory* focuses on how conditions in the womb may influence the risk of adult diseases. For example, researchers have linked low birth weight to an increased risk of heart disease, high blood pressure, obesity, diabetes, and schizophrenia. High birth weight in female infants, however, has been linked to an increased risk of breast cancer in later life.

Although fetal programming theory is not yet embraced by all scientists, these studies emphasize that everything that occurs during pregnancy can have an impact on the developing fetus. In the future, people may be able to use information about their birth weight and other indicators of gestational conditions just as they can now use family history and genetic information—to alert them to special health risks and to help them improve their health.

The Importance of Prenatal Care

Adequate prenatal care—as described in the following sections—is essential to the health of both mother and baby. All physicians recommend that women start getting regular prenatal checkups as soon as they become pregnant. Typically, this means one checkup per month during the first 8 months, then one checkup per week during the final month. About 84% of pregnant women begin receiving adequate prenatal care during the first trimester; about 3.5% wait until the last trimester or receive no prenatal care at all.

Regular Checkups   In the woman's first visit to her obstetrician, she will be asked for a detailed medical history of herself and her family. The physician or midwife will note any hereditary conditions that may assume increased significance during pregnancy. The tendency to develop gestational diabetes (diabetes during pregnancy only), for example, can be inherited; appropriate treatment during pregnancy reduces the risk of serious harm.

The woman is given a complete physical exam and is informed about appropriate diet. She returns for regular checkups throughout the pregnancy, during which her blood pressure and weight gain are measured, her urine is analyzed, and the fetus's size and position are monitored.

Blood Tests   A blood sample is taken during the initial prenatal visit to determine blood type and detect possible anemia or Rh incompatibilities. The **Rh factor** is a blood protein. If an Rh-positive father and an Rh-negative mother conceive an Rh-positive baby, the baby's blood will be incompatible with the mother's. This condition is completely treatable with a serum called Rh-immune globulin, which destroys Rh-positive cells as they enter the mother's body and prevents her from forming antibodies to them. Blood may also be tested for evidence of hepatitis B, syphilis, rubella immunity, thyroid problems, and, with the mother's permission, HIV infection.

Prenatal Nutrition   A nutritious diet throughout pregnancy is essential for both the mother and her unborn baby. Not only does the baby get all its nutrients from the mother, but it also competes with her for nutrients not sufficiently available to meet both their needs. When a

---

TERMS

amniocentesis   A process in which amniotic fluid is removed and analyzed to detect possible birth defects.

chorionic villus sampling (CVS)   Surgical removal of a tiny section of chorionic villi to be analyzed for genetic defects.

quadruple marker screen (QMS)   A measurement of four hormones, used to assess the risk of fetal abnormalities.

Rh factor   A protein found in blood. Rh incompatibility between a mother and fetus can jeopardize the fetus's health.

woman's diet is low in iron or calcium, the fetus receives most of it, and the mother may become deficient in the mineral. To meet the increased nutritional demands of her body, a pregnant woman shouldn't just eat more; she should make sure that her diet is nutritionally adequate.

To maintain her own health and help the fetus grow, a pregnant woman typically needs to consume about 250–500 extra calories per day. Breast-feeding an infant requires even more energy—about 500 or more calories per day. To ensure that she's getting enough calories and nutrients, a pregnant woman should talk to her doctor or a registered dietitian about her dietary habits and determine what changes she should make.

Some physicians prescribe high-potency vitamin and mineral supplements to pregnant and lactating women. Supplements can help boost the levels of nutrients available to mother and child, helping with fetal development while ensuring that the mother doesn't become nutrient deficient. Pregnant and lactating women, however, should not take supplements without the advice of their physician, because some vitamins and minerals are harmful if taken in excess. Pregnant women also should not take herbal dietary supplements without consulting a physician.

Two vitamins—vitamin D and the B vitamin folate—are particularly important to pregnant women. Pregnant women who don't get enough vitamin D are more likely to deliver low-birth-weight babies. Chronic vitamin D deficiency has been linked to other health problems as well, including heart disease.

If woman doesn't get the recommended daily amount of folate, both before and during pregnancy, her child has an increased risk of neural tube defects, including spina bifida. Any woman capable of becoming pregnant should get at least 400 μg (0.4 mg) of folic acid (the synthetic form of folate) daily from fortified foods and/or supplements, in addition to folate from a varied diet. Pregnant women should get 600 μg every day.

Food safety is another special dietary concern for pregnant women because foodborne pathogens can be especially dangerous to them and their unborn children. Germs such as *Listeria monocytogenes* and *Toxoplasma gondii* are both particularly dangerous. Pregnant women should avoid eating undercooked and ready-to-eat meats and should be sure to thoroughly wash produce before eating it. Pregnant women should also follow the FDA's recommendations for consumption of fish and seafood. For complete information on nutrition and food safety, see Chapter 9.

TERMS

teratogen An agent or influence that causes physical defects in a developing fetus.

congenital malformation A physical defect existing at the time of birth, either inherited or caused during gestation.

fetal alcohol syndrome (FAS) A combination of birth defects caused by excessive alcohol consumption by the mother during pregnancy.

Avoiding Drugs and Other Environmental Hazards

In addition to the food the mother eats, the drugs she takes and the chemicals she is exposed to affect the fetus. Everything the mother ingests may eventually reach the fetus in some proportion. Some drugs harm the fetus but not the mother because the fetus is in the process of developing and because the proper dose for the mother is a massive dose for the fetus.

During the first trimester, when the major body structures are rapidly forming, the fetus is extremely vulnerable to environmental factors such as viral infections, radiation, drugs, and other **teratogens,** any of which can cause **congenital malformations,** or birth defects. The most susceptible body parts are those growing most rapidly at the time of exposure. The rubella (German measles) virus, for example, can cause a congenital malformation of a delicate system such as the eyes or ears, leading to blindness or deafness, if exposure occurs during the first trimester, but it does no damage later in the pregnancy. Similarly, the drug thalidomide taken early in pregnancy prevents the formation of arms and legs in fetuses, but taken later, when limbs are already formed, it causes no damage. Other drugs can cause damage throughout prenatal development.

ALCOHOL Alcohol is a potent teratogen. Getting drunk just one time during pregnancy may be enough to cause brain damage in a fetus. A high level of alcohol consumption during pregnancy is associated with miscarriages, stillbirths, and, in live babies, **fetal alcohol syndrome (FAS).** A baby born with FAS is likely to suffer from a small head and body size, unusual facial characteristics, congenital heart defects, defective joints, impaired vision, mental impairment, and abnormal behavior patterns. Researchers now doubt that any level of alcohol consumption is safe, and they recommend total abstinence during pregnancy.

> ## Up to 1.5 in 1000 babies born in the United States have FAS.
> —CDC, 2010

TOBACCO Smoking during pregnancy increases the risk of miscarriage, low birth weight, immune system impairment, and infant death; it may also cause genetic damage or physical deformations. If nicotine levels in a mother's bloodstream are high, fetal breathing rate and movement become more rapid; the fetus may also metabolize cancer-causing by-products of tobacco.

CAFFEINE Caffeine, a powerful stimulant, puts both mother and fetus under stress by raising the level of the hormone epinephrine. Caffeine also reduces the blood supply to the uterus. A pregnant woman should limit her caffeine intake to no more than the equivalent of two cups of coffee per day.

DRUGS Some prescription drugs, such as some blood pressure medications, can harm the fetus, so they should

Physical Activity during Pregnancy

Maintaining a regular routine of moderate-intensity physical activity throughout pregnancy can help a mother-to-be stay healthy and feel her best. Regular exercise can improve posture and decrease common pregnancy-related discomforts, such as backaches and fatigue. There is also evidence that physical activity may prevent gestational diabetes, relieve stress, and build stamina that can be helpful during labor and delivery. Most studies find that a well-managed routine of physical activity results in no significant negative outcomes, such as low birth weight or early labor.

A woman who was physically active before pregnancy should be able to continue her favorite activities in moderation, except for those that carry a risk of trauma (such as basketball or hockey) or falls (such as horseback riding), or unless there is a medical reason to reduce or stop exercise. However, a pregnant woman should adapt her level of exercise to whatever is most comfortable given her condition at the moment. A woman who has never exercised regularly can safely start an exercise program during pregnancy after consulting with her health care provider. A routine of regular walking is considered a safe way to start exercising during pregnancy. The American College of Obstetricians and Gynecologists (ACOG) recommends 30 minutes or more of moderate exercise per day on most if not all days of the week, unless the mother-to-be has a medical or pregnancy complication.

Pregnant women should avoid exercising in the supine position (lying on the back), especially after the first trimester, according to the ACOG. Women should also avoid motionless standing and strenuous lifting throughout pregnancy. Low-impact aerobic activities are safer than high-impact exercise. Pregnant women should not let their heart rate exceed 140 beats per minute and should avoid getting overheated or dehydrated.

Some conditions can restrict a pregnant woman's ability to exercise, such as heart or lung disease, poorly controlled diabetes, carrying multiple fetuses, and experiencing incompetent cervix, ruptured membranes, placenta previa after the 26th week of pregnancy, or persistent vaginal bleeding. The ACOG recommends that a pregnant woman should stop exercising if she experiences vaginal bleeding, dizziness, headache, pain in the chest or calves, weakness, preterm labor, decreased fetal movement, or leakage of amniotic fluid.

SOURCES: ACOG Committee on Obstetric Practice. 2002 (Reaffirmed 2009). Committee opinion: Exercise during pregnancy and the postpartum period. *Obstetrics and Gynecology* 99(1): 171–173; Physical Activity Guidelines Advisory Committee. 2008. *Physical Activity Guidelines Advisory Committee Report, 2008*. Washington, D.C.: U.S. Department of Health and Human Services.

---

be used only under medical supervision. Many babies born to women who use antidepressants during pregnancy suffer withdrawal symptoms after birth. Recreational drugs, such as cocaine, are thought to increase the risk of major birth defects. Marijuana use may also interfere with fertility treatments, and methamphetamine use is associated with underweight babies.

STDS AND OTHER INFECTIONS Infections, including those that are sexually transmitted, are another serious problem for the fetus. Such infections can pose a threat before, during, and after birth. Rubella, syphilis, gonorrhea, hepatitis B, group B streptococcus, herpes, and HIV are among the most dangerous infections for the fetus. Treatment of the mother or immunization of the baby just after birth can help prevent problems from many infections. Women at risk for HIV infection should be tested before or during pregnancy because early treatment can dramatically reduce the chance that the virus will be passed to the fetus; some experts advocate universal HIV screening for pregnant women.

2.3 million
pregnant American women become infected with an STD every year.
—CDC, 2008

Prenatal Activity and Exercise Physical activity during pregnancy contributes to mental and physical wellness (see the box "Physical Activity during Pregnancy"). Women can continue working at their jobs until late in their pregnancy, provided the work isn't so physically demanding that it jeopardizes their health. At the same time, pregnant women need more rest and sleep to maintain their own well-being and that of the fetus.

Kegel exercises, to strengthen the pelvic floor muscles, are recommended for pregnant women. These exercises are performed by alternately contracting and releasing the muscles used to stop the flow of urine. Each contraction should be held for about 5 seconds. Kegel exercises should be done several times a day, for a total of about 50 repetitions daily.

Preparing for Birth Childbirth classes are almost a routine part of the prenatal experience for both mothers and fathers these days. These classes typically teach the details of the birth process as well as relaxation techniques to help deal with the discomfort of labor and delivery. The mother learns and practices a variety of techniques so she will be able to choose what works best for her during labor when the time comes. The father typically acts as a coach, supporting his partner emotionally and helping her with her breathing and relaxing. He remains with her throughout labor and delivery, even when a cesarean section is performed.

Complications of Pregnancy and Pregnancy Loss

About 31% of mothers-to-be suffer complications during pregnancy. Some complications may prevent full-term development of the fetus or affect the health of the infant at birth. As discussed earlier in the chapter, exposure to harmful substances, such as alcohol or drugs, can harm the fetus. Other complications are caused by physiological problems or genetic abnormalities.

Ectopic Pregnancy In an **ectopic pregnancy,** the fertilized egg implants and begins to develop outside of the uterus, usually in an oviduct (Figure 5.5).

Ectopic pregnancies usually occur because the fallopian tube is blocked, most often as a result of pelvic inflammatory disease; smoking also increases a woman's risk for ectopic pregnancy. The embryo may spontaneously abort, or the embryo and placenta may continue to expand until they rupture the oviduct. Sharp pain on one side of the abdomen or in the lower back, usually in about the 7th or 8th week, may signal an ectopic pregnancy, and there may be irregular bleeding.

An ectopic pregnancy is a medical emergency. Surgical removal of the embryo and the oviduct may be necessary to save the mother's life, although microsurgery can sometimes be used to repair the damaged oviduct. If diagnosed early, before the oviduct ruptures, ectopic pregnancy can often be successfully treated without surgery.

Spontaneous Abortion A spontaneous abortion, or miscarriage, is the termination of pregnancy before the 20th week. Most—about 60%—are due to chromosomal abnormalities in the fetus. Certain occupations that involve exposure to chemicals may increase the likelihood of a spontaneous abortion.

> *A miscarriage doesn't mean future pregnancies will fail.* **Up to 90% of women who miscarry get pregnant again.**

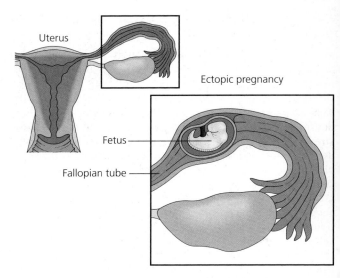

FIGURE 5.5 Ectopic pregnancy in a fallopian tube.

Labels: Uterus · Ectopic pregnancy · Fetus · Fallopian tube

Stillbirth The terms *fetal death, fetal demise, stillbirth,* and *stillborn* all refer to the delivery of a fetus that shows no signs of life. Risk factors for stillbirth include smoking, advanced maternal age, obesity, multiple gestations, and chronic disease. Risk for stillbirth is also correlated with race; black women have twice as many stillbirths as white women.

Preeclampsia A disease unique to human pregnancy, **preeclampsia** is characterized by elevated blood pressure and the appearance of protein in the urine. Symptoms include headache, right upper-quadrant abdominal pain, vision changes (referred to as *scotomata*), and notable increased swelling and weight gain. If preeclampsia is untreated, patients can develop seizures, a condition called **eclampsia.** Other potential complications of preeclampsia are liver and kidney damage, bleeding, fetal growth restriction, and even fetal death.

Women with mild preeclampsia may be monitored closely as outpatients and placed on home bed rest. More severe cases may require hospitalization for close medical management and early delivery.

Placenta Previa In **placenta previa,** the placenta either completely or partially covers the cervical opening, preventing the mother from delivering the baby vaginally. As a result, the baby must be delivered by cesarean section. Risk factors include prior cesarean delivery, multiple pregnancies, intrauterine surgery, smoking, multiple gestations, and advanced maternal age.

Placental Abruption In **placental abruption,** a normally implanted placenta prematurely separates from the uterine wall. Patients experience abdominal pain, vaginal bleeding, and uterine tenderness. The condition increases the risk of fetal death. The risk factors for developing a placental abruption are maternal age, tobacco smoking, cocaine use, multiple gestations, trauma, preeclampsia, hypertension, and preterm premature rupture of membranes.

TERMS

ectopic pregnancy A pregnancy in which the embryo develops outside of the uterus, usually in an oviduct.

preeclampsia A condition of pregnancy characterized by high blood pressure and protein in the urine.

eclampsia A severe, potentially life-threatening form of preeclampsia, characterized by seizures.

placenta previa A complication of pregnancy in which the placenta covers the cervical opening, preventing the mother from delivering the baby vaginally.

placental abruption A complication of pregnancy in which a normally implanted placenta prematurely separates from the uterine wall.

Gestational Diabetes   During gestation, about 4% of all pregnant women develop **gestational diabetes (GDM)**, in which the body loses its ability to use insulin properly. In these women, diabetes occurs only during pregnancy. Women diagnosed with GDM have an increased risk of developing type 2 diabetes later in life. It is important to accurately diagnose and treat GDM as it can lead to preeclampsia, polyhydramnios (increased levels of amniotic fluid), large fetuses, birth trauma, operative deliveries, perinatal mortality, and neonatal metabolic complications.

Preterm Labor   When a pregnant woman goes into labor before the 37th week of gestation, she is said to undergo *preterm labor*. About 30–50% of preterm labors resolve themselves, with the pregnancy continuing to full term. In other cases, interventions may be required to delay labor and allow gestation to continue.

Labor Induction   If pregnancy continues well beyond the baby's due date, it may be necessary to induce labor artificially. This is one of the most common obstetrical procedures and is typically offered to pregnant women who have not delivered and are 7–14 days past their due date. Labor can be artificially induced in several ways.

Low Birth Weight and Premature Birth   A **low-birth-weight (LBW)** baby is one that weighs less than 5.5 pounds at birth. LBW babies may be **premature** (born before the 37th week of pregnancy) or full-term. Babies who are born small even though they're full-term are referred to as *small-for-date* or *small-for-gestational-age* babies. About half of all cases are related to teenage pregnancy, cigarette smoking, poor nutrition, and poor maternal health. Other maternal factors include drug use, stress, depression, and anxiety. Adequate prenatal care is the best way to prevent LBW.

Full-term LBW babies tend to have fewer problems than premature infants. Many of the premature infant's organs are not sufficiently developed. Even mild prematurity increases an infant's risk of dying in the first month or year of life. Premature infants are subject to respiratory problems, infections, and eating difficulties. As they get older, premature infants may have learning difficulties, behavior problems, poor hearing and vision, and physical awkwardness.

Infant Mortality   The U.S. rate of **infant mortality,** the death of a child of less than 1 year of age, is near its lowest point ever; however, it remains far higher than that of most of the developed world. Poverty and inadequate health care are key causes.

Other causes of infant death are congenital problems, infectious diseases, and injuries. In **sudden infant death syndrome (SIDS),** an apparently healthy infant dies suddenly while sleeping. About 2300 infant deaths are attributed to SIDS each year. Research suggests that

abnormalities in the brainstem, the part of the brain that regulates breathing, heart rate, and other basic functions, underlie the risk for SIDS. Risk is greatly increased for infants with these innate differences if they are exposed to environmental risks, such as sleeping face down; being exposed to tobacco smoke, alcohol, or other drugs; or sleeping on a soft mattress or with fluffy bedding, pillows, or stuffed toys. Overbundling a baby or keeping a baby's room too warm also increases the risk of SIDS; because of this, SIDS deaths are more common in the colder months. Several studies have found that the use of a pacifier significantly reduces the risk of SIDS.

CHILDBIRTH

By the end of the 9th month of pregnancy, most women are tired of being pregnant; both parents are eager to start a new phase of their lives. Most couples find the actual process of birth to be an exciting and positive experience.

Choices in Childbirth

Many couples today can choose the type of practitioner and the environment they want for the birth of their child. A high-risk pregnancy is probably best handled by a specialist physician in a hospital with a nursery, but for low-risk births, many options are available.

Parents can choose to have their baby delivered by a physician or by a certified nurse-midwife. In the United States, most babies are delivered in hospitals or freestanding birth centers; in 2006, more than 25,000 babies were delivered at home. Many hospitals have introduced birth centers in response to criticism of traditional hospital routines. These centers provide a comfortable, emotionally supportive environment that is close to up-to-date medical

gestational diabetes (GDM)   A form of diabetes that occurs during pregnancy.

low birth weight (LBW)   Weighing less than 5.5 pounds at birth, often the result of prematurity.

premature   Born before the 37th week of pregnancy.

infant mortality   The death of a child less than 1 year of age.

sudden infant death syndrome (SIDS)   The sudden death of an apparently healthy infant during sleep.

equipment. It is important for prospective parents to discuss all aspects of labor and delivery with their physician or midwife beforehand, so they can learn what to expect and state their preferences.

Labor and Delivery

The birth process occurs in three stages (Figure 5.6). **Labor** begins when hormonal changes in both the mother and the baby cause strong, rhythmic uterine **contractions** to begin. These contractions exert pressure on the cervix and cause the lengthwise muscles of the uterus to pull on the circular muscles around the cervix, causing effacement (thinning) and dilation (opening) of the cervix. The contractions also pressure the baby to descend into the mother's pelvis, if it hasn't already. The entire process of labor and delivery usually takes between 2 and 36 hours, depending on the size of the baby, the baby's position in the uterus, the size of the mother's pelvis, the strength of the uterine contractions, the number of prior deliveries, and other factors. The length of labor is generally shorter for second and subsequent births.

The First Stage of Labor   The first stage of labor averages 13 hours for a first birth, although there is a wide variation among women. It begins with cervical effacement and dilation and continues until the cervix is completely dilated (10 centimeters). Contractions usually last about 30 seconds and occur every 15–20 minutes at first, more often later. The prepared mother relaxes as much as possible during these contractions to allow labor to proceed without being blocked by tension. Early in the first stage, a small amount of bleeding may occur as a plug of slightly bloody mucus that blocked the opening of the cervix during pregnancy is expelled. In some women, the amniotic sac ruptures and the fluid rushes out; this is sometimes referred to as the "water breaking."

The last part of the first stage of labor, called **transition,** is characterized by strong and frequent contractions, much more intense than in the early stages of labor. Contractions may last 60–90 seconds and occur every 1–3 minutes. During transition the cervix opens completely, to a diameter of about 10 centimeters. The head of the fetus usually measures 9–10 centimeters; thus once the cervix has dilated completely, the head can pass through.

(a)

(b)

(c)

FIGURE 5.6   Birth: labor and delivery. (a) The first stage of labor; (b) the second stage of labor: delivery of the baby; (c) the third stage of labor: expulsion of the placenta.

TERMS

labor   The act or process of giving birth to a child, expelling it with the placenta from the mother's body by means of uterine contractions.

contraction   Shortening of the muscles in the uterine wall, which causes effacement and dilation of the cervix and assists in expelling the fetus.

transition   The last part of the first stage of labor, during which the cervix becomes fully dilated; characterized by intense and frequent contractions.

Transition, which normally lasts about 30–60 minutes, is the most difficult part of labor.

The Second Stage of Labor

The second stage of labor begins with complete cervical dilation and ends with the delivery of the baby. The baby is slowly pushed down, through the bones of the pelvic ring, past the cervix, and into the vagina, which it stretches open. The mother bears down with the contractions to help push the baby down and out. The baby's back bends, the head turns to fit through the narrowest parts of the passageway, and the soft bones of the baby's skull move together and overlap as it is squeezed through the pelvis. When the top of the head appears at the vaginal opening, the baby is said to be crowning.

As the head of the baby emerges, the physician or midwife will remove any mucus from the mouth and nose, wipe the baby's face, and check to ensure that the umbilical cord is not around the neck. With a few more contractions, the baby's shoulders and body emerge. As the baby is squeezed through the pelvis, cervix, and vagina, the fluid in the lungs is forced out by the pressure on the baby's chest. Once this pressure is released as the baby emerges from the vagina, the chest expands and the lungs fill with air for the first time. The baby will still be connected to the mother via the umbilical cord, which is not cut until it stops pulsating. The baby will appear wet and often is covered with a cheesy substance. The baby's head may be oddly shaped at first, due to the molding of the soft plates of bone during birth, but it usually takes on a more rounded appearance within 24 hours.

The Third Stage of Labor

In the third stage of labor, the uterus continues to contract until the placenta is expelled. This stage usually takes 5–30 minutes. It is important that the entire placenta be expelled; if part remains in the uterus, it may cause infection or bleeding. Breastfeeding soon after delivery helps control uterine bleeding because it stimulates the secretion of a hormone that makes the uterus contract.

The baby's physical condition is assessed with the **Apgar score**, a formalized system for assessing the baby's need for medical assistance. Heart rate, respiration, color, reflexes, and muscle tone are individually rated with a score of 0–2, and a total score between 0 and 10 is given at 1 and 5 minutes after birth. A score of 7–10 at 5 minutes is considered normal. Most newborns are also tested for 29 specific disorders, some of which are life-threatening. The American Academy of Pediatrics endorses these tests, but they are not routinely performed in every state.

Pain Relief During Labor and Delivery

Women vary in how much pain they experience in childbirth. It is recommended that women and their partners learn about labor and what kinds of choices are available for pain relief. Childbirth preparation courses are a good place to start, and communicating with one's obstetrician or midwife is essential to assessing pain-relief options. Breathing and relaxation techniques such as Lamaze or Bradley have been used effectively.

The most commonly employed medical intervention for pain relief is the epidural. This procedure involves placing a thin plastic catheter between the vertebrae in the lower back. Medication that reduces the transmission of pain signals to the brain is given through this catheter. Local anesthetic drugs are given in low concentration in order to minimize weakening of the leg muscles so that the mother can effectively push during the birth. The amount of medication given is quite low and does not accumulate in the baby or interfere with the baby's transition after birth. The mother is awake and is an active participant in the birth.

Women can also elect to have narcotics, such as fentanyl or demerol, given for pain relief during labor, but these medications usually provide less pain relief than the epidural and, if given shortly before the birth, can cause the baby to be less vigorous at birth.

Cesarean Deliveries

In a **cesarean section**, the baby is removed through a surgical incision in the abdominal wall and uterus. Cesarean sections are necessary when a baby cannot be delivered vaginally—for example, if the baby's head is bigger than the mother's pelvic girdle or if the baby is in an unusual position. If the mother has a serious health condition such as high blood pressure, a cesarean may be safer for her than labor and a vaginal delivery. Cesareans are more common among women who are overweight or have diabetes. Other reasons for cesarean delivery include abnormal or difficult labor, fetal distress, and the presence of a dangerous infection like herpes that can be passed to the baby during delivery.

Repeat cesarean deliveries are also very common. About 90% of American women who have had one child by cesarean have subsequent children delivered the same way. Although the risk of complications from a vaginal delivery after a previous cesarean delivery is low, there is a small (1%) risk of serious complication to the mother and baby if the previous uterine scar opens during labor (uterine rupture). For this reason, women and their doctors may choose to deliver by elective repeat caesarean.

Like any major surgery, cesarean section carries some risk and should be performed only for valid medical

> QUICK STATS
>
> **32.3%** of American babies born in 2008 were delivered by cesarean section.
>
> —CDC, 2010

TERMS

> **Apgar score**   A formalized system for assessing a newborn's need for medical assistance.
>
> **cesarean section**   A surgical incision through the abdominal wall and uterus, performed to deliver a fetus.

reasons (not convenience). Women who have cesarean sections can remain conscious during the operation if they are given a regional anesthetic, and the father may be present.

The Postpartum Period

The **postpartum period**, a stage of about 3 months following childbirth, is a time of critical family adjustments. Parenthood begins literally overnight, and the transition can cause considerable stress.

Breastfeeding **Lactation**, the production of milk, begins about 3 days after childbirth. Prior to that time (sometimes as early as the second trimester), **colostrum** is secreted by the nipples. Colostrum contains antibodies that help protect the newborn from infectious diseases and is also high in protein.

The American Academy of Pediatrics recommends breastfeeding exclusively for 6 months, then in combination with solid food until the baby is 1 year of age, and then for as long after that as a mother and baby desire. Currently, only 11% of U.S. mothers breast-feed exclusively for 6 months. Human milk is perfectly suited to the baby's nutritional needs and digestive capabilities, and it supplies the baby with antibodies. Breastfeeding decreases the incidence of infant ear infections, allergies, anemia, diarrhea, and bacterial meningitis. Preschoolers who were breastfed as babies are less likely to be overweight, and school-age children who were breastfed are less anxious and better able to cope with stress. Breastfeeding even has a beneficial effect on blood pressure and cholesterol levels later in life.

Breastfeeding is also beneficial to the mother. It contributes to postpregnancy weight loss and may reduce the risk of ovarian cancer, breast cancer, and postmenopausal hip fracture. For women who want to breast-feed but who have problems, help is available from support groups, books, or a lactation consultant.

However, bottlefeeding can also provide adequate nutrition, and both breastfeeding and bottlefeeding can be part of loving, secure parent-child relationships.

When a mother doesn't nurse, menstruation usually begins within about 10 weeks. However, ovulation—and pregnancy—can occur before menstruation returns, so breastfeeding is not a reliable contraceptive method.

Postpartum Depression Many women experience fluctuating emotions during the postpartum period as hormone levels change. About 50–80% of new mothers experience "baby blues," characterized by episodes of sadness, weeping, anxiety, headache, sleep disturbances, and irritability. About 5–9% of new mothers experience **postpartum depression**, a more disabling syndrome characterized by despondency, mood swings, guilt, and occasional hostility. Resting, sharing feelings and concerns with others, and relying on supportive relatives and friends for assistance are usually helpful in dealing with mild cases of the baby blues or postpartum depression, which generally lasts only a few weeks. If the depression is serious, professional treatment may be needed.

Attachment Another feature of the postpartum period is the development of attachment—the strong emotional tie that grows between the baby and the adult who cares for the baby. Parents can foster secure attachment relationships in the early weeks and months by responding sensitively to the baby's true needs. A secure attachment relationship helps the child develop and function well socially, emotionally, and mentally.

For most people, the arrival of a child provides a deep sense of joy and accomplishment. However, adjusting to parenthood requires effort and energy. Talking with friends and relatives about their experiences during the first few weeks or months with a baby can help prepare new parents for the period when the baby's needs may require all the energy that both parents have to expend. But the pleasures of nurturing a new baby are substantial, and many parents look back on this time as one of the most significant and joyful of their lives.

TERMS

postpartum period The period of about 3 months after delivering a baby.

lactation The production of milk.

colostrum A yellowish fluid secreted by the mammary glands around the time of childbirth until milk comes in, about the third day.

postpartum depression An emotional low that may be experienced by the mother following childbirth.

Connect to your Choices

Have you ever though about where you get your ideas and plans about having children? Many factors can influence our ideas, some not as obvious as others. Do you assume you will have children one day because it's an expected life path? Are you influenced by media portrayals of parents who do everything successfully—raise children, pursue careers, have active social lives? Do family members say or do things that convey their wish that you eventually have children? Are you influenced by friends who are starting families at this time?

What are the external factors that influence your choices about children? What are your inner motivations and core values, and how do they affect your choices? Based on what you learned in this chapter, will you make some different choices in the future? If so, what will they be?

Go online to Connect to complete this activity.
www.mcgraw-hillconnect.com

TIPS FOR TODAY AND THE FUTURE

Wellness includes understanding your own sexuality and all its components. Preparation for being a parent begins long before pregnancy; it requires prospective parents to make responsible choices.

RIGHT NOW YOU CAN

- Deal with a sexual question or problem you may be avoiding. Unless you're sure it isn't a physical problem, see your physician.
- If you're in a sexual relationship, consider the information you and your partner have shared. Determine whether you know enough about one another to have a safe and healthy sexual relationship.
- Take time to think about whether you really want to have children. Cut through everyone else's expectations, which may stand in the way of making the decision that's best for you.
- Think of things your parents did that you liked when you were a child. Consider how you can do the same things for your children.

IN THE FUTURE YOU CAN

- If you're in a sexual relationship or plan to begin one, open a dialogue with your partner about sex. Make time to talk at length about the responsibilities and consequences of such a relationship.
- Make behavioral changes that can improve your prospects as a parent. For example, you may need to adopt healthier eating habits or start exercising more often.
- If you want to be a parent someday, start looking at the many sources of information on pregnancy, childbirth, and parenting. This is a good idea for anyone—man or woman—who plans to have a family.

SUMMARY

- The female external sex organs are called the vulva; the clitoris plays an important role in sexual arousal and orgasm. The vagina leads to the internal sex organs, including the uterus, oviducts, and ovaries.

- The male external sex organs are the penis and the scrotum; the glans of the penis is an important site of sexual arousal. Internal sexual structures include the testes, vasa deferentia, seminal vesicles, and prostate gland.

- The menstrual cycle has four phases: menses, the estrogenic phase, ovulation, and the progestational phase.

- The ovaries gradually cease to function as women approach age 50 and enter menopause. The pattern of male sexual responses changes with age, and testosterone production gradually decreases.

- The sexual response cycle has four states: excitement, plateau, orgasm, and resolution.

- Physical and psychological problems can both interfere with sexual functioning. Treatment for sexual dysfunction should first address underlying medical conditions and then look at psychological problems.

- Human sexual behaviors include celibacy, erotic fantasy, masturbation, touching, cunnilingus, fellatio, anal intercourse, and vaginal intercourse.

- Responsible sexuality includes open communication, agreed-on sexual activities, sexual privacy, the use of contraception, safer sex practices, sober sex, and taking responsibility for consequences.

- Fertilization is a complex process culminating when a sperm penetrates the membrane of an egg released from the woman's ovary. Infertility affects about 10% of the reproductive-age population of the United States.

- During pregnancy, the uterus enlarges until it pushes up into the rib cage, the breasts enlarge, muscles and ligaments soften and stretch, and other body functions become more efficient.

- The fetal anatomy is almost completely formed in the first trimester of pregnancy, and is refined in the second; during the third trimester, the fetus grows and gains most of its weight.

- Prenatal tests include ultrasound, amniocentesis, chorionic villus sampling, and quadruple marker screening.

- Important elements of prenatal care include regular checkups, good nutrition, avoiding drugs and other harmful environmental agents, and taking childbirth classes.

- Pregnancy usually proceeds without major complications. Problems that can occur include ectopic pregnancy, spontaneous abortion, and low birth weight.

- The first stage of labor begins with contractions that exert pressure on the cervix, causing effacement and dilation. The second stage begins with complete cervical dilation and ends when the baby emerges. The third stage of labor is expulsion of the placenta.

- During the postpartum period, the mother's body begins to return to its prepregnancy state and she may begin to breast-feed. Both mother and father must adjust to their new role as parents.

FOR MORE INFORMATION

BOOKS

American Dietetic Association. 2009. *Expect the Best: Your Guide to Healthy Eating Before, During, and After Pregnancy*. New York: Wiley. *Provides up-to-date dietary information and meal-planning guides for women who want to get pregnant, are pregnant, or have had a baby.*

Beer, A. E., et al. 2006. *Is Your Body Baby-Friendly? Unexplained Infertility, Miscarriage, and IVF Failure Explained and Treated*. Chicago: AJR Publishing. *Covers many issues facing women and couples who are trying to overcome infertility.*

Lees, C., et al. 2007. *Pregnancy and Birth: Your Questions Answered.* London: Dorling Kindersley. *Answers hundreds of common questions about conception, pregnancy, and delivery.*

Marcus, E. 2005. *Is It a Choice? Answers to 300 of the Most Frequently Asked Questions About Gays and Lesbian People,* 3rd ed. San Francisco: Harper. *Candid and informative information on coming out, family roles, and politics.*

Meston, C., and D. Buss. 2009. *Why Women Have Sex.* New York: Times Books. *Fascinating, readable yet scholarly book about all aspects of female sexuality, especially sexual desire.*

Wynbrandt, J. 2008. *Encyclopedia of Genetic Disorders and Birth Defects,* 3rd ed. New York: Facts on File. *A detailed overview of many types of birth defects, both inherited and noninherited.*

ORGANIZATIONS AND WEB SITES

American Association of Sex Educators, Counselors, and Therapists (AASECT). Certifies sex educators, counselors, and therapists and provides listings of local therapists dealing with sexual problems.

> http://www.aasect.org

American College of Obstetricians and Gynecologists (ACOG). Provides written materials relating to many aspects of preconception care, pregnancy, and childbirth.

> http://www.acog.org

American Psychological Association: Information about gender identity and sexual orientation. Question-and-answer format sections on transgender and homosexuality.

> http://www.apa.org/topics/sexuality/transgender.aspx

The American Society for Reproductive Medicine. Provides up-to-date information on all aspects of infertility.

> http://www.asrm.org

Centers for Disease Control and Prevention, National Center on Birth Defects and Developmental Disabilities. Provides information about a variety of topics related to birth defects, including fetal alcohol syndrome and the importance of folic acid.

> http://www.cdc.gov/ncbddd

The Kinsey Institute for Research in Sex, Gender, and Reproduction. One of the oldest and most respected institutions doing research on sexuality.

> http://www.kinseyinstitute.org

National Institute of Child Health and Human Development. Provides information about reproductive and genetic problems; sponsors the "Back to Sleep" campaign to fight SIDS.

> http://www.nichd.nih.gov

Sexuality Information and Education Council of the United States (SIECUS). Provides information on many aspects of sexuality and has an extensive library and numerous publications.

> http://www.siecus.org

U.S. Food and Drug Administration/Consumer Drug Information. Provides information and cautions about the use of drugs to treat sexual dysfunction in men.

> http://www.fda.gov/Drugs/DrugSafety/PostmarketDrugSafety InformationforPatientsandProviders/ucm111085.htm

SELECTED BIBLIOGRAPHY

American College Health Association. 2009. *American College Health Association—National College Health Assessment II: Reference Group Executive Summary Fall 2009.* Linthicum, Md.: American College Health Association.

American Psychological Association. 2010. *Answers to Your Questions about Transgender Individuals and Gender Identity* (http://www.apa.org/topics/sexuality/transgender.aspx; retrieved May 3, 2010).

American Psychological Association. 2010. *Answers to Your Questions for a Better Understanding of Sexual Orientation and Homosexuality* (http://www.apa.org/topics/sexuality/orientation.aspx; retrieved May 3, 2010).

Bruckner, T. A., R. Catalano, and J. Ahern. 2010. Male fetal loss in the U.S. following terrorist attacks of September 11, 2001. *BMC Public Health* 10: 273–279.

Centers for Disease Control and Prevention. 2009. *2007 Assisted Reproductive Technology (ART) Success Rates: National Summary and Fertility Clinic Reports.* Atlanta: Centers for Disease Control and Prevention.

Centers for Disease Control and Prevention. 2009. *Healthy Youth-Sexual Risk Behaviors* (http://www.cdc.gov/HealthyYouth/sexuallbehaviors/index.htm; retrieved March 9, 2010).

Freeman, Ellen. 2007. *Epidemiology and Etiology of Premenstrual Syndromes. Medscape* (http://cme.medscape.com/viewarticle/553603; retrieved March 3, 2010).

Garcia-Falgueras, A., and D. Swaab. 2010. Sexual hormones and the brain: An essential alliance for sexual identity and sexual orientation. *Pediatric Endocrinology* 17:22–35.

Goyal, D., et al. 2010. How much does low socioeconomic status increase the risk of prenatal and postpartum depressive symptoms in first-time mothers? *Women's Health* Issues 20(2): 96–104.

Haggerty, C. L., et al. 2010. Risk of sequelae after *Chlamydia trachomatis* genital infection in women. *The Journal of Infectious Diseases* 201(Suppl. 2): S134–S155.

Ismail, S., et al. 2010. Screening, diagnosing and prevention of fetal alcohol syndrome: Is this syndrome treatable? *Developmental Neuroscience* 32(2): 91–100.

Koning, A. M., et al. 2010. Economic consequences of overweight and obesity in infertility: A framework for evaluating the costs and outcomes of fertility care. *Human Reproduction Update* 16(3): 246–254.

Lee, J. M., et al. 2007. Weight status in young girls and the onset of puberty. *Pediatrics* 119(3): 624–630.

Lindau, S. T., and N. Gavrilova. 2010. Sex, health, and years of sexually active life gained due to good health. *British Medical Journal* 340: c810.

Mayo Clinic. 2009. *Premenstrual Syndrome* (http://www.mayoclinic.com/health/premenstrual-syndrome/DS00134/DSECTION=lifestyle-and-home-remedies; retrieved February 24, 2010).

Mayo Clinic. 2010. *Erectile Dysfunction* (http://www.mayoclinic.com/health/erectile-dysfunction/DS00162; retrieved March 8, 2010).

Meston, Cindy, and David Buss. 2007. Why humans have sex. *Archives of Sexual Behavior,* August 2007.

National Center for Health Statistics. 2009. *Trends in Circumcision Among Newborns* (http://www.cdc.gov/nchs/data/hestat/circumcisions/circumcisions.htm; retrieved March 1, 2010).

National Center for Health Statistics. 2010. Births: Preliminary data for 2008. *National Vital Statistics Reports* 58(16): 1–18.

National Center for Health Statistics. 2010. *Health, United States, 2009: With Special Feature on Medical Technology.* Hyattsville, Md.: National Center for Health Statistics.

North American Menopause Society. 2010. *Estrogen and Progesterone Use in Post-Menopausal Women: 2010 Position Statement* (http://www.menopause.org/PSht10.pdf; retrieved March 4, 2010).

U.S. Department of Health and Human Services. 2009. *Aging Male Syndrome* (http://womenshealth.gov/mens/sexual/arms.cfm; retrieved May 30, 2009).

Wilcox, A. J., et al. 2000. The timing of the "fertile window" in the menstrual cycle: Day-specific estimates from a prospective study. *British Medical Journal* 321(7271): 1259–1262.

World Health Organization. 2010. *Female Genital Mutilation* (http://www.who.int/mediacentre/factsheets/fs241/en/; retrieved March 9, 2010).

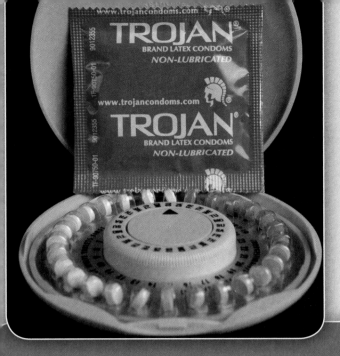

LOOKING AHEAD...

After reading this chapter, you should be able to:

- Explain how contraceptives work and how to interpret information about a contraceptive method's effectiveness, risks, and benefits

- List the most popular contraceptives and discuss their advantages, disadvantages, and effectiveness

- Choose a method of contraception based on the needs of the user and the safety and effectiveness of the method

- Describe the history and current legal status of abortion in the United States

- Describe the methods of abortion available in the United States

6

Contraception and Abortion

People have always had a compelling interest in managing fertility and preventing unwanted pregnancies, a practice commonly known as **birth control**. Records dating to the fourth century B.C. describe the use of foods, herbs, drugs, douches, and sponges to prevent **conception**, which is the fusion of an ovum and sperm that creates a fertilized egg, or *zygote*. Early attempts at **contraception** (blocking conception through the use of a device, substance, or method) were based on the same principle as many modern birth control methods.

Today, women and men can choose from many different types of **contraceptives** to avoid unwanted pregnancies. In addition to preventing pregnancy, many contraceptive products play an important role in protecting against **sexually transmitted diseases**, or STDs. Being informed about the realities and risks and making responsible decisions about sexual and contraceptive behavior are crucial components of lifelong wellness. Because many people's lives are severely affected by unplanned child rearing and because the option of abortion is becoming more restricted, the problem of unplanned, unwanted pregnancies is serious.

PRINCIPLES OF CONTRACEPTION

There are many effective approaches to contraception, including the following:

- **Barrier methods** work by physically blocking the sperm from reaching the egg. Diaphragms, condoms, and several other methods are based on this principle.

- **Hormonal methods,** such as oral contraceptives (birth control pills), alter the biochemistry of the woman's body, preventing ovulation (the release of the egg) and producing changes that make it more difficult for the sperm to reach the egg if ovulation does occur.

- **Natural methods** of contraception are based on the fact that egg and sperm have to be present at the same time if fertilization is to occur.

- **Surgical methods**—female and male sterilization— more or less permanently prevent transport of the sperm or eggs to the site of conception.

All contraceptive methods have advantages and disadvantages that make them appropriate for some people but not for others, or the best choice at one period of life but not at another. Factors that affect the choice of method include effectiveness, convenience, cost, reversibility, side effects and risks, and protection against STDs. This chapter helps you sort through these factors to decide which contraceptive method is best for you.

Contraceptive effectiveness is partly determined by the reliability of the method itself—the failure rate if it were always used exactly as directed ("perfect use"). Effectiveness is also determined by characteristics of the user, including fertility of the individual, frequency of intercourse, and how consistently and correctly the method is used. This "typical use" **contraceptive failure rate** is based on studies that directly measure the percentage of women experiencing an unintended pregnancy in the first year of contraceptive use. For example, the 8% failure rate of oral contraceptives means 8 out of 100 typical users will become pregnant in the first year. This failure rate is likely to be lower for women who are consistently careful in following instructions and higher for those who are frequently careless; the "perfect use" failure rate is 0.3%.

Another measure of effectiveness is the **continuation rate**—the percentage of people who continue to use the method after a specified period of time. This measure is important because many unintended pregnancies occur when a method is stopped and not immediately replaced with another. Thus, a contraceptive with a high continuation rate would be more effective at preventing pregnancy than one with a low continuation rate. A high continuation rate also gives an indication of user satisfaction with a particular method.

REVERSIBLE CONTRACEPTION

Reversibility is an extremely important consideration for young adults when they choose a contraceptive method, because most people either plan to eventually have children or at least want to keep their options open until they're older.

Oral Contraceptives: The Pill

About a century ago, a researcher noted that ovulation does not occur during pregnancy. Further research revealed the hormonal mechanism: During pregnancy, the corpus luteum secretes progesterone and estrogen in amounts high enough to suppress ovulation. **Oral contraceptives (OCs)**, also known as *birth control pills* or "the pill," prevent ovulation by mimicking the hormonal activity of the corpus luteum. The active ingredients in OCs are estrogen and progestins, laboratory-made compounds that are closely related to progesterone.

In addition to preventing ovulation, the birth control pill has other contraceptive effects. It inhibits the movement of sperm by thickening the cervical mucus, alters the rate of ovum transport by means of its hormonal effects on the oviducts, and may prevent implantation by

About 400 eggs are released through ovulation during a woman's fertile life.

—American College of Obstetricians and Gynecologists, 2010

STATS

TERMS

birth control   The practice of managing fertility and preventing unwanted pregnancies.

conception   The fusion of ovum and sperm, resulting in a fertilized egg, or *zygote*.

contraception   The prevention of conception through the use of a device, substance, or method.

contraceptive   Any agent or method that can prevent conception.

sexually transmitted disease (STD)   Any of several contagious diseases contracted through intimate sexual contact.

barrier method   A contraceptive that acts as a physical barrier, blocking the sperm from uniting with the egg.

hormonal method   A contraceptive that alters the biochemistry of a woman's body, preventing ovulation and making it more difficult for sperm to reach an egg if ovulation does occur.

natural method   An approach to contraception that does not use drugs or devices; requires avoiding intercourse during the period of the woman's menstrual cycle when an egg is most likely to be present at the site of conception and the risk of pregnancy is greatest.

surgical method   Sterilization of a male or female, to permanently prevent the transport of sperm or eggs to the site of conception.

contraceptive failure rate   The percentage of women using a particular contraceptive method who experience an unintended pregnancy in the first year of use.

continuation rate   The percentage of people who continue to use a particular contraceptive after a specified period of time.

oral contraceptive (OC)   Hormone compounds (made of estrogen and progestins) in pill form that prevent conception by preventing ovulation; also called the *birth control pill* or "the pill."

Ask Yourself

QUESTIONS FOR CRITICAL THINKING AND REFLECTION

Prior to reading this section, how familiar were you with the principles of contraception? Did you know as much as you thought? Were you aware of the large number of contraceptive options that are currently available?

changing the lining of the uterus in the unlikely event that a fertilized ovum reaches that area.

The most common type of OC is the *combination pill.* Each 1-month packet contains a 3-week supply of pills that combine varying types and amounts of estrogen and progestin. Most packets also include a 1-week supply of inactive pills to be taken following the hormone pills; others simply instruct the woman to take no pills at all for 1 week before starting the next cycle. During the week in which no hormones are taken, a light menstrual period occurs.

Newer use schedules include a variety of extended-cycle regimens. With the pills Seasonale and Seasonique, for example, a woman takes active pills for 84 consecutive days, then inactive pills (Seasonale) or low-dose estrogen pills (Seasonique) for a week. This pattern reduces the number of menstrual periods from 13 per year to just 4 per year. With the pill Lybrel, active pills are taken indefinitely. Several new OCs are specifically packaged for extended use. Other OCs with hormones similar to the prepackaged brands may be used in the same way. The main side effect of those extended-cycle regimens is unpredictable light bleeding (known as *spotting*).

So far, altering the menstrual cycle has not been linked with any major health risks, but some experts are concerned that the suppression of menstruation for most of a woman's reproductive years could become commonplace and may result in unanticipated health problems in the future. Research is ongoing, but it may take many years to fully evaluate the consequences of suppressing menstruation for long periods of a woman's life.

A much less common type of OC is the *minipill,* a small dose of a synthetic progesterone taken every day of the month. Because the minipill contains no estrogen, it has fewer side effects and health risks, but it is associated with more irregular bleeding patterns. It is sometimes prescribed for women who are breast-feeding or have medical problems that make it unsafe for them to take estrogen.

A woman is usually advised to start the first cycle of pills with a menstrual period to increase effectiveness and eliminate the possibility of unsuspected pregnancy. She must take each month's pills completely and according to instructions. Taking a few pills just prior to having sexual intercourse does not provide effective contraception. A backup method is recommended during the first week and any subsequent cycle in which the woman forgets to take any pills.

OC use was once linked to an increased risk of heart attack and stroke. However, these risks have been significantly reduced by the use of lower-dose pills (those with 50 micrograms or less of estrogen) and the identification of women at higher risk for complications.

Advantages   Oral contraceptives are very effective in preventing pregnancy. Nearly all unplanned pregnancies result because the pills were not taken as directed. The pill is relatively simple to use and does not hinder sexual spontaneity. Most women also appreciate the predictable regularity of periods, as well as the reduction in cramps and blood loss. Women who have significant problems associated with menstruation may benefit from menstrual suppression with extended-cycle OCs. For young women, the pill's reversibility is especially important; **fertility**—the ability to reproduce—returns after the pill is discontinued (although not always immediately).

Medical advantages include a decreased incidence of benign breast disease, iron-deficiency anemia, ectopic pregnancy, colon and rectal cancer, endometrial cancer (in the lining of the uterus), and ovarian cancer.

Disadvantages   Although oral contraceptives are effective in preventing pregnancy, they do not protect against STDs. OCs have been associated with an increased risk of cervical chlamydia in some studies but not in others. Regular condom use is strongly recommended for an OC user, unless she is in a long-term, mutually monogamous relationship with an uninfected partner.

The hormones in birth control pills influence many tissues in the body and can lead to a variety of side effects, most of which are minor. The majority of women do not experience any side effects associated with OC use. Among women who experience problems with OCs, the most common issue is bleeding during mid-cycle (called *breakthrough bleeding*), which is usually slight and tends to disappear after a few cycles. Symptoms of early pregnancy—such as morning nausea and swollen breasts—may appear during the first few months of OC use, although these side effects are uncommon with the low-dose pills in current widespread use. Other side effects can include depression, nervousness, changes in sex drive, dizziness, generalized headaches, migraines, and vaginal discharge. *Melasma,* or "mask of pregnancy" (brownish patches on the face), sometimes occurs. Acne may develop or worsen when taking OCs, but most women find their acne improves when they take the pill. In fact, OCs are frequently prescribed as a treatment for acne.

Older OCs with high-dose hormones were sometimes associated with weight gain. However, research shows that currently used low-dose OCs do not, on average, cause weight gain. Most women experience no change in their weight, while a small percentage lose weight and about an equal percentage gain weight while taking OCs. The myth that OCs cause women to gain weight is actually dangerous, because many unintended pregnancies have resulted when women avoided taking OCs due to unfounded fear of weight gain.

Another myth about OCs is that they can cause cancer. Actually, taking the pill greatly reduces a woman's risk for endometrial and ovarian cancers. OC use is associated

fertility   The ability to reproduce.

with little, if any, increase in breast cancer and a slight increase in cervical cancer, but earlier detection and other variables (such as a woman's number of sexual partners) may account for much of this increase.

Serious OC side effects have been reported in a small number of women. These include blood clots, stroke, and heart attack, concentrated mostly in older women who smoke or have a history of circulatory disease. Recent studies have shown no increased risk of stroke or heart attack for healthy, young, nonsmoking women on lower-dose pills. OC users may be slightly more prone to high blood pressure and, very rarely, benign liver tumors.

Birth control pills are not recommended for women with a history of blood clots (or a close family member with unexplained blood clots at an early age), heart disease or stroke, migraines with changes in vision, any form of cancer or liver tumor, or impaired liver function. Women with certain other health conditions or behaviors, including migraines without changes in vision, high blood pressure, cigarette smoking, and sickle-cell disease, require close monitoring when taking the pill.

When deciding whether to use OCs, each woman needs to weigh the benefits against the risks. To make an informed decision, she should begin by getting advice from a health care professional. If you take the pill, you can take several steps to reduce the risks associated with OC use:

1. Request a low-dose pill. (OCs recommended for most new users contain 20–35 micrograms of estrogen.)
2. Stop smoking.
3. Follow the dosage carefully and consistently, making sure to take pills at the same time every day.
4. Be alert to preliminary danger signals, which can be remembered by the word ACHES:

   Abdominal pain (severe)

   Chest pain (severe), cough, shortness of breath or sharp pain on breathing in

   Headaches (severe), dizziness, weakness, or numbness, especially if one-sided

   Eye problems (vision loss or blurring) and/or speech problems

   Severe leg pain (calf or thigh)

5. Make sure your health practitioner knows your personal and family medical history to help determine whether OCs may be unsafe for you.
6. Have regular **Pap tests**, pelvic exams, and breast exams as recommended by your health practitioner.

For the vast majority of young women, the known, directly associated risk of death from taking birth control

Table 6.1 — Risks of Contraception, Pregnancy, and Abortion

CONTRACEPTION	RISK OF DEATH
Oral contraceptives	
Nonsmoker	
Age 15–34	1 in 1,667,000
Age 35–44	1 in 33,300
Smoker	
Age 15–34	1 in 57,800
Age 35–44	1 in 5,200
IUDs	1 in 10,000,000
Barrier methods, spermicides	None
Fertility awareness-based methods	None
Tubal ligation	1 in 66,700
PREGNANCY	RISK OF DEATH
Pregnancy	1 in 8,700
ABORTION	RISK OF DEATH
Spontaneous abortion	1 in 142,900
Medical abortion	1 in 162,500
Surgical abortion	1 in 142,900

SOURCE: Hatcher, R. A., et al. *Contraceptive Technology,* 19th rev. ed. Copyright© 2007 Ardent Media. Reprinted with permission.

pills is much, much lower than the risk of death from pregnancy (Table 6.1). Overall, OC risks are generally very small unless you are over 35, a smoker, and/or have specific medical problems.

Effectiveness Oral contraceptive effectiveness varies substantially because it depends so much on individual factors. If taken exactly as directed, the failure rate is extremely low (0.3%). However, among average users, lapses such as forgetting to take a pill do occur, and a typical first-year failure rate is 8%. The continuation rate for OCs also varies; the average rate is 68% after 1 year. Besides forgetting to take the pill, another reason for OC failure is poor absorption of the drug due to vomiting or diarrhea or to interactions with other medicines (including many antibiotics and the commonly used herb St. John's wort).

Contraceptive Skin Patch

The contraceptive skin patch, Ortho Evra, is a thin, 1¾-inch square patch that slowly releases an estrogen and a progestin into the bloodstream. The patch prevents pregnancy in the same way as combination OCs. Each patch is worn continuously for 1 week and is replaced on the same day of the week for 3 consecutive weeks. The fourth week is patch-free, allowing a woman to have her menstrual period.

The patch can be worn on the upper outer arm, abdomen, buttocks, or upper torso (excluding the breasts); it is designed to stick to skin even during bathing or swimming. If a patch should fall off for more than a day, the FDA advises starting a new 4-week cycle of patches and using a backup method of contraception for the first week. Patches should be discarded according to the manufacturer's directions to avoid leakage of hormones into the environment.

Advantages With both perfect and typical use, the patch is as effective as OCs in preventing pregnancy. Compliance seems to be higher with the patch than with OCs, probably because the patch requires weekly instead of daily action. Medical benefits are likely to be comparable to those of OCs.

Disadvantages Like other hormonal contraceptives, the patch doesn't protect against STDs. Patch users should also use condoms for STD protection unless they are in a long-term monogamous relationship with an uninfected partner. Minor side effects are similar to those of OCs, although breast discomfort may be more common in patch users. Some women also experience skin irritation around the patch. More serious complications are thought to be similar to those of OCs, including an increased risk of side effects among women who smoke. However, because Ortho Evra exposes users to higher doses of estrogen than most OCs, patch use may further increase the risk of blood clots (venus thromboembolis). Recent studies show conflicting results regarding the risk of blood clots, but it is possible that the risk is slightly higher with the patch compared to low-dose OCs.

Effectiveness With perfect use, the patch's failure rate is very low (0.3%) in the first year of use. The typical failure rate is assumed to be lower than the pill's 8%. The product appears to be less effective when used by women weighing more than 198 pounds.

Vaginal Contraceptive Ring

The NuvaRing is a vaginal ring that is molded with a mixture of progestin and estrogen. The 2-inch ring slowly releases hormones and maintains blood hormone levels comparable to those found with OC use; it prevents pregnancy in the same way as OCs. A woman inserts the ring anytime during the first 5 days of her menstrual period and leaves it in place for 3 weeks. During the fourth week, which is ring-free, her next menstrual period occurs. A new ring is then inserted. Rings should be discarded according to the manufacturer's directions to avoid leakage of hormones into the environment. Backup contraception must be used for the first 7 days of the first ring use or if the ring has been removed for more than 3 hours.

Advantages The NuvaRing offers 1 month of protection with no daily or weekly action required. It does not require a fitting by a clinician, and exact placement in the vagina is not critical as it is with a diaphragm. Medical benefits are probably similar to those of OCs.

Disadvantages The NuvaRing gives no protection against STDs. Side effects are roughly comparable to those

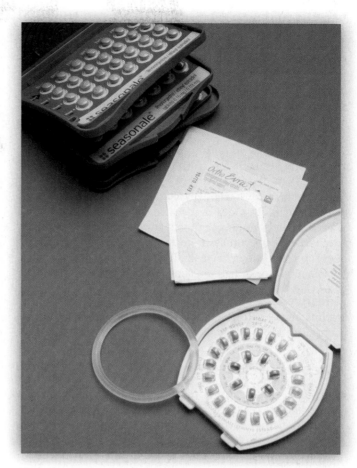

Reversible hormonal contraceptives are available in several forms. Shown here are the patch, the ring, and birth control pills.

seen with OC use, except for a lower incidence of nausea and vomiting. Other side effects may include vaginal discharge, vaginitis, and vaginal irritation. Medical risks also are similar to those found with OC use.

Effectiveness As with the pill and patch, the perfect use failure rate is about 0.3%. The ring's typical use failure rate is likely to be lower than the pill's 8%.

Contraceptive Implants

Contraceptive implants are placed under the skin of the upper arm and deliver a small but steady dose of progestin (a synthetic progesterone) over a period of years. One such implant, called Implanon, is a single implant that was approved for use in the United States in 2006. This device is effective for 3 years.

The progestins in implants have several contraceptive effects. They cause hormonal shifts that may inhibit ovulation and affect development of the uterine lining. The hormones also thicken the cervical mucus, inhibiting the movement of sperm. Contraceptive implants are best suited for women who wish to have continuous, highly effective, and long-term protection against pregnancy.

Advantages Contraceptive implants are highly effective. After insertion of the implants, no further action is required; contraceptive effects are quickly reversed upon removal. Because implants, unlike the combination pill, contain no estrogen, they carry a lower risk of certain side effects, such as blood clots and other cardiovascular complications. Women who are breast-feeding can use Implanon.

Disadvantages Like the pill, an implant provides no protection against STDs. Although the implants are barely visible, their presence may bother some women. Common side effects of contraceptive implants are menstrual irregularities, including longer menstrual periods, spotting between periods, or having no bleeding at all. The menstrual cycle usually becomes more regular after 1 year of use. Less common side effects include headaches, weight gain, breast tenderness, nausea, acne, and mood swings.

Effectiveness The overall failure rate for Implanon is estimated at about 0.1%. It is the most effective method of contraception and also the most discreet.

Injectable Contraceptives

Hormonal contraceptive injections were developed in the 1960s and are currently being used in at least 80 countries throughout the world. The first injectable contraceptive approved for use in the United States was Depo-Provera, which uses long-acting progestins. Injected into the arm or buttocks, Depo-Provera is usually given every 12 weeks, although it actually provides effective contraception for a few weeks beyond that. The product prevents pregnancy in the same ways as implants.

Advantages Injectable contraceptives are highly effective and require little action on the part of the user. Because the injections leave no trace and involve no ongoing supplies, injectables allow women almost total privacy in their decision to use contraception. Depo-Provera has no estrogen-related side effects; it requires only periodic injections rather than the minor surgical procedures of implant insertion and removal.

Disadvantages Injectable contraceptives provide no protection against STDs. A woman must visit a health care facility every 3 months to receive the injections. The side effects of Depo-Provera are similar to those of implants; menstrual irregularities are the most common, and after 1 year of using Depo-Provera many women have no menstrual bleeding at all. Weight gain is a common side effect. After discontinuing the use of Depo-Provera, women may experience temporary infertility for up to 12 months.

Reasons for not using Depo-Provera are similar to those for not using implants. However, Depo-Provera has a unique risk: it can cause a reduction in bone density, especially in women who use it for an extended period. Decreased bone density is a risk factor for osteoporosis and fractures. Women who use Depo-Provera are advised to do weight-bearing exercise and take 1000 mg of calcium daily. A recent study showed that women under age 50 who used Depo-Provera for more than 2 years had a 50% increase in fracture compared with other women. No increase in fractures was found in women who used hormonal contraception that included estrogen. Another recent study showed that smokers who use Depo-Provera are at a higher risk for decreased bone density. Women should use Depo-Provera as a long-term contraceptive (longer than 2 years, for example) only if other methods are inadequate. Some studies have found that bone density rebounds when use of Depo-Provera stops; others have not.

> *It's important to remember that* **hormonal contraceptives provide no protection from STDs.**

Effectiveness The perfect use failure rate is 0.3% for Depo-Provera. With typical use, the failure rate increases to 3% in the first year of use.

Intrauterine Devices (IUDs)

An **intrauterine device (IUD)** is a small plastic object placed in the uterus as a contraceptive. Two IUDs are now available in the United States: the Copper T-380A (also known as the ParaGard), which gives protection for up to 10 years, and the Levonorgestral IUD (Mirena), which releases small amounts of progestin and is effective for up to 5 years.

Researchers do not know exactly how IUDs prevent pregnancy. Current evidence suggests that ParaGard works primarily by preventing fertilization. The copper in this IUD may cause biochemical changes in the uterus and affect the movement of sperm and eggs. ParaGard may also interfere with implantation of fertilized eggs. Mirena slowly releases very small amounts of progestin, disrupting ovulation, fertilization, or implantation.

An IUD must be inserted and removed by a trained professional. The device is threaded into a sterile inserter, which is introduced through the cervix; a plunger pushes the IUD into the uterus. IUDs have two threads attached that protrude from the cervix into the vagina so a woman can feel them to make sure the device is in place. These threads are trimmed so that only 1–1½ inches remain in the upper vagina.

TERMS

intrauterine device (IUD) A device inserted into the uterus as a contraceptive.

Advantages Intrauterine devices are highly reliable and are simple and convenient to use, requiring no attention except for a periodic check of the string position. They do not require the woman to anticipate or interrupt sexual activity. According to the American College of Obstetricians and Gynecologists, IUD use reduces the risk of developing endometrial cancer by as much as 40%. Usually IUDs have only localized side effects, and in the absence of complications they are considered a fully reversible contraceptive.

Disadvantages Heavy menstrual flow and increased menstrual cramping sometimes occur with ParaGard, while Mirena causes a reduction in bleeding and cramping. Most women have light, irregular bleeding during the first few months on Mirena, which tends to decrease over time. Many women stop bleeding altogether after using Mirena for a number of months. Mirena generally reduces menstrual cramps and is often prescribed for that reason. Spontaneous expulsion of the IUD happens to 4–6% of women within the first year, most commonly during the first months after insertion.

A serious but rare complication of IUD use is pelvic inflammatory disease (PID). Most pelvic infections among IUD users occur shortly after insertion, are relatively mild, and can be treated successfully with antibiotics. However, early and adequate treatment is critical—a lingering infection can lead to tubal scarring and subsequent infertility.

Some physicians advise against the use of IUDs by young women who have never been pregnant because of the increased incidence of side effects in this group and the risk of infection with the possibility of subsequent infertility. Early IUD danger signals are abdominal pain, fever, chills, foul-smelling vaginal discharge, and unusual vaginal bleeding. A change in string length may also be a sign of a problem.

Effectiveness The typical first-year failure rate of IUDs is 0.8% for ParaGard and 0.2% for Mirena. Effectiveness can be increased by periodically making sure that the device is in place and by using a backup method for the first few months of IUD use.

Male Condoms

The **male condom** is a thin sheath designed to cover the penis during sexual intercourse. Most brands available in the United States are made of latex, although condoms made of polyurethane and polyisoprene are also now available. Condoms prevent sperm from entering the vagina and provide protection against disease. Condom sales have increased dramatically in recent years, primarily because they are the only method that provides substantial protection against HIV infection as well as some protection against other STDs. At least one-third of all male condoms are bought by women. This

FIGURE 6.1 Use of the male condom. (a) Place the rolled-up condom over the head of the erect penis. Hold the top half-inch of the condom (with air squeezed out) to leave room for semen. (b) While holding the tip, unroll the condom onto the penis. Gently smooth out any air bubbles. (c) Unroll the condom down to the base of the penis. (d) To avoid spilling semen after ejaculation, hold the condom around the base of the penis as the penis is withdrawn. Remove the condom away from your partner, taking care not to spill any semen.

figure will probably increase as more women assume the right to insist on condom use. Many couples combine contraceptives, using condoms for STD protection and another contraceptive method for greater protection against pregnancy.

The man or his partner must put the condom on the penis before it is inserted into the vagina, because the small amounts of fluid that may be secreted unnoticed prior to **ejaculation** often contain sperm capable of causing pregnancy. The rolled-up condom is placed over the head of the erect penis and unrolled down to the base of the penis, leaving a half-inch space (without air) at the tip to collect semen (Figure 6.1). Some brands of condoms have a reservoir tip designed for this purpose. Uncircumcised men must first pull back the foreskin of the penis. Partners must be careful not to damage the condom with fingernails, rings, or other rough objects.

---

male condom A sheath that covers the penis during sexual intercourse; used for contraception and to prevent STDs.

ejaculation An abrupt discharge of semen from the penis after sexual stimulation.

Many condoms are prelubricated with water-based or silicone-based lubricants. These lubricants make the condom more comfortable and less likely to break. Many people find that using extra, non-oil-based lubricants can be helpful. Prelubricated condoms are available containing the **spermicide** nonoxynol-9, the same agent found in many of the contraceptive creams that women use. However, spermicidal condoms are no more effective than condoms without spermicide. They cost more and have a shorter shelf life than most other condoms. Further, condoms with nonoxynol-9 have been associated with urinary tract infections in women and, if they cause tissue irritation, an increased risk of HIV transmission. Planned Parenthood and many other public health agencies advise against the use of condoms lubricated with nonoxynol-9.

If desired, users can lubricate their own condoms with contraceptive foam, creams, or jelly. If vaginal irritation occurs with these products, water-based preparations such as K-Y Jelly or Astroglide can be used. Any products that contain mineral or vegetable oil—including baby oil, many lotions, regular petroleum jelly, cooking oils (corn oil, shortening, butter, and so on), and some vaginal lubricants and anti-fungal or anti-itch creams—should never be used with latex condoms. Such products can cause latex to begin to disintegrate within 60 seconds, thus greatly increasing the chance of condom breakage. (Polyurethane is not affected by oil-based products.)

Advantages   Condoms are easy to purchase and are available without prescription or medical supervision. In addition to being free of medical side effects (other than occasional allergic reactions), latex condoms help protect against STDs. A recent study determined that condoms may also protect women from human papillomavirus (HPV), which causes cervical cancer. Condoms made of polyurethane are appropriate for people who are allergic to latex. However, they are more likely to slip or break than latex condoms, and therefore may give less protection against STDs and pregnancy. Polyurethane condoms are also more expensive than latex condoms. Polyisoprene condoms, marketed under the brand name SKYN, have come on the market recently. They are safe for most people with latex allergies, stretchier, and less expensive than polyurethane condoms. Condoms made of lambskin are also available but permit the passage of HIV and other

disease-causing organisms, so they can be used only for pregnancy prevention, not the prevention of STDs. Except for abstinence, correct and consistent use of latex male condoms offers the most reliable available protection against the transmission of HIV.

Disadvantages   The most common complaints about condoms are that they diminish sensation and interfere with spontaneity. Some people find these drawbacks serious, but others consider them only minor distractions.

Effectiveness   In actual use, the failure rate of condoms varies considerably. During the first year of typical condom use among 100 users, between 10 and 18 pregnancies will occur. With perfect use, the first-year failure rate is about 2%. At least some pregnancies happen because the condom is carelessly removed after ejaculation. Some may also occur because of breakage or slippage, which may happen 1–2 times in every 100 instances of use for latex condoms and up to 10 times in every 100 instances for polyurethane condoms. Breakage is more common among inexperienced users. Other contributing factors include poorly fitting condoms, insufficient lubrication (which increases the risk of breakage), excessively vigorous sex, and improper storage (because heat destroys rubber, latex condoms should not be stored for long periods in a wallet or a car's glove compartment). To help ensure quality, condoms should not be used past their expiration date or more than 5 years past their date of manufacture (2 years for those with spermicide).

If a condom breaks or is carelessly removed, the risk of pregnancy can be reduced somewhat by the immediate use of a vaginal spermicide. A more effective measure is to take an emergency contraceptive (discussed later in the chapter) as soon as possible.

Female Condoms

The female condom is a clear, stretchy, disposable pouch with two rings that can be inserted into a woman's vagina. It is about as effective in preventing pregnancy and the spread of STDs as the male condom.

The first version of the female condom was expensive and did not become very popular as a result. A new, more affordable female condom is now available. Called the FC2, it is a one-size-fits-all, disposable device that consists of a soft, loose-fitting nitrile (synthetic, non-latex rubber) sheath with two flexible rings. The ring at the closed end is inserted into the vagina and placed at the cervix much like a diaphragm. The ring at the open end remains outside the vagina. The female condom protects the inside of the vagina and part of the external genitalia.

The directions that accompany the FC2 should be followed closely. The manufacturer strongly recommends practicing inserting the female condom several times before actually using it for intercourse. Most women find that it is easy to use after they have practiced inserting the

FC2 several times. The FC2 comes prelubricated with a silicone lubricant, but extra lubricant or a spermicide can be used if desired. As with male condoms, users need to take care not to tear the condom during insertion or removal. Following intercourse, the woman should remove the condom before standing up. By twisting and squeezing the outer ring, she can prevent the spilling of semen.

Advantages   Female condoms can be inserted up to 8 hours before sexual activity and are thus less disruptive than male condoms. Because the outer part of the condom covers the area around the vaginal opening as well as the base of the penis during intercourse, it offers potentially better protection against genital warts or herpes. The nitrile pouch can be used by people who are allergic to latex. Because nitrile is thin and pliable, there is little loss of sensation. The FC2 is generously lubricated and the nitrile material conducts heat well, increasing comfort and natural feeling during intercourse. When used correctly, the female condom should theoretically provide protection against HIV transmission and STDs comparable to that of the latex male condom. However, in research involving typical users, the female condom was slightly less effective in preventing both pregnancy and STDs. Effectiveness improves with careful practice and instruction.

Disadvantages   The female condom is unfamiliar to most people and requires some practice to learn to use effectively. The outer ring of the female condom, which hangs visibly outside the vagina, may be bothersome to some couples during foreplay; if so, couples may choose to put the device in just before intercourse. During coitus, both partners must take care that the penis is inserted into the pouch, not outside it, and that the device does not slip inside the vagina. Female condoms, like male condoms, are made for one-time use. A single female condom costs about three to four times as much as a single male condom. Female condoms are harder to find than male condoms. Some pharmacies do not currently carry them, but this will change as the FC2 becomes more popular. You can buy the FC2 at Planned Parenthood and online. Go to the FC2 website (http://www.fc2.us.com/howtogetfc2.html) for more information on where you can buy the FC2.

Effectiveness   The typical first-year failure rate of the female condom is 21%. Having emergency contraception available is recommended.

The Diaphragm with Spermicide

The **diaphragm** is a dome-shaped cup of latex or silicone stretched over a collapsible metal ring. When correctly used with spermicidal cream or jelly, the diaphragm covers the cervix, blocking sperm from the uterus.

Diaphragms are available only by prescription. Because of individual anatomical differences, a diaphragm must

FIGURE 6.2   **The diaphragm properly positioned.**

be carefully fitted by a trained clinician to ensure both comfort and effectiveness. The fit should be checked with each routine annual medical examination, as well as after childbirth, abortion, abdominal or pelvic surgery, or a weight change of more than 10 pounds.

The woman spreads spermicidal jelly or cream on the diaphragm before inserting it and checking its placement (Figure 6.2). If more than 6 hours elapse between the time of insertion and the time of intercourse, additional spermicide must be applied. The diaphragm must be left in place for at least 6 hours after the last act of coitus to give the spermicide enough time to kill all the sperm. With repeated intercourse, a condom should be used for additional protection.

To remove the diaphragm, the woman hooks the front rim down from the pubic bone with one finger and pulls it out. After each use, a diaphragm should be washed with mild soap and water, rinsed, patted dry, and examined for holes or cracks. A diaphragm should be stored in its case.

Advantages   A diaphragm can be inserted up to 6 hours before intercourse. Its use can be limited to times of sexual activity only, and it allows for immediate and total reversibility. The diaphragm is free of medical side effects (other than rare allergic reactions). When used along with spermicidal jelly or cream,

Diaphragms offer protection against STDs such as gonorrhea, which are transmitted only by semen and for which the cervix is the sole site of entry.

diaphragm   A contraceptive device consisting of a flexible, dome-shaped cup that covers the cervix and prevents sperm from entering the uterus.

TERMS

it offers significant protection against gonorrhea and possibly chlamydia, STDs that are transmitted only by semen and for which the cervix is the sole site of entry. Diaphragm use can also protect the cervix from semen infected with the human papillomavirus, which causes cervical cancer. However, the diaphragm is unlikely to protect against STDs that can be transmitted through vaginal or vulvar surfaces (in addition to the cervix), including HIV infection, genital herpes, genital warts, and syphilis.

Disadvantages   Diaphragms must always be used with a spermicide, so a woman must keep both of these supplies with her whenever she anticipates sexual activity. Diaphragms require extra attention because they must be cleaned and stored with care to preserve their effectiveness. Some women cannot wear a diaphragm because of their vaginal or uterine anatomy or frequent bladder infections.

Diaphragms have also been associated with a slightly increased risk of **toxic shock syndrome (TSS)**, an occasionally fatal bacterial infection. To reduce the risk of TSS, a woman should wash her hands carefully with soap and water before inserting or removing the diaphragm, should not use the diaphragm during menstruation or when abnormal vaginal discharge is present, and should never leave the device in place for more than 24 hours.

Effectiveness   With perfect use, the failure rate is about 6%. Typical failure rates are 16% during the first year of use. The main causes of failure are incorrect insertion, inconsistent use, and inaccurate fitting. If a diaphragm slips during intercourse, a woman may choose to use emergency contraception.

FemCap

FemCap, another barrier device, is a small flexible cup that fits snugly over the cervix and is held in place by suction. This cervical cap is a clear silicone cup with a brim around the dome to hold spermicide and trap sperm and a removal strap over the dome. It comes in three sizes and must be fitted by a trained clinician. It is used like a diaphragm, with a small amount of spermicide placed in the cup and on the brim before insertion.

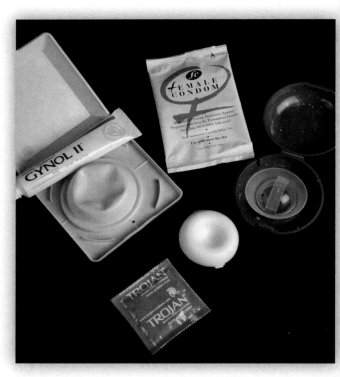

Many contraceptive methods work by blocking sperm from entering the cervix. Barrier methods pictured here are the diaphragm, the female condom, the male condom, the sponge, and the FemCap cervical cap.

Advantages   Advantages of the cervical cap are similar to those associated with diaphragm use and include partial STD protection. It is an alternative for women who cannot use a diaphragm because of anatomical reasons or recurrent urinary tract infections. The cap fits tightly, so it does not require backup condom use with repeated intercourse. It may be left in place for up to 48 hours.

Disadvantages   Along with most of the disadvantages associated with the diaphragm, difficulty with insertion and removal is more common for cervical cap users. Because there may be a slightly increased risk of TSS with prolonged use, the cap should not be left in place for more than 48 hours.

Effectiveness   Studies indicate that the average failure rate for the cervical cap is 16% for women who have never had a child and 32% for women who have had a child. Failure rates drop significantly with perfect use. FemCap is not a commonly used contraceptive; less than 1% of American women have ever used the FemCap.

The Contraceptive Sponge

The **contraceptive sponge** is a round, absorbent device about 2 inches in diameter with a polyester loop on one side (for removal) and a concave dimple on the other side, which helps it fit snugly over the cervix. The sponge is made of polyurethane and is presaturated with the same spermicide that is used in contraceptive creams and foams. The spermicide is activated when moistened with a small amount of water just before insertion. The sponge, which can be used only once, acts as a barrier, as a spermicide, and as a seminal fluid absorbent.

Advantages   The sponge offers advantages similar to those of the diaphragm and cervical cap, including partial protection against some STDs. In addition, sponges can be obtained without a prescription or professional fitting, and they may be safely left in place for 24 hours without the addition of spermicide for repeated intercourse. Most women find the sponge to be comfortable and unobtrusive during sex.

Disadvantages   Reported disadvantages include difficulty with removal and an unpleasant odor if the sponge is left in place for more than 18 hours. Allergic reactions, such as irritation of the vagina, are more common with the sponge than with other spermicide products, probably because the overall dose contained in each sponge is significantly higher than that used with other methods. If irritation of the vaginal lining occurs, the risk of yeast infections and STDs (including HIV) may increase. Because the sponge has also been associated with toxic shock syndrome, the same precautions must be taken as described for diaphragm use.

Effectiveness   The typical effectiveness of the sponge is the same as the diaphragm (16% failure rate during the first year of use) for women who have never experienced childbirth. For women who have had a child, however, sponges are significantly less effective than diaphragms.

Vaginal Spermicides

Spermicidal compounds developed for use with a diaphragm have been adapted for use without a diaphragm by combining them with a bulky base. Foams, creams, and jellies must be placed deep in the vagina near the cervical entrance and must be inserted no more than 60 minutes before intercourse. After an hour, their effectiveness is drastically reduced, and a new dose must be inserted.

The spermicidal suppository is small and easily inserted like a tampon; it is important to wait at least 15 minutes after insertion before having intercourse. The Vaginal Contraceptive Film (VCF) is a paper-thin 2-inch square of film that contains spermicide. It is folded over one or two fingers and placed high in the vagina, as close to the cervix as possible.

Another application of spermicide is required before each repeated act of coitus. If the woman wants to **douche,** she should wait for at least 6 hours after the last intercourse to make sure that there has been time for the spermicide to kill all the sperm; douching is not recommended, however, because it can irritate vaginal tissue and increase the risk of various infections.

Advantages   The use of vaginal spermicides is relatively simple and can be limited to times of sexual activity. They are readily available in most drugstores and do not require a prescription or a pelvic examination. Spermicides allow for complete and immediate reversibility, and the only medical side effects are occasional allergic reactions. Vaginal spermicides may provide limited protection against some STDs but should never be used instead of condoms for reliable protection.

Disadvantages   When used alone, vaginal spermicides must be inserted shortly before intercourse, so their use may be seen as an annoying disruption. Spermicides can alter the balance of bacteria in the vagina and may increase the occurrence of yeast infections and urinary tract infections. Also, this method does not protect against gonorrhea, chlamydia, or HIV. Overuse of spermicides can irritate vaginal tissues; if this occurs, the risk of HIV transmission may increase.

Effectiveness   The typical failure rate is about 29% during the first year of use. Spermicide is generally recommended only in combination with other barrier methods or as a backup to other contraceptives. Plan B provides a better backup than spermicides, however.

Abstinence, Fertility Awareness, and Withdrawal

Millions of people throughout the world do not use any of the contraceptive methods described earlier, because of religious conviction, cultural prohibitions, poverty, or lack of information and supplies. If they use any method at all, they are likely to use one of the following relatively "natural" methods.

Abstinence   The decision not to engage in sexual intercourse for a chosen period of time, or **abstinence,** has been practiced throughout history for a variety of reasons. Until relatively recently, many people abstained because they had no other contraceptive measures. Concern about possible side effects, STDs, and unwanted pregnancy may be factors. For others, the most important reason for choosing abstinence is a moral one, based on cultural or religious beliefs or strongly held personal values. Many people feel that sexual intercourse is appropriate only for married couples or for people in serious, committed relationships. Abstinence may also be considered the wisest choice in terms of one's emotional needs. A period of

douche   To apply a stream of water or other solutions to a body part or cavity such as the vagina; not a contraceptive technique.

abstinence   Avoidance of sexual intercourse; a method of contraception.

abstinence, for example, may be useful as a time to focus on other aspects of one's life.

Couples may choose abstinence to allow time for their relationship to grow. A period of abstinence allows partners to get to know each other better and to develop trust and respect for each other. Many couples who choose to abstain from sexual intercourse in the traditional sense turn to other mutually satisfying alternatives. These may include dancing, massage, hugging, kissing, petting, mutual masturbation, and oral-genital sex.

Fertility Awareness-Based Methods Women who practice a **fertility awareness-based method** of contraception abstain from intercourse during the fertile phase of their menstrual cycle. Ordinarily, only one egg is released by the ovaries each month, and it lives about 24 hours unless it is fertilized. Sperm deposited in the vagina may be capable of fertilizing an egg for up to 6–7 days, so conception can theoretically occur only during 6–8 days of any cycle. Predicting *which* 8 days is difficult. Recent studies show that even in women who have regular menstrual cycles, it is possible to become pregnant at any time during the menstrual cycle. It is even more difficult to predict the fertile time of the cycle in women who have irregular menses, a situation which is very common, especially in teenagers and women who are approaching menopause. Methods that attempt to predict the fertile times of a woman's cycle include calendar methods, temperature methods, and methods that rely on observation of the cyclical changes of the cervical mucus as well as other characteristics of the cervix. Some women use a combination of methods to determine the time of ovulation.

Calendar methods are based on the idea that the average woman releases an egg 14–16 days before her period begins. In order to avoid pregnancy, she should abstain from intercourse for about 8 days during her cycle, beginning several days before and during the time that ovulation is most likely to occur. However, in one recent study, only about 10% of women with regular 28-day cycles actually ovulated 14 days before the next period. The situation is further complicated by the fact that many women have somewhat or very irregular cycles; calendar methods are extremely unreliable for these women.

Temperature methods are based on the knowledge that a woman's body temperature drops slightly just before ovulation and rises slightly after ovulation. A woman using the temperature method records her basal (resting) body temperature (BBT) every morning before getting out of bed and before eating or drinking anything. Once the temperature pattern is apparent (usually after about 3 months), the unsafe period for intercourse can be calculated as the interval from day 5 (day 1 is the first day of the period) until 3 days after the rise in BBT. To arrive at a shorter unsafe period, some women combine the calendar and temperature methods, calculating the first unsafe day from the shortest cycle of the calendar chart and the last unsafe day as the third day after a rise in BBT.

The *mucus method* (or Billings method) is based on changes in the cervical secretions throughout the menstrual cycle. During the estrogenic phase, cervical mucus increases and is clear and slippery. At the time of ovulation, some women can detect a slight change in the texture of the mucus and find that it is more likely to form an elastic thread when stretched between thumb and finger. After ovulation, these secretions become cloudy and sticky and decrease in quantity. Infertile, safe days are likely to occur during the relatively dry days just before and after menstruation. These additional clues have been found to be helpful by some couples who rely on fertility awareness-based methods.

Fertility awareness-based methods are not recommended for women who have very irregular cycles—about 15% of all menstruating women. Any woman for whom pregnancy would be a serious problem should not rely on these methods alone, because the failure rate is high—approximately 25% during the first year of use. Further, fertility awareness-based methods offer no protection against STDs. Some women use fertility awareness in combination with a barrier method to reduce their risk for unwanted pregnancy. Fertility awareness-based methods are recommended by the Catholic Church, since the Church does not approve of other forms of contraception.

Withdrawal In **withdrawal,** or *coitus interruptus,* the male removes his penis from the vagina just before he ejaculates. Withdrawal has a high failure rate because the male has to overcome a powerful biological urge. Further, because preejaculatory fluid may contain viable sperm, pregnancy can occur even if the man withdraws prior to ejaculation. Sexual pleasure is often affected because the man must remain in control and the sexual experience of both partners is interrupted.

5.2% of women who practice some sort of contraception rely on withdrawal as their birth control method.
—Guttmacher Institute, 2010

The failure rate for typical use is about 27% in the first year. Men who are less experienced with sexual intercourse and withdrawal or who have difficulty in foretelling when ejaculation will occur have higher failure rates. Withdrawal does not protect against STDs.

TERMS

fertility awareness-based method A method of preventing conception based on avoiding intercourse during the fertile phase of a woman's cycle.

withdrawal A method of contraception in which the man withdraws his penis from the vagina prior to ejaculation; also called *coitus interruptus.*

Emergency Contraception

Emergency contraception (EC) refers to methods used after unprotected sexual intercourse. An emergency contraceptive may be appropriate if a regularly used method has failed (for example, if a condom breaks) or if unprotected sex has occurred. Sometimes called the "morning-after pill," emergency contraceptives are designed only for emergency use and should not be relied on as a regular birth control method; other methods of birth control are more effective.

When emergency contraceptives were first approved by the FDA, opponents feared that they might act as an **abortifacient**—preventing implantation of a fertilized egg, theoretically causing an abortion. However, recent evidence indicates that emergency contraceptives do not interrupt an established pregnancy. Postcoital pills work primarily by inhibiting or delaying ovulation and by altering the transport of sperm and/or eggs; they do not affect a fertilized egg already implanted in the uterus and thus do not cause abortion.

Until recently, the most frequently used emergency contraceptive was a two-dose regimen of oral contraceptives. Newer products—Plan B, Plan B One-Step, and Next Choice—are now in common use and are more effective, with fewer side effects, than older methods. Plan B One-Step, which replaced Plan B in 2009, contains a single progestin-only pill, while Next Choice has two pills that are taken 12 hours apart. The pills should be taken as soon as possible after inadequately protected sex. If taken within 24 hours after intercourse, emergency contraceptives may prevent as many as 95% of expected pregnancies. Overall, they reduce pregnancy risk by about 89%. They are most effective if initiated in the first 12 hours, but they can be taken up to 120 hours after unprotected intercourse. Possible side effects include nausea, stomach pain, headache, dizziness, and breast tenderness. If a woman is already pregnant, these pills will not interfere with the pregnancy. Current emergency contraceptives are considered very safe.

Plan B One-Step and Next Choice are available as over-the-counter (OTC) drugs (no prescription required) for women and men age 17 and older. They remain prescription drugs for those under age 17. In order to buy an emergency contraceptive, you need to ask for it at the pharmacy counter and show proof of age. It is recommended that you call ahead to your pharmacy to make sure that they have EC on hand. The vast majority of pharmacies, especially the larger chains, currently carry emergency contraceptives.

Some clinicians advise women to keep a package of emergency contraceptives on hand in case their regular contraception method fails or they have unprotected intercourse. Research has found that ready access to emergency contraception does not lead to an increase in unprotected intercourse, unintended pregnancies, or STDs. EC is covered by some health plans as well as by Medicaid in many states. However, many women must pay directly for EC, which costs about $50.

To find out more about emergency contraception and how to obtain it in your area, visit the Emergency Contraception Web site (http://ec.princeton.edu) or the Next Step Web site (http://www.mynextchoice.com) or call the Emergency Contraception Hotline (888-NOT-2-LATE). Plan B One-Step has a Web site (http://www.planbonestep.com) that, as of this printing, contains a card you can print and hand to the pharmacist as an easy way to request EC.

Intrauterine devices can also be used for emergency contraception. If inserted within 5 days of unprotected intercourse, the Copper T ParaGard IUD (discussed earlier) is even more effective than pills for emergency contraception. It has the added benefit of providing up to 10 years of contraception.

A new emergency contraceptive, ulipristal acetate, is currently being used in Europe and has been approved by an advisory panel of the U.S. FDA. (The FDA often takes the advisory panel's recommendations but does not have an obligation to do so.) Sold under the name EllaOne, this drug is effective if taken up to 5 days after unprotected intercourse. Another drug, Meloxicam, is being tested as an EC. Meloxicam is a non-hormonal medicine, currently used to treat arthritis, that has been found to disrupt ovulation.

Combining Methods

Couples can choose to combine the preceding methods in a variety of ways, both to add STD protection and/or to increase contraceptive effectiveness. For example, condoms are strongly recommended along with OCs and other forms of hormonal contraception whenever there is a risk of STDs (Table 6.2). Foam or other forms of spermicides may be added to condom use to increase protection against both STDs and pregnancy. For many couples, and especially for women, the added benefits far outweigh the extra effort and expense of using multiple methods.

Table 6.3 summarizes the effectiveness of available contraceptive methods.

emergency contraception (EC)   A birth control method used after unprotected sexual intercourse has occurred.

abortifacient   An agent or substance that induces abortion.

TERMS

Table 6.2 — Contraceptive Methods and STD Protection

METHOD	LEVEL OF PROTECTION
Hormonal methods	Do not protect against HIV or STDs in lower reproductive tract; may increase risk of cervical chlamydia; provide some protection against PID.
IUD	Does not protect against STDs; associated with PID in first month after insertion.
Latex, polyisoprene, or polyurethane male condom	Best method for protection against STDs (if used correctly); does not protect against infections from lesions that are not covered by the condom. (Lambskin condoms do not protect against STDs.)
Female condom	Reduces STD risk similar to male condom; may provide extra protection for external genitalia.
Diaphragm, sponge, or cervical cap	Provides some protection against cervical infections and PID; should not be relied on for protection against HIV.
Spermicide	Modestly reduces the risk of some vaginal and cervical STDs; does not reduce the risk of HIV, chlamydia, or gonorrhea. If vaginal irritation occurs, infection risk may increase.
Fertility awareness-based methods	Do not protect against STDs.
Sterilization	Does not protect against STDs.
Abstinence	Provides complete protection against STDs (as long as all activities that involve the exchange of body fluids are avoided).

Table 6.3 — Contraceptives: From Most Effective to Least

(Percent of women experiencing unintended pregnancy within the first year of use)

METHOD	TYPICAL USE	PERFECT USE
REVERSIBLE METHODS		
Extremely Effective:		
Complete abstinence	0.0%	0.0%
Implant (Implanon)	0.05%	0.05%
Mirena IUD	0.2%	0.2%
ParaGard IUD	0.8%	0.6%
Injectable (3-month)	3.0%	0.3%
Very Effective:		
Pill	8.0%	0.3%
Patch	8.0%	0.3%
Ring	8.0%	0.3%
Moderately Effective:		
Male condom	15.0%	2.0%
Diaphragm	16.0%	6.0%
Sponge (if never had a child)	16.0%	9.0%
Cervical cap (if never had a child)	16.0%	9.0%
Female condom	21.0%	5.0%
Less Effective		
Periodic abstinence	25.3%	25.3%
Withdrawal	27.0%	4.0%
Spermicides	29.0%	19.0%
Sponge (if have had a child)	32.0%	20.0%
Cervical cap (if have had a child)	32.0%	26.0%
PERMANENT METHODS		
Vasectomy	0.15%	0.1%
Essure	0.2%	0.2%
Tubal sterilization	0.5%	0.5%
NO METHOD*	85.0%	85.0%

*Pregnancy rates for sexually active teens and women in their early 20s who do not use any method of contraception are closer to 90% because younger women have higher fertility rates than older women.

SOURCE: Trussell, J. 2007. Choosing a contraceptive. In *Contraceptive Technology*, 19th ed., ed. R. A. Hatcher, J. Trussell, A. L. Nelson, W. Cates, F. H. Stewart, and D. Kowal. New York: Ardent Media. Also online at http://www.contraceptivetechnology.org/table.html; retrieved October 29, 2010.

PERMANENT CONTRACEPTION

Sterilization is permanent, and it is highly effective at preventing pregnancy. At present it is tied with the pill as the most commonly used method in the United States and is by far the most common method used worldwide. It is especially popular among couples who have been married 10 or more years and have had all the children they intend to have. Sterilization does not protect against STDs.

An important consideration in choosing sterilization is that, in most cases, it cannot be reversed. Some couples choosing male sterilization store sperm to extend the option of childbearing.

Many studies indicate that male sterilization is preferable to female sterilization because the overall cost of a female procedure is about four times that of a male procedure and women are much more likely than men to experience complications following the operation. Furthermore, feelings of regret seem to be more prevalent in women than in men after sterilization.

Male Sterilization: Vasectomy

The procedure for male sterilization, **vasectomy,** involves severing the vasa deferentia, two tiny ducts that transport sperm from the testes to the seminal vesicles. The testes continue to produce sperm, but the sperm are absorbed into the body. Because the testes contribute only about 10% of the total seminal fluid, the actual quantity of ejaculate is only slightly reduced. Hormone production from the testes continues with very little change, and secondary sex characteristics are not altered.

Vasectomy is ordinarily performed in a physician's office and takes about 30 minutes. A local anesthetic is injected into the skin of the scrotum near the vasa. Small incisions are made at the upper end of the scrotum where it joins the body, and the vas deferens on each side is exposed, severed, and tied off or sealed by electrocautery. Some doctors seal each of the vasa with a plastic

Emergency contraceptives do not result in an abortion and do not interfere with an existing pregnancy.

clamp, which is the size of a grain of rice. The incisions are then closed with sutures, and a small dressing is applied. Pain and swelling are usually slight and can be relieved with ice compresses and a scrotal support. Bleeding and infection occasionally develop but are usually easily treated.

Men can have sex again as soon as they feel no further discomfort, usually after about a week. Another method of contraception must be used for at least 3 months after vasectomy, however, because sperm produced before the operation may still be present in the semen. Microscopic examination of a semen sample, called _semen analysis,_ is required to confirm that sperm are no longer present in the ejaculate. Recommendations for semen analysis after vasectomy vary. Most doctors recommend having the first semen analysis about 3 months after surgery, and a second test to confirm the results a few weeks later. Some doctors recommend having another test in a year. Studies show that most men fail to complete follow-up testing after vasectomy. Fortunately, unintended pregnancies following vasectomy are rare, even when follow-up procedures are ignored.

Vasectomy is highly effective. In a small number of cases, a severed vas rejoins itself, so some physicians advise yearly examination of a semen sample. The overall failure rate for vasectomy is 0.2%. About one-half of vasectomy reversals are successful. In at least half of all men who have had vasectomies, the process of absorbing sperm (instead of ejaculating it) results in antisperm antibodies that may interfere with later fertility. The length of time between the vasectomy and the reversal surgery may also be an important predictor of reversal success.

Female Sterilization

The most common method of female sterilization involves severing or blocking the oviducts, thereby preventing eggs from reaching the uterus and sperm from entering the fallopian tubes. Ovulation and menstruation continue, but the unfertilized eggs are released into the abdominal cavity and absorbed. Although progesterone levels in the blood may decline slightly, hormone production by the ovaries and secondary sex characteristics are generally not affected.

Tubal sterilization (also called _tubal ligation)_ is most commonly performed by a method called **laparoscopy.** A laparoscope, a tube containing a small light, is inserted through a small abdominal incision, and the surgeon looks through it to locate the fallopian tubes. Instruments are passed either through the laparoscope or through a second small incision, and the two fallopian tubes are sealed off with ties or staples or by electrocautery. General anesthesia is usually used. The operation takes about 30 minutes, and women can usually leave the hospital 2–4 hours after surgery. Tubal sterilization can also be performed shortly after a vaginal delivery, or in the case of cesarean section immediately after the uterine incision is repaired.

Although tubal sterilization is somewhat riskier than vasectomy, with a rate of minor complications of about 6–11%, it is the more common procedure (see the box "Contraceptive Use Among American Women"). Potential problems include bowel injury, wound infection, and bleeding. Serious complications are rare, and the death rate is low. The failure rate for tubal sterilization is about 0.5%. When pregnancies occur, an increased percentage of them are ectopic (occurring outside the uterus). Ectopic pregnancy is dangerous and can even cause death, so any woman who suspects she might be pregnant after having tubal sterilization should seek medical help. Because reversibility rates are low and the procedure is costly, female sterilization should be considered permanent.

Two new forms of incision-free female sterilization have recently become available. Each of these procedures can be performed with local anesthetic in a doctor's office, and they have very short recovery times. The first, called the Essure System, consists of tiny springlike metallic implants that are inserted through the vagina and into the fallopian tubes, using a special catheter. Within several months, scar tissue forms over the implants, blocking the tubes.

In 2009 the FDA approved a second, somewhat similar method for blocking a woman's fallopian tubes without an incision. The procedure, marketed under the name Adiana, involves using radiofrequency waves to create small lesions just inside the entrance to each fallopian tube. A small silicone insert, the size of a grain of rice, is then placed in each tube. As the lesions heal, healthy new tissue grows on and around the device, eventually blocking the fallopian tube. Adiana's 3-year failure rate is about 1.6%.

Hysterectomy, removal of the uterus, is the preferred method of sterilization for only a small number of women, usually those with preexisting menstrual problems.

---

sterilization   Surgically altering the reproductive system to prevent pregnancy. Vasectomy is the procedure in males; tubal sterilization or hysterectomy is the procedure in females.

vasectomy   The surgical severing of the ducts that carry sperm to the ejaculatory duct.

tubal sterilization   Severing or blocking the oviducts to prevent eggs from reaching the uterus; also called _tubal ligation._

laparoscopy   Examining the internal organs by inserting a tube containing a small light through an abdominal incision.

hysterectomy   Total or partial surgical removal of the uterus.

TERMS

About 62 million women in the United States are in their childbearing years (15–44) and thus face decisions about contraception. About 62% of these women currently use some form of contraception. Most of the remaining 38% are sterile, pregnant, trying to become pregnant, or not sexually active.

Only about 7% of American women are fertile, sexually active, not seeking pregnancy, *and* not using contraceptives. This small group accounts for almost half of the 3 million unintended pregnancies that occur each year. The unintended pregnancies that occur among contraceptive users are usually the result of inconsistent or incorrect use of methods. For example, one-third of barrier method users report not using their method every time they have intercourse.

Oral contraceptives and female sterilization are the two most popular methods among American women. However, choice of contraceptive method and consistency of use vary with age, marital status, and other factors:

- *Age:* Sterilization is much more common among older women, particularly those who are over 35 years of age and/or who have had children. Young women in their teens and twenties are more likely to use the pill or condoms. Older women, however, are more likely to use reversible methods consistently. They are less likely to miss pills and more likely to use barrier methods during every act of intercourse.

- *Marital status:* Women who are or were married have much higher rates of sterilization than women who have never been married. Those who have never been married have high rates of OC and condom usage.

- *Ethnicity:* Overall rates of contraceptive use and use of OCs are highest among white women. Female sterilization, implants, and injectables are more often used by African American women and Latinas, and IUD use is highest among Latinas. Condom use is highest among Asian American women and similar across other ethnic groups. Male sterilization is much more common among white men than among men of other ethnic groups.

- *Socioeconomic status and educational attainment:* Low socioeconomic status and low educational attainment are associated with high rates of female sterilization and low rates of pill and condom use. However, women who are poor or have low educational attainment and who use OCs have higher rates of consistent use than women who are wealthier or have more education. About 20% of women age 15–44 lack adequate health insurance, increasing the cost and difficulty of obtaining contraceptives.

- *New trends:* About 10% of American women have used emergency contraception at least once, up from 4% in 2002. The percentage of women who have ever used the patch rose from 1% to 10% in the last 6 years. Rates of IUD use, especially among women who have already had at least one child, have also risen dramatically.

- *Spotlight on college students:* A 2008 survey of college students showed that about 40% used birth control pills as their method of contraception the last time they had vaginal intercourse; 38% used condoms and 15% used withdrawal. All other methods combined accounted for about 10% of college students. About 4% of students used no method at all the last time they had vaginal intercourse. Nearly one-quarter of college students had never had vaginal intercourse.

- *Racial differences among college students:* Black students were more likely to have used a condom the last time they had vaginal intercourse compared with white students (63% of blacks vs. 58% of whites). On the other hand, white students are far more likely to use hormonal contraception than black students (66% vs. 42%). About 6% of black students reported using no contraception the last time they had vaginal intercourse compared with less than 3% of white students. Unintended pregnancies were nearly four times higher among black college students compared with white students.

Some trends in contraceptive use may also reflect the differing priorities and experiences of women and men. For example, female sterilization is more expensive and carries greater health risks than male sterilization—yet it is more than twice as common. (Worldwide, female sterilization is more than four times as common as male sterilization.) This pattern may reflect culturally defined gender roles and the fact that women are more directly affected by unintended pregnancy. In surveys, women rate pregnancy prevention as the single most important factor when choosing a contraceptive method; in contrast, men rate STD prevention as equally important.

SOURCES: American College Health Association. 2010. *National College Health Assessment Reference Group Data Report Spring 2008* (http://www.pdfdownload.org/pdf2html/view_online.php?url=http%3A%2F%2Fwww.achancha.org%2Fdocs%2FFACHA-NCHA_Reference_Group_Report_Sprin2008.pdf; retrieved October 29, 2010); Buhi, E., et al. 2010. The state of the union: Sexual health disparities in a national sample of U.S. college students. *Journal of American College Health* 58:337–346; Guttmacher Institute. 2008. *Facts in Brief: Facts on Contraceptive Use* (http://www.guttmacher.org/pubs/fb_contr_use.html; retrieved October 29, 2010); Mosher, W. D., and J. Jones. 2010. Use of contraception in the U.S.: 1982–2008. *National Center for Health Statistics* 23(29).

WHICH CONTRACEPTIVE METHOD IS RIGHT FOR YOU?

Each person must consider many variables in deciding which method is most acceptable and appropriate for her or him. Key considerations include those listed here:

1. *Health risks.* When considering any contraceptive method, determine whether it may pose a risk to your health. For example, IUDs are generally not recommended for young women without children because of an increased risk of pelvic infection and subsequent infertility. Hormonal methods should be used only after a clinical evaluation of your medical status and history. Other methods have only minor and local side effects. Talk with your health care provider about the potential health effects of different methods for you. Remember that pregnancy

Talking with a Partner About Contraception

Many people have a difficult time talking about contraception with a potential sex partner. How should you bring it up? And whose responsibility is it, anyway? Talking about the subject may be embarrassing at first, but imagine the possible consequences of *not* talking about it. An unintended pregnancy or a sexually transmitted disease could profoundly affect you for the rest of your life.

Before you talk with your partner, explore your own thoughts and feelings. Find out the facts about different methods of contraception, and decide which one you think would be most appropriate for you.

Pick a good time to bring up the subject. It makes sense to have this discussion before you start having sex, but even if you've already had intercourse with your partner, it's important to be on the same page about contraception. Tell your partner what you know about contraception and how you feel about using it, and talk about what steps you both need to take to get and use a method you can live with. Listen to what your partner has to say, and try to understand his or her point of view. You may need to have more than one discussion, and it may take some time for both of you to feel comfortable with the subject.

If you want your partner to be involved but he or she isn't interested in talking about contraception, or if he or she leaves all the responsibility for it up to you, consider whether this is really a person you want to be sexually involved with. If you decide to go ahead with the involvement, you may want to enlist the support of a friend, family member, or health care provider to help you make and implement decisions about contraception. If you have been involved in hooking up with people you don't know well and are not having an ongoing relationship with, discussions about contraception may seem unrealistic. At a minimum, refuse to have sex with anyone who won't use a condom. If you are a woman, purchase emergency contraception ahead of time, and don't hesitate to use it.

and abortion carry significant health risks that are generally much greater than the risks of any method of contraception.

2. *The implications of an unplanned pregnancy.* Many teens and young adults fail to consider how their life would be affected by an unexpected pregnancy. When considering contraception (or deciding whether to have sex in the first place), think about the potential consequences of your choices.

3. *STD risk.* STDs are another potential consequence of sex. In fact, several activities besides vaginal intercourse (such as oral and anal sex) can put you at risk for an STD. Condom use is of critical importance whenever any risk of STDs is present, even if you are using another contraceptive method to prevent pregnancy. This is especially true whenever you are not in an exclusive, long-term relationship with someone who has never had sex with anyone except you. Abstinence or activities that don't involve intercourse or any other exchange of body fluids can be a satisfactory alternative for some people. Also, consider trying the female condom; although you may be less familiar with it, the female condom has several advantages over male condoms and may be even more effective in STD prevention.

4. *Convenience and comfort level.* The hormonal methods are generally ranked high in this category for most women. If forgetting to take pills is a problem for you, a vaginal ring, contraceptive patch, implant, or injectable method may be a good alternative to the pill. For those who choose a barrier method, the diaphragm, cervical cap, contraceptive sponge, female condom, and spermicides can be inserted before intercourse begins. Some people think condom use disrupts spontaneity, but creative approaches to condom use can decrease these concerns.

5. *Type of relationship.* Barrier methods require more motivation and sense of responsibility from *each* partner than hormonal methods do. When the method depends on the cooperation of one's partner, assertiveness is necessary, no matter how difficult. This is especially true in new relationships, when condom use is most important. When sexual activity is infrequent, a barrier method may make more sense than an IUD or one of the hormonal methods.

6. *Ease and cost of obtaining and maintaining each method.* Investigate the costs of different methods. If you have insurance, find out if it covers any of the costs. Remember that your student health clinic probably provides family planning services, and most communities have low-cost family planning clinics, such as Planned Parenthood.

7. *Religious or philosophical beliefs.* For some, abstinence and/or fertility awareness-based methods may be the only permissible contraceptive methods.

8. *Potential noncontraceptive benefits.* Women with dysmenorrhea, irregular periods, acne, endometriosis, severe PMS, and other medical problems may benefit from using a particular method of contraception. Be sure to discuss these issues with your health care provider so that you can take advantage of the noncontraceptive benefits associated with many methods of birth control.

Whatever your needs, circumstances, or beliefs, *do* make a choice about contraception. Not choosing anything is the one method known *not* to work. This is an area in which taking charge of your health has immediate and profound implications for your future.

Men's Involvement in Contraception

What can be done to increase men's involvement in contraception? Health care professionals are taking the following approaches:

- Develop programs and campaigns that stress the importance of information, counseling, and medical care relating to sexual and reproductive matters from adolescence on. Men are less likely than women to seek regular checkups, but regular care for men would benefit men in their own right and both men and women as individuals, couples, and families.

- Recruit and train male health care workers, who can be important advocates and role models for healthful behaviors.

- Encourage men to take an active role in understanding, selecting, and using contraceptives. Even if a couple chooses to use a female contraceptive, the male partner can share in the responsibility.

- Educate men about the ways in which stereotypical views of male or female sexuality can inhibit good reproductive health for both men and women.

- Develop educational and clinical programs specifically targeted at young men. Men in their early twenties are most likely to engage in risky sexual behaviors and to have adverse reproductive health outcomes. Surveys indicate that most men use a condom the first time they have intercourse, but condom use subsequently declines—and there is much greater reliance on female contraceptive methods.

- Develop new contraceptives for men. Numerous male contraceptives are currently being studied. Future possibilities include hormonal contraceptives, substances that block the vasa deferentia, and a host of other methods, some of which are currently being tested in humans.

What can individuals do? Men can increase their participation in contraception in the following ways:

- Initiate and support communication regarding contraception and STD protection.

- Buy and use condoms whenever appropriate.

- Help pay contraceptive costs.

- Be available for shared responsibility in the resolution of an unintended pregnancy, should one occur.

THE ABORTION ISSUE

Few issues are as complex and emotionally charged as abortion. In the United States, public attention has focused on the legal definition of abortion and the issue of restricting its practice. These far-reaching questions are important, but the most difficult aspects of abortion are personal—especially for women who must decide whether to have an abortion.

The word **abortion**, by strict definition, means the expulsion of an embryo or fetus from the uterus before it is sufficiently developed to survive. As commonly used, however, the term *abortion* refers only to those expulsions that are artificially induced by mechanical means or drugs. The term **miscarriage** is generally used when referring to a *spontaneous abortion*—one that occurs naturally with no causal intervention (see the box "Environmental Hazards and Miscarriage"). In this chapter, *abortion* refers to a deliberately induced expulsion.

Legal Status of Abortion

In the United States, courts began to invalidate state anti-abortion laws on the grounds of constitutional vagueness and violation of the right to privacy beginning in the 1960s (see the box "Key Abortion Decisions and Legislation").

In 1973, the U.S. Supreme Court made abortion legal in the landmark case of *Roe v. Wade*. To replace the restrictions most states still imposed at that time, the justices devised new standards to govern abortion decisions. They divided pregnancy into three parts, or trimesters, giving a woman less choice about abortion as her pregnancy advances toward full term.

In the first trimester, the abortion decision must be left to the judgment of the pregnant woman and her physician. During the second trimester, similar rights remain up to the point when the fetus becomes **viable**—that is, capable of surviving outside of the uterus. Today, most clinicians define this point as 24 weeks of gestation. When the fetus is considered viable, a state may regulate and even bar all abortions except those considered necessary to preserve the mother's life or health.

Although abortion remains legal throughout the United States, subsequent rulings by the Supreme Court allow states to regulate abortion throughout pregnancy as long as no "undue burden" is imposed on women seeking the procedure. As a result, states have passed a variety of laws that have had the effect of reducing women's access to abortion. Between 1995 and 2006, the number of state laws restricting abortion more than quadrupled. Currently, 36 states have laws prohibiting abortion after a certain point in pregnancy, with exceptions, and 17 states provide nonfederal public money to assist some poor women seeking medically necessary abortions. Concerns have been raised that a two-tiered system has been created—one for women with means and another for those without.

TERMS

abortion The artificially induced expulsion of an embryo or fetus from the uterus.

miscarriage A naturally occurring spontaneous abortion.

viable Capable of surviving outside of the uterus.

A miscarriage, or spontaneous abortion, is a pregnancy that ends on its own before the 20th week of gestation. Miscarriage is a common outcome of pregnancy: The American College of Gynecologists and Obstetricians estimates that 15–25% and perhaps even up to 50% of pregnancies end in miscarriage—often before the mother even realizes she is pregnant.

Miscarriages occur for a variety of reasons; among the most common are chromosomal abnormalities in the fetus, maternal health problems, and infections. In many cases, no cause can be identified. But there is also evidence that many miscarriages are associated with exposure to environmental toxins. Although direct cause-and-effect relationships are difficult to establish, scientists have found correlations between environmental hazards and the risk of miscarriage.

Hazards can be both naturally occurring (e.g., arsenic in rock) and of human making (e.g., vehicle exhaust fumes). They can be ingested, inhaled, or absorbed through the skin. Usually, but not always, exposure has to be to a large amount for a long time to cause harm. Environmental hazards interact with other facts in complex ways, such that some women with no known risk factors have miscarriages, and other women who do experience exposure to toxins do not have miscarriages. Innumerable factors may play a role, including the mother's age, her medical history, the duration of exposure, and other individual differences.

Most hazardous substances are found in the workplace, but some are found in the air and water and in chemicals used in the home. Occupational exposure to chemicals that may increase the risk of miscarriage is most prevalent in industrial settings, dry cleaning facilities, semiconductor and electronics plants, agricultural settings, labs, dental offices, and medical settings, especially where chemotherapy drugs and anesthesia are used.

Women whose work involves chemicals may want to consider transferring to another position or locale during their pregnancy. At the least, precautions should be taken, including making sure areas are well ventilated, not eating or drinking in the work area, and wearing protective clothing. Some of the most hazardous substances are described below.

- Carbon monoxide, a poisonous component of air pollution, vehicle exhaust, tobacco smoke, and gas fumes from faulty furnaces or other appliances, increases the risk of miscarriage. A 2009 study found that pregnant women who lived within 55 yards of busy freeways had higher rates of miscarriage.

- Lead was used for many years in gasoline, house paint, and water pipes. It was banned by the EPA in the 1970s but persists in the environment and in older homes. Lead is also present in some crystal glassware, ceramic glazes, and arts and craft supplies. Exposure to high levels of lead during pregnancy contributes to miscarriage, preterm birth, low birth weight, and health problems for the infant.

- Mercury, an element and an industrial by-product, is found in contaminated fish and seafood (especially large fish like swordfish, shark, king mackerel, and tilefish). Repeated exposure to mercury may pose a risk to a fetus or cause miscarriage. The EPA has issued specific cautions regarding fish consumption for pregnant women and children.

- Arsenic can occur naturally in rock and soil and can contaminate drinking water. It is also used in electronics manufacturing and was used in fertilizers until it was banned. Women living near metal smelters, incinerators, or hazardous waste sites may be at increased risk for miscarriage and stillbirth. Another metal, cadmium, used in semiconductor manufacturing and other industries, also poses a risk.

- Pesticides pose a miscarriage risk for women who live in agricultural areas or do agricultural work.

- Volatile organic compounds (VOCs) are carbon-containing compounds that easily become gases or vapors. They are released from burning fuels and from organic solvents, paints, paint thinners, varnishes, glues, nail polish, and other products used and stored in homes and workplaces. Compounds in this category include gasoline, toluene, xylene, glycol ethers, formaldehyde, and perchloroethylene (the main solvent used in dry cleaning). Pregnant women should avoid using these compounds or inhaling their fumes.

- Ionizing radiation (e.g., X rays) poses a danger for pregnant women and should be avoided as much as possible.

Exposure to some hazards during pregnancy is the result of lifestyle choices. Pregnant women who smoke, drink, use recreational drugs, or take prescription or over-the-counter medications may be increasing their risk of miscarriage. Even caffeine—one of the most commonly ingested drugs in America—has been associated with miscarriage and stillbirth. Needed medications can also pose a risk, such as SSRI antidepressants like Paxil and Effexor.

Although everyone is exposed to chemicals and other hazards every day, it makes sense for pregnant women to avoid unnecessary chemical exposures as much as possible. It also makes sense for pregnant women to live a normal life and not become obsessed with exposure to hazardous substances. A balanced, healthy life is the best compromise.

For a detailed discussion of environmental health—how the environment affects you and how you affect the environment—see Chapter 14.

SOURCES: Brown, S. 2008. Miscarriage and its associations. *Seminars in Reproductive Medicine* 26(5): 391–400; Gardella, J. R., and J. A. Hill. 2000. Environmental toxins associated with recurrent pregnancy loss. *Seminars in Reproductive Medicine* 18(4): 407–424; Green, R. S., et al. 2009. Residential exposure to traffic and spontaneous abortion. *Environmental Health Perspectives* 117(12): 1939–1944; Greenwood, D. C., et.al. 2010. Caffeine intake during pregnancy, late miscarriage and stillbirth. *European Journal of Epidemiology* 25(4):275–280.

IN THE NEWS

Mid-1800s to mid-1900s Abortion becomes illegal in all 50 states, with certain exceptions that vary by state (for example, to save the life of the mother). The federal Comstock Act of 1873 outlaws distribution or possession of information about, or devices or medications for, contraception or abortion.

1965 *Griswold v. Connecticut:* The Supreme Court overturns a law prohibiting use of contraceptives by married couples, stating that it violates the Bill of Right's guarantee of marital privacy.

1967–1973 Some states rewrite their abortion laws, including four states that repeal abortion bans.

1972 *Eisenstadt v. Baird:* The Supreme Court overturns a law banning distribution of contraceptives to unmarried adults, stating that the ban violates the Constitution's equal protection clause.

1973 *Roe v. Wade:* The Supreme Court strikes down a Texas law banning abortion and rules that abortion is included in the constitutional right to privacy.

1976 *Planned Parenthood of Central Missouri v. Danforth:* The Supreme Court rules against requiring that married women obtain spousal approval before having an abortion and requiring minors to get written parental consent.

1980 *Harris v. McRae:* The Supreme Court upholds restrictions on Medicaid funding for abortions except as needed to protect the mother's life or in other special circumstances.

1986 *Thornburgh v. American College of Obstetricians and Gynecologists:* The Supreme Court strikes down a law requiring any woman seeking an abortion to receive a state-scripted lecture from her physician about potential risks and possible alternatives.

1989 *Webster v. Reproductive Health Services:* The Supreme Court upholds a state law prohibiting the use of public facilities for abortions that are not medically necessary and requiring physicians to do viability testing on fetuses of more than 20 weeks' gestation.

1991 *Rust v. Sullivan:* The Supreme Court rules that clinics receiving federal Title X (family planning) funding can be prohibited from counseling, referring, or providing information about abortions.

1992 *Planned Parenthood of Southeastern Pennsylvania v. Casey:* The Supreme Court upholds the *Roe* decision but allows states to restrict abortion access as long as the restrictions do not impose an undue burden on women seeking abortions. It upholds a provision requiring minors to obtain consent from one parent or a judge (judicial bypass) to obtain an abortion.

1994 Congress passes the Freedom of Access to Clinics Act, making it a crime to interfere with a woman's right to obtain reproductive health services, including abortion.

2000 The FDA approves mifepristone (RU-486), the abortion pill.

2000 *Stenberg v. Carhart:* The Supreme Court finds a Nebraska law banning partial birth abortion unconstitutional; the law lacked an exception for the mother's health and imposed an undue burden on women seeking abortions.

2003 Congress passes and President Bush signs the Partial Birth Abortion Ban Act with no exception to the ban in cases of risk to a woman's health.

2004 The Partial Birth Abortion Ban Act is declared unconstitutional by federal judges in San Francisco, New York,

and Lincoln, Nebraska. Also, the Freedom of Choice Act (FOCA) is introduced in the Senate. At the federal level, FOCA would prohibit state and federal government entities from denying or interfering with a woman's right to choose to bear a child, to terminate a pregnancy before viability, or to terminate a pregnancy after viability when necessary to protect the mother's life or health.

2007 *Gonzales v. Carhart:* The Supreme Court upholds the Partial Birth Abortion Ban Act and imposes a nationwide ban on a rare but controversial abortion procedure, called intact dilation and extraction (intact D & E).

2008–2010 A number of states, including Michigan, Louisiana, Florida, and Oklahoma, consider or pass legislation requiring women seeking an abortion to undergo an ultrasound procedure, then be given the opportunity to view images of the fetus. Most notably, Oklahoma's law requires the physician to review the images with the woman. The Oklahoma law is not in force pending legal challenges. In June 2010, Florida Governor Charlie Crist vetoed legislation that would require women seeking abortions to pay for an ultrasound procedure prior to an abortion.

SOURCES: Cornell University Legal Information Institute. 2009. *U.S. Supreme Court Decisions* (http://supct.law.cornell.edu/supct/; retrieved, November 3, 2010); CBS News. 2007. *Abortion Timeline* (http://www.cbsnews.com/htdocs/abortion/timeline.html; retrieved November 3, 2010); Guttmacher Institute. 2010. *Abortion* (http://www.guttmacher.org/sections/abortion.php?pub=spib; retrieved November 3, 2010); Planned Parenthood. 2008. *Abortion Issues* (http://www.plannedparenthood.org/issuesaction/abortion-issues-5946.html; retrieved November 3, 2010).

Public Opinion

Some people strongly identify exclusively with either the pro-life or the pro-choice stance, but many have moral beliefs that combine the two. Many people instinctively feel that the fetus gains increasing human value as a pregnancy advances. In this view, first-trimester abortion is acceptable but later-term abortion should be performed only when the mother's health is in jeopardy. Although the most vocal groups in the abortion debate tend to paint

a black-and-white picture, most Americans view abortion as a complex issue without any easy answers.

In general, U.S. public opinion on abortion seems to change depending on the specific situation. Many Americans approve of legal abortion as an option when destructive health or welfare consequences could result from continuing pregnancy, but they do not advocate abortion as a simple way out of an inconvenient situation. Overall, most adults in the United States approve of legal abortion and are opposed to overturning the basic right to abortion

Pro-choice groups believe that the decision to end or continue a pregnancy is a personal matter. Pro-life groups oppose abortion on the basis of their belief that life begins at conception.

established in *Roe v. Wade*. In May, 2010, a Gallup Inc. poll showed that 47% of Americans described themselves as "pro-life" while 45% said they were "pro-choice." Even so, most Americans still say that abortion should be legal in certain situations or under any circumstances (Figure 6.3).

Personal Considerations

For the pregnant woman who is considering abortion, the usual legal and moral arguments may sound meaningless as she attempts to weigh the many short- and long-term ramifications for all those who are directly concerned. If she chooses abortion, can she accept the decision in terms of her own religious and moral beliefs? What are her long-range feelings likely to be regarding this decision? What are her partner's feelings regarding abortion, and how will she deal with his response?

For the woman who decides against abortion and chooses instead to continue the pregnancy, there are other questions. If she decides to raise the child herself, will she have the resources to do it well? Is a supportive, lasting relationship with her partner likely? If not, how does she feel about being a single parent?

If the pregnant woman considers adoption, she will have to try to predict her emotional responses throughout the full-term pregnancy and the adoption process. What are her long-range feelings likely to be? What type of adoption would be most appropriate? (The box "The Adoption Option" addresses some of these questions.)

Abortion Statistics

Abortions are fairly common in the United States. Among American women, about 50% of all pregnancies are unintended; about 40% of such pregnancies end in abortion. About 22% of all pregnancies—wanted and unwanted—end in abortion, not including those that end in miscarriage.

After the Supreme Court's ruling in *Roe v. Wade*, the number of abortions rapidly increased in the United States (Figure 6.4). According to the Guttmacher Institute (a private organization that tracks statistics on contraception and abortion), nearly 750,000 abortions occurred in 1973; the number rose each year after that, until hitting a

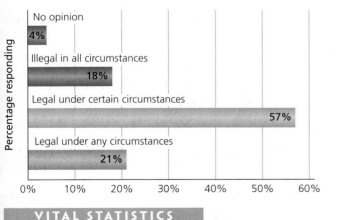

VITAL STATISTICS

FIGURE 6.3 Public opinion about abortion.

SOURCE: Gallup, Inc. 2007. *Public Divided on "Pro-Choice" vs. "Pro-Life" Abortion Labels.* http://www.gallup.com/poll/27628/Public-Divided-ProChoice-vs-ProLife-Abortion-Labels.aspx. Reprinted with permission from Gallup, Inc.

VITAL STATISTICS

FIGURE 6.4 Number of reported abortions in the United States, 1973–2005. (2005 is the most recent year for which there are reliable data.)

SOURCE: Jones, R. K., et al. 2008. Abortion in the United States: Incidence and access to services, 2005. *Perspectives on Sexual and Reproductive Health* 40(1): 6–16.

Before 1977, nearly 9% of unmarried pregnant women gave their children up for adoption. Today only 1% of women choose to place a child for adoption. This decline may be due to a variety of factors, including increased rates of contraceptive use and an easing of the social stigma of single parenthood. The drop in adoption rates in the 1970s probably reflected an increase in the abortion rate following the 1973 legalization of abortion. Since 1990, however, adoption rates have remained steady while the abortion rate has declined, indicating that women are not choosing abortion over adoption.

The decision to go through an unwanted pregnancy and then give the baby to another family is difficult. Adoption is permanent: The adoptive parents will raise the child and have legal authority for his or her welfare. Knowing this, the birth mother should think about her life now and in the future as she weighs alternatives.

Many people can help a pregnant woman consider her options, including her partner, friends, family members, a professional counselor, a crisis pregnancy center, a family planning clinic, or a family services, social services, or adoption agency. A counselor should always be respectful and willing to discuss all the options—keeping the baby, having an abortion, or arranging an adoption.

Adoptions can be confidential or open. In a confidential adoption, the birth parents and the adoptive parents never know each other. Adoptive parents receive any information they might need to take care of the child. A later meeting between the child and the birth parents is possible in confidential adoption, however, if the birth parents leave information with the agency or lawyer who handles the adoption and/or in a national adoption registry.

In an open adoption, the birth parents and adoptive parents know something about each other. There are different levels of openness, ranging from reading a brief description of prospective adoptive parents to meeting them and sharing full information. Birth parents may also be able to stay in touch with the family by visiting, calling, or writing.

In all states, a mother can work with a licensed child-placement (adoption) agency. It may also be possible to work directly with an adopting couple or their attorney; this is called a private or independent adoption.

A woman who gives a child up for adoption should also consider the reaction and rights of the birth father. A woman can choose to have an abortion without the consent or knowledge of the father, but once the baby is born, the father has certain rights. These rights vary from state to state, but at a minimum, most states require that the birth father be notified of the adoption. In some states, the birth father may be able to take the child even if the mother prefers that the child go to an adoptive family.

As with abortion, there are emotional and physical risks associated with pregnancy, childbirth, and adoption. Throughout the adoption process, the mother should make sure that she has the help she needs and that she carefully considers all her options.

SOURCES: Child Welfare Information Gateway. 2010 Update. *Are You Pregnant and Thinking About Adoption?* (http://www.childwelfare.gov/pubs/f_pregna/index.cfm; retrieved November 3, 2010); Child Welfare Information Gateway. 2010 Update. *Voluntary Relinquishment for Adoption: Numbers and Trends* (http://www.childwelfare.gov/pubs/s_place.cfm; retrieved November 18, 2010).

peak of 1.6 million in 1990. The number has steadily declined since then, and the Centers for Disease Control and Prevention reports that 846,000 legal abortions were performed in the United States in 2006, the most recent year for which data are available.

The number of late-term abortions has dropped over time, as well. In 2006, 88% of abortions occurred during the first 12 weeks (the first trimester) of pregnancy; about 1% were performed after the 20th week.

The Guttmacher Institute estimates that about 50% of American women will experience an unintended pregnancy by age 45, and more than one-third will have an abortion. Based on national research, the majority of American women who get abortions share the following characteristics:

- Are under age 25
- Have previously given birth
- Have never been married
- Are poor
- Live in a metropolitan area

Black and Hispanic women are more likely to have an abortion than white women. This disparity is likely due to limited access to and funds for contraception. Figure 6.5 provides some more statistical information about American women who choose to have abortions.

> In the United States, *the number of abortions has declined every year since 1990.*

Methods of Abortion

Abortion methods can be divided into two categories: surgical and medical. Surgical abortion is much more common than medical abortion, in which one or more drugs are used to induce abortion.

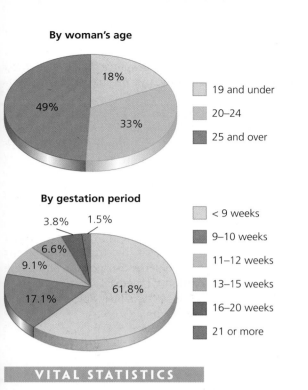

By woman's age

- 18% 19 and under
- 33% 20–24
- 49% 25 and over

By gestation period

- 61.8% < 9 weeks
- 17.1% 9–10 weeks
- 9.1% 11–12 weeks
- 6.6% 13–15 weeks
- 3.8% 16–20 weeks
- 1.5% 21 or more

FIGURE 6.5   Distribution of abortions by the woman's age and by the weeks of gestation: 2006.

SOURCE: Guttmacher Institute. 2010. *In Brief: Facts on Induced Abortion in the United States* (http://www.guttmacher.org/pubs/fb_induced_abortion.html; retrieved November 3, 2010).

First developed in China in 1958, **suction curettage** (commonly known as *dilation and curettage,* or *D & C*) is the most common method for abortions performed from the 6th to the 12th week of pregnancy. It is used in about 90% of all abortions performed in the United States. The procedure can be done quickly, usually on an outpatient basis, and the risk of complications is small.

A sedative may be given, along with a local anesthetic. A speculum is inserted into the vagina, and the cervix is cleansed with a surgical solution. The cervix is dilated and a specially designed tube, called a *suction curette,* is then inserted into the uterus. The curette is attached to the rubber tubing of an electric pump, and suction is applied. In 20–30 seconds, the uterus is emptied. Moderate cramping is common during evacuation. To ensure that no frag-

ments of tissue are left in the uterus, the doctor usually scrapes the uterine lining with a metal curette, an instrument with a spoonlike tip. The entire suction curettage procedure takes 5–10 minutes.

For more than 30 years, gynecologists have used **manual vacuum aspiration (MVA)** to manage incomplete abortions, for endometrial sampling in nonpregnant women, and for elective abortion. During this procedure, as in suction curettage, the woman receives a local anesthetic and her cervix is dilated. A plastic tube attached to a handheld syringe is inserted through the cervix and into the uterus. The syringe provides gentle suction, which empties the uterus.

MVA has several advantages over the traditional D & C. Manual vacuum aspiration may be used earlier in pregnancy, can be performed in the office, and does not require an electric pump or additional equipment. It is also significantly cheaper than suction curettage, does not require electricity, and can be performed by mid-level providers such as midwives and nurses. For these reasons, MVA is ideal for low-resource settings. A number of recent studies have shown that the two techniques have equivalent safety profiles and low rates of complications when done up to 10 weeks of gestation.

Multi-fetal (twin and higher multiple) pregnancies are associated with high fetal morbidity and mortality rates. **Multi-fetal pregnancy reduction (MFPR)** is a procedure that reduces the number of fetuses in a multiple pregnancy. It is usually performed during the first trimester. In the most common method of MFPR, the fetal heart is injected with potassium chloride. The dead fetus is then absorbed by the mother's body. Multi-fetal reduction reduces the risk of preterm delivery for the remaining fetus and improves maternal pregnancy outcomes.

Only about one in ten abortions is performed after the 12th week of pregnancy. The method most commonly used for abortion from 13 to 24 weeks of pregnancy is **dilation and evacuation (D & E).** The

> Only **8%** of U.S. abortion service providers offer abortions at 24 or more weeks of gestation.
>
> —Guttmacher Institute, 2010

QUICK STATS

manual vacuum aspiration (MVA)   The vacuum aspiration of uterine contents shortly after a missed period using a handheld syringe.

multi-fetal pregnancy reduction (MFPR)   A method of abortion used to reduce the number of fetuses in a multiple-fetus pregnancy.

dilation and evacuation (D & E)   The method of abortion most commonly used between 13 and 24 weeks of pregnancy. Following dilation of the cervix, both vacuum aspiration and curettage instruments are used as needed.

TERMS

cervix is opened using dilators, which gradually expand the cervix overnight. The next day, the uterus is emptied using surgical instruments and an aspirating machine.

Intact dilation and extraction (known controversially as *partial birth abortion*) is a surgical abortion wherein an intact fetus is removed from the uterus. Occasionally, the skull is collapsed after fetal limbs and body are delivered to allow it to pass more easily through the cervix. This procedure is performed only rarely, representing 0.17% of all abortions in the United States. Experts say that intact dilation and extraction can be useful when certain fetal anomalies are present, such as severe hydrocephalus (swelling of the fetus's head), and that the procedure may be the safest option for the mother in some circumstances. Intact dilation and extraction became illegal after the 2007 Supreme Court ruling in the case of *Gonzales v. Carhart,* even in situations where the mother's health may be in jeopardy.

Medical abortion is generally used in very early pregnancy, within 49 days of the last menstrual period. The combination of drugs that is given causes the embryo and products of conception to be passed out through the vagina, as in a natural miscarriage. Mifepristone, misoprostol, and methotrexate are three widely used drugs.

Medical abortion is generally safer than surgical abortion because it involves no anesthesia or surgical risks. Some women feel that medical abortion allows them to take more control of the procedure and gives them more privacy than a surgical abortion would. The major disadvantages are that the process takes days or even weeks to complete and that bleeding after the procedure is often heavier and lasts longer than with surgical abortion. Medical abortion also generally requires more clinic visits than surgical abortion. The cost to the patient is generally about the same.

Complications of Abortion

Along with questions regarding the actual procedure of abortion, many people have concerns about possible aftereffects. More information is gradually being gathered on this important subject.

Abortion-related mortality rates have declined substantially since abortion was legalized in 1973.

Possible Physical Effects   The incidence of immediate problems following an abortion (infection, bleeding, trauma to the cervix or uterus, and incomplete abortion requiring repeat curettage) varies widely. The potential for problems is significantly reduced by a woman's good health, early timing of the abortion, use of the suction method, performance by a well-trained clinician, and the availability and use of prompt follow-up care.

Problems related to infection can be minimized through preabortion testing and treatment for gonorrhea, chlamydia, and other infections. Postabortion danger signs are fever above 100°F, abdominal pain or swelling, cramping or backache, abdominal tenderness (to pressure), prolonged or heavy bleeding, foul-smelling vaginal discharge, vomiting or fainting, and delay in resuming menstrual periods (6 weeks or more).

Some cramping and bleeding are an expected part of ending a pregnancy. In rare cases, life-threatening bleeding, infections, or other problems can occur following a miscarriage, surgical abortion, or medical abortion. Prompt medical attention should be sought if heavy bleeding, severe abdominal pain, or fever occurs.

Possible Psychological Effects   After an exhaustive review completed in 1988, then surgeon general C. Everett Koop concluded that the available evidence failed to demonstrate either a negative or a positive long-term impact of abortion on mental health. More recent research has resulted in the same general conclusion. The frequency of any psychiatric diagnoses in women who have undergone an abortion procedure is no higher than in women with no such history.

The psychological side effects of abortion, however, are less clearly defined than the physical ones. Responses vary and depend on the individual woman's psychological makeup, family background, current personal and social relationships, cultural attitudes, and many other factors. A woman who has specific goals with a somewhat structured life may be able to incorporate her decision to have an abortion as the unequivocally best and most acceptable course more easily than a woman who feels uncertain about her future.

Although many women experience great relief after an abortion and virtually no negative feelings, some go through a period of ambivalence. Along with relief, they often feel a mixture of other responses, such as guilt, regret, loss, sadness, and/or anger. For a woman who experiences psychological or emotional effects after an abortion, talking with a close friend or family member can be very

---

TERMS

intact dilation and extraction   A rarely used method of late-term abortion, wherein an intact fetus is removed from the uterus.

Ask Yourself

QUESTIONS FOR CRITICAL THINKING AND REFLECTION

Suppose you are in the position of lending support to a friend who has gone through an abortion. What sort of physical or emotional signals would you look for? What kind of support would you be willing to offer?

TIPS FOR TODAY AND THE FUTURE

Your decisions about contraception are among the most important you will make in your life. You may never have to face an unintended pregnancy, but you should know what choices you would have, as well as where you stand on the issue of abortion.

RIGHT NOW YOU CAN

- If you're sexually active, consider whether you are confident that you're doing everything possible to prevent an unwanted pregnancy. Remember that no method of contraception is 100% effective.
- If you're sexually active, discuss your contraceptive method with your partner. Make sure you are using the method that works best for you.
- Work with your partner to choose a backup contraceptive method to use in case your primary method isn't effective enough.
- Examine your feelings about the possibility of becoming a parent, especially if it were to happen unintentionally.
- Consider your views on the morality of abortion, and whether it is acceptable under certain circumstances.

IN THE FUTURE YOU CAN

- Talk to your physician about contraception and get his or her advice on choosing the best method.
- Occasionally discuss your contraceptive method with your partner to make sure it continues to meet your needs. A change in health status or lifestyle may make a different form of contraception preferable in the future.
- If you are sexually active or plan to become sexually active, talk to your partner about abortion. Do you share similar views and feelings, or are they different? How would you resolve conflicts about this issue?

Connect to Your Choices

Have you ever thought about why you choose the contraceptive methods you use—or choose not to use? Many factors can influence the contraceptive choices we make, some not as obvious as others. Do you choose what's readily available in pharmacies because you don't want to go to a clinic, even if another method might be more appropriate or effective for you? Do you use a method your health care provider recommended, even though you don't like it? Do you go along with your partner's preferences because it's easier than saying what you would like?

What are the external factors that influence your choices about contraception? What are your inner motivations and core values, and how do they affect your choices? Based on what you learned in this chapter, will you make some different choices in the future? If so, what will they be?

Go online to Connect to complete this activity. www.mcgraw-hillconnect.com

helpful. Supportive people can help her feel positive about herself and her decision. If unresolved emotions persist, a woman should seek professional counseling.

SUMMARY

- The choice of contraceptive method depends on effectiveness, convenience, cost, reversibility, side effects and risk factors, protection against STDs, and noncontraceptive benefits.

- Hormonal methods may include a combination of estrogen and progestins or progestins alone. Hormones may be delivered via pills, patch, vaginal ring, implants, or injections. They prevent ovulation, inhibit the movement of sperm, and affect the uterine lining so that implantation is prevented.

- IUDs can provide very effective long-term (5 to 10 years) contraception and are especially useful for women who have already been pregnant and are in monogamous relationships.

- Male condoms are simple to use, immediately reversible, and provide STD protection; female condoms can be inserted hours before intercourse.

- The diaphragm, cervical cap, and contraceptive sponge cover the cervix and block sperm from entering; all are used with or contain spermicide.

- The most commonly used emergency contraceptives are Plan B One-Step and Next Choice, which are now available without a prescription to men and women 17 and older.

- Vaginal spermicides come in the form of foams, creams, jellies, suppositories, and film.

- So-called natural methods include abstinence, withdrawal, and fertility awareness-based methods.

- Vasectomy—male sterilization—involves severing the vasa deferentia. Female sterilization involves severing or blocking the oviducts.

- Issues to be considered in choosing a contraceptive include the individual health risks of each method, the implications of an unplanned pregnancy, STD risk, convenience and comfort level, type of relationship, the cost and ease of obtaining and maintaining each method, and religious or philosophical beliefs.

- The 1973 *Roe v. Wade* Supreme Court case devised new standards to govern abortion decisions; based on the trimesters of pregnancy, it limited a woman's choices as her pregnancy advanced.

- Although the Supreme Court continued to uphold its 1973 decision, later rulings gave states further power to regulate abortion.

- The controversy between pro-life and pro-choice viewpoints focuses on the issue of when life begins. Overall public opinion in the United States supports legal abortion in at least some circumstances and opposes overturning *Roe v. Wade.*

- Methods of abortion include suction curettage, manual vacuum aspiration, dilation and evacuation, and dilation and extraction.

- Physical complications following abortion can be minimized by overall good patient health, early timing, use of the suction method, a well-trained physician, and follow-up care. Psychological aftereffects of abortion vary with the individual.

FOR MORE INFORMATION

BOOKS

Alters, S. M., ed. 2010. *Abortion: An Eternal Social and Moral Issue* (Information Plus Reference Series). Farmington Hills, Mich.: Gale Cengage. *A brief reference outlining legal, political, and ethical issues.*

Glasier, A., and B. Winikoff. 2009. *Fast Facts: Contraception,* 3rd ed. Oxford: Health Press. *Basic facts and figures related to contraceptive methods. Succinct and easy to read.*

Hatcher, R. A., et al. 2008. *Contraceptive Technology,* 19th ed. New York: Ardent Media. *A reliable source of up-to-date information on contraception.*

National Abortion and Reproductive Rights Action League Foundation. 2008. *Who Decides? A State-by-State Review of Abortion and Reproductive Rights.* Washington, D.C.: NARAL Foundation. *An in-depth annual review of the legal status of reproductive rights in the United States.*

Zieman, M., et al. 2010. *A Pocket Guide to Managing Contraception,* 2010–2012 ed. Tiger, Ga.: Bridging the Gap Foundation. *An easy-to-use, reliable source of contraceptive information.*

ORGANIZATIONS AND WEB SITES

Association of Reproductive Health Professionals. Offers educational materials about family planning, contraception, and other reproductive health issues; the Web site includes an interactive questionnaire to help people choose contraceptive methods.
http://www.arhp.org

Emergency Contraception Web Site. Provides extensive information about emergency contraception; sponsored by the Office of Population Research at Princeton University.
http://www.not-2-late.com
http://ec.princeton.edu

The Guttmacher Institute. A nonprofit institute for reproductive health research, policy analysis, and public education.
http://guttmacher.org

Managing Contraception. Provides brief descriptions and tips for using many forms of contraception. Features a detailed survey to help with contraceptive choices.
http://www.managingcontraception.com

MedlinePlus: Abortion. Managed by the National Library of Medicine and the National Institutes of Health, this site provides a list of informational resources on various aspects of abortion.
http://www.nlm.nih.gov/medlineplusl/abortion.html

National Abortion and Reproductive Rights Action League. Provides information on the politics of the pro-choice movement. Also provides information on the abortion laws and politics in each state.
http://www.naral.org

National Abortion Federation. Provides information and resources on the medical and political issues relating to abortion; managed by health care providers.
http://www.prochoice.org

National Adoption Center. A national agency focused on finding adoptive homes for children with special needs or who are currently in foster care.
http://www.adopt.org

National Right to Life Committee. Provides information on alternatives to abortion and the politics of the pro-life movement.
http://www.nrlc.org

Planned Parenthood Federation of America. Provides information on family planning, contraception, and abortion and provides counseling services.
http://www.plannedparenthood.org

SELECTED BIBLIOGRAPHY

American College of Obstetricians and Gynecologists. 2010. *Birth Control Pills* (http://www.acog.org/publications/patient_education/bp021.cfm; retrieved October 29, 2010).

Brohet, R. M., et al. 2007. Oral contraceptives and breast cancer risk in the international BRCA 1/2 carrier cohort study: Areport from EMBRACE, GENEPSO, GEOHEBON, and the IBCCS Collaborating Group. *Journal of Clinical Oncology* 25(25): 3831–3836.

Burkman, R. T. 2007. Transdermal hormonal contraception: Benefits and risks. *American Journal of Obstetrics and Gynecology* 197(2): 134.el–134.e6.

Centers for Disease Control and Prevention. 2010. Abortion surveillance—United States, 2006. *Morbidity and Mortality Weekly Report* 58 (SS08): 1–35.

Coffee, A. L., et al. 2007. Long-term assessment of symptomatology and satisfaction of an extended oral contraceptive regimen. *Contraception* 75(6): 444–449.

Dailey, Kate. 2010. A better female condom. *Newsweek.* March 10, 2010 (http://www.newsweek.com/id/234700/page/1; retrieved October 29, 2010).

Diedrich, J., et al. 2010. Induction of fetal demise before abortion. *Contraception* 81(6): 462–473.

Ely, G. E., and C. N. Dulmus. 2010. Disparities in access to reproductive health options for female adolescents. *Social Work in Public Health* 25(3): 341–351.

Fine, Paul, et al. 2010. Ulipristal acetate taken 48–120 hours after intercourse for emergency contraception. *Obstetrics and Gynecology* 115: 257–263.

Frost, J. J., et al. 2007. Factors associated with contraceptive use and non-use, United States, 2004. *Perspectives on Sexual and Reproductive Health* 39(2): 90–99.

Guttmacher Institute. 2010. *Facts on American Teens' Sexual and Reproductive Health* (http://www.guttmacher.org/pubs/FB-ATSRH.html; retrieved November 3, 2010).

Guttmacher Institute. 2010. *Facts on Induced Abortion in the United States* (http://www.guttmacher.org/pubs/fb_induced_abortion.html; retrieved November 3, 2010).

Guttmacher Institute. 2010. *State Policies in Brief: An Overview of Abortion Laws* (http://www.guttmacher.org/statecenter/spibs/spib_OAL.pdf; retrieved November 3, 2010).

Guttmacher Institute. 2010. *U.S. Teenage Pregnancies, Births and Abortions: National and State Trends and Trends by Race and Ethnicity* (http://www.guttmacher.org/pubs/USTPtrends.pdf; retrieved October 29, 2010).

Hannaford, P. C., et al. 2010. Mortality among contraceptive pill users: Cohort evidence from Royal College of General Practitioners' Oral Contraception Study. *British Medical Journal*, 2010; DOI: 10.1136/bmj.c927.

Leung, V., et al. 2010. Mechanisms of action of hormonal emergency contraceptives. *Pharmacotherapy* 30(2): 158–168.

Macaluso., M., et al. 2007. Efficacy of the male latex condom and of the female polyurethane condom as barriers to semen during intercourse: A randomized clinical trial. *American Journal of Epidemiology* 166(1): 88–96.

MacIsaac, L., and E. Espey. 2007. Intrauterine contraception: The pendulum swings back. *Obstetrics and Gynecology Clinics of North America* 34(1): 91–111.

Moreau, C., et al. 2007. Oral contraceptive tolerance: Does the type of pill matter? *Obstetrics and Gynecology* 109(6): 1277–1285.

Nettleman, M. D., et al. 2007. Reasons for unprotected intercourse: Analysis of the PRAMS survey. *Contraception* 75(5): 361–366.

Planned Parenthood. 2007. *Abortion After the First Trimester in the United States* (http://www.plannedparenthood.org/news-articles-press/politics/policyissues/abortion-access/trimester-abortion-6140.htm; retrieved February 3, 2009).

Roumen, F. J. 2007. The contraceptive vaginal ring compared with the combined oral contraceptive pill: A comprehensive review of randomized controlled trials. *Contraception* 75(6): 420–429.

Sifris, R. 2010. Restrictive regulation of abortion and the right to health. *Medical Law Review* 18(2): 182–212.

Sit, D., et al. 2007. Psychiatric outcomes following medical and surgical abortion. *Human Reproduction* 22(3): 878–884.

Westhoff, C. L., et al. 2007. Oral contraceptive discontinuation: Do side effects matter? *American Journal of Obstetrics and Gynecology* 196(4): 412.e1–412.e6; discussion 412.e6–412.e7.

LOOKING AHEAD...

After reading this chapter, you should be able to:

- Define and discuss the concepts of addictive behavior, substance abuse, and substance dependence

- Explain factors contributing to drug use and dependence

- List the major categories of psychoactive drugs and describe their effects, methods of use, and potential for abuse and dependence

- Discuss social issues related to psychoactive drug use and prevention and treatment

- Evaluate the role of drugs and other addictive behaviors in your life and identify your risk factors for abuse or dependence

7

The Use and Abuse of Psychoactive Drugs

The use of **drugs** for both medical and social purposes is widespread in America (Table 7.1). Many people believe that every problem has or should have a chemical solution. For fatigue, many turn to caffeine; for insomnia, sleeping pills; for anxiety or boredom, alcohol or other recreational drugs. Advertisements, social pressures, and the human desire for quick solutions to life's difficult problems all contribute to the prevailing attitude that drugs can ease all pain. But benefits often come with consequences, and drug use can—and, in many cases, does—pose serious or even life-threatening ones.

The most serious consequences are abuse and **addiction.** The drugs most often associated with abuse are **psychoactive drugs**—those that alter a person's experiences or consciousness. In the short term, psychoactive drugs can cause **intoxication,** a state in which sometimes unpredictable physical and emotional changes occur. A person who is intoxicated may experience serious changes in physical functioning. His or her emotions and judgment may be affected in ways that lead to uncharacteristic and unsafe behavior. In the long term, recurrent drug use can have profound physical, emotional, and social effects.

ADDICTIVE BEHAVIOR

Although addiction is most often associated with drug use, many experts now extend the concept of addiction to other behaviors. **Addictive behaviors** are habits that have gotten out of control, with resulting negative effects on a person's health.

What Is Addiction?

Historically, the term *addiction* was applied only when the habitual use of a drug produced chemical changes in the user's body. One such change is physical **tolerance,** in which the body adapts to a drug so that the initial dose no longer produces the original emotional or psychological effects. This process, caused by chemical changes, means the user has to take larger and larger doses of the drug to achieve the same high. The concept of addiction as a disease process, one based in brain chemistry rather than a moral failing, has led to many advances in the understanding and treatment of drug addiction.

Some scientists think that other behaviors may share some of the chemistry of drug addiction. They suggest

Table 7.1 — Nonmedical Drug Use Among Americans, 2008

	PERCENTAGE USING SUBSTANCE IN THE PAST 30 DAYS		
	COLLEGE-AGE AMERICANS		ALL AMERICANS
	AGE 18–20	AGE 21–25	AGE 12 & OLDER
ILLICIT DRUGS	21.5	18.4	8.0
Marijuana and hashish	18.7	15.0	6.1
Cocaine	1.6	1.5	0.7
Crack	0.2	0.2	0.1
Heroin	0.2	0.2	0.1
Methamphetamine	0.1	0.3	0.1
Hallucinogens	2.3	1.3	0.4
LSD	0.3	0.3	0.1
PCP	0.0	0.0	0.0
Ecstasy	1.3	0.6	0.2
Inhalants	0.5	0.2	0.3
Nonmedical use of psychotherapeutics	6.0	5.8	2.5
Pain relievers	4.8	4.4	1.9
OxyContin	0.4	0.4	0.2
Tranquilizers	1.7	1.7	0.7
Stimulants	1.0	1.1	0.4
Sedatives	0.1	0.3	0.1
TOBACCO (ALL FORMS)	39.6	42.6	28.4
Cigarettes	33.5	37.1	23.9
Smokeless tobacco	5.8	5.1	3.5
Cigars	13.4	9.9	5.3
Pipe tobacco	1.9	1.9	0.8
ALCOHOL	48.7	69.5	51.6
Binge alcohol use	33.7	46.0	23.3

SOURCE: Substance Abuse and Mental Health Services Administration. 2009. *Results from the 2008 National Survey on Drug Use and Health: National Findings.* Rockville, Md.: Office of Applied Studies, NSDUH Series H-36, HHS Publication No. SMA 09-4434.

that activities like gambling, eating, exercising, and sex release brain chemicals that cause a pleasurable rush in much the same way that psychoactive drugs do. The brain's own chemicals thus become the "drug" that can cause addiction. These theorists suggest that all addictions have a common mechanism in the brain. In this view, addiction is partly the result of our own natural wiring. This view does not mean that people are not responsible for their addictive behavior, however.

Characteristics of Addictive Behavior

Experts have identified some general characteristics typically associated with addictive behaviors:

- *Reinforcement.* Addictive behaviors reinforce themselves. The behavior either produces pleasurable physical and/or emotional states, or relieves negative ones.

- *Compulsion or craving.* The addict feels a strong compulsion—a compelling need—to engage in the behavior, often accompanied by obsessive planning for the next opportunity to perform it.

- *Loss of control.* The addict loses control over the behavior and cannot block the impulse to do it.

- *Escalation.* Addiction often involves a pattern of escalation: More and more of the substance or activity is required to produce its desired effects.

- *Negative consequences.* The behavior continues despite serious negative consequences, such as problems with academic or job performance, personal relationships, and health; legal or financial troubles are also typical.

The Development of Addiction

An addiction often starts when a person does something to bring pleasure or avoid pain. The activity may be drinking a beer, using the Internet, playing the lottery, or going shopping. If it works, the person is likely to repeat it. He or she becomes increasingly dependent on the behavior, and tolerance may develop; that is, the person needs more of the behavior to feel the same effect. Eventually, the behavior becomes a central focus of the person's life, and there is a deterioration in other areas, such as school performance or relationships. The behavior no longer brings pleasure, but it is necessary to avoid the pain of going without it. What started as a seemingly innocent way of feeling good becomes a prison.

Although many common behaviors are potentially addictive, most people who engage in them do not develop problems. The reason lies in the combination of factors that are involved in the development of addiction, including personality, lifestyle, heredity, the social and physical environment, and the nature of the substance or behavior in question.

TERMS

drug Any chemical other than food intended to affect the structure or function of the body.

addiction Psychological or physical dependence on a substance or behavior, characterized by a compulsive desire and increasing need for the substance or behavior and by harm to the individual and/or society.

psychoactive drug A drug that can alter a person's consciousness or experience.

intoxication The state of being mentally affected by a chemical (literally, a state of being poisoned).

addictive behavior Any habit that has gotten out of control, resulting in a negative effect on one's health.

tolerance A physical state in which the body adapts to a drug so that the initial dose no longer produces the original emotional or psychological effects.

Many college students have gotten caught up in the poker craze.

Characteristics of People with Addictions

The causes and course of an addiction are extremely varied, but people with addictions (commonly referred to as *addicts*) seem to share some characteristics. Many use a substance or activity as a substitute for healthier coping strategies. People vary in their ability to manage their lives, and those who have the most trouble dealing with stress and painful emotions may be more susceptible to addiction.

Some people may have a genetic predisposition to addiction to a particular substance; such predispositions may involve variations in brain chemistry. People with addictive disorders usually have a distinct preference for a particular addictive behavior. They also often have problems with impulse control and self-regulation, and tend to be risk-takers.

Examples of Addictive Behaviors

Behaviors that are not related to drugs can become addictive for some people, such as eating, watching TV, and playing video games. Any substance or activity that becomes the focus of a person's life at the expense of other needs and interests can be damaging to health.

Compulsive Gambling   Compulsive gamblers cannot control the urge to gamble, even in the face of ruin. The consequences of compulsive gambling are not just financial; the suicide rate of compulsive gamblers is 20 times higher than that of the general population. About 1% of adult Americans are compulsive (pathological) gamblers, and another 2% are "problem gamblers." Some 42% of college students gamble at least once in a year, and about 3% gamble at least once a week.

The American Psychiatric Association (APA) recognizes pathological gambling as a mental disorder and lists ten characteristic behaviors, including preoccupation with gambling, unsuccessful efforts to cut back or quit, and lying to family members to conceal the extent of gambling. Gambling is often linked to other risky behaviors; many compulsive gamblers also have drug and alcohol abuse problems.

Compulsive Exercising   Compulsive exercising is now recognized as a serious departure from normal behavior. It is often accompanied by more severe psychiatric disorders such as anorexia nervosa or bulimia. Traits frequently associated with compulsive exercising include an excessive preoccupation and dissatisfaction with body image, the use of laxatives or vomiting to lose weight, and the development of other obsessive-compulsive symptoms.

Work Addiction   People who are excessively preoccupied with work are often called *workaholics*. Work addiction, however, is actually based on a set of specific symptoms, including: an intense work schedule, the inability to limit one's own work schedule, the inability to relax, even when away from work, and failed attempts at curtailing the intensity of work (in some cases).

Work addicts are likely to neglect other aspects of life. For example, work addicts may tend to exercise less, spend less time with family and friends, and stay away from social activities.

Work addiction typically coincides with a well-known risk factor for cardiovascular disease—the Type A personality. Traits associated with Type A personality include competitiveness, ambition, drive, time urgency, restlessness, hyperalertness, and hostility.

Sex and Love Addiction   Behaviors associated with sex addiction include an extreme preoccupation with sex, a compulsion to have sex repeatedly in a given period of time, spending a great deal of time and energy looking for partners or having sex, using sex as a means of relieving painful feelings, and suffering negative emotional, personal, and professional consequences as a result of sexual activities.

Have you ever repeatedly or compulsively engaged in a behavior that had negative consequences? What was the behavior, and why did you continue? Did you ever worry that you were losing control? Were you able to bring the behavior under control?

Even therapists who challenge the concept of sex addiction recognize that some people become overly preoccupied with sex, cannot seem to control their sex drive, and act in potentially harmful ways in order to stay satisfied. This pattern of sexual behavior seems to meet the criteria for addictive behaviors discussed earlier.

Compulsive Buying or Shopping A compulsive buyer repeatedly gives in to the impulse to buy more than he or she needs or can afford. Compulsive spenders usually buy luxury items rather than daily necessities, even though they are usually distressed by their behavior and its social, personal, and financial consequences. Some experts link compulsive shopping with neglect or abuse during childhood; it also seems to be associated with eating disorders, depression, and bipolar disorder.

Internet Addiction Millions of Americans have become compulsive Internet users—as much as 10% of the U.S. population, by some estimates. To spend more time online, Internet addicts skip other important activities. Compulsive Internet users often spend their work time online, which has led many employers to adopt strict Internet usage policies. Despite negative financial, social, or academic consequences, compulsive Internet users don't feel able to stop. As with other addictive behaviors, online addicts may be using their behavior to alleviate stress or avoid painful emotions.

DRUG USE, ABUSE, AND DEPENDENCE

Drugs are chemicals other than food that are intended to affect the structure or function of the body. They include prescription medicines such as antibiotics and antidepressants; nonprescription or over-the-counter (OTC) substances such as alcohol, tobacco, and caffeine products; and illegal substances such as LSD and heroin.

Drug Abuse and Dependence

The APA's *Diagnostic and Statistical Manual of Mental Disorders* is the authoritative reference for defining all sorts of behavioral disorders, including those related to drugs.

The APA has chosen not to use the term *addiction,* in part because it is so broad and has so many connotations. Instead, the APA refers to two forms of substance (drug) disorders: substance abuse and substance dependence. Both are maladaptive patterns of substance use that lead to significant impairment or distress. Although the APA's definitions are more precise and more directly related to drug use, they clearly encompass the general characteristics of addictive behavior described in the preceding section.

Abuse As defined by the APA, **substance abuse** involves one or more of the following characteristics:

- Recurrent drug use, resulting in a failure to fulfill major responsibilities at work, school, or home
- Recurrent drug use in situations in which it is physically hazardous, such as before or while driving
- Recurrent drug-related legal problems
- Continued drug use despite persistent social or interpersonal problems caused or worsened by the effects of the drug

The pattern of use may be constant or intermittent, and **physical dependence** may or may not be present. For example, a person who smokes marijuana once a week and cuts classes because he or she is high is abusing marijuana, even though he or she is not physically dependent.

Dependence **Substance dependence** is a more complex disorder and is what many people associate with the idea of addiction. The seven specific criteria the APA uses to diagnose substance dependence are listed below. The first two are associated with physical dependence; the final five are associated with compulsive use. To be considered dependent, one must experience a cluster of three or more of these symptoms during a 12-month period.

1. *Developing tolerance to the substance.* When a person requires increased amounts of a substance to achieve the desired effect or notices a markedly diminished effect with continued use of the same amount, he or she has developed tolerance to the substance.

---

substance abuse A maladaptive pattern of using any substance that persists despite adverse social, psychological, or medical consequences. The pattern may be intermittent, with or without tolerance and physical dependence.

physical dependence The result of physiological adaptation that occurs in response to the frequent presence of a drug; typically associated with tolerance and withdrawal.

substance dependence A cluster of cognitive, behavioral, and physiological symptoms that occur in someone who continues to use a substance despite suffering significant substance-related problems, leading to significant impairment or distress; also known as *addiction.*

Drug Use Among College Students

By some measures of substance abuse, double-digit prevalence is the defining characteristic of drug use on college campuses for certain drugs.

According to the most recent survey data from the Substance Abuse and Mental Health Services Administration (SAMHSA), 21.5% of young adults age 18–20 reported using an illicit drug in the past 30 days (see Table 7.1). This number represents a slight decline from 2007. The same survey shows that past-month tobacco use increased slightly and binge drinking decreased significantly, while marijuana and cocaine use remained steady.

Other surveys show that recreational drug use is fairly common among college students. According to the 2009 American College Health Association—National College Health Assessment, more than 12% of college students reported using marijuana at least once in the past 30 days. Another 13% said they had used some other drug at least once in the past 30 days.

Family history, peer pressure, depression, anxiety, low self-esteem, and the dynamics of college life (for example, the drive to compete and distorted perception of drug use among peers) have been suggested as potential explanations for drug use.

Excessive alcohol use often accompanies illicit drug use. In fact, the term *AOD* (Alcohol and Other Drug) has been coined to refer to this type of substance use among college students. Further, AOD use and depression and/or anxiety are generally recognized as coexisting conditions that require a comprehensive approach to prevention and treatment. Despite the growing awareness among college counselors and other health professionals who work with college students, it is not entirely clear whether anxiety and depression precede the onset of alcohol and drug use or whether early pre-college exposure to alcohol and drug use exacerbates more serious psychiatric disorders by the time a student enters college. A third line of research suggests that AOD use, depression, and anxiety share common causes such as genetic predisposition and/or family history.

However, one aspect of drug use among college students remains clear: AOD use has dramatic consequences for the educational, family, and community life of students. Poor academic performance has been linked with AOD use. Further, driving while intoxicated remains one of the most dangerous outcomes associated with AOD use affecting families and communities.

---

2. *Experiencing withdrawal.* In someone who has maintained prolonged, heavy use of a substance, a drop in its concentration within the body can result in unpleasant physical and cognitive **withdrawal** symptoms. For example, nausea, vomiting, and tremors are common for alcohol, opioids, and sedatives. Some drugs have no significant withdrawal symptoms.

3. *Taking the substance in larger amounts or over a longer period than was originally intended.*

4. *Expressing a persistent desire to cut down or regulate substance use.*

5. *Spending a great deal of time getting the substance, using it, or recovering from its effects.*

6. *Giving up or reducing important social, school, work, or recreational activities because of substance use.*

7. *Continuing to use the substance despite the knowledge that it is contributing to a psychological or physical problem.*

If a drug-dependent person experiences either tolerance or withdrawal, he or she is considered physically dependent. However, not everyone who experiences tolerance or withdrawal is drug dependent, and dependence can occur without a physical component, based solely on compulsive use.

Who Uses Drugs?

Drug use and abuse occur at all income and education levels, among all ethnic groups, and across all age groups (see the box "Drug Use Among College Students"). Society is concerned with the casual or recreational use of illegal drugs because it is not really possible to know when it will lead to abuse or dependence. Some casual users develop substance-related problems; others do not. Some drugs are more likely than others to lead to dependence (Table 7.2), but even some heroin or cocaine users do not meet the APA's criteria for substance dependence.

> *Drug dependence can occur without a physical component (tolerance or withdrawal), based solely on compulsive use.*

It isn't possible to accurately predict which drug users will become abusers, but young people at a high risk of *trying* drugs share certain characteristics:

- *Being young.* People who start using drugs when they're very young have a greater risk of dependence and health consequences.

- *Being male.* Males are twice as likely as females to abuse illicit drugs (see the box "Gender Differences in Drug Use").

- *Being a troubled adolescent.* Teens are more likely to try drugs if they have poor self-image or self-control,

Gender Differences in Drug Use

Men are more likely than women to use, abuse, and be dependent on illicit drugs. Rates of use are similar in males and females age 12–17, but among those 18 and older, more men than women use drugs and have problems associated with drug use (see table). Men account for about 80% of arrests for drug abuse violations, 70% of admissions for treatment, and 65% of drug-related deaths.

There are also gender differences in why and how young people use drugs. Young males tend to use alcohol or drugs for sensation seeking or to enhance their social status, factors tied to culturally based gender roles. Young women tend to use drugs to improve mood, increase confidence, and reduce inhibitions. Boys are likelier to receive offers to use drugs in public settings, whereas girls are likelier to receive offers in a private place such as a friend's residence.

Despite overall lower rates of drug use, females may have unique biological vulnerabilities to certain drugs, and they may move more quickly from use to abuse. Major life transitions, including the physical and emotional changes associated with puberty, increase the risk of drug use and abuse for girls more so than for boys. Certain other drug abuse risk factors are also more common in female adolescents, including depression, low self-esteem, eating disorders, and a history of physical or sexual abuse.

Adolescent boys and girls share some protective factors relating to drug abuse, including positive family relationships and extracurricular activities; religious involvement is protective for both boys and girls but may be more protective for girls.

Among older men and women, marriage, children, and employment are associated with lower rates of drug abuse and dependence. Rates of drug abuse and dependence among married adults are less than half of those among unmarried adults. Similar patterns are seen in adults who live with children versus those who do not live with children and adults who are employed versus those who are unemployed.

	National Survey Results: Percent Reporting in Past Year	
	Males	Females
Illicit drug use*	16.4	12.2
Age 12–17	19.0	18.9
Age 18–25	36.9	29.9
Age 26 and older	12.3	8.5
Drove under the influence of an illicit drug	5.5	2.6
Illicit drug or alcohol abuse or dependence	11.5	6.4
Treatment for drug dependence	2.2	1.0

*Illicit drugs include marijuana/hashish, cocaine, heroin, hallucinogens, inhalants, and prescription-type psychotherapeutics used nonmedically.

SOURCE: Substance Abuse and Mental Health Services Administration. 2009. *Results from the 2008 National Survey on Drug Use and Health: National Findings.* Rockville, Md.: Office of Applied Studies, NSDUH Series H-36, HHS Publication No. SMA 09–4434.

Table 7.2	Psychoactive Drugs and Their Potential for Producing Dependence	
	POTENTIAL FOR DEPENDENCE	
DRUG	**PHYSICAL**	**PSYCHOLOGICAL**
Heroin	High	High
Morphine	High	High
Hydrocodone	High	High
Oxycodone	High	High
Codeine	Moderate	Moderate
Gamma hydroxybutric acid	Moderate	Moderate
Benzodiazepines	Moderate	Moderate
Cocaine	Possible	High
Amphetamine/ methamphetamine	Possible	High
Methylphenidate	Possible	High
MDMA (ecstasy)	None	Moderate
LSD	None	Unknown
PCP	Possible	High
Marijuana	Unknown	Moderate
Hashish	Unknown	Moderate
Alcohol	High	High

SOURCE: U.S. Department of Justice, Drug Administration. 2005. *Drugs of Abuse.* Washington, D.C.: U.S. Department of Justice.

use tobacco, or suffer from certain mental or emotional problems.

- *Being a thrill-seeker.* A sense of invincibility is a factor in drug experimentation.
- *Being in a dysfunctional family.* A chaotic home life or parental abuse increases the risk of drug use. The same is true for children from a single-parent home or whose parents didn't complete high school.
- *Being in a peer group that accepts drug use.* Young people who are uninterested in school and earn poor grades are more likely to try drugs.
- *Being poor.* Young people who live in disadvantaged areas are more likely to be around drugs at a young age.
- *Dating young.* Adolescent girls who date boys two or more years older than themselves are more likely to use drugs.

What about people who *don't* use drugs? As a group, nonusers also share some characteristics. Not surprisingly, people who perceive drug use as risky and who disapprove of it are less likely to use drugs than those who believe otherwise. Drug use is also less common among people who have positive self-esteem and self-concept and who are assertive, independent thinkers who are not

Spirituality and Drug Abuse

Although there are diverse religious viewpoints on drug use, many religions infer some link between psychoactive drugs and spirituality. Some religions use drugs in the quest for spiritual transcendence: American Indian, Polynesian, African, and other indigenous religions have used psychoactive drugs such as peyote, khat, alcohol, and hashish for expanding consciousness and developing personal spirituality. Other religions view psychoactive drugs as a threat to spirituality. In Islam, for example, the consumption of alcohol and certain other drugs is strictly forbidden.

In studies of American teens and adults, spiritual or religious involvement is generally associated with a lower risk of trying psychoactive drugs and, for those who do use drugs, a lower risk of heavy use and dependence. Possible reasons include the adoption of a strict code of behavior or set of principles that forbids drug use, the presence of a social support system for abstinence or mod-

eration, and the promotion of values that include avoidance of drug use.

The relationship between religious faith and avoidance of drug use appears to be even stronger in teens than in adults. Teens who attend 25 or more religious services per year are about half as likely to use illicit drugs as teens who attend services less frequently. Overall, people who spend time regularly engaging in spiritual practices such as prayer and transcendental meditation have lower rates of drug abuse.

People with current substance-abuse problems tend to have lower rates of religious affiliation and involvement and lower levels of spiritual wellness, characterized by a lack of a sense of meaning in life. One of the hallmarks of drug dependence is spending increasing amounts of time and energy getting and using drugs. Such a pattern of behavior inevitably reduces the resources one can devote to developing physical, emotional, and spiritual wellness.

Among people in treatment for substance abuse, higher levels of religious faith and spirituality may contribute to the recovery process. A study of people recovering from alcohol or other drug abuse found that spirituality and religiousness were associated with increased coping skills, greater optimism about life, greater resilience to stress, and greater perceived social support. More research is needed to clarify the relationships among spirituality, religion, drug use, and recovery. Although behaviors such as prayer or meditation can be measured, it is more difficult to determine what such practices mean to the individual.

SOURCES: Brown, A. E., et al. 2006. Alcohol recovery and spirituality: Strangers, friends, or partners? *Southern Medical Journal* 99(6): 654–657; Substance Abuse and Mental Health Network. 2004. Religious beliefs and substance use among youths. *NSDUH Report*, January; Dunn, M. S. 2005. The relationship between religiosity, employment, and political beliefs on substance use among high school seniors. *Journal of Alcohol and Drug Education* 49(1): 73.

controlled by peer pressure. Self-control, social competence, optimism, academic achievement, and regular church attendance are also linked to lower rates of drug use. Home environments are also influential: Coming from a strong family, one that has a clear policy on drug use, is another characteristic of people who don't use drugs (see the box "Spirituality and Drug Abuse").

Why Do People Use Drugs?

Young people, especially those from middle-class backgrounds, are frequently drawn to drugs by the allure of the exciting and illegal. They may be curious, rebellious, or vulnerable to peer pressure. Young people may want to imitate adult models in their lives or in the movies. Most people who take illicit drugs do so experimentally, typically trying the drug one or more times but not continuing. The main factors in the initial choice of a drug are whether it is available and whether peers are using it.

Although some people use drugs because they have a desire to alter their mood or are seeking a spiritual experience, others are motivated by a desire to escape boredom, anxiety, depression, feelings of worthlessness, or other distressing symptoms of psychological problems. They use drugs as a way to cope with the difficulties they experience in life. The common practice in our society of seeking a drug solution to every problem is a factor in the widespread reliance on both illicit and prescription drugs.

For people living in poverty in the inner cities, many of these reasons for using drugs are magnified. The problems are more devastating, the need for escape more compelling. Further, the buying and selling of drugs provide access to an unofficial, alternative economy that may seem like an opportunity for success.

Risk Factors for Dependence

Research indicates that some people may be born with a brain chemistry or metabolism that makes them more vulnerable to drug dependence. Psychological risk factors for drug dependence include difficulty in controlling impulses and a strong need for excitement, stimulation, and immediate gratification. Feelings of rejection, hostility, aggression, anxiety, or depression are also associated with drug dependence. People may turn to drugs to blot out their emotional pain. People with mental illnesses have a very high risk of substance dependence.

Other Risks of Drug Use

In 2007, 1.9 million emergency room visits were related to drug misuse or abuse.

Intoxication People who are under the influence of drugs—intoxicated—may act in uncharacteristic and unsafe ways because both their physical and mental functioning are impaired. They are more likely to be injured from a variety of causes, to have unsafe sex, and to be involved in incidents of aggression and violence.

Unexpected Side Effects Psychoactive drugs have many physical and psychological effects beyond the alteration of consciousness. These effects range from nausea and constipation to paranoia, depression, and heart failure. Some drugs also carry the risk of fatal overdose.

Unknown Drug Constituents There is no quality control in the illegal drug market, so the composition, dosage, and toxicity of street drugs are highly variable. Studies indicate that half of all street drugs don't contain their promised primary ingredient. In some cases, a drug may be present in unsafe dosages or mixed with other drugs to boost its effects. Makers of street drugs aren't held to any safety standards, so illicit drugs can be contaminated or even poisonous.

Risks Associated with Injection Drug Use Many injection drug users (IDUs) share or reuse needles, syringes, and other injection supplies, which can easily become contaminated with the user's blood. Small amounts of blood can carry enough human immunodeficiency virus (HIV) and hepatitis C virus (HCV) to be infectious. In 2008, injection drug use accounted for more than 10% of all new HIV/AIDS cases; many more were attributed to sexual contact with IDUs. Injection drug use also accounts for the majority of HCV infections.

The surest way to prevent diseases related to injection drug use is never to inject drugs. Syringe exchange programs (SEPs)—where IDUs can trade a used syringe for a new one—have been advocated to help slow the spread of HIV and reduce the rates and cost of other health problems associated with injection drug use. Getting people off drugs is clearly the best solution, but there are far more IDUs than treatment facilities can currently handle.

> **48%** of confirmed new HCV infections occurred among injection drug users.
> —CDC, 2009

Legal Consequences Many psychoactive drugs are illegal, so using them can result in large fines and/or imprisonment. According to the Federal Bureau of Investigation (FBI), law enforcement officials made 1.7 million arrests for drug abuse violations (12% of all arrests) in 2008—more arrests than for any other offense that year.

Ask Yourself

QUESTIONS FOR CRITICAL THINKING AND REFLECTION

Have you ever tried a psychoactive drug for fun? What were your reasons for trying it? Who were you with, and what were the circumstances? What was your experience like? What would you tell someone else who was thinking about trying a drug?

HOW DRUGS AFFECT THE BODY

The same drug may affect different people differently or the same person in different ways under different circumstances. Beyond a fairly predictable general change in brain chemistry, the effects of a drug may vary depending on drug factors, user factors, and social factors.

Changes in Brain Chemistry

Once a psychoactive drug reaches the brain, it acts on one or more **neurotransmitters,** either increasing or decreasing their concentration and actions. Cocaine, for example, affects dopamine, a neurotransmitter thought to play a key role in the process of reinforcement—the brain's way of telling itself "That's good; do the same thing again." Heroin, nicotine, alcohol, and amphetamines also affect dopamine levels through their effects on the brain.

The duration of a drug's effect depends on many factors and may range from 5 minutes (crack cocaine) to 12 or more hours (LSD). As drugs circulate through the body, they are metabolized by the liver and eventually excreted by the kidneys in urine. Small amounts may also be eliminated in other ways, including in sweat, in breast milk, and via the lungs.

> *Psychoactive drugs work by affecting one or more neurotransmitters in the brain.*

Drug Factors

When different drugs or dosages produce different effects, the differences are usually caused by one or more of five different drug factors:

1. The **pharmacological properties** of a drug are its effects on a person's body chemistry, behavior, and psychology. Pharmacological properties also include

neurotransmitter A brain chemical that transmits nerve impulses.

pharmacological properties The overall effects of a drug on a person's behavior, psychology, and chemistry.

TERMS

the amount of a drug required to exert various effects, the time course of the effects, and other characteristics, such as a drug's chemical composition.

2. The **dose-response function** is the relationship between the amount of drug taken and the type and intensity of its effect. Many psychological effects of drugs reach a plateau in the dose-response function, so that increasing the dose does not increase the effect any further. With LSD, for example, the maximum changes in perception occur at a certain dose, and no further changes in perception take place if higher doses are taken. However, all drugs have more than one effect, and the dose-response functions usually are different for different effects. This means that increasing the dose of any drug may begin to result in additional effects, which are likely to be more unpleasant or dangerous at high doses.

3. The **time-action function** is the relationship between the time elapsed since a drug was taken and the intensity of its effect. A drug's effects are greatest when its concentrations in body tissues are changing fastest, especially if they are increasing.

4. The person's *drug use history* may influence the effects of a drug. A given amount of alcohol, for example, will generally affect a habitual drinker less than an occasional drinker. Tolerance to some drugs, such as LSD, builds rapidly. To experience the same effect, a user has to abstain from the drug for a period of time before that dosage will again exert its original effects.

5. The *method of use* (or *route of administration*) has a direct effect on how strong a response a drug produces. Methods of use include ingestion, inhalation, injection, and absorption through the skin or tissue linings. Drugs are usually injected in one of three ways: intravenously (IV, or mainlining), intramuscularly (IM), or subcutaneously (SC, or skin popping).

User Factors

Certain physical and psychological characteristics help determine how a person will respond to a drug. Body mass is one variable. The effects of a certain dose of a drug on a 100-pound person will be twice as great as on a 200-pound person. Other variables include general health and genetic factors. For example, some people have an inherited ability to rapidly metabolize a cough suppressant called dextromethorphan, which also has psychoactive properties. These people must take a higher-than-normal dose to get a given cough-suppressant effect.

If a person's biochemical state is already altered by another drug, this too can make a difference. Some drugs intensify the effects of other drugs, as is the case with alcohol and sedatives. Some drugs block the effects of other drugs, such as when a tranquilizer is used to relieve anxiety caused by cocaine. Interactions between drugs, including many prescription and OTC medications, can be unpredictable and dangerous.

One physical condition that requires special precautions is pregnancy. It can be risky for a woman to use any drugs at all during pregnancy, including alcohol and common OTC products like cough medicine. The risks are greatest during the first trimester, when the fetus's body is rapidly forming and even small biochemical alterations in the mother can have a devastating effect on fetal development. Even later, the fetus is more susceptible than the mother to the adverse effects of any drugs she takes. The fetus may even become physically dependent on a drug being taken by the mother and suffer withdrawal symptoms after birth.

Sometimes a person's response to a drug is strongly influenced by the user's expectations about how he or she will react (the psychological *set*). With large doses, the drug's chemical properties seem to have the strongest effect on the user's response. But with small doses, psychological (and social) factors are often more important. When people strongly believe that a given drug will affect them a certain way, they are likely to experience those effects regardless of the drug's pharmacological properties. In one study, regular users of marijuana reported a moderate level of intoxication (**high**) after using a cigarette that smelled and tasted like marijuana but contained no THC, the active ingredient in marijuana. This is an example of the **placebo effect**—when a person receives an inert substance yet responds as if it were an active drug. In other studies, subjects who smoked low doses of real marijuana that they believed to be a placebo experienced no effects from the drug. Clearly, the user's expectations had a greater effect on the smokers than the drug itself.

Social Factors

The *setting* is the physical and social environment surrounding the drug use. If a person uses marijuana at home with trusted friends and pleasant music, the effects are likely to be different from the effects if the same dose is taken in an austere experimental laboratory with an impassive research technician. Similarly, the dose of

---

TERMS

dose-response function   The relationship between the amount of a drug taken and the intensity and type of the resulting effect.

time-action function   The relationship between the time elapsed since a drug was taken and the intensity of its effect.

high   The subjectively pleasing effects of a drug, usually felt quite soon after the drug is taken.

placebo effect   A response to an inert or innocuous substance given in place of an active drug.

alcohol that produces mild euphoria and stimulation at a noisy, active cocktail party might induce sleepiness and slight depression when taken at home while alone.

REPRESENTATIVE PSYCHOACTIVE DRUGS

The following sections introduce six representative groups of psychoactive drugs (Figure 7.1): opioids, central nervous system (CNS) depressants, central nervous system stimulants, marijuana and other cannabis products, hallucinogens, and inhalants.

Opioids

Also called *narcotics,* **opioids** are natural or synthetic (laboratory-made) drugs, such as opium, morphine, heroin, methadone, codeine, hydrocodone, oxycodone, meperidine, and fentanyl. Opioids relieve pain, cause drowsiness, and induce **euphoria.** Especially in small doses, opioids have beneficial medical uses, including pain relief and cough suppression. Opioids tend to reduce anxiety and produce lethargy, apathy, and an inability to concentrate. Opioid users become less active and less responsive to frustration, hunger, and sexual stimulation. These effects are more pronounced in novice users; with repeated use, many effects diminish.

Opioids are typically injected. They can also be absorbed into the body through the stomach, intestines, nasal membranes (from snorting or sniffing), or lungs (from smoking). Effects depend on the method of administration. If brain levels of the drug change rapidly, more immediate effects result. Although the euphoria associated with opioids is an important factor in their abuse, many people experience a feeling of uneasiness when they first use these drugs. Users also often feel nauseated and vomit, and they may have other unpleasant sensations. Even so, the abuse of opioids often results in dependence. Tolerance can develop rapidly and be pronounced. Withdrawal symptoms include cramps, chills, sweating, nausea, tremors, irritability, and feelings of panic.

Users who sniff or snort avoid the special disease risks of injection drug use, including HIV infection. Dependence can readily result from sniffing and smoking heroin. In addition, the potentially high but variable purity of street heroin poses a risk of unintentional overdose. Symptoms of overdose include respiratory depression, coma, and constriction of the pupils; death can result.

Nonmedical use of prescription pain relievers that contain oxycodone and hydrocodone, including Oxycontin and Vicodin, has increased in recent years (see the box "Prescription Drug Abuse Among American Teenagers"). When taken as prescribed in tablet form, these drugs treat moderate to severe chronic pain and do not typically lead to abuse. However, as is the case with other opioids, use of prescription painkillers can lead to abuse and dependence. Oxycodone and hydrocodone can be abused orally; the long-acting form of oxycodone is also sometimes crushed and snorted or dissolved and injected, providing a powerful heroin-like high. When taken in large doses or combined with other drugs, oxycodone and hydrocodone can cause fatal respiratory depression.

Central Nervous System Depressants

Central nervous system **depressants,** also known as **sedative-hypnotics,** slow down the overall activity of the **central nervous system (CNS).** The result can range from mild **sedation** to death. CNS depressants include alcohol, barbiturates, and other sedatives.

Types   The various types of barbiturates (downers or downs) are similar in chemical composition and action, but they differ in how quickly and how long they act. Antianxiety agents, also called sedatives or **tranquilizers,** include the benzodiazepines such as Xanax, Valium, Librium, clonazepam (Klonopin), and flunitrazepam (Rohypnol, also called roofies). Other CNS depressants include methaqualone (Quaalude), ethchlorvynol (Placidyl), chloral hydrate ("mickey"), and gamma hydroxy–butyrate (GHB, or "liquid ecstasy").

Effects   CNS depressants reduce anxiety and cause mood changes, impaired muscular coordination, slurring of speech, and drowsiness or sleep. Mental functioning is also affected, but the degree varies from person to person and also depends on the kind of task the person is trying to do. Most people become drowsy with small doses, although a few become more active.

opioid   Any of several natural or synthetic drugs that relieve pain and cause drowsiness and/or euphoria; examples are opium, morphine, and heroin; also called a *narcotic.*

euphoria   An exaggerated feeling of well-being.

depressant, or sedative-hypnotic   A drug that decreases nervous or muscular activity, causing drowsiness or sleep.

central nervous system (CNS)   The brain and spinal cord.

sedation   The induction of a calm, relaxed, often sleepy state.

tranquilizer   A CNS depressant that reduces tension and anxiety.

Ask Yourself

QUESTIONS FOR CRITICAL THINKING AND REFLECTION

Has an over-the-counter medication (such as a decongestant) ever made you feel strange, drowsy, or even high? Did you expect to react to the medication that way? Do such reactions influence the way you use over-the-counter drugs?

Category	Representative drugs	Street names	Appearance	Methods of use	Short-term effects
Opioids	Heroin	Dope, H, junk, brown sugar, smack	White/dark brown powder; dark tar or coal-like substance	Injected, smoked, snorted	Relief of anxiety and pain; euphoria; lethargy, apathy, drowsiness, confusion, inability to concentrate; nausea, constipation, respiratory depression
	Opium	Big O, black stuff, hop	Dark brown or black chunks	Swallowed, smoked	
	Morphine	M, Miss Emma, monkey, white stuff	White crystals, liquid solution	Injected, swallowed, smoked	
	Oxycodone, codeine, hydrocodone	Oxy, O.C., killer, Captain Cody, schoolboy, vike	Tablets, powder made from crushing tablets	Swallowed, injected, snorted	
Central nervous system depressants	Barbiturates	Barbs, reds, red birds, yellows, yellow jackets	Colored capsules	Swallowed, injected	Reduced anxiety, mood changes, lowered inhibitions, impaired muscle coordination, reduced pulse rate, drowsiness, loss of consciousness, respiratory depression
	Benzodiazepines (e.g., Valium, Xanax, Rohypnol)	Candy, downers, tranks, roofies, forget-me pill	Tablets	Swallowed, injected	
	Methaqualone	Ludes, quad, quay	Tablets	Injected, swallowed	
	Gamma hydroxy-butyrate (GHB)	G, Georgia home boy, grievous bodily harm	Clear liquid, white powder	Swallowed	
Central nervous system stimulants	Amphetamine, methamphet-amine	Bennies, speed, black beauties, uppers, chalk, crank, crystal, ice, meth	Tablets, capsules, white powder, white crystals	Injected, swallowed, smoked, snorted	Increased heart rate, blood pressure, metabolism; increased mental alertness and energy; nervousness, insomnia, impulsive behavior; reduced appetite
	Cocaine, crack cocaine	Blow, C, candy, coke, flake, rock, toot	White powder, beige pellets or rocks	Injected, smoked, snorted	
	Ritalin	JIF, MPH, R-ball, Skippy	Tablets	Injected, swallowed, snorted	
Marijuana and other cannabis products	Marijuana	Dope, grass, joints, Mary Jane, reefer, skunk, weed	Dried leaves and stems	Smoked, swallowed	Euphoria, slowed thinking and reaction time, confusion, anxiety, impaired balance and coordination, increased heart rate
	Hashish	Hash, hemp, boom, gangster	Dark, resin-like compound formed into rocks or blocks	Smoked, swallowed	
Hallucinogens	LSD	Acid, boomers, blotter, yellow sunshines	Blotter paper, liquid, gelatin tabs, pills	Swallowed, absorbed through mouth tissues	Altered states of perception and feeling; nausea; increased heart rate, blood pressure; delirium; impaired motor function; numbness, weakness
	Mescaline (peyote)	Buttons, cactus, mesc	Brown buttons, liquid	Swallowed, smoked	
	Psilocybin	Shrooms, magic mushrooms	Dried mushrooms	Swallowed	
	Ketamine	K, special K, cat valium, vitamin K	Clear liquid, white or beige powder	Injected, snorted, smoked	
	PCP	Angel dust, hog, love boat, peace pill	White to brown powder, tablets	Injected, swallowed, smoked, snorted	
	MDMA (ecstasy)	X, peace, clarity, Adam	Tablets	Swallowed	
Inhalants	Solvents, aerosols, nitrites, anesthetics	Laughing gas, poppers, snappers, whippets	Household products, sprays, glues, paint thinner, petroleum products	Inhaled through nose or mouth	Stimulation, loss of inhibition, slurred speech, loss of motor coordination, loss of consciousness

FIGURE 7.1 Commonly abused drugs and their effects.

SOURCES: The Partnership for a Drug-Free America. 2010 *Drug Guide by Name* (http://www.drugfree.org/portal/drug_guide; retrieved November 3, 2010); U.S. Drug Enforcement Agency. 2006. *Photo Library* (http:// www.usdoj.gov/dea/photo_library.html; retrieved November 3, 2010); U.S. Drug Enforcement Agency. 2010. *Drug Information* (http:// www.juistice.gov/dea/concern/concern.htm; retrieved November 3, 2010); National Institute on Drug Abuse. 2010. *Commonly Abused Drugs* (http://www.drugabuse.gov/DrugPages/DrugsofAbuse.html; retrieved November 3, 2010).

According to the 2008 National Survey on Drug Use and Health (NSDUH), nearly 21% of Americans over age 11 have used prescription-type psychotherapeutic drugs for nonmedical reasons at least once in their life, and more than 6 million Americans have done so in the past 30 days. Prescription-type drugs include pain relievers, tranquilizers, stimulants, and sedatives that are legally available only by prescription, as well as similar over-the-counter (OTC) drugs.

Although Americans have been abusing prescription drugs like Valium for decades, the rapidly growing trend of abuse among teenagers is a major source of concern. Over the last decade, the number of middle and high school students who misuse prescription and OTC medications has increased dramatically. The 2008 NSDUH shows that well over a million Americans age 12–20 abused a prescription drug in the past 30 days.

According to another survey, the CDC's Youth Risk Behavior Surveillance for 2009, 20.2% of American high school students have taken prescription drugs at least once without a doctor's prescription. The rate of abuse increases steadily through the grade levels, with 15.1% of freshman and 25.8% of seniors misusing prescription medications. The CDC's study also found that more white students (23.0%) abuse prescription drugs than do Hispanic (17.2%) or black (11.8%) students. Males and females abuse prescription drugs at about the same rate.

Aside from marijuana, prescription-type drugs are the most abused drugs among teenagers. The most commonly abused are painkillers (OxyContin, Vicodin), depressants (sleeping pills, anti-anxiety medications), and stimulants (Ritalin, Adderall). The most commonly abused OTC drugs are cough and cold remedies containing the cough suppressant dextromethorphan, an ingredient in Robitussin and NyQuil. According to the Substance Abuse and Mental Health Services Administration (SAMSHA), 1 million Americans age 12–25 used OTC cough and cold medicines recreationally in 2006.

The primary reason for the increase in abuse of prescription-type drugs is their availability. Teens report getting drugs from relatives and buying them without a prescription over the Internet. They also commonly get them from one another, at school or at parties where drugs are openly exchanged.

In addition, teens apparently choose prescription-type drugs because they believe they are safer than illicit drugs, but this is not the case. Just like their illegal counterparts, these medications carry the risk of dependency, addiction, and lethal overdose, particularly when combined with alcohol. Between 2004 and 2008, emergency room visits due to prescription painkiller abuse increased by more than 110%, and more than 71,000 children are taken to the ER each year for overdoses of OTC medications. In response to the challenge of prescription drug abuse, the government has launched public health campaigns and public service announcements aimed at educating both parents and teens about the dangers of those seemingly innocuous substances.

SOURCES: Centers for Disease Control and Prevention. 2010. Emergency department visits involving nonmedical use of selected prescription drugs—United States, 2004–2008. *Morbidity and Mortality Weekly Report* 59(23): 705–709; Centers for Disease Control and Prevention. 2010. Youth Risk Behavior Surveillance—United States, 2009. *Morbidity and Mortality Weekly Report Surveillance Summaries* 59(SS–5): 1–142; Substance Abuse and Mental Health Services Administration. 2009. *Results from the 2008 National Survey on Drug Use and Health: National Findings*, Rockville, Md.:Office of Applied Studies, NSDUH Series H-36, HHS Publication No. SMA 09-4434.

From Use to Abuse People are usually introduced to CNS depressants either through a medical prescription or through drug-using peers. The use of Rohypnol and GHB is often associated with dance clubs and raves. Most CNS depressants, including alcohol, can lead to physical dependence. Tolerance, sometimes for up to 15 times the usual dose, can develop with repeated use. Tranquilizers have been shown to produce physical dependence even at ordinary prescribed doses. Withdrawal symptoms can be more severe than those accompanying opioid dependence. They may begin as anxiety, shaking, and weakness but may turn into convulsions and possibly cardiovascular collapse and death.

While intoxicated, people on depressants cannot function well. They are confused and are frequently obstinate, irritable, and abusive. Even prescription use of benzodiaze-pines has been associated with an increased risk of automobile crashes. After long-term use, depressants like alcohol can lead to poor health and brain damage, with impaired ability to reason and make judgments.

Too much depression of the central nervous system slows respiration and may stop it entirely. CNS depressants are particularly dangerous in combination with another depressant, such as alcohol. Rohypnol is ten times more potent than Valium and can be fatal if combined with alcohol. GHB is often

20 million Americans used benzodiazepines for nonmedical purposes in 2008.

QUICK STATS

Club Drugs

Some people refer to club drugs as soft drugs because they see them as recreational—for the casual, weekend user—rather than as addictive. But club drugs have many potential negative effects and are particularly potent and unpredictable when mixed with alcohol. Substitute drugs are often sold in place of club drugs, putting users at risk for taking dangerous combinations of unknown drugs.

MDMA (ecstasy, E, X, XTC, Adam, hug drug, lover's speed): Taken in pill form, MDMA (methylenedioxymethamphetamine) is a stimulant with mildly hallucinogenic and amphetamine-like effects. Users may experience euphoria, increased energy, and a heightened sense of belonging. Using MDMA can produce dangerously high body temperature and potentially fatal dehydration; some users experience confusion, depression, anxiety, paranoia, muscle tension, involuntary teeth clenching, blurred vision, nausea, and seizures. Even low doses can affect concentration, judgment, and driving ability. Tolerance can develop, leading users to take the drug more frequently, to use higher doses, or to combine MDMA with other drugs to enhance the drug's effects.

In addition to MDMA, many ecstasy tablets include other drugs such as methamphetamine, ephedrine, or cocaine. At high doses or mixed with other drugs, MDMA is extremely dangerous; most deaths linked to MDMA have occurred as a result of multidrug toxicity or traumatic injuries.

MDMA increases the activity of three neurotransmitters: serotonin, dopamine, and norepinephrine. Increases in serotonin are likely the cause of the drug's mood-elevating effects, but use of MDMA can deplete the brain of serotonin and may cause an emotional letdown (sadness, irritability, etc.) in the days following use.

MDMA users perform worse than non-users on complex cognitive tasks of memory, attention, and general intelligence. Long-term effects may include physical symptoms and psychological problems such as confusion or paranoia. Research suggests that pregnant women who use MDMA are at increased risk for having a baby with congenital malformations and long-term impairment in memory and other cognitive functions.

LSD (acid, boomers, yellow sunshines, red dragon): A potent hallucinogen, LSD (lysergic acid diethylamide) is sold in tablets or capsules, in liquid form, or on small squares of paper called blotters. LSD increases heart rate and body temperature and may cause nausea, tremors, sweating, numbness, and weakness.

Ketamine (special K, vitamin K, K, cat valium, jet): A veterinary anesthetic that can be taken in powdered or liquid form, ketamine may cause hallucinations and impaired attention and memory. At higher doses, ketamine can cause delirium, amnesia, high blood pressure, and potentially fatal respiratory problems. Tolerance to ketamine develops rapidly.

GHB (Georgia home boy, G, grievous bodily harm, liquid ecstasy): GHB (gamma hydroxybutyrate) can be produced in clear liquid, white powder, tablet, and capsule form. GHB is a CNS depressant that in large doses or when taken in combination with alcohol or other depressants can cause sedation, loss of consciousness, respiratory arrest, and death. GHB may cause prolonged and potentially life-threatening withdrawal symptoms.

Some products sold as dietary supplements for bodybuilding, weight loss, or insomnia contain the chemically similar compounds GBL (gamma butyrolactone) or BD (butanediol). It is illegal to sell products containing GHB, GBL, or BD for human consumption. The FDA has issued several warnings to prevent such items from being sold to the public.

Rohypnol (roofies, roche, forget-me pill): Taken in tablet form, Rohypnol (flunitrazepam) is a sedative that is ten times more potent than Valium. Its effects, which are magnified by alcohol, include reduced blood pressure, dizziness, confusion, gastrointestinal disturbances, and loss of consciousness. Users of Rohypnol may develop physical and psychological dependence on the drug.

Several club drugs are used as "date rape drugs." Because they can be added to beverages surreptitiously, these drugs may be unknowingly consumed by intended rape victims. In addition to depressant effects, some drugs also cause anterograde amnesia, the loss of memory of things occurring while under the influence of the drug. Because of concern about such drugs, Congress passed the Drug-Induced Rape Prevention and Punishment Act, which increased federal penalties for use of any controlled substance to aid in sexual assault.

produced clandestinely, resulting in widely varying degrees of purity; it has been responsible for many poisonings and deaths.

Central Nervous System Stimulants

CNS **stimulants** speed up the activity of the nervous or muscular system, causing the heart rate to accelerate, blood pressure to rise, blood vessels to constrict, the pupils and bronchial tubes to dilate, and gastric and adrenal secretions to increase. There is greater muscular tension and sometimes an increase in motor activity. Small doses usually make people feel more awake and alert, less fatigued and bored. The most common CNS stimulants are cocaine, amphetamines, nicotine, ephedrine, and caffeine.

Cocaine Usually derived from the leaves of coca shrubs that grow high in the Andes in South America, cocaine—also known as coke or snow—is a potent CNS stimulant. It is usually snorted and absorbed through the nasal mucosa or injected intravenously, providing rapid increases of the drug's concentration in the blood and therefore fast, intense effects. Another method of use involves processing cocaine with baking soda and water, yielding the ready-to-smoke form of cocaine known as crack. Crack is typically available as small beads or pellets smokable in glass pipes.

EFFECTS   The effects of cocaine are usually intense but short-lived. The euphoria lasts from 5 to 20 minutes and ends abruptly, to be replaced by irritability, anxiety, or slight depression. When cocaine is absorbed via the lungs, by either smoking or inhalation, it reaches the brain in about 10 seconds, and the effects are particularly intense. This is part of the appeal of smoking crack. The effects from IV injections occur almost as quickly—in about 20 seconds. Since the mucous membranes in the nose briefly slow absorption, the onset of effects from snorting takes 2–3 minutes. Heavy users may inject cocaine intravenously every 10–20 minutes to maintain the effects.

The larger the cocaine dose and the more rapidly it is absorbed into the bloodstream, the greater the immediate—and sometimes lethal—effects. Sudden death from cocaine is most commonly the result of excessive CNS stimulation that causes convulsions and respiratory collapse, irregular heartbeat, extremely high blood pressure, blood clots, and possibly heart attack or stroke. Although rare, fatalities can occur in healthy young people; among people age 18–59, cocaine users are seven times more likely than nonusers to have a heart attack. Chronic cocaine use produces inflammation of the nasal mucosa, which can lead to persistent bleeding and ulceration of the septum between the nostrils. The use of cocaine may also cause paranoia and/or aggressiveness.

COCAINE USE DURING PREGNANCY   A woman who uses cocaine during pregnancy is at higher risk for miscarriage, premature labor, and stillbirth. She is more likely to deliver a low-birth-weight baby who has a small head circumference. Her infant may be at increased risk for defects of the genitourinary tract, cardiovascular system, central nervous system, and extremities. It is difficult to pinpoint the effects of cocaine because many women who use cocaine also use tobacco and/or alcohol. Infants whose mothers use cocaine may also be born intoxicated. Cocaine also passes into breast milk and can intoxicate a breastfeeding infant.

Amphetamines   Amphetamines (uppers) are a group of synthetic chemicals that are potent CNS stimulants. Some common drugs in this family are amphetamine (Benzedrine), dextroamphetamine (Dexedrine), and methamphetamine (Methedrine).

EFFECTS   Small doses of amphetamines usually make people feel more alert. Amphetamines generally increase motor activity but do not measurably alter a normal, rested person's ability to perform tasks calling for challenging motor skills or complex thinking. When amphetamines improve performance, it is primarily by counteracting fatigue and boredom. In small doses amphetamines increase heart rate and blood pressure and change sleep patterns. They are sometimes used to curb appetite, but after a few weeks the user develops tolerance and needs higher doses. When people stop taking the drug, their appetite usually returns, and they gain back the weight they lost.

FROM USE TO ABUSE   Much amphetamine abuse begins as an attempt to cope with a temporary situation. A student cramming for an exam or an exhausted long-haul truck driver can go a little longer by taking amphetamines. Unfortunately, the likelihood of making bad judgments significantly increases. The stimulating effects may also wear off suddenly, and the user may precipitously feel exhausted or fall asleep ("crash").

Another problem is **state dependence**, the phenomenon whereby information learned in a certain drug-induced state is difficult to recall when the person is not in that same physiological state. Test performance may deteriorate when students use drugs to study and then take tests in their normal, nondrug state.

DEPENDENCE   Repeated use of amphetamines, even in moderate doses, often leads to tolerance and the need for increasingly larger doses. Long-term use of amphetamines at high doses can cause paranoia, hallucinations, delusions, and incoherence. Methamphetamine is more addictive and dangerous than most forms of amphetamine because it is more toxic and its effects last longer (see the box "Meth and the Environment: A Toxic Impact"). In the short term, meth can cause rapid breathing, increased body temperature, insomnia, tremors, anxiety, and convulsions. Meth use has been linked to high-risk sexual behavior and increased rates of STDs, including HIV infection. In the long term, the effects of meth can include weight loss, severe acne, hallucinations, paranoia, violence, and psychosis. Meth use causes extensive tooth decay and tooth loss, a condition referred to as "meth mouth." Meth takes a toll on the user's heart and can cause heart attack and stroke. Methamphetamine users have signs of brain damage similar to those seen in Parkinson's disease patients that appear to persist even after drug use ceases, causing impaired memory and motor coordination.

Withdrawal from meth causes symptoms that may include muscle aches and tremors, profound fatigue, deep depression, despair, and apathy. Chronic high-dose use is often associated with pronounced psychological cravings and obsessive drug-seeking behavior.

Women who use amphetamines during pregnancy risk premature birth, stillbirth, low birth weight, and early infant death. Babies born to amphetamine-using mothers have a higher incidence of cleft palate, cleft lip, and deformed limbs. They may also experience symptoms of withdrawal from amphetamines.

state dependence   A situation in which information learned in a drug-induced state is difficult to recall when the effect of the drug wears off.

TERMS

Meth and the Environment: A Toxic Impact

Most people know about the toxic effects of methamphetamine on users' health. Fewer people are aware of the toxic effects meth has on the environment.

Although most meth sold in the United States comes from large-scale drug trafficking organizations, the do-it-yourself appeal of meth production has led to the proliferation of small-scale clandestine labs across the country. Users and dealers set up meth labs in kitchens, bathrooms, garages, and abandoned buildings and cook up the drug using commonly available household and automotive chemicals. Although meth labs are found in urban and suburban areas, they are particularly prevalent in rural areas, where it is easier to escape detection.

One meth ingredient, pseudoephedrine, a drug found in cold and allergy medications, is now restricted to behind-the-counter sale in pharmacies, as part of a national attempt to stem the "meth epidemic." Other, more toxic ingredients include engine starter fluid (ether), paint thinner, acetone, Freon, anhydrous ammonia, iodine, red phosphorus (used in matches and road flares), brake cleaner (toluene), drain cleaner (sodium hydroxide/lye), battery acid (sulfuric acid), hydrochloric acid, reactive chemicals (sodium or lithium), and gasoline additives (methanol, alcohol). Because many of these ingredients are volatile and flammable, explosions and fires are common. For every pound of meth produced in a meth lab, about 5 pounds of toxic waste are created. This toxic waste is usually dumped down the drain, in yards or fields, or by back roads, creating toxic waste sites. Poisonous fumes from the waste are released into the air, and toxic chemicals contaminate streams and leach into water supplies. Livestock have been killed by these poisons, as have trees and vegetation. People have stumbled on meth dump sites, which can be recognized by strong chemical odors or the presence of items like empty containers of antifreeze or lye or equipment like rubber tubing or gas cans.

When a waste dump or clandestine lab is discovered, a cleanup has to be undertaken, following EPA regulations. Private contractors with specialized training and equipment provide hazardous waste removal and disposal services to local and state law enforcement agencies and the U.S. Drug Enforcement Administration. The cost of a cleanup ranges from hundreds to thousands of dollars, paid by taxpayers. Additional costs come from property damage, lowered property values, medical care for innocent bystanders (including children), and criminal justice costs. Houses and other structures used as meth labs are often so toxic they have to be destroyed.

Meth isn't the only drug with a negative effect on the environment. An estimated 60% of outdoor marijuana cultivation in the United States takes place on public land, especially the remote parts of national parks and forests. Growers use fertilizers and pesticides to grow the plants and poisons to kill deer and bear that wander too close to the crops. For every acre of forest used to grow marijuana, 10 acres are damaged by toxic chemicals.

In Central and South America, millions of acres of rainforest have been burned and cleared for the production of coca

plants, contributing to soil erosion, air and water pollution, flooding, and global warming. Poisonous chemicals are used to produce cocaine in jungle labs, endangering hundreds of species of mammals, birds, and fish. For every 2 pounds of coca paste produced, 1,300 pounds of trash are generated and 200 gallons of water contaminated.

What can be done to reduce the impact of drug production on the environment? One answer lies in reducing the demand for drugs. In 2010, Mexican President Felipe Calderon blamed the United States for the drug wars in his country, saying Mexico is located next to the country with the highest levels of drug consumption in the world and likening the United States to "the biggest drug addict in the world." Even if the Mexican president was being dramatic, reducing the American addiction to illicit drugs would go a long way toward improving the welfare of the global environment.

SOURCES: U.S. DEA. 2010. *Environmental Impacts of Methamphetamine* (http://www.justice.gov/dea/concern/meth_environment.html; retrieved November 3, 2010); U.S. DEA. 2009. *Demand Reduction, Costs to Society* (http://www.justthinktwice.com/costs/DamagetoEnvironment.cfm; retrieved November 3, 2010); U.S. DEA. 2005. *Comprehensively Combating Methamphetamine: Impact on Health and the Environment* (http://www.justice.gov/dea/speeches/s102005.html; retrieved November 3, 2010); Booth, W. 2010. *Mexico's Deadly Drug Violence Claims Hundreds of Lives in Past 5 Days*. June 6 (http://www.washingtonpost.com; retrieved November 3, 2010).

Ritalin A stimulant with amphetamine-like effects, Ritalin (methylphenidate) is used to treat attention-deficit/hyperactivity disorder (ADHD). When taken orally at prescribed levels, it has little potential for abuse. When injected or snorted, however, dependence and tolerance can rapidly result.

In addition to being one of the most popular psychoactive drugs, caffeine is one of the most ancient.

Caffeine Caffeine is probably the most popular psychoactive drug and also one of the most ancient. It is found in coffee, tea, cocoa, soft drinks, headache remedies, and OTC preparations like NōDōz (Table 7.3). In ordinary doses, caffeine produces greater alertness and a sense of well-being. It also decreases feelings of fatigue or boredom; using caffeine may enable a person to keep at physically tiring or repetitive tasks longer. Such use is usually followed, however, by a sudden letdown. Caffeine does not noticeably influence a person's ability to perform complex mental tasks unless fatigue, boredom, or other factors have already affected normal performance.

Caffeine mildly stimulates the heart and respiratory system, increases muscular tremor, and enhances gastric secretion. Higher doses may cause nervousness, anxiety, irritability, headache, disturbed sleep, and gastric irritation or peptic ulcers. In people with high blood pressure, caffeine can cause blood pressure to rise even more; in people with type 2 diabetes, caffeine may cause glucose and insulin levels to rise after meals. Some people, especially children, are quite vulnerable to the adverse effects of caffeine. They become hyperactive and overly sensitive to any stimulation in their environment.

Drinks containing caffeine are rarely harmful for most people, but some tolerance develops, and withdrawal symptoms of irritability, headaches, and even mild depression do occur. People can usually avoid problems by simply decreasing their daily intake of caffeine.

Marijuana and Other Cannabis Products

Marijuana is the most widely used illegal drug in the United States (cocaine is second). About 47% of Americans have tried marijuana at least once. In 2008, nearly 19% of 18–20-year-olds and 15% of 21–25-year-old Americans reported using marijuana at least once within the past month.

Marijuana is a crude preparation of various parts of the Indian hemp plant *Cannabis sativa,* which grows in most parts of the world. THC (tetrahydrocannabinol) is the main active ingredient in marijuana. Based on THC content, the potency of marijuana preparations varies widely. Marijuana plants that grow wild often have less than 1% THC in their leaves. When selected strains are cultivated by separation of male and female plants (*sinsemilla*), the bud leaves from

Table 7.3	Caffeine Content of Popular Beverages	
	SERVING SIZE	TYPICAL CAFFEINE LEVEL (mg)*
Coffee	8 oz.	
Regular coffee, brewed	8 oz.	95
Regular coffee, instant	1 oz.	93
Espresso	8 oz.	64
Decaffeinated coffee, brewed	8 oz.	5
Decaffeinated coffee, instant	8 oz.	2
Tea		
Regular tea, brewed	8 oz.	47
Decaffeinated tea, brewed	8 oz.	2
Green tea, brewed	8 oz.	Varies
Soda		
Code Red Mountain Dew	12 oz.	54
Mello Yello	12 oz.	53
Diet Coke	12 oz.	47
Dr. Pepper, Diet Dr. Pepper	12 oz.	41
Sunkist Orange Soda	12 oz.	41
Pepsi	12 oz.	38
Coca-Cola Classic, Diet Pepsi	12 oz.	35
Energy Drinks		
No Name	8.4 oz.	280
SoBe No Fear	16 oz.	174
Monster Energy, Rockstar	16 oz.	160
SoBe Adrenaline Rush	16 oz.	152
Full Throttle, Full Throttle Fury	16 oz.	144
AMP Energy Drink	16 oz.	143
Red Bull	8.3 oz.	76
Vault	8 oz.	47

*Caffeine levels vary greatly by brand of product, manner of preparation, and amount consumed. The amounts shown here are averages based on tests conducted by a variety of organizations. The U.S. Food and Drug Administration limits the amount of caffeine in cola and pepper soft drinks to 71 milligrams per 12-ounce serving. To find the exact amount of caffeine in any product, check that product's label.

SOURCES: Center for Science in the Public Interest. 2007. *Caffeine Content of Food & Drugs* (http://www.cspinet.org/new/cafchart.htm; retrieved November 3, 2010); Mayo Clinic. 2008. *Caffeine Content in Tea, Soda, and More* (http://www.mayoclinic.com/health/caffeine/AN01211; retrieved November 3, 2010); U.S. Department of Agriculture, Agricultural Research Service. 2009. *USDA National Nutrient Database for Standard Reference, Release 22* (http://www.ars.usda.gov/ba/bhnrc/ndl; retrieved November 3, 2010).

the flowering tops may contain 7–8% THC. Marijuana is usually smoked, but it can also be ingested.

Short-Term Effects and Uses The effects of a low dose of marijuana are strongly influenced by the user's expectations and past experiences. At low doses, users typically experience euphoria, a heightening of subjective sensory experiences, a slowing down of the perception of passing time, and a relaxed, laid-back attitude. With moderate doses, marijuana's effects become stronger, and the user may have impaired memory function, disturbed

Marijuana is the most widely used illegal drug in the United States.

appetite. These benefits led several states to approve the use of "medical marijuana" by extremely ill patients, with physician monitoring. However, because growing, selling, or possessing marijuana is a federal crime, the Supreme Court has held that state laws permitting medical marijuana use cannot supersede federal law, which means that anyone who uses marijuana for medical reasons—even in a state that approves such use—can still be prosecuted under federal drug laws, although the Obama administration made it known that it would not pursue such prosecutions. Currently, more than 30 states have medical marijuana laws on their books.

Long-Term Effects   The most probable long-term effect of smoking marijuana is respiratory damage, including impaired lung function and chronic bronchial irritation. Although there is no evidence linking marijuana use to lung cancer, it may cause changes in lung tissue that promote cancer growth. Marijuana users may be at increased risk for emphysema and cancer of the head and neck; among people with chronic conditions like cancer and AIDS, marijuana use is associated with increased risk of fatal lung infections. Heavy users may experience learning problems, as well as subtle impairments of attention and memory that may or may not be reversible following long-term abstinence. Long-term use may also decrease testosterone levels and sperm counts and increase sperm abnormalities.

Heavy marijuana use during pregnancy may cause impaired fetal growth and development, low birth weight, and increased risk of ectopic pregnancy. Marijuana may act synergistically with alcohol to increase the damaging effects of alcohol on the fetus. THC rapidly enters breast milk and may impair an infant's early motor development.

Dependence   Regular users of marijuana can develop tolerance; some develop dependence, and researchers estimate that 1.5% of Americans meet the APA criteria for marijuana dependence. Withdrawal symptoms may occur in the majority of dependent or heavy users; common symptoms include anger or aggression, irritability, nervousness or restlessness, sleep difficulties, and decreased appetite or weight loss.

Hallucinogens

Hallucinogens are a group of drugs whose predominant pharmacological effect is to alter the user's perceptions, feelings, and thoughts. Hallucinogens include LSD (lysergic acid diethylamide), mescaline, psilocybin, STP (4-methyl-2,5-dimethoxyamphetamine), DMT (dimethyltryptamine), MDMA (3,4-methylene-dioxymethamphetamine), ketamine, and PCP (phencyclidine). These drugs are most commonly ingested or smoked.

LSD   LSD is one of the most powerful psychoactive drugs. Tiny doses will produce noticeable effects in most people, such as an altered sense of time, visual disturbances,

thought patterns, lapses of attention, and feelings of **depersonalization,** in which the mind seems to be separated from the body.

At higher doses, marijuana's effects are determined mostly by the drug itself rather than by the user's expectations and setting. Very high doses produce marked sensory distortion and changes in body image, causing some users to become anxious or panicky.

Physiologically, marijuana increases heart rate and dilates certain blood vessels in the eyes, which creates the characteristic bloodshot eyes. THC affects parts of the brain controlling balance, coordination, and reaction time; thus marijuana use impairs driving performance. The combination of alcohol and marijuana makes driving even riskier.

According to the Institute of Medicine some compounds in marijuana may have legitimate medical use, such as easing pain, reducing nausea, and increasing

depersonalization   A state in which a person loses the sense of his or her reality or perceives his or her body as unreal.

hallucinogen   Any of several drugs that alter perception, feelings, or thoughts; examples are LSD, mescaline, and PCP.

an improved sense of hearing, mood changes, and distortions in how people perceive their bodies. Dilation of the pupils and slight dizziness, weakness, and nausea may also occur. With larger doses, users may experience a phenomenon known as **synesthesia**, feelings of depersonalization, and other alterations in the perceived relationship between the self and external reality.

Many hallucinogens induce tolerance so quickly that after only one or two doses their effects decrease substantially. The user must then stop taking the drug for several days before his or her system can be receptive to it again. These drugs cause little drug-seeking behavior and no physical dependence or withdrawal symptoms.

The immediate effects of low doses of hallucinogens are largely determined by expectations and setting. Many effects are hard to describe because they involve subjective and unusual dimensions of awareness—the **altered states of consciousness** for which these drugs are famous. For this reason, hallucinogens have acquired a certain aura not associated with other drugs. People have taken LSD in search of a religious or mystical experience or in the hope of exploring new worlds.

> **67%** of inhalant users were under the age of 18 when they first tried it.
>
> —SAMHSA, 2009

A severe panic reaction can result from taking any dose of LSD. Even after the drug's chemical effects have worn off, spontaneous flashbacks and other psychological disturbances can occur. **Flashbacks** are perceptual distortions and bizarre thoughts that occur after the drug has been entirely eliminated from the body.

Other Hallucinogens   Most other hallucinogens have the same general effects as LSD, but there are some variations. For example, a DMT or ketamine high does not last as long as an LSD high; an STP high lasts longer. MDMA (ecstasy) has both hallucinogenic and amphetamine-like properties. Tolerance to MDMA develops quickly, and high doses can cause anxiety, delusions, and paranoia.

PCP reduces and distorts sensory input, especially proprioception, the sensation of body position and movement; it creates a state of sensory deprivation. Because it can be easily made, PCP is often available illegally and is sometimes used as an inexpensive replacement for other psychoactive drugs. The effects of ketamine are similar to those of PCP—confusion, agitation, aggression, and lack of coordination—but they tend to be less predictable. Tolerance to either drug can develop rapidly.

Mescaline, derived from the peyote cactus, is the ceremonial drug of the Native American Church. It causes effects similar to LSD, including altered perception and feeling; increased body temperature, heart rate, and blood pressure; weakness and trembling; and sleeplessness. Mescaline is expensive, so most street mescaline is diluted

LSD or a mixture of other drugs. Hallucinogenic effects can be obtained from certain mushrooms (*Psilocybe mexicana,* or "magic mushrooms"), certain morning glory seeds, nutmeg, jimsonweed, and other botanical products, but unpleasant side effects, such as dizziness, have limited the popularity of these products.

Inhalants

Inhaling certain chemicals can produce effects ranging from heightened pleasure to delirium and death. Inhalants fall into several major groups: (1) volatile solvents, which are found in products such as paint thinner, glue, and gasoline; (2) aerosols, which are sprays that contain propellants and solvents; (3) nitrites, such as butyl nitrite and amyl nitrite; and (4) anesthetics, which include nitrous oxide, or laughing gas.

Inhalant use is difficult to control because inhalants are easy to obtain. They are present in a variety of seemingly harmless products, from dessert-topping sprays to underarm deodorants, that are both inexpensive and legal. Using the drugs also requires no illegal or suspicious paraphernalia. Inhalant users get high by sniffing, snorting, "bagging" (inhaling fumes from a plastic bag), or "huffing" (placing an inhalant-soaked rag in the mouth).

Although different in makeup, nearly all inhalants produce effects similar to those of anesthetics, which slow down body functions. Low doses may cause users to feel slightly stimulated; at higher doses, users may feel less inhibited and less in control. Sniffing high concentrations of the chemicals in solvents or aerosol sprays can cause a loss of consciousness, heart failure, and death. High concentrations of any inhalant can also cause death from suffocation by displacing oxygen in the lungs and central nervous system. Deliberately inhaling from a bag or in a closed area greatly increases the chances of suffocation. Other possible effects of the excessive or long-term use of inhalants include

Ask Yourself

QUESTIONS FOR CRITICAL THINKING AND REFLECTION
Do you know any young teens who may be at risk for using inhalants? If so, would you try to intervene in some way? What would you tell a youngster to convince him or her to stop inhaling chemicals?

synesthesia   A condition in which a stimulus evokes not only the sensation appropriate to it but also another sensation of a different character, such as when a color evokes a specific smell.

altered states of consciousness   Profound changes in mood, thinking, and perception.

flashback   A perceptual distortion or bizarre thought that recurs after the chemical effects of a drug have worn off.

damage to the nervous system; hearing loss; increased risk of cancer; and damage to the liver, kidneys, and bone marrow.

DRUG USE: THE DECADES AHEAD

Drug research will undoubtedly provide new information, new treatments, and new chemical combinations in the decades ahead. Although the use of some drugs, both legal and illegal, has declined dramatically since the 1970s, the use of others has held steady or increased. Mounting public concern has led to great debate and a wide range of opinions about what should be done. Efforts to combat the problem include workplace drug testing, tougher law enforcement and prosecution, and treatment and education.

Drugs, Society, and Families

According to the National Institute on Drug Abuse, the cost to society of illicit drug abuse alone is $181 billion annually. That figure exceeds $500 billion when combined with the costs of alcohol and tobacco use, including health care, criminal justice, and lost productivity. But the costs are more than just financial; they are also paid in human pain and suffering.

The criminal justice system is inundated with people accused of crimes related to drug possession, sale, or use. The FBI reports that more than 1.7 million arrests are made annually for drug violations; at any given time, more than 100,000 people are in jail for violating drug laws. Many assaults and murders are committed when people try to acquire or protect drug territories, settle disputes about drugs, or steal from dealers. Violence and gun use are common in neighborhoods where drug trafficking is prevalent. Addicts commit more robberies and burglaries than criminals not on drugs. People under the influence of drugs, especially alcohol, are more likely to commit violent crimes like rape and murder than people who do not use drugs (see the box "Drug Use and Ethnicity: Risk Factors and Protective Factors").

Drug use is also a health care issue for society. In the United States, illegal drug use leads to more than 800,000 emergency room admissions and nearly 20,000 deaths annually. Although it is in the best interest of society to treat addicts who want help, there is not nearly enough space in treatment facilities to help the millions of Americans who need immediate treatment. Drug addicts who want to quit, especially those among the urban poor, often have to wait a year or more for acceptance into a residential care or other treatment program. Drug abuse also takes a toll on individuals and families. Children born to women who use drugs such as alcohol, tobacco, or cocaine may have long-term health problems. Drug use in families can become a vicious cycle. Observing adults around them using drugs, children assume it is an acceptable way to deal with problems. Abuse, neglect, lack of opportunity, and unemployment become contributing factors to drug use and serve to perpetuate the cycle.

*Many American businesses **require workers to take drugs tests;** a substantial number of employers offer counseling and treatment support for workers who test positive.*

Legalizing Drugs

Pointing out that many social problems associated with drugs are related to prohibition rather than to the effects of the drugs, some people have argued for drug legalization or decriminalization. Proposals range from making drugs such as marijuana and heroin available by prescription to allowing licensed dealers to sell some drugs to adults. Proponents argue that legalizing some currently illicit drugs—but putting controls on them similar to those used for alcohol, tobacco, and prescription drugs—could eliminate many of the problems related to drug use. A measure to legalize marijuana for recreational use and allow it to be sold and taxed was placed on the ballot in California in November 2010; voters defeated that proposition by a significant margin.

Opponents of drug legalization argue that allowing easier access to drugs would expose many more people to possible abuse and dependence. Drugs would be cheaper and easier to obtain, and drug use would be more socially acceptable. Legalizing drugs could cause an increase in drug use among children and teenagers. Opponents point out that alcohol and tobacco are major causes of disease and death in our society and that they should not be used as models for other practices.

Drug Testing

According to data from recent surveys, the majority of substance users hold full-time jobs and constitute a significant public health problem in the workplace. Drug use in the workplace not only creates health problems for individual users, but it has a negative effect on productivity and on safety of coworkers. People who use drugs at work face higher rates of absenteeism, poor health, and a greater likelihood of harming themselves or others in the workplace.

Statistics from the federal government show that 8.4% of full-time workers were illicit drug users in 2007. Illicit drug use is highest among workers in the food industry and construction sectors, while heavy alcohol use is greatest among construction, mining, and repair workers. Premature death, illness, and disability—factors associated with the economic and health burden of lost productivity—are estimated to run as high as $114 billion for drug use and $179 billion for heavy alcohol use.

Surveys of the U.S. population find a variety of trends in drug use and abuse among ethnic groups (see table). In addition to these general trends, there are also trends relating to the use of specific drugs among different groups.

However, as is true for many areas of health, ethnic trends are influenced by a complex interplay of other factors:

- *Educational status:* Adults with four or more years of college are more likely to have *tried* illicit drugs than are people of the same age who never finished high school. *Current* drug use, however, is lower among college graduates than among people with less education. Among teens, poor school performance is associated with a higher risk of drug use.

- *Employment status:* Most adult drug users are employed, but rates of current drug use are much higher among people who are unemployed or who work part-time compared with those who are employed full-time.

- *Parental education and socioeconomic status:* Students from poor families have higher rates of *early* drug use compared with students from wealthier families. By the twelfth grade, the differences disappear. Socioeconomic status and parental education are closely linked.

- *Geographic area:* Current drug use in the United States is highest in the West and Midwest; drug use is also higher in metropolitan and urban areas compared with more rural areas. People living in communities with high rates of poverty, crime, and unemployment have higher than average rates of drug use and abuse. Specific drugs may also be more available—and their abuse more prevalent—in certain regions or communities.

Strong cultural identity is associated with reduced risk of drug use and abuse among all groups. The following factors may contribute to lower rates of drug use among such groups:

- *Parental and community disapproval of drug and alcohol use:* Parents of Asian American children tend to have more restrictive drug and alcohol use norms than African American and white parents. Black parents tend to monitor their children's activities and friendships more closely than white parents. Parental disapproval of drug use is often tied to greater perceived risk of drug use—and lower rates of drug use—among teens.

- *Close family ties:* Asian American teens are the likeliest to come from intact homes. Respect for authority and family loyalty are strongly valued among many Asian American populations. Black teens, although least likely to come from intact homes, often come from single-parent households with close extended family ties. Teens from cohesive and stable families are less likely to use drugs.

- *Focus on schooling and education:* Teens from families who value education and where parents help with homework and limit weeknight time with friends have lower rates of drug use.

SOURCES: Johnston, L. D., et al. 2009. *Monitoring the Future: National Results on Adolescent Drug Use—Overview of Key Findings, 2008.* Bethesda, Md.: National Institute on Drug Abuse, NIH Publication No. 09–7401; Substance Abuse and Mental Health Services Administration, Office of Applied Studies. 2009. *Results from the 2008 National Survey on Drug Use and Health: National Findings.* Rockville, Md.: Office of Applied Studies, NSDUH Series H-36, HHS Publication No. SMA 09–4434.

NATIONAL SURVEY RESULTS, 2009

	LIFETIME DRUG USE	PAST YEAR DRUG USE
White	50.7	14.4
Black or African American	46.1	16.9
Hispanic or Latino	36.4	12.3
Asian American	21.2	7.4
American Indian and Alaska Native	57.6	19.5
Native Hawaiian and Pacific Islander American	N/A	N/A
Two or more races	56.1	22.2

Note: Results shown in percentages of each population group.

N/A = Data not available.

The extent of the problem has given rise to the development of workplace policies to help workers regain their health and well-being such as drug testing and referral services. Despite controversial aspects of drug testing in the workplace, a growing number of U.S. workers recognize the need for such screening. Most drug testing involves a urine test; a test for alcohol involves a blood test or a breath test. If a person tests positive for drugs, the employer may provide drug counseling or treatment, suspend the employee until he or she tests negative, or fire the individual.

Treatment for Drug Dependence

Regardless of the therapeutic approach used for drug dependence, many individuals undergoing treatment will often slide back into their drug habits. Preventing relapse and maintaining long-term cessation of drug use are complex medical goals. Relapse prevention research is increasingly focusing on expanding the repertoire of behavioral skills to overcome dependence. Medications are also used in treating addiction.

Medication-Assisted Treatment Medications can reduce the craving for the abused drug or block or oppose its effects. Perhaps the best-known medication for drug abuse is methadone, a synthetic drug used as a substitute for heroin. Use of methadone prevents withdrawal reactions and reduces the craving for heroin; it enables dependent people to function normally in social and vocational activities, although they remain dependent on methadone. The narcotic buprenorphine, approved for treatment of opioid addiction, also reduces cravings.

Medication therapy is relatively simple and inexpensive and is therefore popular among patients, health care providers, and insurance companies. However, the relapse rate is high. Combining drug therapy with psychological and social services improves success rates, underscoring the importance of psychological factors in drug dependence.

Treatment Centers Treatment centers offer a variety of short-term and long-term services, including hospitalization, detoxification, counseling, and other mental health services. The therapeutic community is a specific type of center, a residential program run in a completely drug-free atmosphere. Administered by ex-addicts, these programs use confrontation, strict discipline, and unre-

lenting peer pressure to attempt to resocialize the addict with a different set of values. Halfway houses, transitional settings between a 24-hour-a-day program and independent living, can be an important phase of treatment.

Self-Help Groups and Peer Counseling Groups such as Alcoholics Anonymous (AA) and Narcotics Anonymous (NA) have helped many people. People treated in drug substitution programs or substance-abuse treatment centers are often urged or required to join a self-help group as part of their recovery. These groups follow a 12-step program. Group members' first step is to acknowledge that they have a problem over which they have no control. Peer support is a critical ingredient of these programs, and members usually meet at least once a week. Each member is paired with a sponsor to call on for advice and support if the temptation to relapse becomes overwhelming. Chapters of AA and NA meet on some college campuses; community-based chapters are listed in the phone book and in local newspapers.

Many colleges also have peer counseling programs, in which students are trained to help other students who have drug problems. A peer counselor's role may be as limited as referring a student to a professional with expertise in substance dependence for an evaluation or as involved as helping arrange a leave of absence from school for participation in a drug-treatment program.

Harm Reduction Strategies Recognizing that many attempts at treatment are at first unsuccessful and that a drug-free society may be an unobtainable goal, some experts advocate the use of harm reduction strategies. The goal of harm reduction is to minimize the negative effects of drug use and abuse; a common example is the use of designated drivers to reduce alcohol-related motor vehicle crashes. In terms of illicit drugs, drug substitution programs such as methadone maintenance are one form of harm reduction; although participants remain drug dependent, the negative individual and social consequences of their drug use are reduced. Syringe exchange programs, designed to reduce transmission of HIV and hepatitis C, are another harm reduction approach. Some experts advocate free testing of street drugs for purity and potency to help users avoid unintentional toxicity or overdose.

Codependency Drug abuse takes a toll on friends and family members, and counseling can help people work through painful feelings of guilt and powerlessness. **Codependency**, in which a person close to the drug

TERMS

codependency A relationship in which a non–substance-abusing partner or family member is controlled by the abuser's behavior; codependent people frequently engage in enabling behaviors.

If Someone You Know Has a Drug Problem . . .

Changes in behavior and mood in someone you know may signal a growing dependence on drugs. Signs that a person's life is beginning to focus on drugs include the following:

- Sudden withdrawal or emotional distance
- Rebellious or unusually irritable behavior
- A loss of interest in usual activities or hobbies
- A decline in school performance
- A sudden change in the chosen group of friends
- Changes in sleeping or eating habits
- Frequent borrowing of money or stealing
- Secretive behavior about personal possessions, such as a backpack or the contents of a drawer
- Deterioration of physical appearance

If you believe a family member or friend has a drug problem, locate information about drug treatment available on campus or in your community. Communicate your concern, provide him or her with information about treatment options, and offer your support during treatment. If the person continues to deny having a problem, talk with an experienced counselor about setting up an intervention—a formal, structured confrontation designed to end denial by having family, friends, and other caring people present their concerns to the drug user.

And finally, examine your relationship with the abuser for signs of codependency. If necessary, get help for yourself; friends and family of drug users can often benefit from counseling.

abuser is controlled by the abuser's behavior, sometimes develops. Codependent people may come to believe that love, approval, and security are contingent on their taking care of the abuser. People can become codependent because they want to help when someone they love becomes dependent on a drug. They may assume their good intentions will persuade the drug user to stop.

Codependent people often engage in behaviors that remove or soften the effects of drug use on the user—so-called *enabling* behaviors. However, the habit of enabling can inhibit a drug abuser's recovery because the person never has to experience the consequences of his or her behavior.

Have you ever been an enabler in a relationship? You may have, if you've ever done any of the following:

- Given someone one more chance to stop abusing drugs, then another, and another . . .
- Made excuses or lied for someone to his or her friends, teachers, or employer
- Joined someone in drug use and blamed others for your behavior
- Loaned money to someone to continue drug use
- Stayed up late waiting for or gone out searching for someone who uses drugs
- Felt embarrassed or angry about the actions of someone who uses drugs
- Ignored the drug use because the person got defensive when you brought it up
- Not confronted a friend or relative who was obviously intoxicated or high on a drug

If you come from a codependent family or see yourself developing codependency relationships or engaging in enabling behaviors, consider acting now to make changes in your patterns of interaction.

Preventing Drug Abuse

Obviously, the best solution to drug abuse is prevention. Government attempts at prevention have historically focused on controlling supply—stopping the production, importation, and distribution of illegal drugs. A new national drug policy announced in 2010, however, redirects federal funding and efforts into lowering demand—developing persuasive antidrug educational programs. Indirect approaches to prevention involve building young people's self-esteem, improving their academic skills, and increasing their recreational opportunities. Direct approaches involve giving information about the adverse effects of drugs and teaching tactics that help students resist peer pressure to use drugs in various situations.

Prevention efforts need to focus on the different motivations individuals have for using and abusing specific drugs at different ages. For example, adolescents in junior or senior high school are often more responsive to peer counselors. Many young adults tend to be influenced by efforts that focus on health education. For all ages, it is important to provide nondrug alternatives—such as recreational facilities, counseling, greater opportunities for leisure activities, and places to socialize—that speak to the individual's or group's specific reasons for using drugs. Reminding young people that most people, no matter what age, do not use drugs is a critical part of preventing substance abuse.

Ask Yourself

QUESTIONS FOR CRITICAL THINKING AND REFLECTION

Do you know someone who may have a drug problem? What steps, if any, have you taken to help that person? If you were using drugs and felt that things had gone out of control, what would you want your friends to do for you?

?

Changing Your Drug Habits

This behavior change strategy focuses on one of the most commonly used drugs—caffeine. If you are concerned about your use of a different drug or another type of addictive behavior, you can devise your own plan based on this one and on the steps outlined in Chapter 1.

Because caffeine supports certain behaviors that are characteristic of our culture, such as sedentary, stressful work, you may find yourself relying on coffee (or tea, chocolate, or cola) to get through a busy schedule. Such habits often begin in college. Fortunately, it's easier to break a habit before it becomes entrenched as a lifelong dependency.

Self-Monitoring

Keep a log of how much caffeine you eat or drink. Use a measuring cup to measure coffee or tea. Using Table 7.3, convert the amounts you drink into an estimate expressed in milligrams of caffeine. Be sure to include all forms, such as chocolate bars and OTC medications, as well as caffeine candy, colas, cocoa or hot chocolate, chocolate cake, tea, and coffee.

Self-Assessment

At the end of the week, add up your daily totals and divide by 7 to get your daily average in milligrams. How much is too much?

At more than 250 mg per day, you may well be experiencing some adverse symptoms. If you are experiencing at least five of the following symptoms, you may want to cut down: restlessness, nervousness, excitement, insomnia, flushed face, excessive sweating, gastrointestinal problems, muscle twitching, rambling thoughts and speech, irregular heartbeat, periods of inexhaustibility, and excessive pacing or movement.

Set Limits

Can you restrict your caffeine intake to a daily total, and stick to this contract? If so, set a cutoff point, such as one cup of coffee. Pegging it to a specific time of day can be helpful, because then you won't confront a decision at any other point (and possibly fail). If you find you cannot stick to your limit, you may want to cut out caffeine altogether; abstinence can be easier than moderation for some people. If you experience caffeine withdrawal symptoms (headache, fatigue), you may want to cut your intake more gradually.

Find Other Ways to Keep Up Your Energy

If you are fatigued, it makes sense to get enough sleep or exercise more, rather than drowning the problem in coffee or tea. Different people need different amounts of sleep; you may also need more sleep at different times, such as during a personal crisis or an illness. Also, exercise raises your metabolic rate for hours afterward—a handy fact to exploit when you need to feel more awake and want to avoid an irritable caffeine jag. And if you've been compounding your fatigue by not eating properly, try filling up on complex carbohydrates such as whole-grain bread or crackers instead of candy bars.

Tips on Cutting Out Caffeine Here are some more ways to decrease your consumption of caffeine:

- Keep some noncaffeinated drinks on hand, such as decaffeinated coffee, herbal teas, mineral water, bouillon, or ice water.
- Alternate between hot and very cold liquids.
- Fill your coffee cup only halfway.
- Avoid the office or school lunchroom or cafeteria and the chocolate sections of the grocery store. (Often people drink coffee or tea and eat chocolate simply because they're available.)
- Read labels of over-the-counter medications to check for hidden sources of caffeine.

Connect to your Choices

Have you ever thought about why you make the choices you do about drugs? Many factors can influence the drug-related choices we make, some not as obvious as others. If you use drugs—or if you don't—have you been influenced by attitudes toward drug use in your family or peer group? Do you take drugs when they're offered at parties because it's easier than saying no? Are you influenced by media portrayals that make drug use look glamorous?

What are the external factors that influence your drug-related choices? What are your inner motivations and core values, and how do they affect your choices? Based on what you learned in this chapter, will you make some different choices in the future? If so, what will they be?

Go online to Connect to complete this activity.
www.mcgraw-hillconnect.com

TIPS FOR TODAY AND THE FUTURE

RIGHT NOW YOU CAN

- If you are a regular caffeine user, look for ways to cut back.
- Consider whether you or someone you know might benefit from drug counseling. Find out what types of services are available on campus or in your area.

IN THE FUTURE YOU CAN

- Investigate the drug-related attitudes of people you know. For example, talk to two older adults and two fellow students about their attitudes toward legalizing marijuana. What are the differences in their opinions, and how do they account for them?
- Analyze media portrayals of drug use. As you watch TV shows and movies, note the way they depict drug use among people of different ages and backgrounds. How realistic are the portrayals, in your view? Think about the influence they have on you and your peers.

SUMMARY

- Addictive behaviors are self–reinforcing. Addicts experience a strong compulsion for the behavior and a loss of control over it; an escalating pattern of abuse with serious negative consequences may result.

- The sources or causes of addiction include heredity, personality, lifestyle, and environmental factors. People may use an addictive behavior as a means of alleviating stress or painful emotions.

- Many common behaviors are potentially addictive, including gambling, shopping, sexual activity, Internet use, eating, and working.

- Drug abuse is a maladaptive pattern of drug use that persists despite adverse social, psychological, or medical consequences.

- Drug dependence involves taking a drug compulsively, which includes neglecting constructive activities because of it and continuing to use it despite experiencing adverse effects resulting from its use. Tolerance and withdrawal symptoms are often present.

- Reasons for using drugs include the lure of the illicit; curiosity; rebellion; peer pressure; and the desire to alter one's mood or escape boredom, anxiety, depression, or other psychological problems.

- Psychoactive drugs affect the mind and body by altering brain chemistry. The effect of a drug depends on the properties of the drug and how it's used (drug factors), the physical and psychological characteristics of the user (user factors), and the physical and social environment surrounding the drug use (social factors).

- Opioids relieve pain, cause drowsiness, and induce euphoria; they reduce anxiety and produce lethargy, apathy, and an inability to concentrate.

- CNS depressants slow down the overall activity of the nerves; they reduce anxiety and cause mood changes, impaired muscular coordination, slurring of speech, and drowsiness or sleep.

- CNS stimulants speed up the activity of the nerves, causing acceleration of the heart rate, a rise in blood pressure, dilation of the pupils and bronchial tubes, and an increase in gastric and adrenal secretions.

- Marijuana usually causes euphoria and a relaxed attitude at low doses; very high doses produce feelings of depersonalization and sensory distortion. The long-term effects may include chronic bronchitis and cancer; use during pregnancy may impair fetal growth.

- Hallucinogens alter perception, feelings, and thought and may cause an altered sense of time, visual disturbances, and mood changes.

- Inhalants are present in a variety of everyday products; they can cause delirium. Their use can lead to loss of consciousness, heart failure, suffocation, and death.

- Economic and social costs of drug abuse include the financial costs of law enforcement, treatment, and health care and the social costs of crime, violence, and family problems. Drug testing and drug legalization have been proposed to address some of the problems related to drug abuse.

- Approaches to treatment include medication, treatment centers, self-help groups, and peer counseling; many programs also offer counseling to family members.

FOR MORE INFORMATION

BOOKS

Aue, P. W. 2007. *Teen Drug Abuse: Opposing Viewpoints.* San Diego: Greenhaven Press. *Explores key issues relating to drug use and abuse by teenagers.*

Hanson, G. R., et al. 2008. *Drugs and Society,* 10th ed. Boston: Jones & Bartlett. *Discusses the impact of drug abuse on individuals' lives and on the broader society.*

Ksir, C., C. L. Hart, and O. S. Ray. 2010. *Drugs, Society, and Human Behavior,* 14th ed. New York: McGraw-Hill. *Examines drugs and behavior from the behavioral, pharmacological, historical, social, legal, and clinical perspectives.*

Lessa, N. R., et al. 2006. *Wiley Concise Guides to Mental Health: Substance Use Disorders.* New York: Wiley. *A clearly written introduction to the diagnosis and treatment of various kinds of substance abuse.*

Murphy, P. J. M., and M. Shlafer. 2006. *Over-the-Counter Drugs of Abuse.* New York: Chelsea House Publications. *An up-to-date discussion of nonprescription medicines and their abuse.*

Rosen Publishing. 2009. *Drug Abuse and Society Series.* New York: Rosen Publishing. *A series of short books, each exploring a different type of drugs—from prescription medicine to club drugs—and their use and abuse.*

ORGANIZATIONS, HOTLINES, AND WEB SITES

ClubDrugs.Gov. Provides information on drugs commonly classified as "club drugs."
http://www.clubdrugs.gov

Do It Now Foundation. Provides youth-oriented information about drugs.
http://www.doitnow.org

Drug Enforcement Administration: Drug Information. Provides basic facts about major drugs of abuse, including penalties for drug trafficking.
http://www.dea.gov/concern/concern.htm

Gamblers Anonymous. Includes questions to help diagnose gambling problems and resources for getting help.
http://www.gamblersanonymous.org

Higher Education Center for Alcohol and Other Drug Abuse and Violence Prevention. Gives information about alcohol and drug abuse on campus and links to related sites.
http://www.higheredcenter.org

Indiana Prevention Resource Center. A clearinghouse of information on substance-abuse topics, including specific psychoactive drugs and issues such as drug testing and drug legalization.
http://www.drugs.indiana.edu

Narcotics Anonymous (NA). Similar to Alcoholics Anonymous, NA sponsors 12-step meetings and provides other support services for drug abusers.

http://www.na.org

There are also 12-step programs that focus on specific drugs:

Cocaine Anonymous

http://www.ca.org

Marijuana Anonymous

http://www.marijuana-anonymous.org

National Center on Addiction and Substance Abuse (CASA) at Columbia University. Provides information about the costs of substance abuse to individuals and society.

http://www.casacolumbia.org

National Clearinghouse for Alcohol and Drug Information. Provides statistics, information, and publications on substance abuse, including resources for people who want to help friends and family members overcome substance-abuse problems.

http://ncadi.samhsa.gov

National Council on Problem Gambling. Provides information and help for people with gambling problems and their families, including a searchable directory of counselors.

http://www.ncpgambling.org

National Drug Information, Treatment, and Referral Hotlines. Sponsored by the SAMHSA Center for Substance Abuse Treatment, these hotlines provide information on drug abuse and on HIV infection as it relates to substance abuse; referrals to support groups and treatment programs are available.

800-662-HELP

800-729-6686 (Spanish)

800-487-4889 (TDD for hearing impaired)

National Institute on Drug Abuse. Develops and supports research on drug-abuse prevention programs.

http://www.drugabuse.gov

Substance Abuse and Mental Health Services Administration (SAMHSA). Provides statistics, information, and other resources related to substance-abuse prevention and treatment.

http://www.samhsa.gov

See also the listings for Chapters 10 and 11.

SELECTED BIBLIOGRAPHY

American Psychiatric Association. 2000. *Diagnostic and Statistical Manual of Mental Disorders,* 4th ed. text revision. (DSM-IV-TR). Washington, D.C.: American Psychiatric Association.

Beers, M. H., et al. 2006. *The Merck Manual of Diagnosis and Therapy,* 18th ed. New York: Wiley.

Centers for Disease Control and Prevention. 2006. Methamphetamine use and HIV risk behaviors among heterosexual men. *Morbidity and Mortality Weekly Report* 55(10): 273–277.

Centers for Disease Control and Prevention. 2006. Surveillance for acute viral hepatitis—United States, 2007. *Morbidity and Mortality Report Surveillance Summaries* 58(SS-3): 1–30.

Centers for Disease Control and Prevention. 2010. *HIV Surveillance Report, 2008,* vol. 20 (http://www.cdc.gov/hiv/topics/surveillance/resources/reports; retrieved November 3, 2010).

Colfax, G., et al. 2005. Longitudinal patterns of methamphetamine, popper (amyl nitrite), and cocaine use and high-risk sexual behavior among a cohort of San Francisco men who have sex with men. *Journal of Urban Health,* 28 February [epub].

Grant, J. E., et al. 2006. Multicenter investigation of the opioid antagonist nalmefene in the treatment of pathological gambling. *American Journal of Psychiatry* 163(2): 303–312.

Hurd, Y. L., et al. 2005. Marijuana impairs growth in mid-gestation fetuses. *Neurotoxicology and Teratology* 27(2): 221–229.

Iannone, M., et al. 2006. Electrocortical effects of MDMA are potentiated by acoustic stimulation in rats. *BMC Neuroscience* 7: 13.

Jefferson, D. J. 2005. America's most dangerous drug. *Newsweek,* 8 August, 41–48.

Johnston, L. D., et al. 2009. *Monitoring the Future: National Results on Adolescent Drug Use: Overview of Key Findings, 2008.* Bethesda, Md.: National Institute on Drug Abuse NIH Publication No. 09–7401.

Kim, S. W., et al. 2006. Pathological gambling and mood disorders: Clinical associations and treatment implications. *Journal of Affective Disorders* 92(1): 109–116.

Mahowald, M. L., J. A. Singh, and P. Majeski. 2005. Opioid use by patients in an orthopedics spine clinic. *Arthritis and Rheumatology* 52(1): 312–321.

Messinis, L., et al. 2006. Neuropsychological deficits in long-term frequent cannabis users. *Neurology* 66(5): 737–739.

National Council on Problem Gambling. 2010. *What Is Problem Gambling?* (http://www.ncpgambling.org/i4a/pages/index.cfm?pageid=1; retrieved November 3, 2010).

National Institute on Drug Abuse. 2008. *Comorbidty: Addiction and Other Mental Illnesses.* Bethesda, Md.: National Institute on Drug Abuse, NIH Publicatoin No. 08–5771.

Office of National Drug Control Policy. 2010. *2010 National Strategy* (http://www.whitehousedrugpolicy.gov/strategy/; retrieved November 3, 2010).

Parrott, A. C. 2005. Chronic tolerance to recreational MDMA (3,4-methylenedioxymethamphetamine) or ecstasy. *Journal of Psychopharmacology* 19(1): 71–83.

Ren, S., et al. 2006. Effect of long-term cocaine use on regional left ventricular function as determined by magnetic resonance imaging. *American Journal of Cardiology* 97(7): 1085–1088.

Savoca, M. R., et al. 2005. Association of ambulatory blood pressure and dietary caffeine in adolescents. *American Journal of Hypertension* 18(1): 116–120.

Substance Abuse and Mental Health Services Administration, Office of Applied Studies. 2009. *Results from the 2008 National Survey on Drug Use and Health: National Findings.* Rockville, Md.: Office of Applied Studies, NSDUH Series H-36, HHS Publication No. SMA 09–4434.

Substance Abuse and Mental Health Services Administration, Office of Applied Studies. 2010. *Drug Abuse Warning Network, 2007: National Estimate of Drug-Related Emergency Department Visits.* Rockville, Md.: Substance Abuse and Mental Health Services Administration.

U.S. Department of Justice, Federal Bureau of Investigation. 2009. *Crime in the United States: 2008* (http://www.fbi.gov/ucr/cius2008/index.html; retrieved November 3, 2010).

Wareing, M., et al. 2005. Visuo-spatial working memory deficits in current and former users of MDMA ("ecstasy"). *Human Psychopharmacology* 20(2): 115–123.

Waska, R. 2006. Addictions and the quest to control the object. *American Journal of Psychoanalysis* 66(1): 43–62.

Zakzanis, K. K., and Z. Campbell. 2006. Memory impairment in now abstinent MDMA users and continued users: A longitudinal follow-up. *Neurology* 66(5): 740–741.

LOOKING AHEAD...

After reading this chapter, you should be able to:

- Explain how alcohol is absorbed and metabolized by the body
- Describe the immediate and long-term effects of drinking alcohol
- Describe the different forms of alcohol abuse and their consequences
- List the reasons people start using tobacco and why they continue to use it
- Explain the short- and long-term health risks associated with tobacco use
- Describe strategies for using alcohol responsibly, and prepare plans to stop using tobacco and to avoid environmental tobacco smoke

Alcohol and Tobacco

8

When we think about drugs, most of us think of either the over-the-counter medications we get for colds and coughs or illicit drugs like marijuana and cocaine. The truth is that the most common and widely used drugs in the United States—and the ones responsible for the most illnesses, injuries, and deaths—are **alcohol** and **tobacco**. Alcohol use is associated with more than 75,000 deaths per year among Americans, and tobacco use is associated with more than 440,000 deaths per year.

Alcohol has a mixed role in human life. Used in moderation, alcohol can enhance social occasions by loosening inhibitions and creating a pleasant feeling of relaxation. But like other drugs, alcohol has physiological effects that can impair functioning in the short term and cause devastating damage in the long term. For some people, alcohol use becomes an addiction, leading to a lifetime of recovery or, for a few, to debilitation and death.

Tobacco use affects the health of people at all stages of life and from all walks of life. On average, a male smoker loses about 13 years from his life; a female smoker loses nearly 15 years. Nonsmokers also suffer, especially the children of parents who smoke. Exposure to environmental tobacco smoke (ETS) kills thousands of nonsmokers every year. Smoking is the leading cause of preventable death in the United States. This chapter examines the complexities of alcohol and tobacco use in the United States.

THE NATURE OF ALCOHOL

If you have ever been around people who are drinking, you probably noticed that alcohol seems to affect different people in different ways. One person may seem to get drunk after just a drink or two, while another appears to tolerate a great deal of alcohol without becoming intoxicated. These differences can be explained by looking at the chemistry of alcohol and how it is absorbed and metabolized by the body.

Alcoholic Beverages

There are several basic types of alcoholic beverages. Ethanol is the psychoactive ingredient in each of them:

- Beer is a mild intoxicant brewed from a mixture of grains. By volume, beer usually contains 3–6% alcohol.

- Ales and malt liquors contain 6–8% alcohol by volume.

- Wines are made by fermenting the juices of grapes or other fruits. In table wines, the concentration of alcohol is about 9–14%. *Fortified wines,* so called because extra alcohol is added to them, include sherry, port, and Madeira. They contain about 20% alcohol.

- Hard liquor—such as gin, whiskey, rum, tequila, vodka, and liqueur—is made by *distilling* brewed or fermented grains or other plant products. Hard liquors usually contain 35–50% alcohol.

The concentration of alcohol in a beverage is indicated by its **proof value,** which is two times the percentage concentration. For example, if a beverage is 100 proof, it contains 50% alcohol by volume. The proof value of hard liquor can usually be found on the bottle's label. When alcohol consumption is discussed, the term **one drink** (or *a standard drink*) means the amount of a beverage that typically contains about 0.6 ounce of alcohol.

Alcohol provides 7 calories per gram, and the alcohol in one drink (14–17 grams) supplies about 100–120 calories. Most alcoholic beverages also contain some carbohydrate so, for example, one beer provides about 150 total calories. The "light" in light beer refers to calories; a light beer typically has close to the same alcohol content as a regular beer and about 100 calories. A 5-ounce glass of red wine has 100 calories; white wine has 96. A 3-ounce margarita supplies 157 calories, a 6-ounce cosmopolitan has 143 calories, and a 6-ounce rum and Coke contains about 180 calories.

Absorption

When a person ingests alcohol, about 20% is rapidly absorbed from the stomach into the bloodstream. About 75% is absorbed through the upper part of the small intestine. Any remaining alcohol enters the bloodstream further along the gastrointestinal tract. Once in the bloodstream, alcohol produces feelings of intoxication.

TERMS

alcohol The intoxicating ingredient in fermented or distilled beverages; a colorless, pungent liquid.

tobacco The leaves of cultivated tobacco plants prepared for smoking, chewing, or use as snuff.

proof value Two times the percentage of alcohol by volume; a "100-proof" beverage is 50% alcohol by volume.

one drink The amount of a beverage that typically contains about 0.6 ounce of alcohol; also called *a standard drink.*

metabolism The chemical transformation of food and other substances in the body into energy and wastes.

blood alcohol concentration (BAC) The amount of alcohol in the blood in terms of weight per unit volume; used as a measure of intoxication.

The rate of absorption is affected by a variety of factors. For example, the carbonation in a beverage like champagne increases the rate of alcohol absorption. Artificial sweeteners (commonly used in drink mixers) have the same effect. Food in the stomach slows the rate of absorption, as does the drinking of highly concentrated alcoholic beverages such as hard liquor.

Metabolism and Excretion

Because alcohol easily moves through most biological membranes, it is rapidly distributed throughout most body tissues via the bloodstream. The main site of alcohol **metabolism** is the liver, though a small amount of alcohol is metabolized in the stomach (see the box "Metabolizing Alcohol: Our Bodies Work Differently"). About 2–10% of ingested alcohol is not metabolized in the liver or other tissues but is excreted unchanged by the lungs, kidneys, and sweat glands. Excreted alcohol causes the telltale smell on a drinker's breath and is the basis of breath and urine analyses for alcohol levels.

Alcohol readily enters the human brain, affecting neurotransmitters, the chemicals that carry messages between brain cells. With chronic heavy usage, however, alcohol's effects become permanent, resulting in permanent disruption of brain function and changes in brain structure.

Alcohol Intake and Blood Alcohol Concentration

Blood alcohol concentration (BAC) is the amount of alcohol in a person's blood, expressed as the percentage of alcohol measured in a deciliter of blood. BAC is affected by the amount of alcohol consumed in a given amount of time and by individual factors:

- *Body weight:* In most cases, a smaller person develops a higher BAC than a larger person after drinking the same amount of alcohol (Figure 8.1). A smaller person has less overall body tissue into which alcohol can be distributed.

- *Percent body fat:* A person with a higher percentage of body fat will usually develop a higher BAC than a more muscular person of the same weight. Alcohol does not concentrate as much in fatty tissue as in muscle and most other tissues, in part because fat has fewer blood vessels.

- *Sex:* Women metabolize less alcohol in the stomach than men do because the stomach enzyme that breaks down alcohol before it enters the bloodstream is four times more active in men than in women. This means that more unmetabolized alcohol is released into the bloodstream in women. Because women are also generally smaller than men and have a higher percentage of body fat, women will have a higher BAC than men after consuming the same amount of alcohol. Hormonal fluctuations

Metabolizing Alcohol: Our Bodies Work Differently

Do you notice that you react differently to alcohol than some of your friends? If so, you may be witnessing genetic differences in alcohol metabolism that are associated with ethnicity. Alcohol is metabolized mainly in the liver, where it is converted by an enzyme (alcohol dehydrogenase) to a toxic substance called acetaldehyde. Acetaldehyde is responsible for many of alcohol's noxious effects. Ideally, it is quickly broken down by another enzyme (acetaldehyde dehydrogenase).

But some people, primarily those of Asian descent, have inherited ineffective or inactive variations of the latter enzyme. Other people, including some of African descent and some Jewish population groups, have forms of alcohol dehydrogenase that metabolize alcohol to acetaldehyde unusually quickly. In either case, the result is a buildup of acetaldehyde when these people drink alcohol. They experience a reaction called *flush-ing syndrome*. Their skin feels hot, their heart and respiration rates increase, and they may get a headache, vomit, or break out in hives. The severity of their reaction is affected by the inherited form of their alcohol-metabolizing enzymes. Drinking makes some people so uncomfortable that it's unlikely they could ever become addicted to alcohol.

The body's response to acetaldehyde is the basis for treating alcohol abuse with the drug disulfiram (Antabuse), which inhibits the action of acetaldehyde dehydrogenase. When a person taking disulfiram ingests alcohol, acetaldehyde levels increase rapidly, and he or she develops an intense flushing reaction along with weakness, nausea, vomiting, and other disagreeable symptoms.

How people behave in relation to alcohol is influenced in complex ways by many factors, including social and cultural ones. But in this case at least, individual choices and behavior are strongly influenced by a specific genetic characteristic.

may also affect the rate of alcohol metabolism, making a woman more susceptible to high BACs at certain times during her menstrual cycle (usually just prior to the onset of menstruation).

BAC also depends on the balance between the rate of alcohol absorption and the rate of alcohol metabolism. A man who weighs 150 pounds and has normal liver function metabolizes about 0.3 ounce of alcohol per hour, the equivalent of about half a 12-ounce bottle of beer or half a 5-ounce glass of wine. The rate of alcohol metabolism varies among individuals and is largely determined by genetic factors and drinking behavior. Although the rate of alcohol absorption can be slowed by factors like food, the metabolic rate *cannot* be influenced by exercise, breathing deeply, eating, drinking coffee, or taking other drugs. The rate of alcohol metabolism is the same whether a person is asleep or awake.

If a person absorbs slightly less alcohol each hour than he or she can metabolize in an hour, the BAC remains low. People can drink large amounts of alcohol this way over a long period of

79,000 American deaths are related to excessive alcohol use each year.

—CDC, 2010

QUICK STATS

FIGURE 8.1 Approximate blood alcohol concentration and body weight. This chart illustrates the BAC an average person of a given weight would reach after drinking the specified number of drinks in the time shown. The legal limit for BAC in all states is 0.08%; for drivers under 21 years of age, many states have zero-tolerance laws that set BAC limits of 0.01% or 0.02%.

Dealing with an Alcohol Emergency

Remember: Being very drunk is potentially life-threatening. Helping a drunken friend could save a life.

- Be firm but calm. Don't engage the person in an argument or discuss her drinking behavior while she is intoxicated.

- Get the person out of harm's way. Don't let her drive, wander outside, or drink any more alcohol.

- If the person is unconscious, don't assume she is just "sleeping it off." Place her on her side with her knees up. This position helps prevent choking if she should vomit.

- Stay with the person. You need to be ready to help if she vomits or stops breathing.

- Don't try to give the person anything to eat or drink, including coffee or other drugs. Don't give cold showers or try to make her walk around. None of these things help anyone to sober up, and they can be dangerous.

Call 911 immediately in any of the following instances:

- You can't wake the person even with shouting or shaking.

- The person is taking fewer than 8 breaths per minute or her breathing seems shallow or irregular.

- You think the person took other drugs with alcohol.

- The person has had an injury, especially a blow to the head.

- The person drank a large amount of alcohol in a short period of time and then became unconscious. Death caused by alcohol poisoning most often occurs when the blood alcohol level rises very quickly due to rapid ingestion of alcohol.

If you aren't sure what to do, call 911. You may save a life.

---

time without becoming noticeably intoxicated. Regardless, they run the risk of long-term health hazards. If a person drinks alcohol more quickly than it can be metabolized, the BAC will steadily increase, and he or she will become more and more drunk.

ALCOHOL AND HEALTH

The effects of alcohol consumption on health depend on the individual, the circumstances, and the amount of alcohol consumed.

The Immediate Effects of Alcohol

Alcohol is a CNS depressant, and its effects vary because body systems are affected to different degrees at different BACs. At any given BAC, the effects of alcohol are more pronounced when the BAC is rapidly increasing than when it is slowly increasing, steady, or decreasing. The effects of alcohol are more pronounced if a person drinks on an empty stomach, because alcohol is absorbed more quickly and the BAC rises more quickly.

The effects of alcohol can first be felt at a BAC of about 0.03–0.05% and may include light-headedness, relaxation, and a release of inhibitions. Most drinkers experience mild euphoria and become more sociable. When people drink in social settings, alcohol often seems to act as a stimulant, enhancing conviviality or assertiveness. This apparent stimulation occurs because alcohol depresses inhibitory centers in the brain.

At higher concentrations, the pleasant effects tend to be replaced by more negative ones: interference with motor coordination, verbal performance, and intellectual functions. (See page T1-2 of the color transparency insert "Touring Lifestyle Behaviors" in this chapter.)

Alcohol Hangover Alcohol's effects wear off slowly. The symptoms of a hangover include headache, shakiness, nausea, diarrhea, fatigue, and impaired mental functioning. During a hangover, heart rate and blood pressure increase, making some individuals more vulnerable to heart attacks. Electroencephalography (brain wave measurement) shows diffuse slowing of brain waves for up to 16 hours after BAC drops to 0.0%. Studies of pilots, drivers, and skiers all indicate that coordination and cognition are impaired in a person with a hangover, increasing the risk of injury.

Alcohol Poisoning Drinking large amounts of alcohol in a short time can rapidly raise the BAC into the lethal range. Death from alcohol poisoning may be caused either by central nervous system and respiratory depression or by inhaling fluid or vomit into the lungs. The amount of alcohol it takes to make a person unconscious is dangerously close to a fatal dose. Although passing out may prevent someone from drinking more, BAC can keep rising during unconsciousness, because the body continues absorbing ingested alcohol into the bloodstream. Special care should be taken to ensure the safety of anyone who has been drinking heavily, especially if he or she passes out (see the box "Dealing with an Alcohol Emergency").

Using Alcohol with Other Drugs Alcohol-drug combinations are a leading cause of drug-related deaths. Using alcohol while taking a medication that causes CNS depression increases the effects of both drugs, potentially leading to coma, respiratory depression, and death. Such drugs include barbiturates, Valium-like drugs, narcotics such as codeine, and OTC antihistamines such as Benadryl. For people who consume 3 or more drinks per day, use of OTC pain relievers like aspirin, ibuprofen, or acetaminophen increases the risk of stomach bleeding or liver damage.

Caffeinated Alcoholic Beverages: The Dangers of Being "Drunk and Wide Awake"

Over the past decade, the practice of blending alcoholic beverages with highly caffeinated energy drinks has grown increasingly popular, particularly among young adults and underage drinkers. A 2007 study showed that 31% of 12- to 17-year-olds and 34% of 18- to 24-year-olds regularly drink caffeinated alcoholic beverages (CABs), also known as alcoholic energy drinks (AEDs). The caffeine in a CAB masks the depressant effects of the alcohol, producing a "drunk and wide awake" state of alert intoxication, potentially leading the drinker to consume more alcohol than he or she would otherwise. Caffeine does nothing to speed the metabolism of the alcohol.

Cashing in on the lucrative energy drink market and the CAB trend, alcoholic beverage manufacturers have flooded the market with commercial, pre-mixed CABs, and by the end of 2009, at least 30 manufacturers were marketing dozens of varieties, with names like Rockstar 21, Sparks, and Torque. CABs makers target a youth market and associate their product with extreme sports and activities like skateboarding and snowboarding, emphasizing the "energy boost" the products can provide.

Commercial CABs are typically malt- or distilled-spirits based and have higher alcohol content than beer (5–12% alcohol by volume compared to 4–5% for beer). The amount of caffeine and other stimulants in a CAB is usually not reported by the manufacturer. Health officials are concerned that many CABs contain much higher levels of caffeine than are found in soft drinks,

which is limited by the FDA to 200 parts per million. This amount meets criteria for being "generally regarded as safe (GRAS)" for human consumption.

A growing body of evidence highlights the risks associated with the use of caffeinated alcoholic beverages. For example, studies cited by the CDC have reported the following:

- Being in a "drunk/awake" state can lead to risky behaviors such as drunk driving, unplanned sex or sexual assault, and aggression.

- CAB drinkers are three times as likely as non-CAB drinkers to binge drink.

- CAB drinkers are about twice as likely as non-CAB drinkers to report being taken

advantage of sexually, taking advantage of someone sexually, or riding with a driver who was under the influence of alcohol.

- Emerging evidence indicates that CAB use, especially by adolescents, may lead to an increased risk of alcohol or drug dependence later in life.

These concerns and others led the FDA to launch an investigation into the safety, and even the legality, of commercial CABs. In 2009, the FDA sent letters to nearly 30 CAB manufacturers, asking them to prove that their products met GRAS criteria. Manufacturers that could not provide sufficient evidence of their products' safety risked having their products removed from the marketplace. The FDA investigation is ongoing.

Prior to the investigation, two manufacturers of CABs voluntarily removed their products from the market and committed to discontinuing production of such beverages permanently. In light of this development, and skepticism among scientists that CABs can be proven safe, the CAB market may start to shrink—if not disappear altogether—in the near future. By late 2010, several states had banned the sale of CABs.

SOURCES: Arria, A. M., et al. 2009. *Letter to the FDA Regarding the Use of Caffeine in Alcoholic Beverages* (http://www.fda.gov/downloads/food/foodingredientspackaging/ucm190372.pdf; retrieved July 8, 2010); Centers for Disease Control and Prevention. 2010. *Alcohol and Public Health: Caffeinated Alcoholic Beverages* (http://www.cdc.gov/alcohol/caff-alcohol-bev.htm; retrieved July 8, 2010); U.S. Food and Drug Administration. 2010. *Caffeinated Alcoholic Beverages* (http://www.fda.gov/food/foodingredientspackaging/ucm190366.htm; retrieved July 8, 2010).

Some antibiotics and diabetes medications can also interact dangerously with alcohol. Many illegal drugs are especially dangerous when combined with alcohol. Life-threatening overdoses occur at much lower doses when heroin and other narcotics are combined with alcohol. A recent trend among young drinkers is mixing alcoholic beverages with caffeinated ones, especially highly caffeinated energy drinks (see the box "Caffeinated Alcoholic Beverages: The Dangers of Being 'Drunk and Wide Awake'").

Alcohol-Related Injuries and Violence The combination of impaired judgment, weakened sensory perception, reduced inhibitions, impaired motor coordination, and increased aggressiveness and hostility that characterizes alcohol intoxication can be dangerous. Through homicide, suicide, automobile crashes, and other traumatic incidents, alcohol use is linked to more than 79,000 American deaths each year. Among successful suicides, alcohol use is common as well. Alcohol use more than triples the risk of fatal injuries during leisure activities such as swimming and boating. More than 50% of fatal falls and serious burns happen to people who have been drinking.

Alcohol and Aggression   In 2008, more than 2,720,000 arrests were made for alcohol-related offenses (driving under the influence of alcohol, public drunkenness, and liquor-law violations). Alcohol use contributes to over 50% of all murders, assaults, and rapes. Alcohol is frequently found in the bloodstream of victims as well as perpetrators. However, only some people become violent under alcohol's influence. These people are often predisposed to aggressive behavior and are highly impulsive. Some may have an underlying psychiatric condition called *antisocial personality disorder.* Alcohol is an important component of gang life, affirming masculinity and male togetherness and contributing to gang violence.

Alcohol abuse can wreak havoc on home life. Marital discord and domestic violence often occur in the presence of excess alcohol. Heavy drinking by parents is associated with child abuse, typically emotional or psychological abuse.

Alcohol and Sexual Decision Making   Alcohol seriously affects a person's ability to make wise decisions about sex. Heavy drinkers are more likely to have multiple sex partners and to engage in other forms of high-risk sexual behavior. Rates of sexually transmitted infections (including HIV) and unwanted pregnancy are higher among people who drink heavily than among people who drink moderately or not at all. Women who binge-drink are at increased risk of rape and other forms of nonconsensual sex.

Drinking and Driving

In 2008, 11,773 Americans were killed in accidents involving drivers with a BAC of 0.08% or higher—about 32% of all traffic fatalities for the year. This figure represents a 10% decrease in alcohol-related traffic fatalities from 2007; even so, the National Highway Transportation Safety Administration (NHTSA) estimates that someone is killed in an alcohol-related crash every 45 minutes. Each year, more than 275,000 people are injured in alcohol-related car crashes—an average of 1 person injured every 2 minutes. In the 2008 National Survey on Drug Use and Health, 13.4% of

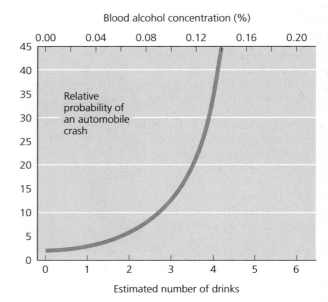

FIGURE 8.2   The dose-response relationship between BAC and automobile crashes.

Americans age 18 and older admitted driving under the influence of alcohol.

People who drink and drive are unable to drive safely because their judgment is impaired, their reaction time is slower, and their coordination is reduced. Some driving skills are affected at BACs of 0.02% and lower. The *dose-response function* is the relationship between the amount of alcohol or drug consumed and the type and intensity of the resulting effect. Higher doses of alcohol are associated with a much greater probability of automobile crashes (Figure 8.2). A person driving with a BAC of 0.14% is more than 40 times more likely to be involved in a crash than someone with no alcohol in his or her blood. For those with a BAC above 0.14%, the risk of a fatal crash is estimated to be 380 times higher.

In addition to an increased risk of injury and death, driving while intoxicated can have serious legal consequences. Since 2003, the legal limit for BAC has been 0.08% in all states, the District of Columbia, and Puerto Rico. There are stiff penalties for drunk driving, including fines, loss of license, confiscation of vehicle, and jail time. Under current zero-tolerance laws in many states, drivers under age 21 who have consumed *any* alcohol may have their license suspended. If you are out of your home and drinking, find alternative transportation or have a *designated driver* who doesn't drink and can provide safe transportation home.

It's more difficult to protect yourself against someone else who drinks and drives. Learn to be alert to the erratic driving that signals an impaired driver. Warning signs include wide, abrupt, and illegal turns; straddling the center line or lane marker; driving against traffic; driving on the shoulder; weaving, swerving, or nearly striking an object or another vehicle; following too closely; erratic

Central nervous system: Impaired reaction time and motor coordination; impaired judgment and sedation; coma and death at high BACs

Senses: Less acute vision, smell, taste, and hearing

Stomach: Nausea, inflammation, and bleeding

Skin: Flushing; sweating; heat loss and hypothermia; formation of broken capillaries

Sexual functioning: In men, reduced erection response

Brain: Damaged/destroyed brain cells; impaired memory; loss of sensation in limbs; brain atrophy

Cardiovascular system: Weakened cardiac muscle; elevated blood pressure; irregular heartbeat; increased risk of stroke

Breast: Increased risk of breast cancer

Immune system: Lowered resistance to disease

Digestive system: Cirrhosis of the liver; hepatitis; inflammation of stomach and pancreas; increased risk of cancers of the lip, mouth, larynx, esophagus, liver, rectum, stomach, and pancreas

Kidney: Kidney failure associated with end-stage liver disease

Nutrition: Nutrient deficiencies; obesity

Reproductive system: In women, menstrual irregularities and increased risk of having children with fetal alcohol syndrome (FAS); in men, impotence and impaired sperm production

Bone: Increased risk of osteoporosis; increased risk of fractures from frequent falls

FIGURE 8.3 The immediate and long-term effects of alcohol abuse.

speed; driving with headlights off at night; and driving with the window down in very cold weather. If you see any of these signs, try the following strategies:

- If the driver is ahead of you, maintain a safe following distance. Don't try to pass.

- If the driver is behind you, turn right at the nearest intersection, and let the driver pass.

- If the driver is approaching your car, move to the shoulder and stop. Avoid a head-on collision by sounding your horn or flashing your lights.

- When approaching an intersection, slow down and stay alert for vehicles that don't slow.

- Make sure your safety belt is fastened and children are in approved safety seats.

- Report suspected impaired drivers to the nearest police station by phone.

The Effects of Chronic Use

Because alcohol is distributed throughout most of the body, it can affect many different organs and tissues (Figure 8.3).

The Digestive System   Even in the short term, alcohol can alter the functioning of the liver. Within just a few days of heavy alcohol consumption, fat begins to accumulate in liver cells, resulting in the development of "fatty liver." If drinking continues, inflammation of the liver can occur, resulting in alcoholic hepatitis, a frequent cause of hospitalization and death in alcoholics. With continued alcohol use, liver cells are progressively damaged and then permanently destroyed. The destroyed cells are replaced by fibrous scar tissue, a condition known as **cirrhosis.** People with cirrhosis who continue to drink have only a 50% chance of surviving 5 or more years.

Alcohol can inflame the pancreas, causing nausea, vomiting, abnormal digestion, and severe pain. Unlike cirrhosis, which usually occurs after years of fairly heavy alcohol use, pancreatitis can occur after one or two severe binge-drinking episodes. Acute pancreatitis is often fatal; in survivors it can become a chronic condition.

cirrhosis   A disease in which the liver is severely damaged by alcohol, other toxins, or infection.

TERMS

The Cardiovascular System   The effects of alcohol on the cardiovascular system depend on the amount of alcohol consumed. Moderate doses of alcohol—one drink or less a day for women and one to two drinks a day for men—may reduce the risk of heart disease and heart attack in some people. However, higher doses of alcohol have harmful effects on the cardiovascular system. In some people, more than two drinks a day will elevate blood pressure, making stroke and heart attack more likely. Some alcoholics show a weakening of the heart muscle, a condition known as **cardiac myopathy.** Binge drinking can cause "holiday heart," a syndrome characterized by serious abnormal heart rhythms, which usually appear within 24 hours of a binge episode.

Cancer   The U.S. Department of Health and Human Services lists alcoholic beverages as human carcinogens. Chronic alcohol consumption is a clear risk factor for cancers of the mouth, throat, larynx, and esophagus. Five or six daily drinks, especially combined with smoking, increase risk of these cancers by a factor of 50 or more. Alcohol also is largely responsible for the most common form of liver cancer. Recent studies show that breast cancer risk, although still small, begins to increase at two to three drinks per day, and continues to rise with increasing numbers of daily drinks. Research conducted in 2009 indicates that even moderate drinking may encourage the recurrence of breast cancer in women who have survived the disease before.

> *The U.S. Department of Health and Human Services has listed alcohol as a known human carcinogen.*

Brain Damage   Imaging studies document that many alcoholics experience brain shrinkage with loss of both grey and white matter, reduced blood flow, and slowed metabolic rates in some brain regions. About half of the alcoholics in the United States have cognitive impairments, ranging from mild to severe. These include memory loss, dementia, and compromised problem-solving and reasoning abilities. Malnutrition, particularly thiamine deficiency, contributes to severe brain damage.

Mortality   Excessive alcohol consumption is a factor in several of the leading causes of death for Americans. Average life expectancy among alcoholics is about 15 years less than among nonalcoholics. About half the deaths caused by alcohol are due to chronic conditions such as cirrhosis and cancer; the other half are due to acute conditions or events such as car crashes, falls, and suicide.

TERMS

cardiac myopathy   Weakening of the heart muscle through disease.

The Effects of Alcohol Use During Pregnancy

During pregnancy, alcohol and its metabolic product acetaldehyde readily cross the placenta, potentially harming the developing fetus. Damage to the fetus depends on the amount of alcohol consumed and the stage of the pregnancy. Early in pregnancy, heavy drinking can cause spontaneous abortion or miscarriage. Alcohol in early pregnancy can also cause a collection of birth defects known as fetal alcohol syndrome (FAS). Children with FAS have a characteristic mixture of deformities, and their physical and mental growth is slower than normal.

FAS is a permanent, incurable condition that causes lifelong disability; it is among the most common preventable causes of mental retardation in the Western world. Full-blown FAS occurs in up to 15 out of every 10,000 live births

> **12.2%** of **pregnant women drink alcohol, and almost 2% are binge drinkers.**
>
> —CDC, 2009

Experts warn that there is no safe level of alcohol consumption during pregnancy.

in the United States. About three times as many babies are born with **alcohol-related neurodevelopmental disorder (ARND).** Children with ARND appear physically normal but often have significant learning and behavioral disorders. The whole range of FAS and ARND is commonly called *fetal alcohol spectrum disorder (FASD).*

No one is sure exactly how much alcohol causes FASD or ARND, but a recent study found that children born to mothers who drank as little as one and a half drinks per week during their pregnancy weighed less and were shorter at age 14 than children of mothers who drank nothing during pregnancy. Such evidence has led experts to assert that no amount of alcohol during pregnancy is safe.

Women who are trying to conceive, or who are sexually active without using effective contraception, are also advised to abstain from alcohol to avoid inadvertently harming their baby in the first few days or weeks of pregnancy. And because alcohol quickly enters breast milk, many physicians advise mothers to abstain from drinking alcohol if they are breast-feeding.

Possible Health Benefits of Alcohol

Numerous studies have shown that, on average, light to moderate drinkers live longer than either abstainers or heavy drinkers. Alcohol consumption appears to confer health benefits primarily to middle-aged or older individuals.

If you are 35 or younger, your odds of dying *increase* in direct proportion to the amount of alcohol you drink. Among people under age 35, even light drinkers have slightly higher mortality rates than nondrinkers. In other words, young adults who drink *any* amount of alcohol are more likely to die than nondrinkers of the same age.

Alcohol's benefits relate to heart health. The lowest rates of coronary heart disease (CHD) deaths occur with moderate alcohol use, which in studies had a positive effect on both healthy people and individuals at risk for CHD. In a 2006 study of men age 50 and over, those who drank moderately each day reduced their risk of CHD by about 40%, compared to men who never drank. The difference was not as great in women. Moderate drinking may improve heart health by raising blood levels of HDL (the beneficial form of cholesterol), by thinning the blood, and by reducing inflammation and the risk of dangerous blood clots, all of which can contribute to the risk of a heart attack. Some evidence also suggests that moderate drinkers may be less likely to develop or better able to

manage a variety of other conditions, including diabetes, high blood pressure, strokes, arterial blockages in the legs, cognitive decline (including Alzheimer's disease), and benign prostate enlargement.

ALCOHOL ABUSE AND DEPENDENCE

The CDC estimates that about 60% of Americans age 18 and older drink alcohol routinely or infrequently. Approximately 15% of Americans are former drinkers, and 25% are lifetime abstainers. According to the National Survey on Drug Abuse and Health for 2008, almost 7% of Americans were classified as heavy alcohol users. Excessive alcohol use is responsible for 79,000 deaths per year among Americans and is the third leading lifestyle-related cause of death.

Abuse Versus Dependence

Alcohol abuse is recurrent alcohol use that has negative consequences, such as drinking in dangerous situations (before driving, for instance), or drinking patterns that result in academic, professional, interpersonal, or legal difficulties. **Alcohol dependence**, or **alcoholism**, involves more extensive problems with alcohol use, usually involving physical tolerance and withdrawal. Alcoholism is discussed in greater detail later in the chapter.

How can you tell if you or someone you know is becoming alcohol-dependent? Look for the following warning signs:

- Drinking alone or secretively
- Using alcohol deliberately and repeatedly to perform or get through difficult situations
- Feeling uncomfortable on certain occasions when alcohol is not available
- Escalating alcohol consumption beyond an already established drinking pattern
- Consuming alcohol heavily in risky situations, such as before driving
- Getting drunk regularly or more frequently than in the past
- Drinking in the morning or at other unusual times

Ask Yourself

QUESTIONS FOR CRITICAL THINKING AND REFLECTION

Have you ever witnessed or been involved in an alcohol emergency? Did you think the situation was urgent at the time? What were the circumstances surrounding the event? How did the people involved deal with it?

College Binge Drinking

College binge drinking, a serious problem for decades, has recently come under a harsh spotlight due largely to highly publicized alcohol-related tragedies on campus. Deaths from alcohol overdose, alcohol-related injuries (including motor vehicle crashes), violent crimes, student riots, and serious vandalism have all drawn attention to the epidemic of heavy drinking on college campuses.

Drinking on campus is pervasive. Approximately 61% of college students report having drunk alcohol at least once in the past month. According to the 2008 National Survey on Drug Use and Health, nearly 41% of college students reported binge drinking at least once in the past month, and 16% reported being heavy drinkers.

Every year, an estimated 1700 college students age 18–24 die from overdoses and alcohol-related injuries. Another 600,000 sustain unintentional alcohol-related injuries, 700,000 are assaulted by other students who have been drinking, and 100,000 are victims of alcohol-related date rape or sexual assault.

These statistics have shocked many students, administrators, and parents into demanding changes in college attitudes and policies regarding alcohol. In response, the Task Force of the National Advisory Council on Alcohol Abuse and Alcoholism was formed. Its report documents the extent of the alcohol problem and is a call to action for colleges and their surrounding communities to re-examine their alcohol policies and overhaul the campus drinking culture. These efforts, according to the Task Force, must focus on three levels:

1. Ultimately, *individual students* must take responsibility for their own behavior, but programs that encourage and support development of healthy attitudes toward alcohol are often needed. These programs should target students at increased risk of developing alcohol problems.

2. The *student body as a whole* must work to discourage alcohol abuse. This effort might include promoting alcohol-free activities, reducing the availability of alcohol, and avoiding social and commercial promotion of alcohol on campus. Fraternities, sororities, eating clubs, and other campus organiza-

tions should be held accountable if underage or otherwise inappropriate alcohol use takes place on their premises.

3. *Colleges and surrounding communities* must cooperate to discourage excessive drinking. Those who enable students to drink irresponsibly must be held accountable.

In 2007, the U.S. Surgeon General's Call to Action to Prevent and Reduce Underage Drinking suggested eliminating alcohol sponsorship of athletic events and other social activities. Working together, students, faculty, administrators, parents, and the community have begun to put an end to the destructive culture of heavy drinking on college campuses. At some schools, there is an effort to shift classes to Fridays and even Saturdays, after it was found that binge drinking increases when students don't have Friday classes. Increasingly, incoming students are required to take a 3-hour online class about alcohol. And there is stricter punishment for underage drinking and public drunkenness on some campuses, with the likelihood of suspension for repeat offenders.

Binge Drinking

The National Institute on Alcohol Abuse and Alcoholism defines **binge drinking** as a pattern of alcohol use that brings a person's BAC up to 0.08% or above (typically four drinks for men or three drinks for women), consumed within about 2 hours. The National Survey on Drug Use and Health defines binge drinking as having five or more drinks within about 2 hours, at least once within 30 days; the 2007 survey estimated that 23% of people over the age of 12 were binge drinkers. Almost 7% were heavy drinkers, defined as having five or more drinks on the same occasion on each of 5 or more days in the past 30 days.

Among Americans under 21 years old, most drinking is in the form of binging. However, a sizeable number of those 25 years or older are binge drinkers, and about 75% of the alcohol consumed by adults in the United States meets the definition of binge drinking.

Binge drinking has a profound effect on students' lives (see the box "College Binge Drinking"). Frequent binge

drinkers were found to be three to seven times more likely than non–binge drinkers to engage in unplanned or unprotected sex, to drive after drinking, and to get hurt or injured (Table 8.1). Binge drinkers were also more likely to miss classes, get behind in schoolwork, and argue with friends. The more frequent the binges, the more problems the students encountered. Despite their experiences, fewer than 1% of the binge drinkers identified themselves as problem drinkers.

Alcoholism

As mentioned earlier, alcoholism, or alcohol dependence, is usually characterized by tolerance to alcohol and withdrawal symptoms.

Patterns and Prevalence   Alcoholism occurs among people of all ethnic groups and at all socioeconomic levels. There are different patterns of alcohol dependence, including these four common ones: (1) regular daily intake of large amounts, (2) regular heavy drinking limited to weekends, (3) long periods of sobriety interspersed with binges of daily heavy drinking lasting for weeks or months, and (4) heavy drinking limited to periods of stress.

Table 8.1 — The Effects of Binge Drinking on College Students

ALCOHOL-RELATED PROBLEM	PERCENTAGE OF STUDENTS EXPERIENCING PROBLEMS	
	NON–BINGE DRINKERS	FREQUENT BINGE DRINKERS
Drove after drinking alcohol	18	58
Did something they regretted	17	62
Argued with friends	10	43
Engaged in unplanned sex	9	41
Missed a class	9	60
Got behind in schoolwork	9	42
Had unprotected sex	4	21
Got hurt or injured	4	28
Got into trouble with police	2	14
Had five or more of these problems since school year began	4	48

SOURCE: Wechsler, H., and B. Wuethrich. 2003. *Dying to Drink: Confronting Binge Drinking on College Campuses*, reprint ed. Emmaus, Pa.: Rodale.

More than 17 million

Americans are heavy drinkers.

—SAMHSA, 2009

Health Effects *Tolerance* means that a drinker needs more alcohol to achieve intoxication or the desired effect, that the effects of continued use of the same amount of alcohol are diminished, or that the drinker can function adequately at doses or a BAC that would produce significant impairment in a casual user. Heavy users of alcohol may need to consume about 50% more than they originally needed in order to experience the same degree of intoxication.

Withdrawal symptoms include trembling hands (shakes or jitters), a rapid pulse and accelerated breathing rate, insomnia, nightmares, anxiety, and gastrointestinal upset. More severe withdrawal symptoms occur in about 5% of alcoholics. These include seizures (sometimes called rum fits), confusion, and **hallucinations.** Still less common is **delirium tremens (the DTs),** a medical emergency characterized by severe disorientation, confusion, epileptic-like seizures, and vivid hallucinations, often of vermin and small animals. The mortality rate from DTs can be as high as 15%.

Alcoholics face all the physical health risks associated with intoxication and chronic drinking described earlier. Some of the damage is compounded by nutritional deficiencies that often accompany alcoholism. A mental problem associated with alcohol use is profound memory gaps (commonly known as blackouts).

Social and Psychological Effects Alcohol use causes more serious social and psychological problems than all other forms of drug abuse combined. For every person who is an alcoholic, another three or four people are directly affected.

Alcoholics frequently suffer from mental disorders in addition to their substance dependence. Alcoholics are much more likely than nonalcoholics to suffer from clinical depression, panic disorder, schizophrenia, and antisocial personality disorders. People with anxiety or panic attacks may try to use alcohol to lessen their anxiety, even though alcohol often makes these disorders worse.

Causes of Alcoholism The precise causes of alcoholism are unknown, but many factors are probably involved. Some studies suggest that as much as 50–60% of a person's risk for alcoholism is determined by genetic factors, but not all children of alcoholics become alcoholic, and it is clear that other factors are involved. A person's risk of developing alcoholism may be increased by certain personality disorders, having grown up in a violent or otherwise troubled household, and imitating the alcohol abuse of peers and other role models. People who begin drinking excessively in their teens are especially prone to binge drinking and alcoholism later in life. Certain social factors have also been linked with alcoholism, including urbanization, disappearance of the extended family, a general loosening of kinship ties, increased mobility, and changing values.

Treatment Some alcoholics recover without professional help. How often this occurs is unknown, but possibly as many as one-third stop drinking on their own or reduce their drinking enough to eliminate problems. Often these spontaneous recoveries are linked to an alcohol-related crisis, such as a blackout or alcohol-related automobile crash, a health problem, or the threat of being fired. Most alcoholics, however, require a treatment program of some kind in order to stop drinking. Many different

*Alcohol-treatment programs achieve extended **sobriety for about 50% of alcoholics** who participate.*

hallucination A false perception that does not correspond to external reality, such as seeing visions or hearing voices that are not there.

delirium tremens (the DTs) A state of confusion brought on by the reduction of alcohol intake in an alcohol-dependent person; other symptoms are sweating, trembling, anxiety, hallucinations, and seizures.

kinds of programs exist. No single treatment works for everyone, so a person may have to try different programs before finding the right one.

One of the oldest and best-known recovery programs is Alcoholics Anonymous (AA). AA consists of self-help groups that meet several times each week in many communities and follow a 12-step program. Important steps for people in these programs include recognizing that they are "powerless over alcohol" and must seek help from a "higher power" in order to regain control of their lives. By verbalizing these steps, the alcoholic directly addresses the denial that is often prominent in alcoholism and other addictions. Many AA members have a sponsor of their choosing who is available by phone 24 hours a day for individual support and crisis intervention.

Other recovery approaches are available. Some, like Rational Recovery and Women for Sobriety, deliberately avoid any emphasis on higher spiritual powers. A more controversial approach to problem drinking is offered by the group Moderation Management, which encourages people to manage their drinking behavior by limiting intake or abstaining.

Al-Anon is a companion program to AA for families and friends of alcoholics. In Al-Anon, spouses and others explore how they enabled the alcoholic to drink by denying, rationalizing, or covering up his or her drinking and how they can change this codependent behavior.

Employee assistance programs and school-based programs represent another approach to alcoholism treatment. Inpatient hospital rehabilitation is useful for some alcoholics, especially if they have serious medical or mental problems or if life stressors threaten to overwhelm them.

There are also several medical treatments for alcoholism:

- *Disulfiram* (Antabuse) inhibits the metabolic breakdown of acetaldehyde and causes patients to flush and feel ill when they drink, thus theoretically inhibiting impulse drinking.
- *Naltrexone* reduces the craving for alcohol and decreases its pleasant, reinforcing effects without making the user feel ill.
- *Injectable naltrexone* is a single monthly shot administered by a health professional.
- *Acamprosate* (Campral) helps people maintain abstinence after they have stopped drinking by acting on brain pathways related to alcohol abuse.

In people who abuse alcohol and have significant depression or anxiety, the use of antidepressant or anti-anxiety medication can improve both mental health and drinking behavior. In addition, drugs such as diazepam (Valium) are sometimes prescribed to replace alcohol during initial stages of withdrawal. Such chemical substitutes are usually useful for only a week or so, because alcoholics are at particularly high risk for developing dependence on other drugs.

Table 8.2 Users and Abusers of Alcohol in the U.S., by Demographic Characteristics: 2008

	PAST YEAR PREVALENCE (PERCENTAGE)	
	ALCOHOL USE	ALCOHOL ABUSE OR DEPENDENCE
Gender		
Men	70.1	9.7
Women	62.3	5.1
Ethnicity		
White	70.4	7.5
Black or African American	56.9	6.6
American Indian and Alaska Native	55.3	8.4
Native Hawaiian and other Pacific Islander	N/A	N/A
Asian American	52.3	3.5
Hispanic or Latino	58.6	8.0
Two or more races	60.7	7.2
Total Population	**66.1**	**7.5**

SOURCE: Substance Abuse and Mental Health Services Administration. 2009. *Results from the 2008 National Survey on Drug Use and Health: National Findings.* Rockville, Md.: Office of Applied Studies, NSDUH Series H–36, HHS Publication No. SMA 09–4434.

Gender and Ethnic Differences

Alcohol abusers come from all socioeconomic levels and cultural groups, but there are notable differences in patterns of drinking between men and women and among different ethnic groups (Table 8.2).

Men Among white American men, excessive drinking often begins in the teens or twenties and progresses gradually through the thirties until the individual is clearly identifiable as an alcoholic by the time he is in his late thirties or early forties (see the box "Drinking Behavior and Responsibility"). Other men remain controlled drinkers until later in life, sometimes becoming alcoholic in association with retirement, the loss of friends and loved ones, boredom, illness, or psychological disorders.

Ask Yourself

QUESTIONS FOR CRITICAL THINKING AND REFLECTION

Do you know anyone with a serious alcohol problem? From what you have read in this chapter, would you say that person abuses alcohol or is dependent on it? What effects, if any, has this person's problem had on your life? Have you thought about getting support or help?

Drinking Behavior and Responsibility

Examine Your Attitudes and Behavior

Think about how you really feel about drinking: Is it of little consequence to you or perhaps even an intrusion into your college experience? Or is alcohol the key ingredient for any and all fun activities? How do you perceive nondrinkers at a party where others are drinking?

Also consider the sources of your ideas about alcohol. How was alcohol used in your family when you were growing up? How is it used—or how do you think it's used—by students at your school? And how is alcohol use portrayed in advertisements you're exposed to? What effect do they have on you and your attitudes about drinking?

Finally, carefully examine your drinking behavior. If you drink alcohol, what are your reasons for doing so? Is your drinking behavior moderate and responsible? Or do you frequently overindulge and suffer negative consequences? Try tracking your alcohol use in your health journal for a week or two to help evaluate your drinking behavior.

Drinking Moderately and Responsibly

- *Drink slowly and space your drinks.* Sip your drinks, and alternate them with nonalcoholic choices. Don't drink alcoholic beverages to quench your thirst, and avoid drinks made with carbonated mixers.

- *Eat before and while drinking.* Don't drink on an empty stomach. Food in your stomach will slow the rate at which alcohol is absorbed.

- *Know your limits and your drinks.* Learn how different BACs affect you and how to keep your BAC and behavior under control.

- *Be aware of the setting.* In dangerous situations, abstinence is the only appropriate choice.

- *Use designated drivers.* Arrange carpools to and from parties or events where alcohol will be served. Rotate the responsibility for acting as a designated driver.

- *Learn to enjoy activities without alcohol.* If you can't have fun without drinking, you may have a problem with alcohol.

Encourage Responsible Drinking in Others

- *Encourage responsible attitudes.* Learn to express disapproval about someone who has drunk too much. Don't treat the choice to abstain as strange. The majority of American adults drink moderately or not at all.

- *Be a responsible host.* Serve only enough alcohol for each guest to have a moderate number of drinks, and serve lots of nonalcoholic choices. Always serve food along with alcohol, and stop serving alcohol an hour or more before people will leave. Insist that a guest who drinks too much take a taxi, ride with someone else, or stay overnight rather than drive.

- *Hold drinkers fully responsible for their behavior.* Pardoning unacceptable behavior fosters the attitude that the behavior is due to the drug rather than the person.

- *Take community action.* Find out about prevention programs on your campus or in your community. Consider joining an action group such as Students Against Destructive Decisions (SADD) or Mothers Against Drunk Driving (MADD); visit www.sadd.org and www.madd.org.

Women Women tend to become alcoholic at a later age and with fewer years of heavy drinking. It is not unusual for women in their forties or fifties to become alcoholic after years of controlled drinking. Women alcoholics develop cirrhosis and other medical complications somewhat more often than men. Women alcoholics may have more medical problems because they are less likely to seek early treatment. In addition, there may be an inherently greater biological risk for women who drink.

African Americans Although as a group African Americans use less alcohol than most other groups (including whites), they face disproportionately high levels of alcohol-related birth defects, cirrhosis, cancer, hypertension, and other medical problems. In addition, blacks are more likely than members of other ethnic groups to be victims of alcohol-related homicides, criminal assaults, and injuries. AA groups of predominantly African Americans are effective, perhaps because essential elements of AA—sharing common experiences, mutual acceptance of one another as human beings, and trusting a higher power—are already a part of African American culture.

Latinos Drinking patterns among Latinos vary significantly, depending on their specific cultural background and how long they and their families have lived in the United States. Drunk driving and cirrhosis are the most common causes of alcohol-related death and injury among Hispanic men. Hispanic women are more likely to abstain from alcohol than white or black women, but those who do drink are at special risk for problems. Treating the entire family as a unit is an important part of treatment because family pride, solidarity, and support are important aspects of Latino culture. Some Hispanics may do better if treatment efforts are integrated with the techniques of folk healers and spiritists.

Asian Americans As a group, Asian Americans have lower-than-average rates of alcohol abuse. However, acculturation may somewhat weaken the generally strong Asian taboos and community sanctions against alcohol misuse. For many Asian Americans, though, the genetically based physiological aversion to alcohol remains a deterrent to abuse. Ethnic agencies, health care professionals, and ministers seem to be the most effective sources of treatment, when needed.

American Indians and Alaska Natives Alcohol abuse is one of the most widespread and severe health problems among American Indians and Alaska Natives, especially for adolescents and young adults. The rate of alcoholism among American Indians is twice that of the general population, and the death rate from alcohol-related causes is about eight times higher. Treatment may be more effective if it reflects tribal values.

Helping Someone with an Alcohol Problem

Helping a friend or relative with an alcohol problem requires skill and tact. Start by making sure you are not enabling someone to continue excessively using alcohol. Enabling takes many forms, such as making excuses for the alcohol abuser—for example, saying "he has the flu" when it is really a hangover. Another important step is open, honest labeling—"I think you have a problem with alcohol." Such explicit statements usually elicit emotional rebuttals and may endanger a relationship. However, you are not helping your friends by allowing them to deny their problems with alcohol or other drugs. Taking action shows that you care. Even when problems are acknowledged, there is usually reluctance to get help. Your best role might be to obtain information about the available resources and persistently encourage their use.

WHO USES TOBACCO?

In spite of the known health hazards—and despite increasing public and private efforts to restrict smoking—nearly 71 million Americans currently smoke, and thousands more join their ranks every day, the vast majority of them teenagers. In 2008, about 23% of men and 18% of women smoked cigarettes. Rates of smoking varied based on gender, age, ethnicity, and education level (Table 8.3).

QUICK STATS

2.8 million
Americans age 12–17 are current tobacco users.

—SAMHSA, 2009

Table 8.3	Who Smokes?		
	PERCENTAGE OF SMOKERS		
	MEN	WOMEN	TOTAL
Ethnic Group (age ≥ 18)			
White	23.5	20.6	22.0
Black	25.6	17.8	21.3
Asian	15.7	4.7	9.9
American Indian/Alaskan Native	42.3	22.4	32.4
Latino	20.7	10.7	15.8
Education (age ≥ 25)			
≤ 8 years	24.2	13.0	19.0
9–11 years	38.1	36.6	35.7
12 years (no diploma)	33.8	19.0	26.4
GED	45.2	37.5	41.3
12 years (diploma)	30.0	21.5	25.5
Associate degree	21.8	17.3	19.3
Undergraduate degree	11.5	9.7	10.6
Graduate degree	5.6	5.9	5.7
Total	**23.1**	**18.3**	**20.6**

SOURCE: Centers for Disease Control and Prevention. 2009. Cigarette smoking among adults—United States, 2008. *Morbidity and Mortality Weekly Report* 58(44): 1227–1232.

Most adult smokers began smoking as teenagers.

As of June 2010, new federal regulations made it a federal crime to sell tobacco products to anyone under 18 years of age. Even so, minors smoke an estimated 800 million packs of cigarettes each year; more than half of these cigarettes are purchased at retail stores. Each day, roughly 1000 teenagers become regular smokers; at least one-third of them will die prematurely because of tobacco. According to the 2008 Monitoring the Future survey, one-fifth of American teens become current smokers (meaning they smoke at least one cigarette per month) by the time they leave high school.

Men and women with other drug-abuse problems frequently use tobacco. Smoking also is more prevalent among people with mental disorders than among the rest of the population: 40% of people with major depression, social phobias, and generalized anxiety disorder are smokers, as are 80% of people with schizophrenia. Such findings suggest that underlying psychological or physiological traits may predispose people to drug use, including tobacco.

WHY PEOPLE USE TOBACCO

Although people start smoking for a variety of reasons, they usually become long-term smokers after becoming addicted to nicotine—the key psychoactive ingredient in tobacco smoke.

Nicotine Addiction

The primary reason people continue to use tobacco is that they have become addicted to a powerful psychoactive drug: **nicotine.** Many researchers consider nicotine to be the most physically addictive of all the psychoactive drugs.

Some neurological studies indicate that nicotine acts on the brain in much the same way as cocaine and heroin. Nicotine reaches the brain via the bloodstream seconds after it is inhaled or, in the case of spit tobacco, absorbed through membranes of the mouth or nose. It triggers the release of powerful chemical messengers in the brain, including epinephrine, norepinephrine, and dopamine. But unlike street drugs, most of which are used to achieve a high, nicotine's primary attraction seems to lie in its ability to modulate everyday emotions.

At low doses, nicotine acts as a stimulant. It increases heart rate and blood pressure. In adults, nicotine can enhance alertness, concentration, rapid information processing, memory, and learning. In some circumstances, nicotine acts as a mild sedative. Most commonly, nicotine relieves symptoms such as anxiety, irritability, and mild depression in tobacco users who are experiencing withdrawal. Nicotine addiction fulfills the criteria for substance dependence, including loss of control, tolerance, and withdrawal.

Loss of Control About 70% of smokers say they want to quit completely, and about 40% of smokers try to quit each year. Regular tobacco users live according to a rigid cycle of need and gratification. On average, they can go no more than 40 minutes between doses of nicotine; otherwise, they begin feeling edgy and irritable and have trouble concentrating. If ignored, nicotine cravings build until getting tobacco becomes a paramount concern, crowding out other thoughts. Tobacco users become adept at keeping a steady amount of nicotine circulating in the blood and going to the brain. They may plan their daily schedule around opportunities to satisfy their nicotine cravings; this loss of control and personal freedom can affect all the dimensions of wellness (see the box "Tobacco Use and Religion: Global Views").

Tolerance and Withdrawal Using tobacco builds up tolerance. Where one cigarette may make a beginning smoker nauseated and dizzy, a long-term smoker may have to chain-smoke a pack or more to experience the same effects. For most regular tobacco users, sudden abstinence from nicotine produces predictable withdrawal symptoms, which come on several hours after the last dose of nicotine and can include severe cravings, insomnia, confusion, tremors, difficulty concentrating, fatigue, muscle pains, headache, nausea, irritability, anger, and depression. Although most of these symptoms of physical dependence pass in 2 or 3 days, many ex-smokers report intermittent urges to smoke for years after quitting.

Social and Psychological Factors

Social and psychological forces combine with physiological addiction to maintain the tobacco habit. Many people, for example, have established habits of smoking while doing something else—while talking, working, drinking, and so on. The spit tobacco habit is also associated with certain situations, such as studying or playing sports. It is difficult for these people to break their habits because the activities they associate with tobacco use continue to trigger their urge.

---

nicotine A poisonous, addictive substance found in tobacco and responsible for many of the effects of tobacco.

TERMS

Religious traditions can best assist adult smokers by reminding them of two principles: one, the value of liberation from any form of slavery, and two, respect for life and the body.

Tobacco Use as a Violation of Religious Principles

All religions condemn tobacco use for its damaging effects on the body. Most religions regard the human body as the dwelling place of the spirit; as such, it deserves care and respect.

The Baha'i faith, for example, strongly discourages smoking as unclean and unhealthy. Some Protestant churches consider tobacco use a violation of the body. For Hindus, smoking goes against one of the primary spiritual practices, the care of the body. The Roman Catholic Church endorses the age-old adage "a sound mind in a sound body." For Muslims, one of the five essential principles on which religious law is based is protection of the integrity of the individual. In Judaism, people are urged to "choose life" and to choose whatever strengthens the capacity to live. Buddhists believe that the body doesn't belong to the person at all—even suicide is considered murder—and one must do nothing to harm it.

Most religions also contend that dependence and addiction run counter to ideas of freedom, choice, and human dignity. Buddhism teaches a path of freedom—a way of life without dependence on anything. Hindus regard tobacco use as a dependence that is not necessary for health. Protestant churches caution that any form of dependence is contrary to the notion of Christian freedom.

Another argument against tobacco use is the immorality of imposing secondhand smoke on nonsmokers, which is seen as inflicting harm on others.

The Role of Individual Responsibility

Most religions focus on the role of individual responsibility in overcoming dependence on tobacco. In Buddhism, for example, people must assume responsibility for their habits; they practice introspection to understand the cause of problems within themselves and the effects of their actions on others. The principles of Islam are based on notions of responsibility and protection; you are responsible for your body and health.

Religion and Tobacco Control

Different religions share common views on how the problem of tobacco use should be approached. The Islamic view is that the campaign to control tobacco use must be based on awareness, responsibility, and justice. According to the Geneva Interreligious Platform (a project involving Hindus, Buddhists, Jews, Christians, Muslims, and Baha'is), the best approach is prevention. Here, the rights of nonsmokers clearly prevail over the freedom of smokers. In support of this position, the common religious exhortation not to do unto others what you would not have them do unto you can be invoked.

Why Start in the First Place?

In the United States, nearly 90% of all adult smokers started smoking before age 18. The average age for starting smokers and smokeless tobacco users is around 15. The earlier people begin smoking, the more likely they are to become heavy smokers—and to die of tobacco-related disease.

Young people start using tobacco for a variety of reasons. Many young, white, male athletes, for example, begin using spit tobacco to emulate professional athletes. Young women often take up smoking because they think it will help them lose weight or stay thin. Most often, however, young people start smoking simply because their peers are already doing it.

*Nicotine **addiction** can start within a few days of **smoking** and after just a few cigarettes.*

Rationalizing the Dangers Making the decision to smoke requires minimizing or denying both the health risks of tobacco use and the tremendous pain, disability, emotional trauma, family stress, and financial expense involved in tobacco-related diseases such as cancer and emphysema. A sense of invincibility, characteristic of many adolescents and young adults, also contributes to the decision to use tobacco.

Many teenagers believe they can stop smoking when they want. In fact, adolescents are more vulnerable to nicotine than are older tobacco users. Compared with older smokers, adolescents become heavy smokers and develop dependence after fewer cigarettes.

Emulating Smoking in the Media Both the Institute of Medicine and the National Cancer Institute have identified media portrayals of smoking as a key influence on young people who start smoking. In fact, studies by the National Cancer Institute have concluded that a direct causal relationship exists between media portrayals of smoking and actual smoking initiation by young moviegoers. One study found that more than 50% of young people surveyed began smoking after watching repeated favorable portrayals of smoking in movies.

In general, the portrayal of smoking in films does not reflect U.S. patterns of tobacco use. The prevalence of smoking among lead characters is three to four times that among comparable Americans. Films typically show the smoker as white, male, well educated, successful, and attractive. In reality, smokers tend to be poor and to

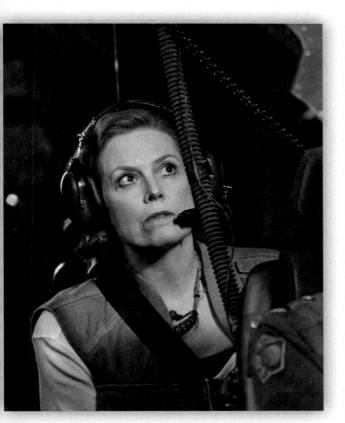

Antismoking advocates criticized the 2009 movie *Avatar* for its cigarette-smoking character Dr. Grace Augustine, portrayed by Sigourney Weaver. Director James Cameron responded that Grace was not intended as an inspirational role model for teenagers.

Ask Yourself

QUESTIONS FOR CRITICAL THINKING AND REFLECTION

What has influenced your decision to smoke, not to smoke, or to quit smoking? Have you ever felt that images or messages in the media were encouraging you to use tobacco? How do you react to such messages?

have less education. Public campaigns to reduce images of smoking in movies have succeeded to an extent; smoking is shown less often in films and television shows now than even just a few years ago. Still, antismoking advocates stay that films continue to be a critical and highly successful form of advertising for the tobacco industry.

HEALTH HAZARDS

Tobacco adversely affects nearly every part of the body, including the brain, stomach, mouth, and reproductive organs.

Tobacco Smoke: A Toxic Mix

Tobacco smoke contains hundreds of damaging chemical substances, including acetone (nail polish remover), ammonia, hexamine (lighter fluid), and toluene (industrial solvent). Smoke from a typical unfiltered cigarette contains about 5 billion particles per cubic millimeter—50,000 times as many as are found in an equal volume of smoggy urban air. These particles, when condensed, form a brown, sticky mass called **cigarette tar.**

Carcinogens and Poisons At least 43 chemicals in tobacco smoke are linked to the development of cancer. Some, such as benzo(a)pyrene and urethane, are **carcinogens**; that is, they directly cause cancer. Other chemicals, such as formaldehyde, are **cocarcinogens**; they do not themselves cause cancer but combine with other chemicals to stimulate the growth of certain cancers, at least in laboratory animals. Tobacco also contains poisonous substances, including arsenic and hydrogen cyanide. In addition to being an addictive psychoactive drug, nicotine is also a poison and can be fatal in high doses. Many cases of nicotine poisoning occur each year in toddlers and infants who eat cigarette butts they find at home or on the playground.

Cigarette smoke contains carbon monoxide, the deadly gas in automobile exhaust, in concentrations 400 times greater than is considered safe in industrial workplaces. Carbon monoxide displaces oxygen in red blood cells, depleting the body's supply of oxygen needed for extra work. Carbon monoxide also impairs visual acuity, especially at night.

QUICK STATS

High-tar cigarettes (up to 15 mg of tar per cigarette) made up 93% of the domestic cigarette market in 2006.

—Federal Trade Commission, 2009

Additives Tobacco manufacturers use additives to manipulate the taste and effect of cigarettes and other tobacco products.

Additives include sugars as flavor enhancers to mask the harsh, bitter taste of tobacco, so smokers can inhale more smoke and absorb more nicotine. Other flavor components, such as theobromine and glycyrrhizin, act as bronchodilators, opening the lungs' airways and making it easier for nicotine to get into the bloodstream.

> **cigarette tar**   A brown, sticky mass created when the chemical particles in tobacco smoke condense.
>
> **carcinogen**   Any substance that causes cancer.
>
> **cocarcinogen**   A substance that works with a carcinogen to cause cancer.

TERMS

Ammonia boosts the amount of addictive nicotine delivered by cigarettes. Some additives are intended to make **sidestream smoke** (the uninhaled smoke from a burning cigarette) less obvious and objectionable.

Nearly 600 chemicals, approved as safe when used as food additives, are used in manufacturing cigarettes, but some form cancer-causing agents when heated or burned.

"Reduced Harm" Cigarettes   Some smokers switch to low-tar, low-nicotine, or filtered cigarettes because they believe them to be healthier alternatives. The tobacco industry has long promoted such products as "reduced harm" cigarettes, meaning they are supposedly less damaging to their users' health. But there is no such thing as a safe cigarette, and smoking behavior is a more important factor in tar and nicotine intake than the type of cigarette smoked. Smokers who switch to a low-nicotine brand often compensate by smoking more cigarettes, inhaling more deeply, taking larger or more frequent puffs, or blocking ventilation holes with lips or fingers to offset the effects of filters.

> As of June 2010, federal law prohibited the use of terms such as "Light" and "Mild" on cigarette packaging.

Studies have found that people who smoke "light" cigarettes inhale up to eight times as much tar and nicotine as printed on the label. Studies also show that smokers of light cigarettes are less likely to quit than smokers of regular cigarettes, probably due to the misperception that light cigarettes are safer.

As of June 2010, new federal regulations prohibit cigarette manufacturers from labeling their products with descriptors such as "light," "mild," or "low"—terms that have effectively convinced many consumers that such cigarettes are safer alternatives to higher-tar cigarettes. In the future, manufacturers who want to apply such labels will have to receive special permission from the U.S. Food and Drug Administration.

Menthol Cigarettes   About 70% of African American smokers smoke menthol cigarettes, as compared to 30% of whites. Studies have found that blacks absorb more nicotine than other groups and metabolize it more slowly; they also have lower rates of successful quitting. The anesthetizing effect of menthol, which may allow smokers to inhale more deeply and hold smoke in their lungs for a longer period, may be partly responsible for these differences.

The Immediate Effects of Smoking

The beginning smoker often has symptoms of mild nicotine poisoning: dizziness; faintness; rapid pulse; cold, clammy skin; and sometimes nausea, vomiting, and diarrhea. The effects of nicotine on smokers vary, depending greatly on the size of the nicotine dose and how much tolerance one has built up through previous smoking. Nicotine can either excite or tranquilize the nervous system, depending on dosage. (For an illustration of both the immediate and long-term effects of smoking, see page T1-3 of the color transparency insert "Touring Lifestyle Behaviors" in this chapter.)

Nicotine has many other immediate effects. It stimulates the part of the brain called the **cerebral cortex.** It also stimulates the adrenal glands to discharge adrenaline. Nicotine inhibits the formation of urine; constricts the blood vessels, especially in the skin; accelerates the heart rate; and elevates blood pressure. Higher blood pressure, faster heart rate, and constricted blood vessels require the heart to pump more blood. Smoking depresses hunger contractions and dulls the taste buds. Smokers who quit often notice that food tastes much better.

The Long-Term Effects of Smoking

Smoking is linked to many deadly and disabling diseases. Total amount of tobacco smoke inhaled is a key factor contributing to disease. People who smoke more cigarettes per day, inhale deeply, puff frequently, smoke cigarettes down to the butts, or begin smoking at an early age run a greater risk of disease than do those who smoke more moderately or who do not smoke at all.

Cardiovascular Disease   Although lung cancer tends to receive the most publicity, **coronary heart disease (CHD)** is actually the most widespread single cause of death for cigarette smokers. CHD often results from **atherosclerosis,** a condition in which fatty deposits called **plaques** form on the inner walls of heart arteries, causing them to narrow and stiffen. Smoking and exposure to environmental tobacco smoke (ETS) permanently accelerate the rate of plaque accumulation in the coronary arteries—50% for smokers, 25% for ex-smokers, and 20% for people regularly exposed to ETS. If the plaque completely blocks the flow of blood to a portion of the heart, a heart attack (**myocardial infarction**) occurs. CHD can also interfere with the heart's electrical activity, resulting in disturbances of the normal heartbeat rhythm.

Smokers have a death rate from CHD that is 70% higher than that of nonsmokers. The risks of CHD decrease rapidly when a person stops smoking; this is particularly true for younger smokers, whose coronary arteries have not yet been extensively damaged. Cigarette smoking has also been linked to other cardiovascular diseases, including the following:

- *Stroke,* a sudden interference with the circulation of blood in a part of the brain, resulting in the destruction of brain cells
- *Aortic aneurysm,* a bulge in the aorta caused by a weakening in its walls
- *Pulmonary heart disease,* a disorder of the right side of the heart, caused by changes in the blood vessels of the lungs

Lung Cancer and Other Cancers Cigarette smoking is the primary cause of lung cancer. Those who smoke two or more packs of cigarettes a day have lung cancer death rates 12–25 times greater than those of nonsmokers. The dramatic rise in lung cancer rates among women in the past 40 years clearly parallels the increase of smoking in this group; lung cancer now exceeds breast cancer as the leading cause of cancer deaths among women. The risk of developing lung cancer increases with the number of cigarettes smoked each day, the number of years of smoking, and the age at which the person started smoking. Evidence suggests that after 1 year without smoking, the risk of lung cancer decreases substantially. After 10 years, the risk of lung cancer among ex-smokers is 50% lower than that of continuing smokers.

Research has also linked smoking to cancers of the trachea, mouth, pharynx, esophagus, larynx, pancreas, bladder, kidney, breast, cervix, stomach, liver, colon, and skin.

Chronic Obstructive Pulmonary Disease The lungs of a smoker are constantly exposed to dangerous chemicals and irritants, and they must work harder to function adequately. The stresses placed on the lungs by smoking can permanently damage lung function and lead to *chronic obstructive pulmonary disease (COPD),* also known as chronic obstructive lung disease (COLD), or chronic lower respiratory disease. COPD is the fourth leading cause of death in the United States. This progressive and disabling disorder consists of several different but related diseases; emphysema and chronic bronchitis are two of the most common. **Emphysema** is a disabling condition in which the walls of the lungs' air sacs lose their elasticity and are gradually destroyed. The lungs' ability to take in oxygen and expel carbon dioxide is impaired. A person with emphysema is breathless, is constantly gasping for air, and has the feeling of drowning. The heart must pump harder and may become enlarged. People with emphysema often die from a damaged heart. There is no known way to reverse this disease. In its advanced stage, the victim is bedridden and severely disabled. **Chronic bronchitis** is a persistent, recurrent inflammation of the bronchial tubes. When the cell lining of the bronchial tubes is irritated, it secretes excess mucus. Bronchial congestion is followed by a chronic cough, which makes breathing more and more difficult. If smokers have chronic bronchitis, they face a greater risk of lung cancer, no matter how old they are or how many cigarettes they smoke. Chronic bronchitis seems to be a shortcut to lung cancer.

Even when a smoker shows no signs of lung impairment or disease, cigarette smoking causes other respiratory damage. Normally the cells lining the bronchial tubes secrete mucus, a sticky fluid that collects particles of soot, dust, and other substances in inhaled air. Mucus is carried up to the mouth by the continuous motion of *cilia,* hairlike structures that protrude from the inner surface of the bronchial tubes. If the cilia are destroyed or impaired, or if inhaled air contains more pollutants than the system can remove, the protection provided by cilia is lost.

Cigarette smoke first slows and then stops the action of the cilia. Eventually it destroys them, leaving delicate membranes exposed to injury from substances inhaled in cigarette smoke or from the polluted air. This interference with the functioning of the respiratory system often leads rapidly to the conditions known as smoker's throat and smoker's cough, as well as to shortness of breath. Other respiratory effects of smoking include a worsening of allergy and asthma symptoms and an increase in the smoker's susceptibility to colds.

Additional Health, Cosmetic, and Economic Concerns People who smoke are more likely to develop peptic ulcers and heartburn, raising the risk of esophageal cancer. Smokers are twice as likely as nonsmokers to experience erectile dysfunction (impotence), and smoking is linked to reduced fertility in both men and women. Smokers are at increased risk for tooth decay and gum and periodontal diseases, with symptoms appearing by the mid-20s. Smoking dulls the senses of taste and smell

TERMS

myocardial infarction   A heart attack caused by the complete blockage of a main coronary artery.

emphysema   A disease characterized by a loss of lung tissue elasticity and breakup of the air sacs, impairing the lungs' ability to take in oxygen and expel carbon dioxide.

chronic bronchitis   Recurrent, persistent inflammation of the bronchial tubes.

Gender and Tobacco Use

American men are currently more likely than women to smoke, but women younger than age 23 are becoming smokers at a faster rate than any other population segment. As the rate of smoking among women approaches that of men, so do rates of tobacco-related illness and death. More American women now die each year from lung cancer than from breast cancer.

Although overall risks of tobacco-related illness are similar for women and men, sex appears to make a difference in some diseases. Women, for example, are more at risk for smoking-related blood clots and strokes than are men, and the risk is even greater for women using oral contraceptives. Among men and women with the same smoking history, the odds for developing three major types of cancer, including lung cancer, is 1.2–1.7 times higher in women.

For both men and women, tobacco use is associated with increased incidence of sex-specific health problems. Men who smoke increase their risk of erectile dysfunction and infertility due to reduced sperm density and motility. Women who smoke have higher rates of osteoporosis, thyroid-related diseases, and depression.

Women who smoke also have risks associated with reproduction and the reproductive organs. Smoking is associated with greater menstrual bleeding, longer duration of painful menstrual cramps, and more variability in menstrual cycle length. Smokers have a more difficult time becoming pregnant, and they reach menopause on average a year or two earlier than nonsmokers. They face increased chances of miscarriage or placental disorders that lead to bleeding and premature delivery; rates of ectopic pregnancy, preeclampsia, and stillbirth are also higher among women who smoke. Smoking is a risk factor for cervical cancer.

When women decide to try to stop smoking, they are more likely than men to join a support group. Overall, though, women are less successful than men in quitting. Women report more severe withdrawal symptoms and are more likely than men to report cravings in response to social and behavioral cues associated with smoking.

For men, relapse to smoking is often associated with work or social pressure; women are more likely to relapse when sad or depressed or concerned about weight gain. Nicotine replacement therapy appears to work better for men, whereas the non-nicotine medication bupropion appears to work better for women.

QUICK STATS

The total health care and productivity costs of smoking amount to **$193 billion** annually.

—American Cancer Society, 2010

and increases the risk for hearing loss and blindness. Smokers have higher rates of motor vehicle crashes, fire-related injuries, and back pain. Smoking can cause premature skin wrinkling, premature baldness, stained teeth, discolored fingers, and a persistent tobacco odor in clothes and hair. In July 2010, the average per-pack price of cigarettes was $5.33. A pack-a-day habit costs more than $1900 per year for cigarettes alone. In addition, smoking contributes to osteoporosis, increases the risk of complications from diabetes, and accelerates the course of multiple sclerosis.

Cumulative Effects The cumulative effects of tobacco use fall into two general categories. The first category is reduced life expectancy. A male who takes up smoking before age 15 and continues to smoke is only half as likely to live to age 75 as a male who never smokes. Females who have similar smoking habits also have a reduced life expectancy.

The second category involves quality of life. A national health survey begun in 1964 shows that smokers spend one-third more time away from their jobs because of illness than nonsmokers. Both men and women smokers show a greater rate of acute and chronic disease than people who have never smoked (see the box "Gender and Tobacco Use"). Smokers become disabled at younger ages than nonsmokers and have more years of unhealthy life as well as a shorter life span.

Other Forms of Tobacco Use

Many smokers have switched from cigarettes to other forms of tobacco, such as spit (smokeless) tobacco, cigars and pipes, and clove cigarettes and bidis. These alternatives, however, are far from safe.

Spit (Smokeless) Tobacco More than 8.1 million adults and about 9% of all high school students are current spit tobacco users. Spit tobacco comes in two major forms: snuff and chewing tobacco (chew). In snuff, the tobacco leaf is processed into a coarse, moist powder and mixed with flavorings. Snuff is usually sold in small tins. Users place a "pinch," "dip," or "quid" between the lower lip or cheek and gum and suck on it. In chewing tobacco, the tobacco leaf may be shredded ("leaf"), pressed into bricks or cakes ("plugs"), or dried and twisted into rope-like strands ("twists"). Chew is usually sold in pouches. Users place a wad of tobacco in their mouth and then chew or suck it to release the nicotine. All types of smokeless tobacco cause an increase in saliva production, and the resulting tobacco juice is spit out or swallowed.

The nicotine in spit tobacco—along with flavorings and additives—is absorbed through the gums and lining of the mouth. Holding an average-size dip in the mouth

Cigars contain more tobacco than cigarettes and so produce more tar when smoked. Cigar smokers face an increased risk of cancer even if they don't inhale the smoke.

Cigars and Pipes

The popularity of cigars is highest among white males age 18–44 with higher-than-average income and education, but women are also smoking cigars in record numbers. Cigar use is also growing among young people: In government surveys, 12% of American high school students reported having smoked at least one cigar in the previous month. Less than 1% of Americans, mostly males who also smoke cigarettes, are pipe smokers.

Cigars are made from rolled whole tobacco leaves; pipe tobacco is made from shredded leaves and often flavored. Users absorb nicotine through the gums and lining of the mouth. Cigars contain more tobacco than cigarettes and so contain more nicotine and produce more tar when smoked. Large cigars may contain as much tobacco as a whole pack of cigarettes and take 1–2 hours to smoke.

The smoke from cigars contains many of the same toxins and carcinogens as the smoke from cigarettes, some in much higher quantities. The health risks of cigars depend on the number of cigars smoked and whether the smoker inhales. Because most cigar and pipe users do not inhale, they have a lower risk of cancer and cardiovascular and respiratory diseases than cigarette smokers. However, their risks are substantially higher than those of nonsmokers.

Nicotine addiction is another concern. Most adults who smoke cigars do so only occasionally, and there is little evidence that use of cigars by adults leads to addiction. The recent rise in cigar use among teens has raised concerns, however, because nicotine addiction almost always develops in the teen or young adult years.

Clove Cigarettes and Bidis

Clove cigarettes, also called "kreteks" or "chicartas," are made of tobacco mixed with chopped cloves; they are imported primarily from Indonesia and Pakistan. Clove cigarettes contain almost twice as much tar, nicotine, and carbon monoxide as conventional cigarettes and so have all the same health hazards. Some chemical constituents of cloves may also be dangerous. For example, eugenol, an anesthetic compound found in cloves, may impair the respiratory system's ability to detect and defend against foreign particles. There have been a number of serious respiratory injuries and deaths from the use of clove cigarettes.

Bidis, or "beadies," are small cigarettes imported from India that contain species of tobacco different from those used by U.S. cigarette manufacturers. The tobacco in bidis is hand-rolled in Indian ebony leaves (tendu) and then often flavored; clove, mint, chocolate, and fruit varieties are available. Bidis contain up to four times more nicotine than U.S. cigarettes and twice as much tar.

E-Cigarettes

The electronic cigarette, or *e-cig,* is a battery-powered device that resembles a real cigarette. Instead of containing tobacco, the device uses a changeable filter that contains one or more chemicals, such as nicotine, flavorings, and other compounds. The user "smokes" an e-cig by sucking the filtered end; the device's battery heats the

for 30 minutes delivers about the same amount of nicotine as two or three cigarettes. Because of its nicotine content, spit tobacco is highly addictive. Some users keep it in their mouth even while sleeping.

Although not as dangerous as smoking cigarettes, the use of spit tobacco carries many health risks. Changes can occur in the mouth after only a few weeks of use. Gums and lips become dried and irritated and may bleed. White or red patches may appear inside the mouth; this condition, known as *leukoplakia,* can lead to oral cancer. About 25% of regular spit tobacco users have *gingivitis* (inflammation) and recession of the gums and bone loss around the teeth, especially where the tobacco is usually placed. The senses of taste and smell are usually dulled.

One of the most serious effects of spit tobacco is an increased risk of oral cancer—cancers of the lip, tongue, cheek, throat, gums, roof and floor of the mouth, and larynx. Spit tobacco contains at least 28 chemicals known to cause cancer, and long-term snuff use may increase the risk of oral cancer by as much as 50 times. Surgery to treat oral cancer is often disfiguring and may involve removing parts of the face, tongue, cheek, or lip.

chemicals to create an inhalable vapor. During use, the device's tip even glows like the burning end of a real cigarette.

Marketers of e-cigs have claimed that the devices deliver only nicotine, making them a safe cigarette that does not cause cancer and can serve as an alternative to other nicotine replacement products such as gum and patches. According to the FDA, however, not all e-cigs actually contain nicotine. Further, the FDA has warned consumers not to purchase or use e-cigs, after analysis of nearly 20 e-cig cartridges revealed they contained carcinogens, including at least one of the same carcinogens found in real cigarettes. Several samples contained a toxic chemical used in antifreeze.

In issuing its warning, the FDA noted that some varieties of e-cigs are flavored, apparently to make them appeal to youngsters and other first-time smokers. The products do not carry the same types of warnings required on tobacco products.

THE EFFECTS OF SMOKING ON THE NONSMOKER

Tens of thousands of nonsmokers die each year because of exposure to secondhand smoke. Further, the medical and societal costs of tobacco use are enormous.

Environmental Tobacco Smoke

The U.S. Environmental Protection Agency (EPA) has designated **environmental tobacco smoke (ETS)**—more commonly called *secondhand smoke*—a Class A carcinogen. The Surgeon General has concluded that there is no safe level of exposure to ETS.

Environmental tobacco smoke consists of mainstream smoke and sidestream smoke. Smoke exhaled by smokers is referred to as **mainstream smoke.** Sidestream smoke enters the atmosphere from the burning end of a cigarette, cigar, or pipe. Nearly 85% of the smoke in a room where someone is smoking comes from sidestream smoke. Undiluted sidestream smoke, because it is not filtered through either a cigarette filter or a smoker's lungs, has twice as much tar and nicotine, three times as much benzo(a)pyrene, almost three times as much carbon monoxide, and three times as much ammonia.

In rooms where people are smoking, levels of carbon monoxide can exceed those permitted by Federal Air Quality Standards for outside air. The carcinogens in the secondhand smoke from a single cigar exceeds that of three cigarettes, and cigar smoke contains up to 30 times more carbon monoxide (see the box "Tobacco Use and the Environment").

ETS Effects   Nonsmokers subjected to ETS frequently develop coughs, headaches, nasal discomfort, and eye irritation. Other symptoms range from breathlessness to sinus problems. People with allergies tend to suffer the most.

ETS causes 3400 lung cancer deaths and about 46,000 deaths from heart disease each year in people who do not smoke. ETS also aggravates asthma and increases the risk for breast and cervical cancers. Scientists have been able to measure changes that contribute to lung tissue damage and potential tumor promotion in the bloodstreams of healthy young test subjects who spend just 3 hours in a smoke-filled room. After just 30 minutes of exposure to ETS, the function in the coronary arteries of healthy nonsmokers is reduced to the same level as that of smokers. And nonsmokers can still be affected by the harmful effects of ETS hours after they have left a smoky environment. Carbon monoxide, for example, lingers in the bloodstream 5 hours later.

Infants, Children, and ETS   Infants exposed to smoke are more likely to die of sudden infant death syndrome (SIDS) than babies not exposed to ETS. ETS causes up to 18,600 cases of low birth weight each year. Children under 5 whose primary caregiver smokes ten or more cigarettes per day have measurable blood levels of nicotine and

According to the U.S. Surgeon General, there is no safe level of exposure to secondhand smoke.

environmental tobacco smoke (ETS)   Smoke that enters the atmosphere from the burning end of a cigarette, cigar, or pipe, as well as smoke that is exhaled by smokers; also called *secondhand smoke.*

mainstream smoke   Smoke that is inhaled by a smoker and then exhaled into the atmosphere.

Millions of American infants and children are regularly exposed to environmental tobacco smoke.

Worldwide, an estimated 600,000 people die every year because of exposure to secondhand tobacco smoke, according to a recent report from the World Health Organization (WHO). The WHO also states that about 1 in 10 smoking-related deaths is caused by exposure to ETS. The World Lung Foundation (WLF) estimates that 40% of the world's children are exposed to secondhand tobacco smoke in their homes; globally, more than 30% of those who die prematurely from ETS exposure are children.

Tobacco use and its by-products also add to the pollution of the natural environment. In 2006, the California Air Resources Board identified secondhand tobacco smoke as a toxic air contaminant that pollutes outside air as well as inside air. The board estimated that, in California alone, ETS accounts for the release of 40 tons of nicotine, 365 tons of inhalable particulate matter, and 1900 tons of carbon monoxide into the atmosphere each year. ETS also releases smaller but measurable amounts of poisonous contaminants such as arsenic and benzene into the air. These pollutants are dangerous to all living things, including animals and plants. Particulate matter and carbon monoxide also contribute to the greenhouse effect and global warming.

In addition to the tons of air pollutants released in the form of ETS, smoking creates other forms of pollution as well. For example, billions of cigarette butts and cigar stubs are discarded on the ground and in open waters every year. Although each one contains only minute amounts of tobacco and additives, together they release untold amounts of toxins and carcinogens into the environment. Cigarette butts are commonly eaten by animals and are known to have negative effects on the health of wildlife.

These problems have been recognized by the U.S. Environmental Protection Agency (EPA), as well as many state and local agencies. A few states, with California in the lead, have initiated programs to clean up cigarette butts in roadside and natural areas, and many municipalities levy fines on people who dispose of cigarette butts in the open. Such measures may increase awareness of the dangers posed by tobacco use not just to people but to the planet.

SOURCES: Environment News Service. 2006. *California Identifies Secondhand Smoke as a Toxic Air Contaminant* (http://www.ens-newswire.com/ens/jan2006/2006-01-27-04.html; retrieved November 3, 2010); U.S. Environmental Protection Agency. 2008. *U.S. EPA's 2008 Report on the Environment (Final Report)*. Washington D.C.: U.S. Environmental Protection Agency; World Health Organization. 2009. *WHO Report on the Global Tobacco Epidemic, 2009: Implementing Smoke-Free Environments*. Geneva: World Health Organization.

tobacco carcinogens. Chemicals in tobacco smoke also show up in breast milk, and breastfeeding may pass more chemicals to the infant of a smoking mother than does direct exposure. ETS triggers 150,000–300,000 cases of bronchitis, pneumonia, and other respiratory infections in infants and toddlers up to age 18 months each year.

Older children suffer, too. ETS is a risk factor for asthma in children who have not previously displayed symptoms of the disease, and it aggravates the symptoms of children who already have asthma. ETS is also linked to reduced lung function and fluid buildup in the middle ear, a contributing factor in middle-ear infections, a leading reason for childhood surgery. Later in life, people exposed to ETS as children are at increased risk for lung cancer, emphysema, and chronic bronchitis.

Smoking and Pregnancy

Smoking almost doubles a pregnant woman's chance of having a miscarriage, and it significantly increases her risk of ectopic pregnancy. Maternal smoking causes hundreds of infant deaths in the United States each year, primarily due to premature delivery and smoking-related problems with the placenta. Maternal smoking is a major factor in low birth weight, which puts newborns at high risk for infections and other serious problems. If a nonsmoking mother is regularly exposed to ETS, her infant is also at greater risk for low birth weight.

Babies born to mothers who smoke more than two packs a day perform poorly on developmental tests in the first hours after birth, compared to babies of nonsmoking mothers. Later in life, obesity, hyperactivity, short attention span, and lower scores on spelling and reading tests all occur more frequently in children whose mothers smoked during pregnancy than in those born to nonsmoking mothers. Prenatal tobacco exposure has also been associated with behavioral problems in children.

WHAT CAN BE DONE?

There are many ways to act against this public health threat.

Action at Many Levels

Thousands of local ordinances across the nation restrict or ban smoking in restaurants, stores, workplaces, and even public outdoor areas. An assessment made in 2010 found that 75% of Americans live in municipalities that restrict or ban smoking in public buildings, workplaces, restaurants, and bars. At least 260 colleges and universities now have totally smoke-free campuses or prohibit smoking in residential buildings. As local nonsmoking laws proliferate, evidence mounts that environmental restrictions are effective in encouraging smokers to quit.

At the state level, many tough anti-tobacco laws have been passed. As of January 2010, comprehensive smoke-free air laws were in effect in 35 states, the District of Columbia, and Puerto Rico. California has one of the most aggressive—and successful—tobacco control programs, combining taxes on cigarettes, graphic advertisements, and bans on smoking in bars and restaurants.

Ask Yourself

QUESTIONS FOR CRITICAL THINKING AND REFLECTION

What are your views on the government's role in regulating tobacco products? Is there currently enough regulation, or should the government go further in controlling the production and marketing of these products? What events or experiences have shaped your views on this issue?

QUICK STATS

Smoking-related health costs amount to $10.47 per pack of cigarettes consumed by Americans.

—CDC, 2010

Smoking is also banned on many international air flights, as well as in many restaurants and hotels and on public transportation in some countries. The World Health Organization has taken the lead in international anti-tobacco efforts by sponsoring the Framework Convention on Tobacco Control. Another international activity is the annual commemoration of World No Tobacco Day (May 31), on which smokers are encouraged to stop smoking for 1 day.

Such local, state, national, and international efforts represent progress, but health activists warn that tobacco industry influence remains strong. The tobacco industry contributes heavily to sympathetic legislative officeholders and candidates. Since 1999, tobacco interests have spent more than $115 million on federal lobbying activities.

Individual Action

Nonsmokers have the right not only to breathe clean air but also to take action to help solve one of society's most serious public health threats. Here are a few actions you can take: When a smoker violates a no-smoking designation, complain. If your favorite restaurant or shop doesn't have a nonsmoking policy, ask the manager to adopt one. If you see children buying tobacco, report this illegal activity to the facility manager or the police. Learn more about addiction and tobacco cessation so you can better support the tobacco users you know. Vote for candidates who support anti-tobacco measures; contact local, state, and national representatives to express your views.

You can also cancel your subscriptions to magazines that carry tobacco advertising and send a letter to the publisher explaining your decision. Voice your opinion about other positive representations of tobacco use. (A recent study found that more than two-thirds of children's animated feature films have featured tobacco or alcohol use with no clear message that such practices were unhealthy.) Volunteer with the American Lung Association, the American Cancer Society, or the American Heart Association.

HOW A TOBACCO USER CAN QUIT

Giving up tobacco is a long-term process. Research shows that tobacco users move through predictable stages—from being uninterested in stopping, to thinking about change, to making a concerted effort to stop, to finally maintaining abstinence. But most attempt to quit several times before they finally succeed. Relapse is a normal part of the process.

The Benefits of Quitting

Giving up tobacco provides immediate health benefits to men and women of all ages (Table 8.4). The younger people are when they stop smoking, the more pronounced

Different remedies work for different people!! [handwritten annotation]

Table 8.4	Benefits of Quitting Smoking

Within 20 minutes of your last cigarette:
- You stop polluting the air
- Blood pressure drops to normal
- Pulse rate drops to normal
- Temperature of hands and feet increases to normal

8 hours:
- Carbon monoxide level in blood drops to normal
- Oxygen level in blood increases to normal

24 hours:
- Chance of heart attack decreases

48 hours:
- Nerve endings start regrowing
- Ability to smell and taste is enhanced

2–3 months:
- Circulation improves
- Walking becomes easier
- Lung function increases up to 30%

1–9 months:
- Coughing, sinus congestion, fatigue, and shortness of breath all decrease

1 year:
- Heart disease death rate is half that of a smoker

5 years:
- Stroke risk drops nearly to the risk for nonsmokers

10 years:
- Lung cancer death rate drops to 50% of that of continuing smokers
- Incidence of other cancers (mouth, throat, larynx, esophagus, bladder, kidney, and pancreas) decreases
- Risk of ulcer decreases

15 years:
- Risk of lung cancer is about 25% of that of continuing smokers
- Risks of heart disease and death are close to those for nonsmokers

Smoking Cessation Products

Each year, millions of Americans visit their doctors in the hope of finding a drug that can help them stop smoking. Although pharmacological options are limited, the few available drugs have proved successful.

Chantix (Varinicline)

The newest smoking cessation drug, marketed under the name Chantix, works in two ways: It reduces nicotine cravings, easing the withdrawal process, and it blocks the pleasant effects of nicotine. The drug acts on neurotransmitter receptors in the brain.

Unlike most smoking cessation products currently on the market, Chantix is not a nicotine replacement. For this reason, smokers may be advised to continue smoking for the first few days of treatment, to avoid withdrawal and to allow the drug to build up in their system. The approved course of treatment is 12 weeks, but the duration and recommended dosage depend on several factors, including the smoker's general health and the length and severity of his or her nicotine addiction.

Side effects reported with Chantix include nausea, headache, vomiting, sleep disruptions, and change in taste perception. Chantix is not recommended for women who are pregnant or nursing.

Zyban (Bupropion)

Bupropion is an antidepressant (prescribed under the name Wellbutrin) as well as a smoking cessation aid (prescribed under the name Zyban). As a smoking cessation aid, bupropion eases the symptoms of nicotine withdrawal and reduces the urge to smoke. Like Chantix, it acts on neurotransmitter receptors in the brain.

Bupropion users have reported an array of side effects, but they are rare. Side effects may be reduced by changing the dosage, taking the medicine at a different time of day, or taking it with or without food. Zyban and Wellbutrin should not be taken together.

Nicotine Replacement Products

The most widely used smoking cessation products replace the nicotine that the user would normally get from tobacco, reducing withdrawal symptoms and cravings. Although still harmful, nicotine replacement products provide a cleaner form of nicotine, without the thousands of poisons and tars produced by burning tobacco. Less of the product is used over time, as the need for nicotine decreases.

Nicotine replacement products come in several forms, including patches, gum, lozenges, nasal sprays, and inhalers. They are available in a variety of strengths and can be worked into many different smoking cessation strategies. Most are available without a prescription.

The nicotine patch is popular because it can be applied and forgotten until it needs to be removed or changed, usually every 16 or 24 hours. Placed on the upper arm or torso, it releases a steady stream of nicotine, which is absorbed through the skin. The main side effects are skin irritation and redness. Nicotine gum and nicotine lozenges have the advantage of allowing the smoker to use them whenever he or she craves nicotine. Side effects of nicotine gum include mouth sores and headaches; nicotine lozenges can cause nausea and heartburn. Nicotine nasal sprays and inhalers are available only by prescription.

Although all these products have proved to be effective in helping users stop smoking, experts recommend them only as one part of a complete smoking cessation program. Such a program should include regular professional counseling and physician monitoring.

---

the health improvements. And these improvements gradually but invariably increase as the period of nonsmoking lengthens. It's never too late to quit, though. According to a U.S. Surgeon General's report, people who quit smoking, regardless of age, live longer than people who continue to smoke.

Options for Quitting

Most tobacco users—76% in a recent survey—want to quit, and half of those who want to quit will make an attempt this year. What are their options? No single method works for everyone, but each does work for some people some of the time. Choosing to quit requires developing a strategy for success. Some people quit cold turkey, whereas others taper off slowly. There are over-the-counter and prescription products that help many people (see the box "Smoking Cessation Products" for more on these options). Behavioral factors that have been shown to increase the chances of a smoker's permanent smoking cessation are support from others and regular exercise. Support can come from friends and family and/or formal group programs sponsored by organizations such as the American Cancer Society and the American Lung Association or by your college health center or community hospital.

Free telephone quitlines are emerging as a popular and effective strategy to help stop smoking. Quitlines are staffed by trained counselors who help each caller plan a personal quitting strategy, usually including a combination of nicotine replacement therapy, changes in daily habits, and emotional support. In 2004, the Department of Health and Human Services established a national toll-free number, 1-800-QUITNOW (1-800-784-8669), to serve as a single access point for smokers seeking information and assistance in quitting.

Most smokers in the process of quitting experience both physical and psychological effects of nicotine withdrawal, and exercise can help with both. For many smokers, their tobacco use is associated with certain times and places—following a meal, for example. Resolving to walk after dinner instead of lighting up provides a distraction from cravings and eliminates the cues that trigger a desire to smoke. In addition, many people worry about weight

> *It's never too late to stop smoking, and smokers have a variety of options for quitting.*

gain associated with quitting. Although most ex-smokers do gain a few pounds, at least temporarily, incorporating exercise into a new tobacco-free routine lays the foundation for healthy weight management. The health risks of adding a few pounds are far outweighed by the risks of continued smoking; it's estimated that a smoker would have to gain 75–100 pounds to equal the health risks of smoking a pack a day.

As with any significant change in health-related behavior, giving up tobacco requires planning, sustained effort, and support. It is an ongoing process, not a one-time event. The Behavior Change Strategy describes the steps that successful quitters follow.

SUMMARY

- After being absorbed into the bloodstream in the stomach and small intestine, alcohol is transported throughout the body. The liver metabolizes alcohol as blood circulates through it.

- Alcohol is a CNS depressant. At low doses, it tends to make people feel relaxed.

- Alcohol use increases the risk of injury and violence; drinking before driving is particularly dangerous, even at low doses.

- Continued alcohol use has negative effects on the digestive and cardiovascular systems and increases cancer risk and overall mortality.

- Pregnant women who drink risk giving birth to children with a cluster of birth defects known as fetal alcohol syndrome (FAS). Even occasional drinking during pregnancy can cause brain injury in the fetus.

- Alcohol abuse involves drinking in dangerous situations or drinking to a degree that causes academic, professional, interpersonal, or legal difficulties.

- Alcohol dependence, or alcoholism, is characterized by more extensive problems with alcohol, usually involving tolerance and withdrawal.

- Binge drinking is a common form of alcohol abuse on college campuses that has negative effects on both drinking and nondrinking students.

- Physical consequences of alcoholism include the direct effects of tolerance and withdrawal, as well as all the problems associated with chronic drinking. Psychological problems include memory loss and additional mental disorders such as depression.

- Treatment approaches include mutual support groups like AA, job- and school-based programs, inpatient hospital programs, and pharmacological treatments.

Kicking the Tobacco Habit

You can look forward to a longer and healthier life if you join the 48 million Americans who have quit using tobacco. The steps for quitting described below are discussed in terms of the most popular tobacco product in the United States—cigarettes—but they can be adapted for all forms of tobacco.

Gather Information

Collect personal smoking information in a detailed journal about your smoking behavior. Write down the time you smoke each cigarette of the day, the situation you are in, how you feel, where you smoke, and how strong your craving for the cigarette is, plus any other information that seems relevant. Part of the job is to identify patterns of smoking that are connected with routine situations (for example, the coffee break smoke, the after-dinner cigarette, the tension-reduction cigarette). Use this information to discover the behavior patterns involved in your smoking habit.

Make the Decision to Quit

Choose a date in the near future when you expect to be relatively stress-free and can give quitting the energy and attention it will require. Don't choose a date right before or during finals week, for instance. Consider making quitting a gift: Choose your birthday as your quit date, for example, or make quitting a Father's Day or Mother's Day present. You might also want to coordinate your quit date with a buddy—a fellow tobacco user who wants to quit or a nonsmoker who wants to give up another bad habit or begin an exercise program. Tell your friends and family when you plan to quit. Ask them to offer encouragement and help hold you to your goal.

Decide what approach to quitting will work best for you. Will you go cold turkey, or will you taper off? Will you use nicotine patches or gum? Will you join a support group or enlist the help of a buddy? Prepare a contract for quitting, as discussed in Chapter 1. Set firm dates and rewards, and sign the contract. Post it in a prominent place.

Prepare to Quit

One of the most important things you can do to prepare to quit is to develop and practice nonsmoking relaxation techniques. Many smokers find that they use cigarettes to help them unwind in tense situations or to relax at other times. If this is true for you, you'll need to find and develop effective substitutes. It takes time to become proficient at relaxation techniques, so begin practicing before your quit date. Refer to the detailed discussion of relaxation techniques in Chapter 2.

Other things you can do to help prepare for quitting include the following:

- Make an appointment to see your physician. Ask about OTC and prescription aids for tobacco cessation and whether one or more might be appropriate for you.

- Make a dentist's appointment to have your teeth cleaned the day after your target quit date.

- Start an easy exercise program, if you're not exercising regularly already.

- Buy some sugarless gum. Stock your kitchen with low-calorie snacks.

- Clean out your car, and air out your house. Send your clothes out for dry cleaning.

- Throw away all your cigarette-related paraphernalia (ashtrays, lighters, etc.).

- The night before your quit day, get rid of all your cigarettes. Have fun with this—get your friends or family to help you tear them up.

- Make your last few days of smoking inconvenient: Smoke only outdoors and when alone. Don't do anything else while you smoke.

Quitting

Your first few days without cigarettes will probably be the most difficult. It's hard to give up such a strongly ingrained habit, but remember that millions of Americans have done it—and you can, too. Plan and rehearse the steps you will take when you experience a powerful craving. Avoid or control situations that you know from your journal are powerfully associated with your smoking. If your hands feel empty without a cigarette, try holding or fiddling with a small object such as a paper clip or pencil.

Social support can also be a big help. Arrange with a buddy to help you with your weak moments, and call him or her whenever you feel overwhelmed by an urge to smoke. Tell people you've just quit. You may discover many inspiring former smokers who can encourage you and reassure you that it's possible to quit and lead a happier, healthier life. Find a formal support group to join if you think it will help.

Maintaining Nonsmoking

The lingering smoking urges that remain once you've quit should be carefully tracked and controlled because they can cause relapses if left unattended. Keep track of these urges in your journal to help you deal with them. If certain situations still trigger the urge for a cigarette, change something about the situation to break past associations. If stress or boredom causes strong smoking urges, use a relaxation technique, take a brisk walk, have a stick of gum, or substitute some other activity for smoking.

Don't set yourself up for a relapse. If you allow yourself to get overwhelmed at school or work or to gain weight, it will be easier to convince yourself that now isn't the right time to quit. This *is* the right time. Continue to practice time-management and relaxation techniques. Exercise regularly, eat sensibly, and get enough sleep. These habits will not only ensure your success at remaining tobacco-free but also serve you well in stressful times throughout your life. In fact, former smokers who have quit for at least 3 months report reduced stress levels, probably because quitting smoking lowers overall arousal.

Watch out for patterns of thinking that can make nonsmoking more difficult. Focus on the positive aspects of not smoking, and give yourself lots of praise—you deserve it. Stick with the schedule of rewards you developed for your contract.

Keep track of the emerging benefits that come from having quit. Items that might appear on your list include improved stamina, an increased sense of pride at having kicked a strong addiction, a sharper sense of taste and smell, no more smoker's cough, and so on. Keep track of the money you're saving by not smoking, and spend it on things you really enjoy. And if you do lapse, be gentle with yourself. Lapses are a normal part of quitting. Forgive yourself, and pick up where you left off.

- Smoking is the largest preventable cause of ill health and death in the United States. Nevertheless, millions of Americans continue to use tobacco.

- People who begin smoking are usually imitating others or responding to seductive advertising. Smoking is associated with low education level and the use of other drugs.

- Tobacco smoke is made up of hundreds of different chemicals, including some that are carcinogenic or poisonous or that damage the respiratory system.

- Nicotine acts on the nervous system as a stimulant or a depressant. It can cause blood pressure and heart rate to increase, straining the heart.

- Cardiovascular disease is the most widespread cause of death for cigarette smokers. Cigarette smoking is the primary cause of lung cancer and is linked to many other cancers and respiratory diseases.

- The use of spit tobacco leads to nicotine addiction and is linked to oral cancers.

- Cigars, pipes, clove cigarettes, and bidis are not safe alternatives to cigarettes.

- Environmental tobacco smoke (ETS) contains high concentrations of toxic chemicals and can cause headaches, eye and nasal irritation, and sinus problems. Children whose parents smoke are especially susceptible to respiratory diseases.

- Smoking during pregnancy increases the risk of miscarriage, stillbirth, congenital abnormalities, premature birth, and low birth weight. SIDS, behavior problems, and long-term impairments in development are also risks.

- Giving up smoking is a difficult and long-term process. Although most ex-smokers quit on their own, some smokers benefit from stop-smoking programs, OTC and prescription medications, and support groups.

FOR MORE INFORMATION

BOOKS

Dean, Michael. 2007. *Empty Cribs: The Impact of Smoking on Child Health.* New York: Arts & Sciences Publishing. *Examines the effects of smoking on children, before and after birth.*

Gilman, S. L., ed. 2004. *Smoke: A Global History of Smoking.* London: Reaktion Books. *A look at smoking and its effects, including history and issues related to culture, art, and gender.*

Herrick, C. 2007. *100 Questions & Answers About Alcoholism & Drug Addiction.* Boston: Jones and Bartlett. *Answers a range of specific questions about alcohol abuse, dependence, and treatment options.*

How to Quit Smoking Without Gaining Weight. 2004. New York: American Lung Association.

Kinney, J. 2009. *Loosening the Grip: A Handbook of Alcohol Information*, 9th ed. New York: McGraw-Hill. *A fascinating book about alcohol, including information on physical effects, abuse, alcoholism, and cultural aspects of alcohol use.*

Seaman, B. 2006. *Binge: Campus Life in an Age of Disconnection and Excess.* New York: Wiley. *An exploration of campus life at 12 residential colleges and universities, with discussions on the effects of student isolation, peer pressure, and drinking on today's students.*

Wholey, D. 2007. *Why Do I Keep Doing That?* Deerfield Beach, Fla.: Health Communications. *An optimistic approach to breaking self-destructive habits.*

ORGANIZATIONS, HOTLINES, AND WEB SITES

Action on Smoking and Health (ASH). An advocacy group that provides statistics, news briefs, and other information.
   http://ash.org

Al-Anon Family Group Headquarters. Provides information and referrals to local Al-Anon and Alateen groups. The Web site includes a self-quiz to determine if you are affected by someone's drinking.
   888-4AL-ANON
   http://www.al-anon.alateen.org

Alcoholics Anonymous (AA) World Services. Provides general information on AA, literature on alcoholism, and information about AA meetings and related 12-step organizations.
   212-870-3400
   http://www.aa.org

Alcohol Treatment Referral Hotline. Provides referrals to local intervention and treatment providers.
   800-ALCOHOL

American Cancer Society (ACS). Sponsor of the annual Great American Smokeout; provides information on the dangers of tobacco, as well as tools for prevention and cessation for both smokers and users of spit tobacco.
   http://www.cancer.org

American Lung Association. Provides information on lung diseases, tobacco control, and environmental health.
   http://www.lungusa.org

Bacchus and Gamma Peer Education Network. An association of college- and university-based peer education programs that focus on prevention of alcohol abuse.
   http://www.bacchusgamma.org

CDC's Tobacco Information and Prevention Source (TIPS). Provides research results, educational materials, and tips on how to quit smoking; Web site includes special sections for kids and teens.
   http://www.cdc.gov/tobacco

The College Alcohol Study. Harvard School of Public Health. Provides information about and results from the recent studies of binge drinking on college campuses.
   http://www.hsph.harvard.edu/cas

College Drinking Prevention. Includes information about alcohol, including myths about alcohol use and an interactive look at how alcohol affects the body.
   http://www.collegedrinkingprevention.gov

Environmental Protection Agency Indoor Air Quality/ETS. Provides information and links about secondhand smoke.
   http://www.epa.gov/smokefree

Mothers Against Drunk Driving (MADD). Supports efforts to develop solutions to the problems of drunk driving and underage drinking; provides news, information, and brochures about many topics, including a guide for giving a safe party.
   http://www.madd.org

National Association for Children of Alcoholics (NACoA). Provides information and support for children of alcoholics.
   888-554-COAS
   http://www.nacoa.net

Touring Lifestyle Behaviors

Alcohol Use: Stages of Intoxication

Tobacco Use: Immediate Effects and Long-Term Health Risks

Exercise: Immediate Effects and Long-Term Health Benefits

The Greenhouse Effect, Climate Change, and You

GOALS OF THE TOUR

1. **Alcohol Use.** Describe the stages of intoxication and the effects experienced in each stage.

2. **Tobacco Use.** Identify and describe the immediate effects and long-term health risks of tobacco use.

3. **Exercise.** Identify and describe the immediate effects and long-term health benefits of exercise.

4. **The Greenhouse Effect.** Explain the greenhouse effect and describe actions individuals can take to reduce their carbon footprint.

Alcohol Use: Stages of Intoxication

1 Describe the stages of intoxication and the effects experienced at each stage.

Blood alcohol concentration (BAC) rises quickly with alcohol consumption, but alcohol is metabolized at a relatively slow rate—about 1 drink per hour. Note that rate of alcohol metabolism varies widely depending on sex, body weight, ethnicity, age, food in the stomach, genetics, and other factors—so the effects at different BACs also vary.

One drink =

a 12-ounce beer

or

a 1.5-ounce shot

or

a 5-ounce glass of wine

Number of drinks in 1 hour before the legal BAC limit of 0.08 is reached

Weight in pounds	Drinks in 1 hour
90–109	1
110–129	1
130–149	2
150–169	2
170–189	2
190–200+	3

150 lbs 130 lbs 180 lbs 170 lbs 102 lbs 200 lbs

BAC 0.00 0.02 0.05 0.08 0.10 0.15

effects

BAC: 0.01–0.05
Relaxation; mild euphoria; reduced inhibition; decreased alertness; impaired motor coordination and judgment.
Approximate time to metabolize: 2–3 hours

BAC: 0.10–0.15
Mood swings; aggression; staggering gait; impaired balance; slurred speech.
Approximate time to metabolize: 7–10 hours

BAC: 0.05–0.10
Emotional instability; exaggerated feelings and behaviors; impaired reasoning, judgment, and visual tracking; slowed information processing, reflexes, and reaction time; sleepiness; nausea. Legally intoxicated at 0.08% in all 50 states.
Approximate time to metabolize: 3–6 hours

Tobacco Use: Immediate Effects and Long-Term Health Risks

Identify and describe the immediate effects and long-term health risks of tobacco use. **2**

Immediate Effects

Brain
- Nicotine triggers release of sedating and stimulating chemicals in brain

Skin
- Nicotine constricts blood vessels, reducing blood flow to skin

Heart
- Nicotine increases heart rate, elevates blood pressure
- Heart must work harder to deliver oxygen to cells

Lungs, bronchi
- Smoke is absorbed into bloodstream and carried throughout the body
- Oxygen delivery to cells is impaired

Liver
- Nicotine causes liver to convert glycogen to glucose and release it into bloodstream, raising blood sugar levels

Adrenal glands
- Nicotine triggers release of adrenaline, causing stimulating effects throughout the body and reduced body temperature in extremities

Kidneys
- Nicotine inhibits production of urine

Digestive system
- Nicotine depresses appetite and hunger contractions

Reproductive system
- In pregnant women, nicotine and chemicals are passed to fetus

Exercise: Immediate Effects and Long-Term Health Benefits

3 Identify and describe the immediate effects and long-term health benefits of exercise.

Immediate Effects

Brain
- Increased oxygen and nutrients to brain
- Increased levels of neurotransmitters

Heart
- Increased heart rate
- Greater volume of blood pumped to body

Lungs
- Increased breathing rate
- Increased oxygen consumption

Stomach
- Reduced blood flow to digestive system

Muscles
- Increased blood flow to muscles
- Increased energy production in muscles

Skin
- Increased blood flow to skin
- Increased sweating to maintain safe body temperature

The Greenhouse Effect, Climate Change, and You

Explain the greenhouse effect and describe actions individuals can take to reduce their carbon footprint.

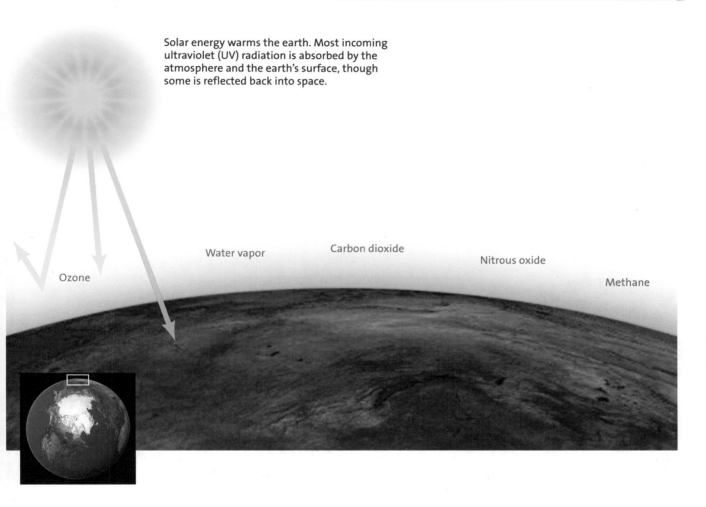

Solar energy warms the earth. Most incoming ultraviolet (UV) radiation is absorbed by the atmosphere and the earth's surface, though some is reflected back into space.

Water vapor

Carbon dioxide

Nitrous oxide

Ozone

Methane

National Clearinghouse for Alcohol and Drug Information/Prevention Online. Provides statistics and information on alcohol abuse, including resources for people who want to help friends and family members overcome alcohol-abuse problems.

http://ncadi.samhsa.gov

National Council on Alcoholism and Drug Dependence (NCADD). Provides information and counseling referrals.

212-269-7797; 800-NCA-CALL (24-hour Hope Line)
http://www.ncadd.org

National Institute on Alcohol Abuse and Alcoholism (NIAAA). Provides booklets and other publications on a variety of alcohol-related topics, including fetal alcohol syndrome, alcoholism treatment, and alcohol use and minorities.

http://www.niaaa.nih.gov

Nicotine Anonymous. A 12-step program for tobacco users.

http://www.nicotine-anonymous.org

Rational Recovery. A free self-help program that offers an alternative to 12-step programs; the emphasis is on learning the skill of abstinence.

http://www.rational.org

Smokefree.Gov. Provides step-by-step strategies for quitting as well as expert support via telephone or instant messaging.

http://www.smokefree.gov

World Health Organization Tobacco Free Initiative. Promotes the goal of a tobacco-free world.

http://www.who.int/tobacco/en

SELECTED BIBLIOGRAPHY

American Cancer Society. 2010. *Cancer Facts and Figures, 2010.* Atlanta, Ga.: American Cancer Society.

American Lung Association. 2010. *State of Tobacco Control 2009.* New York: America Lung Association.

American Lung Association. 2010. *Trends in Tobacco Use* (http://www.lungusa.org/finding-cures/our-research/trend-reports/Tobacco-Trend-Report.pdf; retrieved November 3, 2010).

Campaign for Tobacco-Free Kids. 2010. *Enforcing Laws Prohibiting Cigarette Sales to Kids Reduces Youth Smoking.* Washington, D.C.: Campaign for Tobacco-Free Kids.

Campaign for Tobacco-Free Kids. 2010. *State Cigarette Excise Tax Rates and Rankings.* Washington, D.C.: Campaign for Tobacco-Free Kids.

Centers for Disease Control and Prevention. 2008. Surveillance for cancers associated with tobacco use—United States, 1999–2004. *Morbidity and Mortality Weekly Report* 57(SS-08): 1–33.

Centers for Disease Control and Prevention. 2008. Youth risk behavior surveillance—United States, 2007. *Morbidity and Mortality Weekly Report* 57(SS-04): 1–131.

Centers for Disease Control and Prevention. 2009. Alcohol use among pregnant and nonpregnant women of childbearing age: United States, 1991–2005. *Morbidity and Mortality Weekly Report* 58(19): 529–532.

Centers for Disease Control and Prevention. 2009. Cigarette smoking among adults and trends in smoking cessation—United States, 2008. *Morbidity and Mortality Weekly Report* 58(44): 1227–1232.

Centers for Disease Control and Prevention. 2010. *Alcohol and Public Health* (http://www.cdc.gov/alcohol/index.htm; retrieved November 3, 2010).

Centers for Disease Control and Prevention. 2010. *Public Health Impact of Tobacco Control Law* (http://www.fda.gov/TobaccoProducts/NewsEvents/ucm217158.htm; retrieved November 3, 2010).

Centers for Disease Control and Prevention. 2010. *Smoking and Tobacco Use Fact Sheet: Tobacco-Related Mortality* (http://www.cdc.gov/tobacco/data_statistics/fact_sheets/health_effects/tobacco_related_mortality; retrieved November 3, 2010).

Centers for Disease Control and Prevention. 2010. Youth risk behavior surveillance—United States, 2009. *Morbidity and Mortality Weekly Report* 59(SS–05): 1–148.

College Drinking Prevention. 2007. *A Snapshot of Annual High-Risk College Drinking Consequences* (http://www.collegedrinkingprevention.gov/StatsSummaries/snapshot.aspx; retrieved November 3, 2010).

Department of Health and Human Services. 2007. *The Surgeon General's Call to Action to Prevent and Reduce Underage Drinking.* Washington, D.C.: Department of Health and Human Services, Office of the Surgeon General.

Federal Trade Commission. 2009. *Federal Trade Commission Cigarette Report for 2006.* Washington, D.C.: Federal Trade Commission.

Fiore, M. C., et al. 2008. *Treating Tobacco Use and Dependence: 2008 Update. Clinical Practice Guideline.* Rockville, Md.: U.S. Department of Health and Human Services, Public Health Service.

Food and Drug Administration. 2008. *Consumer Update: New Safety Warnings for Chantix* (http://www.fds.gov/consumer/updates/chantix020508.html; retrieved November 3, 2010).

Hingson, R. W., et al. 2006. Age at drinking onset and alcohol dependence: Age at onset, duration, and severity. *Archives of Pediatrics and Adolescent Medicine* 160(7): 739–746.

Mannino, D. M., and A. S. Buist. 2007. Global burden of COPD: Risk factors, prevalence, and future trends. *Lancet* 370(9589): 765–773.

National Center for Health Statistics. 2010. Deaths: Final data for 2007. *National Vital Statistics Reports* 58(19): 1–21.

National Highway Traffic Safety Administration. 2009. *Traffic Safety Facts 2008: Alcohol-Impaired Driving.* Washington, D.C.: National Highway Traffic Safety Administration. DOT Pub. 811 155.

National Institute on Alcohol Abuse and Alcoholism. 2006. *Young Adult Drinking.* Alcohol Alert No. 68. Bethesda, Md.: National Institute on Alcohol Abuse and Alcoholism.

Perreira, K. M., and K. E. Cortes. 2006. Explaining race/ethnicity and nativity differences in alcohol and tobacco use during pregnancy. *American Journal of Public Health,* 27 July [epub].

Substance Abuse and Mental Health Services Administration. 2009. *Results from the 2008 National Survey on Drug Use and Health: National Findings.* Rockville, Md.: Office of Applied Studies, NSDUH Series H–36, HHS Publication No. SMA 09–4434.

Titus-Ernstoff, L., et al. 2008. Longitudinal study of viewing smoking in movies and initiation of smoking by children. *Pediatrics* 121(1): 15–21.

U.S. Food and Drug Administration Center for Tobacco Products. 2010. *2009–2010: Inaugural Year in Review.* Washington, D.C.: U.S. Food and Drug Administration.

U.S. Surgeon General. 2006. *The Health Consequences of Involuntary Exposure to Tobacco Smoke* (http://www.surgeongeneral.gov/library/secondhandsmoke/ report/; retrieved November 3, 2010).

WebMD Health News. 2009. *Alcohol Raises Risk of Breast Cancer Recurrence: Study Shows Drinking More Than 3 Drinks a Week Is Linked to Return of Cancer* (http://www.webmd.com/breast-cancer/news/20091210/alcohol-raises-risk-of-breast-cancer-recurrence; retrieved November 3, 2010).

World Health Organization. 2010. *WHO Report on the Global Tobacco Epidemic, 2009* (http//www.who.int/tobacco/mpower/2009/en/index.html; retrieved November 3, 2010).

LOOKING AHEAD...

After reading this chapter, you should be able to:

- List the essential nutrients, and describe the functions they perform in the body

- Describe the guidelines that have been developed to help people choose a healthy diet, avoid nutritional deficiencies and reduce their risk of diet-related chronic diseases

- Discuss nutritional guidelines for vegetarians and for special population groups

- Explain how to use food labels and other consumer tools to make informed choices about foods

- Put together a personal nutrition plan based on affordable foods that you enjoy and that will promote wellness, today as well as in the future

Nutrition Basics

9

n your lifetime, you'll spend about 6 years eating—about 70,000 meals and 60 tons of food. What you eat can have profound effects on your health and well-being. Your nutritional habits help determine your risk of major chronic diseases, including heart disease, cancer, stroke, and diabetes. Choosing foods that provide the nutrients you need while limiting the substances linked to disease should be an important part of your daily life.

Choosing a healthy diet is a two-part process. First, you have to know which nutrients you need and in what amounts. Second, you have to translate those requirements into a diet consisting of foods you like that are both available and affordable. Once you know what constitutes a healthy diet for you, you can adjust your current diet to bring it into line with your goals.

This chapter explains the basic principles of **nutrition.** It introduces the six classes of essential nutrients, explaining their roles in the functioning of the body. It also provides guidelines that you can use to design a healthy diet plan.

NUTRITIONAL REQUIREMENTS: COMPONENTS OF A HEALTHY DIET

You probably think about your diet in terms of the foods you like to eat. What's important for your health, though, are the nutrients contained in those foods. Your body requires proteins, fats, carbohydrates, vitamins, minerals, and water—about 45 **essential nutrients.** In this context, the word *essential* means that you must get these substances from food because your body is unable to manufacture them, or at least do so fast enough to meet your physiological needs.

The body needs some essential nutrients in relatively large amounts; these *macronutrients* include protein, fat, carbohydrate, and water. *Micronutrients,* such as vitamins and minerals, are required in much smaller amounts. Your body obtains nutrients through the process of **digestion,** in which the foods you eat are broken down into compounds your gastrointestinal tract can absorb and your body can use (Figure 9.1).

Salivary glands

Tongue

Trachea (*to lungs*)

Esophagus
(*to stomach*)

Liver

Gallbladder

Pancreas

Stomach

Large intestine
(colon)

Small
intestine

Appendix

Rectum

Anus

FIGURE 9.1 **The digestive system.** Food is partially broken down by being chewed and mixed with saliva in the mouth. After traveling to the stomach via the esophagus, food is broken down further by stomach acids and other secretions. As food moves through the digestive tract, it is mixed by muscular contractions and broken down by chemicals. Most absorption of nutrients occurs in the small intestine, aided by secretions from the pancreas, gallbladder, and intestinal lining. The large intestine reabsorbs excess water; the remaining solid wastes are collected in the rectum and excreted through the anus.

The energy in foods is expressed as **kilocalories.** One kilocalorie represents the amount of heat it takes to raise the temperature of 1 liter of water 1°C. A person needs about 2000 kilocalories per day to meet his or her energy needs. In common usage, people usually refer to kilocalories as *calories*, which is technically a much smaller energy unit (1 kilocalorie contains 1000 calories). This text uses the familiar word *calorie* to stand for the larger energy unit; you'll also find the word *calorie* used on food labels.

Of the six classes of essential nutrients, three supply energy:

- Fat = 9 calories per gram
- Protein = 4 calories per gram
- Carbohydrate = 4 calories per gram

Alcohol, though not an essential nutrient, also supplies energy, providing 7 calories per gram. The high caloric content of fat is one reason experts often advise against high fat consumption. Most people do not need the extra calories to meet energy needs. Regardless of their source, calories consumed in excess of energy needs are converted

to fat and stored in the body. Just meeting energy needs is not enough, however. Your body needs enough of the essential nutrients to grow and function properly.

Proteins—The Basis of Body Structure

Proteins form important parts of the body's main structural components: muscles and bones. Proteins also form important parts of blood, enzymes, some hormones, and cell membranes. When consumed, proteins also provide energy (4 calories per gram) for the body.

Amino Acids The building blocks of proteins are called **amino acids.** Twenty common amino acids are found in food; nine of these are essential (indispensable). The other eleven amino acids can be produced by the body, given the presence of the needed components supplied by foods.

Complete and Incomplete Proteins Individual protein sources are considered *complete* if they supply all the essential amino acids in adequate amounts and *incomplete* if they do not. Meat, fish, poultry, eggs, milk, cheese, and soy provide complete proteins. Incomplete proteins, which come from other plant sources such as legumes and nuts, are good sources of most essential amino acids but are usually low in one or two.

Certain combinations of vegetable proteins, such as wheat and peanuts in a peanut butter sandwich, allow each vegetable protein to make up for the amino acids missing in the other protein. The combination yields a complete protein. Many traditional

nutrition The science of food and how the body uses it in health and disease.

essential nutrients Substances the body must get from foods because it cannot manufacture them at all or fast enough to meet its needs. These nutrients include proteins, fats, carbohydrates, vitamins, minerals, and water.

digestion The process of breaking down foods in the gastrointestinal tract into compounds the body can absorb.

kilocalorie A measure of energy content in food; 1 kilocalorie represents the amount of heat needed to raise the temperature of 1 liter of water 1°C; commonly referred to as *calorie*.

protein An essential nutrient; a compound made of amino acids that contains carbon, hydrogen, oxygen, and nitrogen.

amino acids The building blocks of proteins.

TERMS

food pairings, such as beans and rice or corn and beans, emerged as dietary staples because they are complementary proteins. Vegetarians should include a variety of vegetable protein sources in their diets to make sure they get all the essential amino acids in adequate amounts. About two-thirds of the protein in the American diet comes from animal sources (meat and dairy products); therefore, the American diet is rich in essential amino acids.

Recommended Protein Intake   Adequate daily intake of protein for adults is 0.8 gram per kilogram (0.36 gram per pound) of body weight, corresponding to 50 grams of protein per day for someone who weighs 140 pounds and 65 grams of protein for someone who weighs 180 pounds. Most Americans meet or exceed the protein intake needed for adequate nutrition. If you consume more protein than your body needs, the extra protein is synthesized into fat for energy storage or burned for energy requirements. A little extra protein is not harmful, but it can contribute fat to the diet because protein-rich foods are often fat-rich as well. A very high protein intake can also strain the kidneys.

A fairly broad range of protein intakes is associated with good health, and the Food and Nutrition Board recommends that the amount of protein adults eat should fall within the range of 10–35% of total daily calorie intake, depending on the individual's age. The average American diet includes about 15–16% of total daily calories as protein.

Fats—Essential in Small Amounts

Fats, also known as *lipids*, are the most concentrated source of energy, at 9 calories per gram. The fats stored in your body represent usable energy, they help insulate your body, and they support and cushion your organs. Fats in the diet help your body absorb fat-soluble vitamins, and add important flavor and texture to foods. Fats are the major fuel for the body during rest and light activity. Two fats, linoleic acid and alpha-linolenic acid, are essential components of the diet.

Types and Sources of Fats   Most of the fats in foods are fairly similar in composition, generally including a molecule of glycerol (an alcohol) with three fatty acid

chains attached to it. The resulting structure is called a *triglyceride*. Animal fat, for example, is primarily made of triglycerides. Within a triglyceride, differences in the fatty acid structure result in different types of fats. Depending on this structure, a fat may be unsaturated, monounsaturated, polyunsaturated, or saturated. (The essential fatty acids—linoleic and alpha-linolenic acids—are both polyunsaturated.) The different types of fatty acids have different characteristics and different effects on your health.

Food fats are usually composed of both saturated and unsaturated fatty acids; the dominant type of fatty acid determines the fat's characteristics. Food fats containing large amounts of saturated fatty acids are usually solid at room temperature; they are generally found naturally in animal products. The leading sources of saturated fat in the American diet are red meats (hamburger, steak, roasts), whole milk, cheese, hot dogs, and lunch meats. Food fats containing large amounts of monounsaturated and polyunsaturated fatty acids usually come from plant sources and are liquid at room temperature. Olive, canola, safflower, and peanut oils contain mostly monounsaturated fatty acids. Soybean, corn, and cottonseed oils contain mostly polyunsaturated fatty acids.

Hydrogenation   There are notable exceptions to these generalizations. When unsaturated vegetable oils undergo the process of **hydrogenation**, a mixture of saturated and unsaturated fatty acids is produced. Hydrogenation also changes some unsaturated fatty acids to **trans fatty acids**, unsaturated fatty acids with an atypical shape that affects their behavior in the body. Food manufacturers use hydrogenation to increase the stability of an oil so it can be reused for deep frying, to improve the texture of certain foods, and to extend the shelf life of foods made with oil. Hydrogenation also transforms a liquid oil into margarine or vegetable shortening.

Leading sources of trans fats in the American diet are fried fast foods such as french fries and fried chicken (typically fried in vegetable shortening rather than oil), baked and snack foods, and stick margarine. In general, the more solid a hydrogenated oil is, the more saturated and trans fats it contains; for example, stick margarines typically contain more saturated and trans fats than do tub or squeeze margarines. Small amounts of trans fatty acids are found naturally in meat and milk.

Hydrogenated vegetable oils are not the only plant fats that contain saturated fats. Palm and coconut oils, although derived from plants, are also highly saturated. However, fish oils, derived from an animal source, are rich in polyunsaturated fats.

Fats and Health   Different types of fats have very different effects on health. Many studies have examined the effects of dietary fat intake on blood **cholesterol** levels and the risk of heart disease. Saturated and trans fatty acids raise blood levels of **low-density lipoprotein (LDL)**, or "bad" cholesterol, thereby increasing a person's

---

TERMS

hydrogenation   A process by which hydrogens are added to unsaturated fats, increasing the degree of saturation and turning liquid oils into solid fats.

trans fatty acid   A type of unsaturated fatty acid produced during the process of hydrogenation; trans fats have an atypical shape that affects their chemical activity.

cholesterol   A waxy substance in the blood and cells, needed for synthesis of cell membranes, vitamin D, and hormones.

low-density lipoprotein (LDL)   Blood fat that transports cholesterol to organs and tissues; excess amounts result in the accumulation of deposits on artery walls.

risk of heart disease. (However, a recent study concluded that saturated fat is not associated with an increased risk of certain forms of heart disease and that the benefits of a diet low in saturated fat may come from the larger amounts of polyunsaturated fats that these diets provide.)

Unsaturated fatty acids lower LDL. Monounsaturated fatty acids, such as those found in olive and canola oils, may also increase levels of **high-density lipoproteins (HDL)**, or "good" cholesterol, providing even greater benefits for heart health. In large amounts, trans fatty acids may lower HDL. Saturated fats have been found to impair the ability of HDLs to prevent inflammation of the blood vessels, one of the key factors in vascular disease; they have also been found to reduce the ability of the blood vessels to react normally to stress. Thus, to reduce the risk of heart disease, it is important to choose unsaturated fats instead of saturated and trans fats.

Most Americans consume four to five times as much saturated fat as trans fat (8–10% versus 2% of total daily calories). However, health experts are particularly concerned about trans fats because of their double negative effect on heart health—they both raise LDL and lower HDL. Since January 2006, food labels have included trans fat content. Consumers can also check for trans fats by looking for partially hydrogenated oil or vegetable shortening on the label.

Although saturated and trans fats pose health hazards, other fats can be beneficial. When used in place of saturated fats, monounsaturated fatty acids—as found in avocados, most nuts, and olive, canola, peanut, and safflower oils—improve cholesterol levels and may help protect against some cancers. **Omega-3 fatty acids,** a form of polyunsaturated fat found primarily in fish, may be even more healthful. Omega-3s and the compounds the body makes from them have a number of heart-healthy effects. Nutritionists recommend that Americans increase the proportion of omega-3s in their diet by eating fish two or more times a week. Salmon, tuna, trout, mackerel, herring, sardines, and anchovies are all good sources of omega-3s. Lesser amounts are found in plant foods, including dark-green leafy vegetables; walnuts; flaxseeds; and canola, walnut, and flaxseed oils.

Most of the polyunsaturated fats currently consumed by Americans are omega-6 fatty acids, primarily from corn oil and soybean oil. However, some nutritionists recommend that people reduce the proportion of omega-6s they consume in favor of omega-3s. The American Heart Association recommends consuming 5–10% of energy from omega-6 fatty acids. To make this adjustment, use canola oil rather than corn oil in cooking, and check for corn, soybean, or cottonseed oil in products such as mayonnaise, margarine, and salad dressing.

In addition to its effects on heart disease risk, dietary fat can affect health in other ways. Diets high in fatty red meat are associated with an increased risk of certain forms of cancer, especially colon cancer. A high-fat diet can also make weight management more difficult. The types of fatty acids and their effects on health are summarized in Table 9.1.

Recommended Fat Intake　To meet the body's demand for essential fats, adult men need about 17 grams per day of linoleic acid and 1.6 grams per day of alpha-linolenic acid; adult women need 12 grams of linoleic acid and 1.1 grams of alpha-linolenic acid. It takes only 3–4 teaspoons (15–20 grams) of vegetable oil per day incorporated into your diet to supply the essential fats. Most Americans consume sufficient amounts of the essential fats; limiting unhealthy fats is a much greater health concern.

Limits for total fat, saturated fat, and trans fat intake have been set by a number of government and research organizations. The Food and Nutrition Board recommends that fats make up 20–35% of total calories consumed daily. Although they are more difficult for consumers to monitor, guidelines have also been set for omega-6 fatty acids (5–10%) and omega-3 fatty acids (0.6–1.2%) as part of total fat intake. Because any amount of saturated and trans fats increases the risk of heart disease, the Food and Nutrition Board recommends that saturated fat and trans fat intake be kept as low as possible; most fat in a healthy diet should be unsaturated.

For advice on setting individual intake goals, see the box "Setting Intake Goals for Protein, Fat, and Carbohydrate." To determine how close you are to meeting your personal intake goals for fat, keep a running total over the course of the day. For prepared foods, food labels list the number of grams of fat, protein, and carbohydrate. Nutrition information is also available in many grocery stores, in inexpensive published nutrition guides, and online. By checking these resources, you can keep track of the total grams of fat, protein, and carbohydrate you eat and assess your current diet. You can still eat high-fat foods as long as you limit the size of your portions and balance your intake with low-fat foods.

Carbohydrates—An Ideal Source of Energy

Carbohydrates are needed in the diet primarily to supply energy for body cells. Some cells, such as those found in the brain and other parts of the nervous system and in

high-density lipoprotein (HDL)　Blood fat that helps transport cholesterol out of the arteries, thereby protecting against heart disease.

omega-3 fatty acids　Polyunsaturated fatty acids commonly found in fish oils; beneficial to cardiovascular health.

carbohydrate　An essential nutrient, required for energy for cells; sugars, starches, and dietary fiber are all carbohydrates.

TERMS

Table 9.1 Types of Fatty Acids and Their Possible Effects on Health

	TYPE OF FATTY ACID	FOUND IN[a]	POSSIBLE EFFECTS ON HEALTH
Keep Intake Low	SATURATED	• Animal fats (especially fatty meats and poultry fat and skin) • Butter, cheese, and other high-fat dairy products • Palm and coconut oils	• Raises total cholesterol and LDL cholesterol • May increase risk of heart disease • May increase risk of colon and prostate cancers
	TRANS	• Deep-fried fast foods • Stick margarines, shortening • Packaged cookies and crackers • Processed snacks and sweets	• Raises total cholesterol and LDL cholesterol • Lowers HDL cholesterol • May increase risk of heart disease and breast cancer
Choose Moderate Amounts	MONOUNSATURATED	• Olive, canola, and safflower oils • Avocados, olives • Peanut butter (without added fat) • Many nuts, including almonds, cashews, pecans, and pistachios	• Lowers total cholesterol and LDL cholesterol • May reduce blood pressure and lower triglycerides (a risk factor for heart disease) • May reduce risk of heart disease, stroke, and some cancers
	POLYUNSATURATED (two groups)[b]		
	Omega-3	• Fatty fish, including salmon, white albacore tuna, mackerel, anchovies, and sardines • Lesser amounts in walnut, flaxseed, canola, and soybean oils; tofu; walnuts; flaxseeds; and dark green leafy vegetables	• Reduces blood clotting and inflammation and inhibits abnormal heart rhythms • Lowers triglycerides • May lower blood pressure in some people • May reduce risk of fatal heart attack, stroke, and some cancers
	Omega-6	• Corn, soybean, and cottonseed oils (often used in margarine, mayonnaise, and salad dressings)	• Lowers total cholesterol and LDL cholesterol • May lower HDL cholesterol • May reduce risk of heart disease • May slightly increase risk of cancer if omega-6 intake is high and omega-3 intake is low

[a] Food fats contain a combination of types of fatty acids in various proportions. For example, canola oil is composed mainly of monounsaturated fatty acids (62%) but also contains polyunsaturated (32%) and saturated (6%) fatty acids. Food fats are categorized here according to their predominant fatty acid.
[b] The essential fatty acids are polyunsaturated: Linoleic acid is an omega-6 fatty acid and alpha-linolenic acid is an omega-3 fatty acid.

blood, use only carbohydrates for fuel. During high-intensity exercise, muscles also use primarily carbohydrates for fuel.

Simple and Complex Carbohydrates Carbohydrates are classified into two groups: simple and complex. *Simple carbohydrates* are sugars; they include sucrose (table sugar), fructose (fruit sugar, honey), maltose (malt sugar), and lactose (milk sugar). Simple carbohydrates add sweetness in foods and are found naturally in fruits and milk and are added to soft drinks, fruit drinks, candy, and sweet desserts. There is no evidence that any type of simple carbohydrate is more nutritious than others.

Complex carbohydrates include starches and most types of dietary fiber. Starches are found in a variety of plants, especially grains (wheat, rye, rice, oats, barley, millet), legumes (dry beans, peas, and lentils), and tubers (potatoes and yams). Most other vegetables contain a mixture of complex and simple carbohydrates.

During digestion in the mouth and small intestine, your body breaks down carbohydrates into simple sugar molecules, such as **glucose,** for absorption. Once glucose is in the bloodstream, the pancreas releases the hormone insulin, which allows cells to take up glucose and use it for energy. The liver and muscles also take up glucose to provide carbohydrate storage in the form of **glycogen.** Some people have problems controlling blood glucose levels, a disorder called *diabetes mellitus.*

Refined Carbohydrates Versus Whole Grains Complex carbohydrates can be further divided between refined, or processed, carbohydrates and unrefined carbohydrates, or **whole grains.** Before they are processed, all grains are whole grains, consisting of an inner layer, germ; a middle layer, the endosperm; and an outer layer, bran. During processing, the germ and bran are often removed, leaving just the starchy endosperm. The refinement of whole grains transforms whole-wheat flour to white flour, brown rice to white rice, and so on.

TERMS

glucose A simple sugar that is the body's basic fuel.

glycogen A starch stored in the liver and muscles.

whole grain The entire edible portion of a grain such as wheat, rice, or oats, consisting of the germ, endosperm, and bran. During milling or processing, parts of the grain are removed, often leaving just the endosperm.

Setting Intake Goals for Protein, Fat, and Carbohydrate

Goals have been established by the Food and Nutrition Board to help ensure adequate intake of the essential amino acids, fatty acids, and carbohydrate. Here are the daily goals for adults:

	Men	Women
Protein	56 grams	46 grams
Fat: Linoleic acid	17 grams	12 grams
Alpha-linolenic acid	1.6 grams	1.1 grams
Carbohydrate	130 grams	130 grams

Protein intake goals can be calculated more specifically by multiplying your body weight in kilograms by 0.8 or your body weight in pounds by 0.36. (Refer to the Nutrition Resources section at the end of the chapter for information for specific age groups and life stages.)

To meet your daily energy needs, you need to consume more than the minimally adequate amounts of the energy-providing nutrients listed above, which alone supply only about 800–900 calories. The Food and Nutrition Board provides additional guidance in the form of Acceptable Macronutrient Distribution Ranges (AMDRs). The ranges can help you balance your intake of the energy-providing nutrients in ways that ensure adequate intake while reducing the risk of chronic disease. The AMDRs for protein, total fat, and carbohydrate are as follow:

Protein	10–35% of total daily calories
Total fat	20–35% of total daily calories
Carbohydrate	45–65% of total daily calories

To set individual goals, begin by estimating your total daily energy (calorie) needs; if your weight is stable, your current energy intake is the number of calories you need to maintain your weight at your current activity level. Next, select percentage goals for protein, fat, and carbohydrate. You can allocate your total daily calories among the three classes of macronutrients to suit your preferences; just make sure that the three percentages you select total 100% and that you meet the minimum intake goals listed.

To translate your own percentage goals into daily intake goals expressed in calories and grams, multiply the appropriate percentages by total calorie intake and then divide the results by the corresponding calories per gram. For example, a fat limit of 35% applied to a 2200-calorie diet would be calculated as follows: 0.35 × 2200 = 770 calories of total fat; 770 ÷ 9 calories per gram = 86 grams of total fat. (Remember that fat has 9 calories per gram and that protein and carbohydrate have 4 calories per gram.)

SOURCE: Food and Nutrition Board, Institute of Medicine, National Academies. 2010. *Dietary Reference Intakes: The Essential Guide to Nutrient Requirements*. Washington, DC: National Academies Press. http://www.iom.edu/Activities/Nutrition/SummaryDRIs/DRI-Tables.aspx. Reprinted with permission from the National Academies Press, Copyright 2010, National Academy of Sciences.

42% of Americans never eat any whole grains.

—USDA, 2005

Refined carbohydrates usually retain all the calories of their unrefined counterparts, but they tend to be much lower in fiber, vitamins, minerals, and other beneficial compounds. Unrefined carbohydrates tend to take longer to chew and digest than refined ones; they also enter the bloodstream more slowly. This slower digestive pace tends to make people feel full sooner and for a longer period. Also, a slower rise in blood glucose levels following consumption of complex carbohydrates may help in the management of diabetes. Whole grains are also high in dietary fiber and so have all the benefits of fiber (discussed later).

Consumption of whole grains has been linked to a reduced risk of heart disease, diabetes, high blood pressure, stroke, and certain forms of cancer. For all these reasons, whole grains are recommended over those that have been refined (see the box "Choosing More Whole-Grain Foods").

Glycemic Index Insulin and glucose levels rise and fall following a meal or snack containing any type of carbohydrate. Some foods cause a quick and dramatic rise in glucose and insulin levels—these foods are said to have a high **glycemic index.** Other foods have a slower, more moderate effect. For people with particular health concerns, such as diabetes, glycemic index may be an important consideration in choosing foods. However, it should not be the sole criterion for food choices. Although unrefined complex carbohydrates and high-fiber foods generally tend to have a low glycemic index, patterns are less clear for other types of foods. The fat content of a food also affects its glycemic index, with higher fat foods having a lower effect on glucose levels. Ripeness, storage time, processing, and food preparation are other factors that can affect a food's glycemic index. In addition, what other foods are consumed at the same time makes a difference, as does the individual's fitness status.

Unrefined grains, fruits, vegetables, and legumes are rich in nutrients, have a relatively low energy density, and have a low to moderate glycemic index. Your best bet, therefore, is to choose a variety of vegetables daily and limit foods that are high in added sugars but low in other nutrients.

> **glycemic index** A measure of how a particular food affects blood glucose levels.

TERMS

Choosing More Whole-Grain Foods

Because whole-grain foods offer so many health benefits, federal dietary guidelines recommend six or more servings of grain products every day, with at least half of those servings from whole grains.

What Are Whole Grains?

The first step in increasing your intake of whole grains is to correctly identify them. The following are whole grains:

whole wheat	whole-grain corn
whole rye	popcorn
whole oats	brown rice
oatmeal	whole-grain barley

More unusual choices include bulgur (cracked wheat), millet, kasha (roasted buckwheat kernels), quinoa, wheat and rye berries, amaranth, wild rice, graham flour, whole-grain kamut, whole-grain spelt, and whole-grain triticale.

Wheat flour, unbleached flour, enriched flour, and degerminated corn meal are not whole grains. Wheat germ and wheat bran are also not whole grains, but they are the constituents of wheat typically left out when wheat is processed and so are healthier choices than regular wheat flour, which typically contains just the grain's endosperm.

Checking Packages for Whole Grains

To find packaged foods rich in whole grains, read the list of ingredients and check for special health claims related to whole grains. The *first* item on the list of ingredients should be one of the whole grains listed above. The FDA allows manufacturers to include special health claims for foods that contain 51% or more whole-grain ingredients. Such products may display a statement such as the following on their packaging: "Rich in whole grain," "Made with 100% whole grain," or "Diets rich in whole-grain foods may help reduce the risk of heart disease and certain cancers." However, many whole-grain products will not carry such claims—another reason to check the ingredient list for whole grains.

Recommended Carbohydrate Intake On average, Americans consume 200–300 grams of carbohydrate per day, well above the 130 grams needed to meet the body's requirement for essential carbohydrate. A range of intakes is associated with good health, and experts recommend that adults consume 45–65% of total daily calories as carbohydrate (about 225–325 grams of carbohydrate for someone consuming 2000 calories per day). The focus should be on consuming a variety of foods rich in complex carbohydrates, especially whole grains.

Although the Food and Nutrition Board set an AMDR for added sugars of 25% or less of total daily calories, many health experts recommend an even lower intake. World Health Organization guidelines suggest a limit of 10% of total daily calories from added sugars. Limits set by the USDA are even lower, with a maximum of about 8 teaspoons (32 grams) suggested for someone consuming 2000 calories per day. Foods high in added sugar are generally high in calories and low in nutrients and fiber, thus providing empty calories. The simple carbohydrates in your diet should come mainly from fruits, which are excellent sources of vitamins and minerals, and from low-fat or fat-free milk and other dairy products, which are high in protein and calcium.

dietary fiber Nondigestible carbohydrates and lignin that are intact in plants.

functional fiber Nondigestible carbohydrates either isolated from natural sources or synthesized; these may be added to foods and dietary supplements.

total fiber The total amount of dietary fiber and functional fiber in the diet.

Fiber—A Closer Look

Fiber is the term given to nondigestible carbohydrates provided by plants. Instead of being digested, like starch, fiber passes through the intestinal tract and provides bulk for feces in the large intestine, which in turn facilitates elimination. In the large intestine, some types of fiber are broken down by bacteria into acids and gases, which explains why consuming too much fiber can lead to intestinal gas. Even though humans cannot digest fiber, it is necessary for good health.

Types of Fiber The Food and Nutrition Board has defined two types of fiber:

• **Dietary fiber** refers to the nondigestible carbohydrates (and the noncarbohydrate substance *lignin*) that are present naturally in plants such as grains, legumes, and vegetables.

• **Functional fiber** refers to nondigestible carbohydrates that have been either isolated from natural sources or synthesized in a lab and then added to a food product or dietary supplement.

Total fiber is the sum of dietary and functional fiber. Fibers have different properties that lead to different physiological effects in the body. For example, *soluble (viscous) fiber* such as that found in oat bran or legumes can delay stomach emptying, slow the movement of glucose into the blood after eating, and reduce absorption of cholesterol. *Insoluble fiber,* such as that found in wheat bran or psyllium seed, increases fecal bulk and helps prevent constipation, hemorrhoids, and other digestive disorders. A diet high in fiber can help reduce the risk of type 2 diabetes, heart disease, and pulmonary disease as well as improve gastrointestinal health and aid in weight management. Some studies have linked high-fiber diets with a reduced risk of colon and rectal cancer; other studies have suggested that other characteristics of diets rich in fruits, vegetables, and whole grains may be responsible for this reduction in risk.

Sources of Fiber   All plant foods contain some dietary fiber. Fruits, legumes, oats (especially oat bran), and barley all contain the viscous types of fiber that help lower blood glucose and cholesterol levels. Wheat (especially wheat bran), other grains and cereals, and vegetables are good sources of cellulose and other fibers that help prevent constipation. Psyllium, which is often added to cereals or used in fiber supplements and laxatives, improves intestinal health and also helps control glucose and cholesterol levels. The processing of packaged foods can remove fiber, so it is important to rely on fresh fruits and vegetables and foods made from whole grains as your main sources of fiber.

> A cup of black or pinto beans has more than **15 grams** of fiber.
> —USDA, 2009

Recommended Fiber Intake   To reduce the risk of chronic disease and maintain intestinal health, the Food and Nutrition Board recommends a daily fiber intake of 38 grams for adult men and 25 grams for adult women. Americans currently consume about half this amount. Fiber should come from foods, not supplements, which should be used only under medical supervision.

Vitamins—Organic Micronutrients

Vitamins are organic (carbon-containing) substances required in small amounts to regulate various processes within living cells (Table 9.2). Humans need 13 vitamins; 4 are fat-soluble (A, D, E, and K), and 9 are water-soluble (C and the B-complex vitamins: thiamin, riboflavin, niacin, vitamin B-6, folate, vitamin B-12, biotin, and pantothenic acid).

Functions of Vitamins   Many vitamins help chemical reactions take place. They provide no energy to the body directly but help unleash the energy stored in carbohydrates, proteins, and fats. Vitamins are critical in the production of red blood cells and the maintenance of the nervous, skeletal, and immune systems. Some vitamins act as **antioxidants**, which help preserve the health of cells in the body. Key vitamin antioxidants include vitamin E, vitamin C and the vitamin A precursor beta-carotene.

Sources of Vitamins   The human body does not manufacture most of the vitamins it requires and must obtain them from foods. Vitamins are abundant in fruits, vegetables, and grains. In addition, many processed foods, such as flour and breakfast cereals, contain added vitamins. A few vitamins are made in certain parts of the body: The skin makes vitamin D when it is exposed to sunlight, and intestinal bacteria make vitamin K.

Vitamin Deficiencies   If your diet lacks a particular vitamin, characteristic symptoms of deficiency can develop. (Table 9.2 lists the signs of certain vitamin deficiencies.) For example, *scurvy* is a potentially fatal illness caused by a long-term lack of vitamin C. Children who do not get enough vitamin D can develop *rickets,* which leads to potentially disabling bone deformations. Vitamin A deficiency may cause blindness, and seizures can develop in people whose diet lacks vitamin B-6. Low intake of folate and vitamins B-6 and B-12 has been linked to an increased risk of heart disease.

New research is tying vitamin deficiencies with other health risks as well. For example, experts once thought that vitamin D was the only vitamin that played a role in bone health. Now scientists know that vitamins C and K and several B vitamins are also important in the prevention of osteoporosis. A great deal of recent research has focused on vitamin D, with surprising results. A systematic review of 17 studies suggests that vitamin D supplementation can reduce the risk of cardiovascular disease. Other studies also link low vitamin D levels to an increased risk of several cancers.

Vitamin deficiency diseases are most often seen in developing countries and are relatively rare in the United States because vitamins are readily available from our food supply. Still, many Americans consume lower than recommended amounts of several vitamins, including A, C, and E. Even in the face of new findings, however, experts warn that there is not yet enough evidence to prove that everyone should begin taking vitamin supplements.

Extra vitamins in the diet can also be harmful, especially when taken as supplements. Megadoses of fat-soluble vitamins are particularly dangerous because the excess is stored in the body rather than excreted, increasing the risk of toxicity. Even when vitamins are not taken in

vitamins   Carbon-containing substances needed in small amounts to help promote and regulate chemical reactions and processes in the body.

antioxidant   A substance that can lessen the breakdown of food or body constituents by free radicals; actions include binding oxygen, donating electrons to free radicals, and repairing damage to molecules.

TERMS

Table 9.2   Facts About Vitamins

VITAMIN	IMPORTANT DIETARY SOURCES	MAJOR FUNCTIONS	SIGNS OF PROLONGED DEFICIENCY	TOXIC EFFECTS OF MEGADOSES
Fat-Soluble				
Vitamin A	Liver, milk, butter, cheese, fortified margarine, carrots, spinach, orange and deep-green vegetables and fruits	Maintenance of immune function and vision, skin, linings of the nose, mouth, digestive and urinary tracts	Night blindness, scaling skin, increased susceptibility to infection, loss of appetite, anemia, kidney stones	Liver damage, miscarriage, birth defects, headache, vomiting, diarrhea, vertigo, double vision, bone abnormalities
Vitamin D	Fortified milk and margarine, fish oils, butter, egg yolks (sunlight on skin also produces vitamin D)	Development and maintenance of bones and teeth, promotion of calcium absorption	Rickets (bone deformities) in children; bone softening, loss, and fractures in adults	Kidney damage, calcium deposits in soft tissues, depression, death
Vitamin E	Vegetable oils, whole grains, nuts and seeds, green leafy vegetables, asparagus, peaches	Protection and maintenance of cellular membranes	Red blood cell breakage and anemia, weakness, neurological problems, muscle cramps	Relatively nontoxic, but may cause excess bleeding or formation of blood clots
Vitamin K	Green leafy vegetables; smaller amounts widespread in other foods	Production of factors essential for blood clotting and bone metabolism	Hemorrhaging	None reported
Water-Soluble				
Biotin	Cereals, yeast, egg yolks, soy flour, liver; widespread in foods	Synthesis of fat, glycogen, and amino acids	Rash, nausea, vomiting, weight loss, depression, fatigue, hair loss	None reported
Folate	Green leafy vegetables, yeast, oranges, whole grains, legumes, liver	Amino acid metabolism, synthesis of RNA and DNA, new cell synthesis	Anemia, weakness, fatigue, irritability, shortness of breath, swollen tongue	Masking of vitamin B-12 deficiency
Niacin	Eggs, poultry, fish, milk, whole grains, nuts, enriched breads and cereals, meats, legumes	Conversion of carbohydrates, fats, and protein into usable forms of energy	Pellagra (symptoms include diarrhea, dermatitis, inflammation of mucous membranes, dementia)	Flushing of the skin, nausea, vomiting, diarrhea, liver dysfunction, glucose intolerance
Pantothenic acid	Animal foods, whole grains, broccoli, potatoes; widespread in foods	Metabolism of fats, carbohydrates, and proteins	Fatigue, numbness and tingling of hands and feet, gastrointestinal disturbances	None reported
Riboflavin	Dairy products, enriched breads and cereals, lean meats, poultry, fish, green vegetables	Energy metabolism, maintenance of skin, mucous membranes, and nervous system structures	Cracks at corners of mouth, sore throat, skin rash, hypersensitivity to light, purple tongue	None reported
Thiamin	Whole-grain and enriched breads and cereals, organ meats, lean pork, nuts, legumes	Conversion of carbohydrates into usable forms of energy, maintenance of appetite and nervous system function	Beriberi (symptoms include muscle wasting, mental confusion, anorexia, enlarged heart, nerve changes)	None reported
Vitamin B-6	Eggs, poultry, fish, whole grains, nuts, soybeans, liver, kidney, pork	Metabolism of amino acids and glycogen	Anemia, convulsions, cracks at corners of mouth, dermatitis, nausea, confusion	Neurological abnormalities and damage
Vitamin B-12	Meat, fish, poultry, fortified cereals	Synthesis of blood cells, other metabolic reactions	Anemia, fatigue, nervous system damage, sore tongue	None reported
Vitamin C	Peppers, broccoli, spinach, brussels sprouts, citrus fruits, strawberries, tomatoes, potatoes, cabbage, other fruits and vegetables	Maintenance and repair of connective tissue, bones, teeth, and cartilage; promotion of healing; iron absorption	Scurvy, anemia, reduced resistance to infection, loosened teeth, joint pain, poor wound healing, hair loss, poor iron absorption	Urinary stones in some people, acid stomach from ingesting supplements in pill form, nausea, diarrhea, headache, fatigue

SOURCES: Food and Nutrition Board, Institute of Medicine. 2006. *Dietary Reference Intakes: The Essential Guide to Nutrient Requirements.* Washington, D.C.: The National Academies Press. The complete Dietary Reference Intake reports are available from the National Academy Press (http://www.nap.edu); Shils, M. E., et al., eds. 2005. *Modern Nutrition in Health and Disease,* 10th ed. Baltimore: Lippincott Williams & Wilkins.

Table 9.3   Facts About Selected Minerals

MINERAL	IMPORTANT DIETARY SOURCES	MAJOR FUNCTIONS	SIGNS OF PROLONGED DEFICIENCY	TOXIC EFFECTS OF MEGADOSES
Calcium	Milk and milk products, tofu, fortified orange juice and bread, green leafy vegetables, bones in fish	Formation of bones and teeth, control of nerve impulses, muscle contraction, blood clotting	Stunted growth in children, bone mineral loss in adults, urinary stones	Kidney stones, calcium deposits in soft tissues, inhibition of mineral absorption, constipation
Fluoride	Fluoridated water, tea, marine fish eaten with bones	Maintenance of tooth and bone structure	Higher frequency of tooth decay	Increased bone density, mottling of teeth, impaired kidney function
Iodine	Iodized salt, seafood, processed foods	Essential part of thyroid hormones, regulation of body metabolism	Goiter (enlarged thyroid), cretinism (birth defect)	Depression of thyroid activity, hyperthyroidism in susceptible people
Iron	Meat and poultry, fortified grain products, dark green vegetables, dried fruit	Component of hemoglobin, myoglobin, and enzymes	Iron-deficiency anemia, weakness, impaired immune function, gastrointestinal distress	Nausea, diarrhea, liver and kidney damage, joint pains, sterility, disruption of cardiac function, death
Magnesium	Widespread in foods and water (except soft water); especially found in grains, legumes, nuts, seeds, green vegetables, milk	Transmission of nerve impulses, energy transfer, activation of many enzymes	Neurological disturbances, cardiovascular problems, kidney disorders, nausea, growth failure in children	Nausea, vomiting, diarrhea, central nervous system depression, coma, death in people with impaired kidney function
Phosphorus	Present in nearly all foods, especially milk, cereal, peas, eggs, meat	Bone growth and maintenance, energy transfer in cells	Impaired growth, weakness, kidney disorders, cardiorespiratory and nervous system dysfunction	Drop in blood calcium levels, calcium deposits in soft tissues, bone loss
Potassium	Meats, milk, fruits, vegetables, grains, legumes	Nerve function and body water balance	Muscular weakness, nausea, drowsiness, paralysis, confusion, disruption of cardiac rhythm	Cardiac arrest
Selenium	Seafood, meat, eggs, whole grains	Defense against oxidative stress, regulation of thyroid hormone action	Muscle pain and weakness, heart disorders	Hair and nail loss, nausea and vomiting, weakness, irritability
Sodium	Salt, soy sauce, salted foods, tomato juice	Body water balance, acid-base balance, nerve function	Muscle weakness, loss of appetite, nausea, vomiting; deficiency is rarely seen	Edema, hypertension in sensitive people
Zinc	Whole grains, meat, eggs, liver, seafood (especially oysters)	Synthesis of proteins, RNA, and DNA; wound healing; immune response; ability to taste	Growth failure, loss of appetite, impaired taste acuity, skin rash, impaired immune function, poor wound healing	Vomiting, impaired immune function, decline in blood HDL levels, impaired copper absorption

SOURCES: Food and Nutrition Board, Institute of Medicine. 2006. *Dietary Reference Intakes: The Essential Guide to Nutrient Requirements*. Washington, D.C.: The National Academies Press. The complete Dietary Reference Intake reports are available from the National Academy Press (http://www.nap.edu); Shils, M. E., et al., eds. 2005. *Modern Nutrition in Health and Disease*, 10th ed. Baltimore: Lippincott Williams & Wilkins.

excess, relying on supplements for an adequate intake of vitamins can be a problem. There are many substances in foods other than vitamins and minerals, and some of these compounds may have important health effects.

Minerals—Inorganic Micronutrients

Minerals are inorganic (non–carbon-containing) elements you need in relatively small amounts to help regulate body functions, aid in the growth and maintenance of body tissues, and help release energy (Table 9.3). There

are about 17 essential minerals. The major minerals, those that the body needs in amounts exceeding 100 milligrams per day, include calcium, phosphorus, magnesium, sodium, potassium, and chloride. The essential trace minerals, those that you need in minute amounts, include copper, fluoride, iodide, iron, selenium, and zinc.

minerals   Inorganic compounds needed in relatively small amounts for regulation, growth, and maintenance of body tissues and functions.

TERMS

Eating for Healthy Bones

Osteoporosis is a condition in which the bones become dangerously thin and fragile over time. An estimated 10 million Americans over age 50 have osteoporosis, and another 34 million are at risk. Women account for about 80% of osteoporosis cases. Most bone mass is built by age 18. After bone density peaks between ages 25 and 35, bone mass is lost over time. To prevent osteoporosis, the best strategy is to build as much bone as possible during your youth and do everything you can to maintain it as you age. Up to 50% of bone loss is determined by controllable lifestyle factors. Key nutrients for bone health include the following:

- **Calcium.** Getting enough calcium is important throughout life to build and maintain bone mass. Milk, yogurt, and calcium-fortified orange juice, bread, and cereals are all good sources.

- **Vitamin D.** Vitamin D is necessary for bones to absorb calcium; a daily intake of 5 micrograms is recommended for adults age 19–50. Vitamin D can be obtained from foods and is manufactured by the skin when exposed to sunlight.

Candidates for vitamin D supplements include people who don't eat many foods rich in vitamin D; those who don't expose their face, arms, and hands to the sun (without sunscreen) for 5–15 minutes a few times each week; and people who live north of an imaginary line roughly between Boston and the Oregon–California border (where the sun is weaker).

- **Vitamin K.** Vitamin K promotes the synthesis of proteins that help keep bones strong. Broccoli and leafy green vegetables are rich in vitamin K.

- **Other nutrients.** Other nutrients that may play an important role in bone health include vitamin C, magnesium, potassium, phosphorus, fluoride, manganese, zinc, copper, and boron.

Several dietary substances that may have a *negative* effect on bone health, especially if consumed in excess: alcohol, sodium, caffeine, and retinol (a form of vitamin A).

In addition, weight-bearing aerobic exercise helps maintain bone mass throughout life, and strength training improves bone density, muscle mass, strength, and balance.

Characteristic symptoms develop if an essential mineral is consumed in a quantity too small or too large for good health. The minerals commonly lacking in the American diet are iron, calcium, potassium, and magnesium. Iron-deficiency **anemia** is a problem in many age groups, and researchers fear poor calcium intakes in childhood are sowing the seeds for future **osteoporosis**, especially in women (see the box "Eating for Healthy Bones").

Water—Vital but Often Ignored

Water is the major component in both foods and the human body: You are composed of about 50–60% water. Your need for other nutrients, in terms of weight, is much less than your need for water. You can live up to 50 days without food, but only a few days without water.

Water is distributed all over the body, among lean and other tissues and in blood and other body fluids. Water is used in the digestion and absorption of food and is the medium in which most of the chemical reactions take place within the body. Some water-based fluids, like blood, transport substances around the body, whereas other fluids serve as lubricants or cushions. Water also helps regulate body temperature.

Water is contained in almost all foods, particularly in liquids, fruits, and vegetables. The foods and fluids you consume provide 80–90% of your daily water intake; the remainder is generated through metabolism. You lose water each day in urine, feces, and sweat and through evaporation from your lungs.

Most people can maintain a healthy water balance by consuming beverages at meals and drinking fluids in response to thirst. The Food and Nutrition Board has set levels of adequate water intake to maintain hydration. All fluids, including those containing caffeine, can count toward your total daily fluid intake. Under these guidelines, men need about 3.7 total liters of water daily, with 3.0 liters (about 13 cups) coming from beverages; women need 2.7 total liters, with 2.2 liters (about 9 cups) coming from beverages. (See Table 1 in the Nutrition Resources section at the end of the chapter for information on specific age groups.) If you exercise vigorously or live in a hot climate, you need to consume additional fluids to maintain a balance between water consumed and water lost.

Other Substances in Food

Many substances in food are not essential nutrients but may influence health.

Antioxidants When the body uses oxygen or breaks down certain fats or proteins as a normal part of metabolism, it gives rise to substances called **free radicals.** Environmental factors such as cigarette smoke, exhaust fumes, radiation, excessive sunlight, certain drugs, and stress can increase free radical production. A free radical is a

anemia A deficiency in the oxygen-carrying material in the red blood cells.

osteoporosis A condition in which the bones become extremely thin and brittle and break easily.

free radical An electron-seeking compound that can react with fats, proteins, and DNA, damaging cell membranes and mutating genes in its search for electrons.

Berries are rich in antioxidants, vitamins, and dietary fiber.

chemically unstable molecule that reacts with fats, proteins, and DNA, damaging cell membranes and mutating genes. Free radicals have been implicated in aging, cancer, cardiovascular disease, and other degenerative diseases like arthritis.

Antioxidants found in foods can help protect the body from damage by free radicals in several ways. Some prevent or reduce the formation of free radicals; others remove free radicals from the body; still others repair some types of free radical damage after it occurs. Some antioxidants, such as vitamin C, vitamin E, and selenium, are also essential nutrients. Others—such as the carotenoids found in yellow, orange, and deep-green vegetables—are not. Some of the top antioxidant-containing foods and beverages include blackberries, walnuts, strawberries, artichokes, cranberries, brewed coffee, raspberries, pecans, blueberries, cloves, grape juice, unsweetened baking chocolate, sour cherries, and red wine. Also high in antioxidants are brussels sprouts, kale, cauliflower, and pomegranates.

Phytochemicals Antioxidants fall into the broader category of **phytochemicals,** substances found in plant foods that may help prevent chronic disease. In the past 20 years, researchers have begun to identify and study all the different compounds found in foods, and many findings are promising. For example, certain substances found in soy foods may help lower cholesterol levels. Sulforaphane, a compound isolated from broccoli and other **cruciferous vegetables,** may render some carcinogenic compounds harmless. Allyl sulfides, a group of chemicals found in garlic and onions, appear to boost the activity of cancer-fighting immune cells. Carotenoids found in green vegetables may help preserve eyesight with age.

If you want to increase your intake of phytochemicals, it is best to eat a variety of fruits, vegetables, and grains rather than relying on supplements. Like many vitamins and minerals, isolated phytochemicals may be harmful if taken in high doses. In addition, it is likely that their health benefits are the result of chemical substances working in combination.

NUTRITIONAL GUIDELINES: PLANNING YOUR DIET

Various tools have been created by scientific and government groups to help people design healthy diets. The **Dietary Reference Intakes (DRIs)** are standards for nutrient intake designed to prevent nutritional deficiencies and reduce the risk of chronic disease. **Dietary Guidelines for Americans** have been established to promote health and reduce the risk of major chronic diseases through diet and physical activity. **MyPyramid** provides daily food intake patterns that meet the DRIs and are consistent with the Dietary Guidelines for Americans.

Dietary Reference Intakes (DRIs)

The Food and Nutrition Board establishes dietary standards, or recommended intake levels, for Americans of all

phytochemical A naturally occurring substance found in plant foods that may help prevent and treat chronic diseases like cancer and heart disease; *phyto* means plant.

cruciferous vegetables Vegetables of the cabbage family, including cabbage, broccoli, brussels sprouts, kale, and cauliflower; the flower petals of these plants form the shape of a cross, hence the name.

Dietary Reference Intakes (DRIs) An umbrella term for four types of nutrient standards: Estimated Average Requirement (EAR), Adequate Intake (AI), Recommended Dietary Allowance (RDA), Tolerable Upper Intake Level (UL).

Dietary Guidelines for Americans Recommendations for good nutrition intended to help prevent certain diet-related diseases; issued by the US DHHS and USDA.

MyPyramid A food-group plan that provides practical advice to ensure a balanced intake of the essential nutrients.

Ask Yourself

QUESTIONS FOR CRITICAL THINKING AND REFLECTION

Experts say that two of the most important factors in a healthy diet are eating the "right" kinds of carbohydrates and eating the "right" kinds of fats. Based on what you've read so far in this chapter, which are the "right" carbohydrates and fats? How would you say your own diet stacks up when it comes to carbs and fats?

ages. The current set of standards, called Dietary Reference Intakes (DRIs), is relatively new, having been introduced in 1997. The DRIs are frequently reviewed and are updated as substantial new nutrition-related information becomes available. The DRIs present different categories of nutrients in easy-to-read table format. An earlier set of standards, called the Recommended Dietary Allowances (RDAs), focused on preventing nutritional deficiency diseases such as anemia. The DRIs have a broader focus because of research that looked not just at the prevention of nutrient deficiencies but also at the role of nutrients in promoting health and preventing chronic diseases.

The DRIs include standards for both recommended intakes and maximum safe intakes. The recommended intake of each nutrient is expressed as either *Recommended Dietary Allowance (RDA)* or *Adequate Intake (AI)*. An AI is set when there is not enough information available to set an RDA value; regardless of the type of standard used, however, the DRI represents the best available estimate of intake for optimal health. The *Tolerable Upper Intake Level (UL)* is the maximum daily intake that is unlikely to cause health problems in a healthy person.

Because of lack of data, ULs have not been set for all nutrients. This does not mean that people can tolerate chronic intakes of these vitamins and minerals above recommended levels. Like all chemical agents, nutrients can produce adverse effects if intakes are excessive. There is no established benefit from consuming nutrients at levels above the RDA or AI. The DRIs can be found in the Nutrition Resources section at the end of the chapter.

Because the DRIs are too cumbersome to use as a basis for food labels, the U.S. Food and Drug Administration (FDA) uses another set of dietary standards, the **Daily Values.** The Daily Values are based on several different sets of guidelines and include standards for fat, cholesterol, carbohydrate, dietary fiber, and selected vitamins and minerals. The Daily Values represent appropriate intake levels for a 2000-calorie diet. The percent Daily Value shown on a food label shows how well that food contributes to your recommended daily intake.

Dietary Guidelines for Americans

To provide general guidance for choosing a healthy diet, the U.S. Department of Agriculture (USDA) and the U.S. Department of Health and Human Services (DHHS) issue Dietary Guidelines for Americans, revising them every 5 years. These guidelines are intended for all healthy Americans, including children age 2 and older. Following these guidelines promotes health and reduces risk for chronic disease, including heart disease, cancer, diabetes, stroke, osteoporosis, and obesity. Each of the guidelines is supported by an extensive review of scientific and medical evidence.

Although the official 2010 Dietary Guidelines were not released until the end of 2010, the Dietary Guidelines Advisory Committee issued its recommendations for updates to the 2005 guidelines in June 2010 and invited public comment. The advisory committee notes that the report is different from previous guidelines in the following ways:

- It addresses an American population of whom two-thirds are overweight or obese and yet undernourished in several key nutrients.
- It focuses on the total diet and how to integrate the recommendations into a practical eating pattern that is nutrient dense and calorie balanced.
- It includes findings on the broad environmental and societal aspects of the American diet—that is, the "food environment."

The report points out the large disconnect between the recommendations and the actual American diet, which includes too few vegetables, fruits, high-fiber whole grains, low-fat milk and milk products, and seafood and too much added sugar, solid fat, refined grain, and sodium. Several dietary patterns from around the world can help Americans meet the recommendations, including the DASH-style pattern, the Mediterranean-style pattern, and the USDA Food Pattern.

General Guidelines

Overall recommendations to Americans include the following:

- Reduce overweight and obesity by reducing calorie intake and increasing physical activity.
- Shift food intake patterns to a more plant-based diet that emphasizes vegetables, cooked dry beans and peas, fruits, whole grains, nuts, and seeds; increase the intake of seafood and fat-free and low-fat milk and milk products; consume only moderate amounts of lean mean, poultry, and eggs.
- Significantly reduce intake of foods with solid fats and added sugars ("SoFAS"); reduce sodium intake, and lower intake of refined grains, especially those that are coupled with added sugar, solid fat, and sodium.
- Meet the 2008 Physical Activity Guidelines for Americans.

The report acknowledges the barriers that make it difficult for Americans to reach these goals, and it calls for a coordinated strategic plan that includes all sectors of society, from families to food producers and restaurants to policy makers. According to the report, adopting such a plan will go a long way toward reducing health disparities among racial and ethnic minorities and among different socioeconomic groups. The report also calls for a focus on children, because obesity begins in childhood.

The advisory committee report makes specific recommendations in eight topic areas, as described in the following sections.

Energy Balance and Weight Management

The obesity epidemic is fueled by the overconsumption of total calories and especially of energy-dense (high-calorie), nutrient-poor foods and beverages, along with very low levels of physical activity and too much sedentary time. Americans get too many of their calories from foods high in solid fats and added sugars that offer few or no nutrients. Other behaviors that promote weight gain are eating out frequently (especially at fast-food restaurants) and consuming large portions. In addition to increased physical activity, the report recommends self-monitoring and mindful eating, so that people can become more conscious of what, when, and how much they eat.

Nutrient Adequacy

Energy-dense foods should be replaced with nutrient-dense foods—that is, high-calorie, low-nutrient foods should be replaced with low-calorie, high-nutrient foods—to increase intakes of nutrients lacking in the American diet, especially vitamin D, calcium, potassium, and dietary fiber. Women of reproductive age should consume foods rich in folate and iron, and older adults should make sure they get enough vitamin B-12. A daily multivitamin/mineral supplement is not recommended for healthy Americans, although some population groups can benefit from supplements.

Fatty Acids and Cholesterol

To reduce the risk and incidence of cardiovascular disease (CVD) and type 2 diabetes, Americans are advised to limit intake of saturated fatty acids to less than 7% of total calories, cholesterol to less than 300 milligrams per day (200 mg for people at high risk for CVD or diabetes), and trans fatty acids from natural sources to less than 0.5% of calories. Trans fatty acids from hydrogenation should be avoided (see the box "Reducing Your Trans Fat Intake"). The report recommends that people consume two servings of seafood per week for their heart-healthy omega-3 fatty acids, favoring fish such as salmon, mackerel, and trout.

Protein

The highest-quality proteins come from animal sources, including meat, poultry, seafood, milk, and eggs. Plant proteins can form complete proteins if legumes and grains are combined. Well-planned plant-based diets can meet protein requirements.

Carbohydrates

Carbohydrates are the primary energy source for active people. Sedentary people should decrease consumption of energy-dense carbohydrates to balance energy needs and maintain ideal weight. Carbohydrate staples in the diet should be whole grains, vegetables, fruits, and cooked dry beans, along with fat-free and low-fat milk and milk products. Carbohydrate sources that should be avoided include sugar-sweetened beverages and desserts, including grain-based desserts (cake, pie, pastries, etc.). Consumers should watch out for the extra calories from sugar in specialty coffee drinks, sports drinks, and regular soda.

Sodium and Potassium

Americans currently consume too much sodium and not enough potassium, contributing to high rates of hypertension and heart disease. In 2005, the Dietary Guidelines recommended a daily sodium intake of less than 2300 milligrams for the general adult population and 1500 milligrams for people with hypertension, African Americans, and middle-aged and older adults. Because these three groups now comprise 70% of American adults, the 2010 report recommends a limit of 1500 milligrams for the entire general population. Given the current excessive intake of sodium, the report advises that this reduction occur over time to allow for adjustments in taste perception.

Food manufacturers should gradually lower the sodium content of their products, and consumers should check food labels, lower their intake of processed and prepared foods, and limit their use of high-sodium condiments like soy sauce, ketchup, mustard, pickles, and olives.

Individuals should also increase their consumption of dietary potassium, which helps lower blood pressure. Potassium-rich foods include leafy green vegetables, potatoes, bananas, tomato sauce, and orange juice.

Alcohol

For middle-aged and older adults, an average daily intake of one or two alcoholic beverages is associated

Reducing Your Trans Fat Intake

In 2004, the Center for Science in the Public Interest petitioned the FDA to ban trans fat as a food ingredient. That same year, restaurants in Tiburon, CA, voluntarily stopped using cooking oils containing trans fat. The grassroots effort in Tiburon served as a model for regulations around the United States, leading New York City, Philadelphia, and numerous other cities to enact similar laws restricting the amount of trans fat served in restaurant food. In 2010, California began banning the use of trans fats in restaurants and in the preparation of food for retail sale. On the international level, Denmark has made it illegal for any food to contain more than 2% trans fat, and Canada is considering a nationwide ban on trans fat in restaurant food.

What Are Trans Fats?

Trans fats are unsaturated fatty acids that have a physical structure more like a saturated fatty acid. Although small amounts of trans fat occur naturally in some meat and dairy products, most trans fats are formed through hydrogenation, the industrial process of converting liquid oils into solid or semisolid fats, like margarine and shortening. Partially hydrogenated oils have a longer shelf life and physical properties that make them desirable for use in baked goods. They also have a longer fry life and are more cost effective for deep fat frying than nonhydrogenated oils.

The use of partially hydrogenated oils grew throughout the 1960s, 1970s, and 1980s in response to public health recommendations to reduce saturated fat intake from animal fats and tropical oils (such as palm and coconut oil). In the 1990s, however, studies began to show that trans fats affect the body in some of the same ways as saturated fats. Further research found that trans fats are actually worse than saturated fats because they raise LDL ("bad") cholesterol while lowering HDL ("good") cholesterol. A recent study found that a 2% increase in dietary intake from trans fat was associated with a 23% increase in heart disease. Trans fats also increase the risk for type 2 diabetes.

Can We Eliminate Trans Fats from Our Diet?

Trans fats are not an essential part of our diet. In fact, health organizations recommend that trans fat intake be as low as possible. For example, the American Heart Association recommends limiting trans fat intake to less than 1% of your daily calories, and the report of the 2010 Dietary Guidelines Advisory Committee recommends limiting intake to less than 0.5% of daily calories, only from natural sources.

Luckily, more and more products in the grocery store are available in trans fat-free form, and as consumer interest in trans fat-free food in restaurants grows, it will get easier to limit trans fat when eating out. According to the Center for Science in the Public Interest, the amount of trans fat added to our food has declined by more than 50% since 2005.

Reducing Your Trans Fat Intake

Because some trans fats occur naturally, it's important to avoid partially hydrogenated oils, which are still abundant in many restaurant items and prepared and packaged foods. Get in the habit of reading food labels, which list trans fat. A product is allowed to contain up to 0.5 gram of trans fat and still list 0 on the label and claim to be "trans fat free," so check the ingredient list for partially hydrogenated oil. Also check the calories—if a food is trans fat free but has more calories from saturated fat or added sugars, it's not a healthy choice. As part of the 2010 health care reform legislation, national chain restaurants were required to provide information about calorie content of their foods, and this will also help consumers make smart choices.

SOURCES: Mozaffarian, D., et al. 2006. Trans fatty acids and cardiovascular disease. *New England Journal of Medicine* 354(15): 1601–1613; Eckel, R. H., et al. 2006. Understanding the complexity of trans fatty acid reduction in the American diet. American Heart Association Trans Fat Conference 2006. Report of the Trans Fat Conference Planning Group. *Circulation* 115(16): 2231–2246; American Heart Association. 2009. *Trans Fats* (http://www.americanheart.org/presenter.jhtml?identifier=3045792; retrieved November 5, 2010); Center for Science in the Public Interest. 2010. *Trans Fat* (http://www.cspinet.org/transfat; retrieved November 5, 2010); U.S. Food and Drug Administration. 2010. *Trans Fat Now Listed with Saturated Fat and Cholesterol on the Nutrition Facts Label* (http://www.fda.gov/Food/LabelingNutrition/Consumer Information/ucm109832.thm; retrieved November 5, 2010).

with the lowest all-cause mortality and a low risk of diabetes and coronary heart disease. Despite this benefit, the Dietary Guidelines Advisory Committee recommends that alcohol be consumed only in moderation and only by adults. Moderation means, for women, up to one drink per day and no more than three drinks in a single day and, for men, up to two drinks per day and no more than four drinks in a single day. Among younger people, alcohol provides little if any health benefit, and heavy drinking is associated with heart problems, stroke, liver disease, violence, and injuries and death. Alcohol supplies 7 calories per gram but no nutrients.

Food Safety and Technology According to the report, food safety concerns have escalated since the 2005 Dietary Guidelines were released, with numerous recalls of contaminated foods and widespread cases of foodborne illness. Consumers have to take more responsibility for carrying out safe food practices at home, and the food industry has to ensure a safe food supply for the nation.

The report asserts that the health benefits of consuming a variety of cooked seafood outweigh the risks associated with exposure to methyl mercury and persistent organic pollutants, as long as the types and sources of seafood to be avoided are clearly communicated to consumers. Local

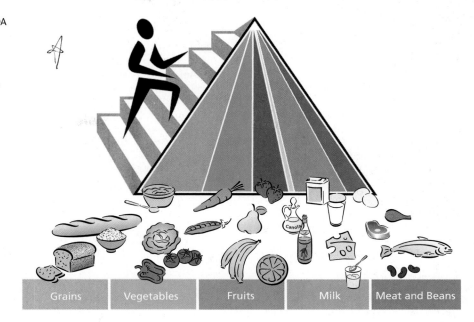

FIGURE 9.2 USDA's MyPyramid. The USDA food guidance system, called MyPyramid, can be personalized based on several factors. Visit MyPyramid.gov to obtain a food plan appropriate for you. MyPyramid contains five main food groups plus oils (yellow band). Key consumer messages include the following:
- Grains: Make half your grains whole
- Vegetables: Vary your veggies
- Fruits: Focus on fruits
- Oils: Know your fats
- Milk: Get your calcium-rich foods
- Meat and Beans: Go lean with protein

SOURCE: U.S. Department of Agriculture. 2005. *MyPyramid* (http://www.mypyramid.gov; retrieved November 5, 2010).

Grains | Vegetables | Fruits | Milk | Meat and Beans

and federal advisories should be followed, particularly by pregnant women, nursing mothers, and children 12 and younger.

Food safety and guidelines for fish consumption are covered in detail later in this chapter.

USDA's MyPyramid

Many Americans are familiar with the USDA Food Guide Pyramid, the food guidance system that was first released in 1992. Since the initial release of the Pyramid, scientists have updated both nutrient recommendations (the DRIs) and the Dietary Guidelines for Americans. The USDA also reassessed its overall food guidance system and released MyPyramid in April 2005 (Figure 9.2). For updates to MyPyramid made in 2010 and later, visit www.MyPyramid.gov.

A variety of experts have proposed other food-group plans. Some of these address perceived shortcomings in the USDA plans, and some adapt the basic 1992 Pyramid to special populations. The USDA Center for Nutrition Policy and Promotion (www.usda.gov/cnpp) has more on alternative food plans for special populations such as young children, older adults, and people choosing particular ethnic diets. MyPyramid is available in Spanish, and there are special adaptations of MyPyramid for preschoolers age 2–5, children age 6–11, pregnant women, and breastfeeding women (www.MyPyramid.gov).

Besides MyPyramid, two other dietary patterns are recommended in the report of the 2010 Dietary Guidelines Advisory Committee—the DASH-style pattern and the Mediterranean-style pattern. The DASH (Dietary Approaches to Stop Hypertension) diet, developed for people with high blood pressure, is a low-sodium diet that emphasizes whole grains; fruits and vegetables; low-fat and nonfat dairy products; lean meats, fish, and poultry; and nuts, seeds, and legumes. The Mediterranean-style diet also emphasizes whole grains, fruits, and vegetables, along with daily servings of beans, legumes, and nuts; moderate consumption of fish, poultry, and dairy products; and the use of olive oil over other types of fat, especially saturated fat. The Mediterranean diet has been associated with lower rates of heart disease and cancer and a reduced risk of Alzheimer's disease.

Key Messages of MyPyramid MyPyramid is designed to remind consumers to make healthy food choices and to be active every day. Key messages include the following:

- *Personalization* is represented by the person on the steps and the MyPyramid.gov site, which includes individualized recommendations, interactive assessments of food intake and physical activity, and tips.
- *Daily physical activity,* represented by the person climbing the steps, is important for maintaining a healthy weight and reducing the risk of chronic disease.
- *Moderation* of food intake is represented by the narrowing of each food group from bottom to top.
- *Proportionality* is represented by the different widths of the food group bands.
- *Variety* is represented by the six color bands; foods from all groups are needed daily for good health.
- *Gradual improvement* is a good strategy; people can benefit from taking small steps each day.

The MyPyramid chart in Figure 9.3 shows the food intake patterns recommended for different levels of calorie

Daily Amount of Food from Each Group

Food group amounts shown in cups (c) or ounce-equivalents (oz-eq), with number of daily servings (srv) shown in parentheses; vegetable subgroup amounts are per week

Calorie level	1600	1800	2000	2200	2400	2600	2800	3000
Grains	5 oz-eq	6 oz-eq	6 oz-eq	7 oz-eq	8 oz-eq	9 oz-eq	10 oz-eq	10 oz-eq
Whole grains	3 oz-eq	3 oz-eq	3 oz-eq	3.5 oz-eq	4 oz-eq	4.5 oz-eq	5 oz-eq	5 oz-eq
Other grains	2 oz-eq	3 oz-eq	3 oz-eq	3.5 oz-eq	4 oz-eq	4.5 oz-eq	5 oz-eq	5 oz-eq
Vegetables	2 c (4 srv)	2.5 c (5 srv)	2.5 c (5 srv)	3 c (6 srv)	3 c (6 srv)	3.5 c (7 srv)	3.5 c (7 srv)	4 c (8 srv)
Dark green	2 c/wk	3 c/wk	3 c/wk	3 c/wk	3 c/wk	3 c/wk	3 c/wk	3 c/wk
Orange	1.5 c/wk	2 c/wk	2 c/wk	2 c/wk	2 c/wk	2.5 c/wk	2.5 c/wk	2.5 c/wk
Legumes	2.5 c/wk	3 c/wk	3 c/wk	3 c/wk	3 c/wk	3.5 c/wk	3.5 c/wk	3.5 c/wk
Starchy	2.5 c/wk	3 c/wk	3 c/wk	6 c/wk	6 c/wk	7 c/wk	7 c/wk	9 c/wk
Other	5.5 c/wk	6.5 c/wk	6.5 c/wk	7 c/wk	7 c/wk	8.5 c/wk	8.5 c/wk	10 c/wk
Fruits	1.5 c (3 srv)	1.5 c (3 srv)	2 c (4 srv)	2 c (4 srv)	2 c (4 srv)	2 c (4 srv)	2.5 c (5 srv)	2.5 c (5 srv)
Milk	3 c	3 c	3 c	3 c	3 c	3 c	3 c	3 c
Lean meat and beans	5 oz-eq	5 oz-eq	5.5 oz-eq	6 oz-eq	6.5 oz-eq	6.5 oz-eq	7 oz-eq	7 oz-eq
Oils	5 tsp	5 tsp	6 tsp	6 tsp	7 tsp	8 tsp	8 tsp	10 tsp

The discretionary calorie allowances shown below are the calories remaining at each level after nutrient-dense foods in each food group are selected. Those trying to lose weight may choose not to use discretionary calories. For those wanting to maintain weight, discretionary calories may be used to increase the amount of food from each food group; to consume foods that are not in the lowest fat form or that contain added sugars; to add oil, fat, or sugars to foods; or to consume alcohol. The amounts below show how discretionary calories may be divided between solid fats and added sugars.

Discretionary calories	132	195	267	290	362	410	426	512
Solid fats	11 g	15 g	18 g	19 g	22 g	24 g	24 g	29 g
Added sugars	12 g (3 tsp)	20 g (5 tsp)	32 g (8 tsp)	38 g (9 tsp)	48 g (12 tsp)	56 g (14 tsp)	60 g (15 tsp)	72 g (18 tsp)

FIGURE 9.3 MyPyramid food intake patterns. To determine an appropriate amount of food from each group, find the column with your approximate daily energy intake. That column lists the daily recommended intake from each food group. Visit MyPyramid.gov for a personalized intake plan and for intakes for other calorie levels.

SOURCE: U.S. Department of Agriculture. 2005. *MyPyramid Food Intake Patterns* (www.mypyramid.gov; retrieved November 5, 2010).

intake. Table 9.4 provides guidance for determining an appropriate calorie intake for weight maintenance. Use the table to identify an energy intake that is about right for you. Then refer to the appropriate column in Figure 9.3. A personalized version of MyPyramid recommendations can also be found at www.MyPyramid.gov. Each food group is described briefly in the following sections. Past experiences have shown that many Americans have trouble identifying serving sizes, so recommended daily intakes are given in terms of cups and ounces (see the box "Judging Portion Sizes").

Grains Foods from this group are usually low in fat and rich in complex carbohydrates, dietary fiber (if grains are unrefined), and vitamins and minerals, including thiamin, riboflavin, iron, niacin, folic acid (if enriched or fortified), and zinc. Someone eating 2000 calories a day should include 6 ounce-equivalents each day, with half of

Judging Portion Sizes

Studies have shown that most people underestimate the size of their food portions, in many cases by as much as 50%. If you need to retrain your eye, try using measuring cups and spoons and an inexpensive kitchen scale when you eat at home. For quick estimates, use the following equivalents:

- 1 teaspoon of margarine = the tip of your thumb
- 1 ounce of cheese = your thumb, four dice stacked together, or an ice cube
- 3 ounces of chicken or meat = a deck of cards
- 1 cup of pasta = a small fist or a tennis ball

- ½ cup of rice or cooked vegetables = an ice cream scoop or one-third of a can of soda
- 2 tablespoons of peanut butter = a ping-pong ball or large marshmallow
- 1 medium potato = a computer mouse
- 2-ounce muffin or roll = a plum or a large egg
- 2-ounce bagel = a hockey puck or a yo-yo
- 1 medium fruit (apple or orange) = a baseball
- ¼ cup nuts = a golf ball
- Small cookie or cracker = a poker chip

those servings from whole grains such as whole-grain bread. The following items count as 1 ounce-equivalent:

- 1 slice of bread
- 1 small (2½-inch diameter) muffin
- 1 cup ready-to-eat cereal flakes

- ½ cup cooked cereal, rice, grains, or pasta
- 1 6-inch tortilla

Choose foods that are typically made with little fat or sugar (bread, rice, pasta) over those that are high in fat and sugar (croissants, chips, cookies, doughnuts).

Vegetables   Vegetables contain carbohydrates, dietary fiber, carotenoids, vitamin C, folate, potassium, and other nutrients. They are also naturally low in fat. In a 2000-calorie diet, 2½ cups (5 servings) of vegetables should be included daily. Each of the following counts as 1 serving (½ cup or equivalent) of vegetables:

- ½ cup raw or cooked vegetables
- 1 cup raw leafy salad greens
- ½ cup vegetable juice

Because vegetables vary in the nutrients they provide, it is important to consume a variety of vegetables. MyPyramid recommends that servings from five different subgroups be consumed each week (see Figure 9.3).

Only 14% of adult Americans eat the recommended amount of fruits and vegetables.

—CDC, 2009

QUICK STATS

Fruits   Fruits are rich in carbohydrates, dietary fiber, and many vitamins, especially vitamin C. For someone eating a 2000-calorie diet, 2 cups (4 servings) of fruits are recommended daily. Each of the following counts as 1 serving (½ cup or equivalent) of fruit:

- ½ cup fresh, canned, or frozen fruit
- ½ cup fruit juice (100% juice)
- 1 small whole fruit
- ¼ cup dried fruit

Table 9.4	MyPyramid Daily Calorie Intake Levels		
AGE (YEARS)	SEDENTARY[a]	MODERATELY ACTIVE[b]	ACTIVE[c]
Child			
2–3	1000	1000–1400	1000–1400
Female			
4–8	1200–1400	1400–1600	1400–1800
9–13	1400–1600	1600–2000	1800–2200
14–18	1800	2000	2400
19–30	1800–2000	2000–2200	2400
31–50	1800	2000	2200
51+	1600	1800	2000–2200
Male			
4–8	1200–1400	1400–1600	1600–2000
9–13	1600–2000	1800–2200	2000–2600
14–18	2000–2400	2400–2800	2800–3200
19–30	2400–2600	2600–2800	3000
31–50	2200–2400	2400–2600	2800–3000
51+	2000–2200	2200–2400	2400–2800

[a]A lifestyle that includes only the light physical activity associated with typical day-to-day life.
[b]A lifestyle that includes physical activity equivalent to walking about 1.5 to 3 miles per day at 3 to 4 miles per hour (30–60 minutes a day of moderate physical activity), in addition to the light physical activity associated with typical day-to-day life.
[c]A lifestyle that includes physical activity equivalent to walking more than 3 miles per day at 3 to 4 miles per hour (60 or more minutes a day of moderate physical activity), in addition to the light physical activity associated with typical day-to-day life.

SOURCE: U.S. Department of Agriculture. 2005. *MyPyramid Food Intake Pattern Calorie Levels* (http://www.mypyramid.gov; retrieved November 5, 2010).

Choose whole fruits often—they are higher in fiber and often lower in calories than fruit juices. Fruit *juices* typically contain more nutrients and less added sugar than fruit *drinks*. For canned fruits, choose those packed in 100% fruit juice or water rather than in syrup.

Milk   This group includes all milk and milk products, such as yogurt, cheeses (except cream cheese), and dairy desserts, as well as lactose-free and lactose-reduced products. Foods from this group are high in protein, carbohydrate, calcium, riboflavin, and vitamin D (if fortified). Those consuming 2000 calories per day should include 3 cups of milk or the equivalent daily. Each of the following counts as the equivalent of 1 cup:

- 1 cup milk or yogurt
- ½ cup ricotta cheese
- 1½ ounces natural cheese
- 2 ounces processed cheese

Cottage cheese is lower in calcium than most other cheeses; ½ cup is equivalent to ¼ cup milk. Ice cream is also lower in calcium and higher in sugar and fat than many other dairy products; one scoop counts as ⅓ cup milk. To limit calories and saturated fat in your diet, it is best to choose servings of low-fat and fat-free items from this group.

Meat and Beans   This group includes meat, poultry, fish, dry beans and peas, eggs, nuts, and seeds. These foods provide protein, niacin, iron, vitamin B-6, zinc, and thiamin. The animal foods in the group also provide vitamin B-12. A 2000-calorie diet should include 5½ ounce-equivalents daily. Each of the following counts as equivalent to 1 ounce:

- 1 ounce cooked lean meat, poultry, or fish
- ¼ cup cooked dry beans (legumes) or tofu
- 1 egg
- 1 tablespoon peanut butter
- ½ ounce nuts or seeds

Choose lean meat and skinless poultry, and watch your serving sizes carefully. Choose at least one serving of plant proteins, such as black beans, lentils, or tofu, every day.

Oils   This group includes oils that are added to foods during processing, cooking, or at the table. Oils and soft margarines include vegetable oils and soft vegetable oil table spreads that have no trans fats. These are major sources of vitamin E and unsaturated fatty acids, including the essential fatty acids. For a 2000-calorie diet, 6 teaspoons of oils per day are recommended. One teaspoon is the equivalent of the following:

- 1 teaspoon vegetable oil or soft margarine
- 1 tablespoon salad dressing or light mayonnaise

Foods that are mostly oils include nuts, olives, avocados, and some fish. The following portions include about 1 teaspoon of oil: 8 large olives, ⅙ medium avocado, ½ tablespoon peanut butter, and ⅓ ounce roasted nuts. Food labels can help you identify the type and amount of fat in various foods.

Discretionary Calories, Solid Fats, and Added Sugars
MyPyramid assumes that you choose nutrient-dense forms of foods from each food group. Nutrient-dense forms are those that are fat-free or low-fat and that contain no added sugars. If this pattern is followed, then a small amount of additional calories can be consumed—the *discretionary calorie allowance*. Figure 9.3 shows the discretionary calorie allowance at each calorie level in MyPyramid.

People who are trying to lose weight may choose not to use discretionary calories. For those wanting to maintain weight, discretionary calories may be used to increase the amount of food from a food group; to consume foods that are not in the lowest fat form or that contain added sugars; to add oil, fat, or sugars to foods; or to consume alcohol. The amounts shown in Figure 9.3 show how discretionary calories may be divided between solid fats and added sugars. The values for additional fat target no more than 30% of total calories from fat and less than 10% of calories from saturated fat. Examples of discretionary solid fat calories include choosing higher-fat meats such as sausages, or chicken with skin, or whole milk instead of fat-free milk and topping foods with butter. For example, a cup of whole milk has 60 calories more than a cup of fat-free milk; these 60 calories would be counted as discretionary calories.

The suggested amounts of added sugars may be helpful limits for including some sweetened foods or beverages in the daily diet without exceeding energy needs or underconsuming other nutrients. For example, in a 2000-calorie diet, MyPyramid suggests 32 grams (8 teaspoons) for discretionary intake of added sugars. In the American diet, added sugars are often found in sweetened beverages, dairy products, and refined grain products. For example, a 20-ounce regular soda has 260 calories from added sugars that would be counted as discretionary calories. The current American diet includes higher-than-recommended levels of sugar intake.

The Vegetarian Alternative

Vegetarians choose a diet in which foods of animal origin (meat, poultry, fish, eggs, milk) are eliminated or restricted. Many vegetarians follow their diet for health reasons, because vegetarian diets tend to be lower in saturated fat, cholesterol, and animal protein and higher in complex carbohydrates, dietary fiber, folate, vitamins C and E, carotenoids, and phytochemicals. Some people adopt a vegetarian diet out of concern for the environment, for financial considerations, or for reasons related to ethics or religion.

How Different Are the Nutritional Needs of Women and Men?

When it comes to nutrition, men and women have a lot in common. Both sexes need the same essential nutrients, and the Dietary Guidelines for Americans apply equally to both. But beyond the basics, men and women need different amounts of essential nutrients and have different nutritional concerns.

Women tend to be smaller and weigh less than men and thus have lower energy requirements and need to consume fewer calories than men to maintain a healthy weight. For most nutrients, women need the same or slightly lower amounts than men. But because women consume fewer calories, they may have more difficulty getting adequate amounts of all essential nutrients and need to focus on nutrient-dense foods.

Two nutrients of special concern to women are calcium and iron. Low calcium intake may be linked to the development of osteoporosis in later life. The *Healthy People 2010* report sets a goal of increasing from 40% to 75% the proportion of women age 20–49 who meet the dietary recommendation for calcium. Fat-free and low-fat dairy products and fortified cereal, bread, and orange juice are good choices for calcium-rich foods.

Menstruating women also have higher iron needs than other groups, and low iron intake can lead to iron-deficiency anemia. Lean red meat, green leafy vegetables, and fortified breakfast cereals are good sources of iron. All women capable of becoming pregnant should consume adequate folic acid from fortified foods and/or supplements.

Men are seldom thought of as having nutritional deficiencies because they generally have high-calorie diets. However, many men have a diet that does not follow recommended food intake patterns and includes more red meat and fewer fruits, vegetables, and whole grains than recommended. This dietary pattern is linked to heart disease and some types of cancer. A high intake of calories can lead to weight gain over time if a man's activity level decreases as he ages. To reduce chronic disease risk, men should focus on increasing their consumption of fruits, vegetables, and whole grains to obtain vitamins, minerals, fiber, and phytochemicals.

The "Fruits & Veggies—More Matters" initiative (www.fruitsandveggies-morematters.org) is the result of a

partnership of health organizations led by the CDC and the Produce for Better Health Foundation. The goal is to increase consumption of fruits and vegetables. Information found in stores, online, and on packaging will help both men and women make healthful choices.

Types of Vegetarian Diets   There are various vegetarian styles; the wider the variety of the diet eaten, the easier it is to meet nutritional needs. *Vegans* eat only plant foods. *Lacto-vegetarians* eat plant foods and dairy products. *Lacto-ovo-vegetarians* eat plant foods, dairy products, and eggs. Others can be categorized as partial vegetarians, semivegetarians, or pescovegetarians. These individuals eat plant foods, dairy products, eggs, and usually a small selection of poultry, fish, and other seafood.

A Food Plan for Vegetarians   MyPyramid can be adapted for use by vegetarians with only a few key modifications. For the meat and beans group, vegetarians can focus on the nonmeat choices of dry beans, nuts, seeds, eggs, and soy foods like tofu. Vegans and other vegetarians who do not consume any dairy products must find other sources of calcium. Fruits, vegetables, and whole grains are healthy choices for people following all types of vegetarian diets.

A healthy vegetarian diet emphasizes a wide variety of plant foods. Although plant proteins are generally of lower quality than animal proteins, choosing a variety of plant foods will supply all of the essential amino acids. Choosing minimally processed and unrefined foods will maximize nutrient value and provide ample dietary fiber. Daily consumption of a variety of plant foods in amounts that meet total energy needs can provide all needed nutrients, except vitamin B-12 and possibly vitamin D.

Dietary Challenges for Special Population Groups

The Dietary Guidelines for Americans and MyPyramid can help nearly everyone to create a healthy diet. However, some population groups face special dietary challenges (see the box "How Different Are the Nutritional Needs of Women and Men?").

Children and Teenagers   Perhaps the best thing a parent can do for younger children is to provide them with a variety of foods. Allowing children to help prepare meals

Eating Strategies for College Students

In General

- Eat a colorful, varied diet. The more colorful your diet is, the more varied and rich in fruits and vegetables it will be. Fruits and vegetables are typically inexpensive, delicious, and low in fat and calories.

- Eat breakfast. You'll have more energy in the morning and be less likely to grab an unhealthy snack later on.

- Choose healthy snacks—fruits, vegetables, whole grains, and cereals.

- Drink water, nonfat milk, or 100% fruit juice more often than soft drinks or other sweetened beverages.

- Pay attention to portion sizes.

- Combine physical activity with healthy eating.

Eating in the Dining Hall

- Choose a meal plan that includes breakfast.

- Decide what you want to eat before you get in line, and stick to your choices.

- Build your meals around grains and vegetables.

- Choose leaner poultry, fish, or bean dishes rather than high-fat meats and fried entrees.

- Ask that gravies and sauces be served on the side.

- Choose broth-based or vegetable soups, not cream soups.

- At the salad bar, load up on leafy greens, beans, and fresh vegetables. Avoid mayonnaise-coated salads, bacon, croutons, and high-fat dressings. Put dressing on the side, and dip your fork into it rather than pouring it over the salad.

- Choose fruit for dessert rather than pastries or cookies.

Eating in Fast-Food Restaurants

- Look for the calorie content of items on the menu and select lower-calorie items when you can.

- Order small single burgers with no cheese instead of double burgers with many toppings.

- Ask for items to be prepared without mayonnaise, tartar sauce, sour cream, or other high-fat sauces. Ketchup, mustard, and fat-free mayonnaise or sour cream are better choices and are available at many fast-food restaurants.

- Choose whole-grain bread for burgers and sandwiches.

- Choose chicken items made from chicken breast, not processed chicken.

- Order vegetable pizzas without extra cheese.

- Get fruit or a salad as a side dish.

- If you order french fries or onion rings, get the smallest size and/or share them with a friend. Better yet, get a salad or fruit cup instead.

Eating on the Run

- Carry healthy snacks in your backpack or a small insulated lunch sack (with a frozen gel pack).

- Include fresh fruits or veggies, snack-size cereal bars, small whole-wheat bagels, pretzels, rice cakes, popcorn, or water.

---

is another good way to increase variety and develop a child's interest in eating well. Many children and teenagers enjoy eating at fast-food restaurants; they should be encouraged to select the healthiest choices and balance the day's diet with low-fat, nutrient-rich foods.

College Students   Convenient foods are not always the healthiest choices. Students who eat in buffet-style dining halls or food courts can easily overeat, and the foods offered are not necessarily high in nutrients and low in fat. The same is true of meals at fast-food restaurants. See the box "Eating Strategies for College Students" for tips on healthy, inexpensive choices.

Older Adults   Nutrient needs do not change much as people age, but because older adults tend to become less active, they require fewer calories to maintain body weight. At the same time, the absorption of nutrients tends to be lower in older adults because of age-related changes in the digestive tract. Thus, they must consume nutrient-dense foods in order to meet their nutritional

requirements. Foods fortified with vitamin B-12 and/or B-12 supplements are recommended for people over age 50. Because constipation is a common problem, consuming foods high in fiber and getting adequate fluids are important goals.

Athletes   Key dietary concerns for athletes are meeting their increased energy requirements and drinking enough fluids during practice and throughout the day to remain fully hydrated. Endurance athletes may also benefit from increasing the amount of carbohydrate in the diet to 60–70% of total daily calories; this increase should come in the form of complex, rather than simple, carbohydrates. Athletes for whom maintaining low body weight and body fat is important—such as skaters, gymnasts, and wrestlers—should consume adequate nutrients and avoid falling into unhealthy patterns of eating.

People with Special Health Concerns   Many Americans have special health concerns that affect their dietary needs. For example, women who are pregnant or breast-feeding require extra calories, vitamins, and minerals. People with diabetes benefit from a well-balanced diet that is low in simple sugars, high in complex carbohydrates, and rich in monounsaturated fats. People with high blood pressure need to control their weight and limit their sodium consumption. If you have a health concern that may require a special diet, discuss your situation with a physician or registered dietitian.

A PERSONAL PLAN: MAKING INFORMED CHOICES ABOUT FOOD

Understanding the basics of good nutrition should get you started on creating a diet that works for you. But eating well involves other skills too, including knowing how to read food labels and dietary supplement labels, knowing how to handle and prepare food safely, and understanding food industry practices so you can make informed choices about what you ingest.

Reading Food Labels

All processed foods regulated by either the FDA or the USDA include standardized nutrition information on their labels. Every food label shows serving sizes and the amount of fat, saturated fat, trans fat, cholesterol, sodium, total carbohydrate, dietary fiber, sugars, and protein in each serving. To make intelligent choices about food, learn to read and *understand* food labels (see the box "Using Food Labels").

Dietary Supplements

The aim of the Dietary Reference Intakes (DRIs) is to guide you in meeting your nutritional needs primarily with food, rather than with vitamin and mineral supplements. Supplements lack the fiber and potentially beneficial phytochemicals that are found only in whole foods. Most Americans can get the vitamins and minerals they need by eating a nutritionally balanced diet of various foods. The use of supplements to reduce heart disease or cancer risk remains controversial, so experts suggest that you avoid taking any nutrient at a level exceeding the Tolerable Upper Intake Level (UL).

The question of whether to take supplements is a serious one. Some vitamins and minerals are dangerous when taken in excess. Large doses of particular nutrients can also cause health problems by affecting the absorption of certain vitamins or minerals. For this reason, ask your doctor or a dietitian before taking any high-dose supplement.

People Who Benefit from Supplements In setting the DRIs, the Food and Nutrition Board recommended supplements of particular nutrients for specific groups:

- Women who are capable of getting pregnant should get 400 μg per day of folic acid (the synthetic form

of the vitamin folate) from fortified foods and/or supplements in addition to folate from a varied diet. This level of folate can reduce the risk of neural tube defects in a developing fetus. Enriched breads, flours, cornmeal, rice, noodles, and other grain products are fortified with folic acid. Folate is found naturally in leafy green vegetables, legumes, oranges, and strawberries.

- People over age 50 should eat foods fortified with vitamin B-12, take a B-12 supplement, or combine the two to meet the RDA of 2.4 μg daily. Up to 30% of people over 50 may have trouble absorbing protein-bound B-12 in foods.

- Because of the oxidative stress caused by smoking, smokers should get 35 mg more vitamin C per day than the RDA set for their age and sex. Supplements aren't usually necessary, however, because this extra vitamin C can easily be found in foods. For example, an 8-ounce glass of orange juice has about 100 mg of vitamin C.

Supplements may be recommended in other cases. Women with heavy menstrual flows, for example, may need extra iron. Older adults, people with dark skin, and people exposed to little sunlight may need extra vitamin D. Some vegetarians may need supplemental calcium, iron, zinc, and B-12, depending on their food choices. Other people may benefit from supplementation based on their physical condition, the medicines they take, or their dietary habits.

Before deciding whether to take a vitamin or mineral supplement, consider whether you already eat a fortified breakfast cereal every day. Many breakfast cereals contain almost as many nutrients as a multivitamin pill. If you elect to take a supplement, choose one that contains 50–100% of the Daily Value for vitamins and minerals. Avoid supplements containing large doses of particular nutrients.

Reading Supplement Labels Dietary supplements include vitamins, minerals, amino acids, herbs, glandular extracts, enzymes, and other compounds. They are available as tablets, capsules, liquids, and powders. Although dietary supplements are often thought to be safe and "natural," they contain powerful bioactive chemicals that have the potential for harm. About one-quarter of all pharmaceutical drugs are derived from botanical sources— morphine from poppies and digoxin from foxglove, for example. And, as described earlier, even essential vitamins and minerals can have toxic effects if consumed in excess.

In the United States, supplements are not legally considered drugs and are not regulated the same way drugs are. Before a drug is approved by the FDA and put on the market, it must undergo clinical studies to determine safety, effectiveness, side effects and risks, possible interactions with other substances, and appropriate dosages.

Using Food Labels

Food labels are designed to help consumers make food choices based on the nutrients that are most important to good health. In addition to listing nutrient content by weight, the label puts the information in the context of a daily diet of 2000 calories that includes no more than 65 grams of fat (approximately 30% of total calories). For example, if a serving of a particular product has 13 grams of fat, the label will show that the serving represents 20% of the daily fat allowance. If your daily diet contains fewer or more than 2000 calories, you need to adjust these calculations accordingly.

Food labels contain uniform serving sizes. This means that if you look at different brands of salad dressing, for example, you can compare calories and fat content based on the serving amount. (Food label serving sizes may be larger or smaller than MyPyramid serving size equivalents, however.) Regulations also require that foods meet strict definitions if their packaging includes the terms *light, low-fat,* or *high-fiber* (see below). Health claims such as "good source of dietary fiber" or "low in saturated fat" on packages are signals that those products can wisely be included in your diet. Overall, the food label is an important tool to help you choose a diet that conforms to MyPyramid and the Dietary Guidelines.

Selected Nutrient Claims and What They Mean

Healthy A food that is low in fat, is low in saturated fat, has no more than 360–480 mg of sodium and 60 mg of cholesterol, *and* provides 10% or more of the Daily Value for vitamin A, vitamin C, protein, calcium, iron, or dietary fiber.

Light or lite One-third fewer calories or 50% less fat than a similar product.

Reduced or fewer At least 25% less of a nutrient than a similar product; can be applied to fat ("reduced fat"), saturated fat, cholesterol, sodium, and calories.

Extra or added 10% or more of the Daily Value per serving when compared to what a similar product has.

Good source 10–19% of the Daily Value for a particular nutrient per serving.

High, rich in, or excellent source of 20% or more of the Daily Value for a particular nutrient per serving.

Low calorie 40 calories or less per serving.

High fiber 5 g or more of fiber per serving.

Good source of fiber 2.5–4.9 g of fiber per serving.

Fat-free Less than 0.5 g of fat per serving.

Low-fat 3 g of fat or less per serving.

Saturated fat-free Less than 0.5 g of saturated fat and 0.5 g of trans fatty acids per serving.

Low saturated fat 1 g or less of saturated fat per serving and no more than 15% of total calories.

Cholesterol-free Less than 2 mg of cholesterol and 2 g or less of saturated fat per serving.

Low cholesterol 20 mg or less of cholesterol and 2 g or less of saturated fat per serving.

Low sodium 140 mg or less of sodium per serving.

Very low sodium 35 mg or less of sodium per serving.

Lean Cooked seafood, meat, or poultry with less than 10 g of fat, 4.5 g or less of saturated fat, and less than 95 mg of cholesterol per serving.

Extra lean Cooked seafood, meat, or poultry with less than 5 g of fat, 2 g of saturated fat, and 95 mg of cholesterol per serving.

Note: The FDA has not yet defined nutrient claims relating to carbohydrates, so foods labeled low- or reduced-carbohydrate do not conform to any approved standard.

1. Serving size: Determine how many servings there are in the food package and compare it to how much you actually eat. You may need to adjust the rest of the nutrient values based on your typical serving size.

2. Calories and calories from fat: Note whether a serving is high in calories and fat. The sample food shown here is low in fat, with only 30 of its 235 calories from fat.

3. Daily Values: Based on a 2000-calorie diet, Daily Value percentages tell you whether the nutrients in a serving of food contribute a lot or a little to your total daily diet.
　　5% or less is low
　　20% or more is high

4. Limit these nutrients: Look for foods low in fat, saturated fat, trans fat, cholesterol, and sodium.

5. Get enough of these nutrients: Look for foods high in dietary fiber, vitamin A, vitamin C, calcium, and iron.

Nutrition Facts

Serving Size 1 cup (265g)
Servings per Container 2

Amount per Serving

Calories 235　Calories from Fat 30

	% Daily Value*
Total Fat 3g	5%
Saturated Fat 1g	5%
Trans Fat 0.5g	
Cholesterol 30mg	10%
Sodium 775mg	32%
Total Carbohydrate 34g	11%
Dietary Fiber 9g	36%
Sugars 5g	
Protein 18g	

Vitamin A 25%	•	Vitamin C 0%
Calcium 12%	•	Iron 20%

*Percent Daily Values are based on a 2,000 calorie diet. Your daily values may be higher or lower depending on your calorie needs:

	Calories	2,000	2,500
Total Fat	Less than	65g	80
Sat Fat	Less than	20g	25g
Cholesterol	Less than	300mg	300mg
Sodium	Less than	2,400mg	2,400mg
Total Carbohydrate		300g	375g
Dietary Fiber		25g	30g

Calories per gram:
Fat 9 • Carbohydrate 4 • Protein 4

Footnote: This section shows recommended daily intake for two levels of calorie consumption and values for dietary calculations; it's the same on all labels.

The FDA does not authorize or test dietary supplements, and supplements are not required to demonstrate either safety or effectiveness prior to marketing. Although dosage guidelines exist for some of the compounds in dietary supplements, dosages for many are not well established.

There are also key differences in how drugs and supplements are manufactured. FDA-approved medications are standardized for potency, and quality control and proof of purity are required. Dietary supplement manufacture is not as closely regulated, and there is no guarantee that a product even contains a given ingredient, let alone in the appropriate amount. The potency of herbal supplements tends to vary widely due to differences in growing and harvesting conditions, preparation methods, and storage. In addition, herbs can be contaminated or misidentified at any stage from harvest to packaging. To provide consumers with more reliable and consistent information about supplements, the FDA requires supplements to have labels similar to those found on foods (see the box "Using Dietary Supplement Labels").

Protecting Yourself Against Foodborne Illness

Many people worry about additives or pesticide residues in their food, but a greater threat comes from microorganisms that cause foodborne illnesses. Raw or undercooked animal products, such as chicken, hamburger, and oysters, pose the greatest threat, although in recent years contaminated fruits and vegetables have been catching up.

Symptoms of foodborne illness include diarrhea, vomiting, fever, pain, headache, and weakness. Although the effects of foodborne illnesses are usually not serious, some groups, such as children, pregnant women, and the elderly, are more at risk for severe complications.

Most cases of foodborne illness are caused by pathogens, disease-causing microorganisms. The most common contaminants are *Campylobacter jejuni* (found in contaminated water, raw milk, and raw or undercooked poultry, meat, or shellfish); *Salmonella* bacteria (found in raw or undercooked eggs, poultry, and meat; milk and dairy products; seafood; fruits and vegetables, including sprouts; and inadequately refrigerated and reheated leftovers); *Shigella* bacteria (found in the human intestinal tract and usually transmitted via fecal contamination of food and water); *Escherichia coli* bacteria (found in the intestinal tracts of humans and animals, most commonly contaminate water, raw milk, raw to rare ground beef, unpasteurized juices, and fruits and vegetables); *Listeria monocytogenes* (found in soft cheeses, raw milk, improperly processed ice cream, raw leafy vegetables, hot dogs

and lunch meats, and other meat, poultry, and processed foods); *Clostridium botulinum* (found in improperly canned foods, garlic in oil, sausages and other meat products, and vacuum-packed and tightly wrapped foods); and *Norovirus* (found in contaminated water, raw or insufficiently cooked shellfish, and salads contaminated by food handlers).

Another potential threat from food is bovine spongiform encephalopathy (BSE), or "mad cow disease," a fatal degenerative neurological disease caused by an abnormal protein that forms deposits in the brain. Visit the USDA Web site for more information (www.usda.gov).

Foodborne illness outbreaks associated with food-processing plants make headlines, but most cases of illness trace back to poor food handling in the home or in food-service establishments. To decrease your risk of food-borne illness, follow the guidelines in the box "Safe Food Handling."

Organic Foods

Some people who are concerned about pesticides and other environmental contaminants choose to buy foods that are **organic.** To be certified as organic by the USDA, foods must meet strict production, processing, handling, and labeling criteria. Organic crops must meet limits on pesticide residues; for meat, milk, eggs, and other animal products to be certified organic, animals must be given organic feed and access to the outdoors and may not be given antibiotics or growth hormones. The use of genetic engineering, ionizing radiation, and sewage sludge is prohibited. Products can be labeled "100% organic" if they contain all organic ingredients and "organic" if they contain at least 95% organic ingredients; all such products may carry the USDA organic seal. A product with at least 70% organic ingredients can be labeled "made with organic ingredients" but cannot use the USDA seal.

Some experts recommend that consumers who want to buy organic produce spend their money on those fruits and vegetables that have the highest levels of pesticide residue when grown conventionally (the "dirty dozen"): apples, bell peppers, celery, cherries, imported grapes, nectarines, peaches, pears, potatoes, red raspberries, spinach, and strawberries. Experts also recommend buying organic beef, poultry, eggs, dairy products, and baby food. Fruits and vegetables that carry little pesticide residue whether grown conventionally or organically include asparagus, avocadoes, bananas, broccoli, cauliflower, corn,

organic A designation applied to foods grown and produced according to strict guidelines limiting the use of pesticides, nonorganic ingredients, hormones, antibiotics, irradiation, genetic engineering, and other practices.

TERMS

Using Dietary Supplement Labels

Since 1999, specific types of information have been required on the labels of dietary supplements. In addition to basic information about the product, labels include a "Supplement Facts" panel, modeled after the "Nutrition Facts" panel used on food labels (see the label below). Under the Dietary Supplement Health and Education Act (DSHEA) and food labeling laws, supplement labels can make three types of health-related claims.

● *Nutrient-content claims,* such as "high in calcium," "excellent source of vitamin C," or "high potency." The claims "high in" and "excellent source of" mean the same as they do on food labels. A "high potency" single-ingredient supplement must contain 100% of that nutrient's Daily Value; a "high potency" multi-ingredient product must contain 100% or more of the Daily Value of at least two-thirds of the nutrients present for which Daily Values have been established.

● *Health claims,* if they have been authorized by the FDA or another authoritative scientific body. The association between adequate calcium intake and lower risk of osteoporosis is an example of an approved health claim. Since 2003, the FDA has also allowed so-called *qualified* health claims for situations in which there is emerging but as yet inconclusive evidence for a particular claim. Such claims must include qualifying language such as "scientific evidence suggests but does not prove" the claim.

● *Structure-function claims,* such as "antioxidants maintain cellular integrity" or "this product enhances energy levels." Because these claims are not reviewed by the FDA, they must carry a disclaimer (see the sample label).

Tips for Choosing and Using Dietary Supplements

● Check with your physician before taking a supplement. Many are not meant for children, elderly people, women who are pregnant or breast-feeding, people with chronic illnesses or upcoming surgery, or people taking prescription or OTC medications.

● Choose brands made by nationally known food and drug manufacturers or house brands from large retail chains. Due to their size and visibility, such sources are likely to have high manufacturing standards.

● Look for the USP verification mark on the label, indicating that the product meets minimum safety and purity standards developed under the Dietary Supplement Verification Program by the United States Pharmacopeia (USP). The USP mark means that the product (1) contains the ingredients stated on the label, (2) has the declared amount and strength of ingredients, (3) will dissolve effectively, (4) has been screened for harmful contaminants, and (5) has been manufactured using safe, sanitary, and well-controlled procedures. The National Nutritional Foods Association (NNFA) has a self-regulatory testing program for its members; other associations and labs, including ConsumerLab.Com, also test and rate dietary supplements.

● Follow the label's cautions, directions, and dosage.

● If you experience side effects, discontinue use of the product and contact your physician. Report any serious reactions to the FDA's MedWatch monitoring program (800-FDA-1088; http://www.fda.gov/medwatch).

For More Information About Dietary Supplements

ConsumerLab.Com: http://www.consumerlab.com

Food and Drug Administration: http://www.fda.gov/food/DietarySupplements/default.htm

National Institutes of Health, Office of Dietary Supplements: http://dietary-supplements.info.nih.gov

Natural Products Association: http://www.naturalproductsassoc.org

U.S. Department of Agriculture: http://fnic.nal.usda.gov/nal_display/index.php?info_center=4&tax_level=1&tax_subject=274

U.S. Pharmacopeia: http://www.usp.org/USPVerified/dietarySupplements

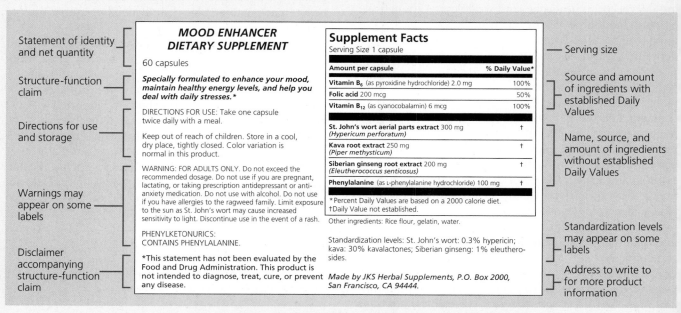

Statement of identity and net quantity

Structure-function claim

Directions for use and storage

Warnings may appear on some labels

Disclaimer accompanying structure-function claim

MOOD ENHANCER DIETARY SUPPLEMENT

60 capsules

Specially formulated to enhance your mood, maintain healthy energy levels, and help you deal with daily stresses. *

DIRECTIONS FOR USE: Take one capsule twice daily with a meal.

Keep out of reach of children. Store in a cool, dry place, tightly closed. Color variation is normal in this product.

WARNING: FOR ADULTS ONLY. Do not exceed the recommended dosage. Do not use if you are pregnant, lactating, or taking prescription antidepressant or anti-anxiety medication. Do not use with alcohol. Do not use if you have allergies to the ragweed family. Limit exposure to the sun as St. John's wort may cause increased sensitivity to light. Discontinue use in the event of a rash.

PHENYLKETONURICS: CONTAINS PHENYLALANINE.

*This statement has not been evaluated by the Food and Drug Administration. This product is not intended to diagnose, treat, cure, or prevent any disease.

Supplement Facts
Serving Size 1 capsule

Amount per capsule	% Daily Value*
Vitamin B₆ (as pyroxidine hydrochloride) 2.0 mg	100%
Folic acid 200 mcg	50%
Vitamin B₁₂ (as cyanocobalamin) 6 mcg	100%
St. John's wort aerial parts extract 300 mg (Hypericum perforatum)	†
Kava root extract 250 mg (Piper methysticum)	†
Siberian ginseng root extract 200 mg (Eleutherococcus senticosus)	†
Phenylalanine (as L-phenylalanine hydrochloride) 100 mg	†

*Percent Daily Values are based on a 2000 calorie diet.
†Daily Value not established.

Other ingredients: Rice flour, gelatin, water.

Standardization levels: St. John's wort: 0.3% hypericin; kava: 30% kavalactones; Siberian ginseng: 1% eleutherosides.

Made by JKS Herbal Supplements, P.O. Box 2000, San Francisco, CA 94444.

Serving size

Source and amount of ingredients with established Daily Values

Name, source, and amount of ingredients without established Daily Values

Standardization levels may appear on some labels

Address to write to for more product information

Safe Food Handling

- Don't buy food in containers that leak, bulge, or are severely dented. Refrigerated foods should be cold, and frozen foods should be solid.

- Refrigerate perishable items as soon as possible after purchase. Use or freeze fresh meats within 3–5 days and fresh poultry, fish, and ground meat within 1–2 days.

- Thaw frozen food in the refrigerator or in the microwave oven, not on the kitchen counter. Cook foods immediately after thawing.

- Thoroughly wash your hands with warm soapy water for 20 seconds before and after handling food, especially raw meat, fish, shellfish, poultry, or eggs.

- Make sure counters, cutting boards, dishes, utensils, and other equipment are thoroughly cleaned before and after use using hot soapy water. Wash dishcloths and kitchen towels frequently.

- If possible, use separate cutting boards for meat, poultry, and seafood and for foods that will be eaten raw. Replace cutting boards once they become worn or develop hard-to-clean grooves.

- Thoroughly rinse and scrub fruits and vegetables with a brush, if possible, or peel off the skin.

- Cook foods thoroughly, especially beef, poultry, fish, pork, and eggs; cooking kills most microorganisms. Use a food thermometer to ensure that foods are cooked to a safe temperature. Hamburgers should be cooked to 160°F. Turn or stir microwaved food to make sure it is heated evenly throughout.

- Keep hot foods hot (140°F or above) and cold foods cold (40°F or below). Harmful bacteria can grow rapidly between these two temperatures. Refrigerate foods within 2 hours of purchase or preparation, and within 1 hour if the air temperature is above 90°F. Refrigerate foods at or below 40°F and freeze at or below 0°F. Use refrigerated leftovers within 3–4 days.

- Don't eat raw animal products, including raw eggs in homemade hollandaise sauce or eggnog. Use only pasteurized milk and juice.

- Cook eggs until they're firm, and fully cook foods containing eggs. Store eggs in the coldest part of the refrigerator, not in the door, and use them within 3–5 weeks.

- Avoid raw sprouts. Even sprouts grown under clean conditions in the home can be risky because bacteria may be present in the seeds. Cook sprouts before eating them.

- According to the USDA, "When in doubt, throw it out." Even if a food looks and smells fine, it may not be safe. If you aren't sure that a food has been prepared, served, and stored safely, don't eat it.

Additional precautions are recommended for people at particularly high risk for foodborne illness—pregnant women, young children, older persons, and people with weakened immune systems or certain chronic illnesses. If you are a member of one of these groups, don't eat or drink any of the following products: unpasteurized juices; raw sprouts; unpasteurized (raw) milk and products made from unpasteurized milk; raw or undercooked meat, poultry, eggs, fish, and shellfish; and soft cheeses such as feta, Brie, Camembert, or blue-veined cheeses. To protect against *Listeria*, it's also important to avoid ready-to-eat foods such as hot dogs, luncheon meats, and cold cuts unless they are reheated until they are steaming hot.

---

kiwi, mangoes, onions, papaya, pineapples, and peas. All foods are subject to strict pesticide limits; the debate about the health effects of small amounts of residue is ongoing.

Whether organic foods are better for your health or not, organic farming is better for the environment (see the box "Organic Farming, Organic Food").

Guidelines for Fish Consumption

A specific area of concern has been mercury contamination in fish. Overall, fish and shellfish are healthy sources of protein, omega-3 fats, and other nutrients, and the report of the 2010 Dietary Guidelines Advisory Committee recommends that Americans consume two servings of fish per week. However, the FDA and Environmental Protection Agency (EPA) recommend that pregnant women and nursing mothers not eat shark, swordfish, king mackerel, or tilefish; limit consumption of other fish to 12 ounces per week and albacore tuna to 6 ounces per week; and check advisories about locally caught fish. The same recommendations apply to young children but in smaller servings. (For more information, visit the FDA and EPA

Web sites.) There is also concern about levels of toxic chemicals like PCBs in lakes and reservoirs, and some researchers suggest that consumers limit their consumption of farmed salmon to 8 ounces per month.

Additives in Food

Today, some 2800 substances are intentionally added to foods to maintain or improve nutritional quality, to maintain freshness, to help in processing or preparation, or to alter taste or appearance. Additives make up less than 1% of our food. The most widely used are sugar, salt, and corn syrup; these three plus citric acid, baking soda, vegetable colors, mustard, and pepper account for 98% by weight of all food additives used in the United States.

Some additives may be of concern for certain people, either because they are consumed in large quantities or because they cause some type of reaction.

To avoid potential problems, eat a variety of foods in moderation. If you are sensitive to an additive, check food labels when you shop, and ask questions when you eat out.

Organic Farming, Organic Foods

Since the mid-20th century, agriculture in the United States and other developed countries has been industrialized, with huge, corporate-owned farms producing billions of tons of produce and millions of animals for food. Industrial farming vastly improves productivity, but it takes an enormous toll on the environment. Although traditional, nonindustrial farming is as old as civilization itself, organic farming as we know it now developed in reaction to this industrialized form of agriculture. Americans interested in buying safer foods grown in environmentally friendly ways are buying organic foods in ever-increasing numbers. According to USDA statistics, organic products now account for about 3% of all food purchases—about $21 billion in sales during 2008.

Organic agriculture is a food production and management system that promotes and enhances ecological harmony, biodiversity, natural biological cycles, and sustainability over the long term. Where industrial agriculture applies massive amounts of chemical and synthetic products to the soil, plants, and air, in the form of fertilizers, pesticides, and herbicides, organic agriculture uses natural means—compost, crop rotation, beneficial insects and birds, and other natural practices—to enrich the soil and control pests and weeds. And where industrial agriculture treats animals as commodities, organic agriculture takes animal welfare into account.

Here are a few of the environmental benefits of organic farming as compared with industrial farming:

Sustainability   Where industrial farming is geared toward the greatest yield and highest profits in the short term, organic farming aims to produce food while establishing an ecological balance, maintaining soil fertility, and preventing pest problems. It puts back into the environment what it takes out and replenishes the earth's resources.

Biodiversity   Where industrial agriculture favors one or two strains or varieties of a crop species, selected or engineered for desired traits, and large single-crop farms, organic farming favors variety and diversity of species. Biodiversity is critical as the basis for the evolution of species as they adapt to changing environmental conditions. Cultivating a variety of plant and animal species makes farms more resistant to unpredictable weather patterns and pest outbreaks, as are predicted with climate change.

Soil   Where industrial farming causes soil degradation, contamination, and erosion, organic farming uses soil-building practices such as crop rotation, intercropping, symbiotic associations, cover crops, organic fertilizers, and minimum tillage to enhance the health, integrity, and productivity of the soil.

Water   Industrial farming pollutes surface and ground water with the toxic runoff from chemicals. Organic farming conserves water and protects water supplies by using organic fertilizers (compost, animal manure) that degrade naturally.

Air and climate   Compared to industrial farming, which uses petroleum-based fertilizers and gasoline to run farm machinery, organic farming reduces the need for fossil fuels and thus reduces the release of greenhouse gases, which contribute to global warming. Humus, the well-composted part of organic soil matter, helps mitigate climate change by removing carbon from the atmosphere and fixing it in the soil.

Animal welfare   Commercially raised livestock commonly spend most of their lives in crowded, stressful conditions that encourage the spread of disease. Animals are treated with antibiotics, growth hormone, steroids, and other drugs to prevent disease and spur growth. Organic farming regulations prohibit the use of any of these treatments. Animals must be fed organic feed and given access to the outdoors. Preventive measures like rotational grazing, a balanced diet, and clean housing are used to minimize disease.

Ecosystems   Industrial farming causes the death of insects, birds, and beneficial soil organisms; organic farming supports the maintenance of natural areas within and around organic fields. The absence of chemicals creates suitable habitats for wildlife and attracts new species to the area.

Food   Organic foods are free of antibiotics and artificial hormones and contain little or no pesticide residue. There is no evidence that organic foods are more nutritious than conventionally grown foods, although some fans of organic foods claim they contain more essential minerals and taste better. Some people worry that organic foods are more likely to cause foodborne illness, but recent outbreaks of foodborne illness have occurred as a result of practices within the industrial food

Food Irradiation

Food irradiation is the treatment of foods with gamma rays, X rays, or high-voltage electrons to kill potentially harmful pathogens, including bacteria, parasites, insects, and fungi that cause foodborne illness. It also reduces spoilage and extends shelf life. Few irradiated foods are currently on the market due to consumer resistance and skepticism. All primary irradiated foods (meat, vegetables, and so on) are labeled with the flowerlike radura symbol and a brief information label. Although irradiation kills most pathogens, proper handling of irradiated foods is still critical for preventing foodborne illness.

Genetically Modified Foods

Genetic engineering involves altering the characteristics of a plant, animal, or microorganism by adding, rearranging, system. The recall of half a billion eggs contaminated with *Salmonella* in August 2010 demonstrated this flaw in the agribusiness system. The eggs all came from two Iowa egg farms.

Farm worker safety Industrial farming exposes farm workers to toxic chemicals; organic farming does not.

The growing popularity of organic foods has attracted commercial corporations in recent years. Large companies like Dean Foods and Heinz now own many popular organic food brands, and supermarket chains like Safeway and Wal-Mart have added their own organic lines. These corporations comply with specific organic certification requirements but sometimes at a minimal level. For example, "access to the outdoors" may mean that animals are housed near screened windows or where there is an open door leading to a cement patio. These companies also maintain some industrial farming practices, such as large-scale operations and nationwide food distribution, using fossil fuels to truck organic foods thousands of miles.

In response to these developments, advocates of organic farming have suggested that consumers also consider the *sustainability* of the farming practices used to produce the organic foods they buy. Sustainability is more a philosophy or way of life than a certifiable set of farming practices. Sustainable organic farming is done by families who live on the land, planting crops in small mixed plots as a form of pest control. Animals are given outdoor space to behave naturally, whether that means grazing, pecking, rooting, or another behavior. Sustainable food is distributed and sold close to the farm.

In support of sustainability, consumers are encouraged to buy locally grown foods, for example, at farmers' markets or even directly from the farmer. In 2009, the Obama administration called for a reinvigoration of local food systems, and the USDA launched an initiative called "Know Your Farmer, Know Your Food" to promote sustainable local and regional food systems that support farmers and ranchers, strengthen rural communities, promote healthy eating, and protect natural resources (www.usda.gov/knowyourfarmer). Another initiative is community-supported agriculture (CSA), in which consumers pledge support to a farm operation and share in the farm's output during the growing season, typically receiving a box of produce on a weekly basis. In many areas, community gardens are flourishing, where participants plant a variety of crops together and share the bounty.

What can you do to support food production that benefits and sustains the environment?

- Buy organic. Any kind of organic agriculture, even large-scale corporate organic agriculture, is better for the environment than industrial agriculture. Organic food products are available at natural or whole food markets around the country and in three out of four conventional grocery stores.

- Buy locally grown food. Buy directly from an organic producer, shop at farmers' markets, or join a CSA.

- Join a community garden, or plant your own vegetables if you have a little plot of land or even a planter on a patio. You can enjoy the taste of a homegrown tomato while knowing your eating habits aren't harming the planet or contributing to global warming.

For a detailed discussion of environmental health—how the environment affects you and how you affect the environment—see Chapter 14.

SOURCES: U.S. Department of Agriculture, Economic Research Service. 2009. *Organic Agriculture* (http://www.ers.usda.gov/briefing/organic; retrieved November 5, 2010); U.S. Environmental Protection Agency. 2009. *Agriculture: Organic Farming* (http://www.epa.gov/agriculture/torg.html; retrieved November 5, 2010); *Sustainable Table, The Issues: Organic* (www.sustainabletable.orga/issues/organic; retrieved November 5, 2010); Food and Agriculture Organization of the United Nations. *What Are the Environmental Benefits of Organic Agriculture?* (www.fao.org/organicag/oa-faq/oa-faq6/en; retrieved November 5, 2010).

or replacing genes in its DNA; the result is a **genetically modified (GM) organism.** New DNA may come from related species or from entirely different types of organisms.

In 2010, a biotech company sought FDA approval for a genetically modified Atlantic salmon that grows to market size about twice as fast as conventional salmon. The GM organism contains an extra growth hormone gene from another species that allows it to produce growth hormone all year long rather than just during the warm season.

Many GM crops are already grown in the United States: About 75% of the current U.S. soybean crop has been genetically modified to be resistant to an herbicide used to kill weeds, and about 34% of the U.S. corn crop carries genes for herbicide resistance or pest resistance. The FDA does not require special labeling for foods from genetically modified sources. The only foods guaranteed not to contain GM ingredients are those certified as organic.

genetically modified (GM) organism A plant, animal, or microorganism in which genes have been added, rearranged, or replaced through genetic engineering.

TERMS

The potential benefits of GM foods cited by supporters include improved yields overall and in difficult growing conditions, increased disease resistance, improved nutritional content, lower prices, and less pesticide use. Critics of biotechnology argue that unexpected effects may occur: Gene manipulation could elevate levels of naturally occurring toxins or allergens, permanently change the gene pool and reduce biodiversity, and produce pesticide-resistant insects. Experience has shown that GM products are difficult to keep separate from non-GM products; animal escapes, cross-pollination, and contamination during processing are just a few ways GM organisms could potentially appear unexpectedly in the food supply or the environment.

Food Allergies and Food Intolerances

For some people, consuming a particular food causes symptoms such as itchiness, swollen lips, or abdominal pain. Adverse reactions like these may be due to a food allergy or a food intolerance, and symptoms may range from annoying to life-threatening.

A true **food allergy** is a reaction of the body's immune system to a food or food ingredient, usually a protein. This immune reaction can occur within minutes of ingesting the food, resulting in symptoms that affect the skin (hives), gastrointestinal tract (cramps or diarrhea), respiratory tract (asthma), or mouth (swelling of the lips or tongue). The most severe response is a systemic reaction called *anaphylaxis,* which involves a potentially life-threatening drop in blood pressure.

Although numerous food allergens have been identified, just eight foods account for more than 90% of the food allergies in the United States: cow's milk, eggs, peanuts, tree nuts (walnuts, cashews, and so on), soy, wheat, fish, and shellfish. Food labels are now required to state the presence of these eight allergens in plain language in the ingredient list. Individuals with food allergies, especially those prone to anaphylaxis, must diligently avoid trigger foods.

A **food intolerance** is a much more common source of adverse food reactions. In this case, the problem usually lies with metabolism rather than with the immune system. Lactose intolerance is a fairly common food intolerance. A more serious condition is intolerance of gluten, a protein component of some grains; in affected individuals, consumption of gluten damages the lining of the small intestine. Sulfite, a common food additive, can produce severe asthmatic reactions in sensitive individuals.

Many people with food intolerances can consume small amounts of the food that affects them; exceptions

Improving Your Diet by Choosing Healthy Beverages

This Behavior Change Strategy focuses on choosing healthy beverages to increase intake of nutrients and decrease intake of empty calories from added sugars and fat. However, this model of dietary change can be applied to any modification you'd like to make to your diet.

Gather Data and Establish a Baseline

Begin by tracking your beverage consumption in a journal. Write down the types and amounts of beverages you drink, including water. Also note where you were at the time and whether you obtained the beverage there or brought it with you. At the same time, investigate your options. Find out what other beverages you can easily find over the course of your daily routine. This information will help you put together a successful plan for change.

Analyze Your Data and Set Goals

Evaluate your beverage consumption by dividing your typical daily consumption between healthy and less healthy choices. Use the following guide as a basis, and add other beverages to the lists as needed.

Choose less often:

- Regular soda
- Sweetened bottled iced tea
- Fruit beverages made with little fruit juice (usually labeled fruit drinks, punches, beverages, blends, or ades)
- Flavored water sweetened with sugar
- Coffee drinks with milk and sugar
- Whole milk

Choose more often:

- Water—plain, mineral, or sparkling
- Low-fat or fat-free milk
- Fruit juice (100% juice)
- Unsweetened herbal tea

How many beverages do you consume daily from each category? What would be a healthy and realistic goal for change? For example, if your beverage consumption is currently evenly divided between the "choose more often" and "choose less often" categories (four from each list), you might set a final goal for your behavior change program of increasing your healthy choices by two (to six from the "more often" list and two from the "less often" list).

Develop a Plan for Change

Once you've set your goal, you need to develop strategies that will help you choose healthy beverages more often. Consider the following possibilities:

- Keep healthy beverages on hand; if you live in a dorm, rent a small refrigerator or keep healthy choices in the dorm kitchen's refrigerator.
- Plan ahead, and put a bottle of water or 100% juice in your backpack every day.
- Check food labels on beverages for serving sizes, calories, and nutrients; comparison shop to find the healthiest choices, and watch your serving sizes.

Use this information to make your "choose more often" list longer and more specific.

- If you eat out frequently, examine all the beverages available at the places you typically eat your meals. You'll probably find that healthy choices are available; if not, bring along your own drink or find somewhere else to eat.
- For a snack, try water and a piece of fruit rather than a heavily sweetened beverage.
- Create healthy beverages that appeal to you; for example, try adding slices of citrus fruit to water or mixing 100% fruit juice with sparkling water.

You may also need to make changes in your routine to decrease the likelihood that you'll make unhealthy choices. For example, you might discover from your health journal that you always buy a soda after class when you pass a particular vending machine. If this is the case, try another route that allows you to avoid the machine. And try to guard against impulse buying by carrying water or a healthy snack with you every day.

To complete your plan, try some of the other behavior change strategies described in Chapter 1: Develop and sign a contract, set up a system of rewards, involve other people in your program, and develop strategies for challenging situations. Once your plan is complete, take action. Keep track of your progress by continuing to monitor and evaluate your beverage consumption.

---

are gluten and sulfite, which must be avoided by sensitive individuals. Through trial and error, most people with food intolerances can adjust their intake of the trigger food to an appropriate level.

SUMMARY

- To function at its best, the human body requires about 45 essential nutrients in specific proportions. People get the nutrients needed to fuel their bodies and maintain tissues and organ systems from foods; the body cannot synthesize most of them.

- Proteins, made up of amino acids, form muscles and bones and help make up blood, enzymes, hormones, and cell membranes. Foods from animal sources provide complete proteins; plants provide incomplete proteins.

- Fats, a concentrated source of energy, also help insulate the body and cushion the organs; 1 tablespoon of vegetable oil per day supplies the essential fats. Dietary fat intake should be 20–35% of total daily calories. Unsaturated fats should be favored over saturated and trans fats.

- Carbohydrates supply energy to the brain and other parts of the nervous system as well as to red blood cells. The body needs about 130 grams of carbohydrates a day, but more is recommended.

- Fiber includes nondigestible carbohydrates provided mainly by plants. Adequate intake of fiber (38 grams per day for men and 25 grams per day for women) can help people manage diabetes and high cholesterol levels and improve intestinal health.

- The 13 vitamins needed in the diet are organic substances that promote specific chemical and cell processes within living tissue. Deficiencies or excesses can cause serious illnesses and even death.

- The approximately 17 minerals needed in the diet are inorganic substances that regulate body functions, aid in the growth and maintenance of body tissues, and help in the release of energy from foods.

- Water is used to digest and absorb food, transport substances around the body, and regulate body temperature.

- Foods contain other substances such as phytochemicals, which may not be essential nutrients but which reduce chronic disease risk.

- Dietary Reference Intakes (DRIs) are recommended intakes for essential nutrients that meet the needs of healthy people.

- The Dietary Guidelines for Americans address the prevention of diet-related diseases such as CVD, cancer, and diabetes. The 2010 Dietary Guidelines Advisory Committee report advises us to reduce overweight and obesity by reducing calorie intake and increasing physical activity; shift to a more plant-based diet, increasing consumption of seafood and fat-free and low-fat dairy products and consuming only moderate amounts of lean meat; reduce consumption of foods with solid fats and added sugars; and meet the 2008 Physical Activity Guidelines for Americans. The report also includes specific recommendations in eight topic areas.

- Choosing foods from each group in MyPyramid every day helps ensure that people get necessary nutrients.

- A vegetarian diet can meet human nutritional needs.

- Almost all foods have labels that show how much fat, cholesterol, protein, fiber, and sodium they contain. Dietary supplements also have uniform labels.

- Foodborne illnesses are a greater threat to health than additives and environmental contaminants. Other dietary issues of concern to some people include organic foods, food irradiation, genetic modification of foods, and food allergies and intolerances.

FOR MORE INFORMATION

BOOKS

Byrd-Bredbenner, C., et al. 2009. *Wardlaw's Perspectives in Nutrition,* 8th ed. New York: McGraw-Hill. *An easy-to-understand review of major concepts in nutrition.*

Duyff, R. L. 2006. *ADA Complete Food and Nutrition Guide,* 3rd ed. Hoboken, N.J.: Wiley. *An excellent review of current nutrition information.*

Insel, P. 2009. *Discovering Nutrition,* 4th ed. Sudbury, Mass.: Jones & Bartlett. *An introductory nutrition textbook covering a variety of key topics.*

Nestle, M. 2007. *What to Eat.* New York: North Point Press. *A nutritionist examines the marketing of food and explains how to interpret food-related information while shopping.*

Selkowitz, A. 2005. *The College Student's Guide to Eating Well on Campus,* revised ed. Bethesda, Md.: Tulip Hill Press. *Provides practical advice for students, including how to make healthy choices when eating in a dorm or restaurant and how to stock a first pantry.*

NEWSLETTERS

Environmental Nutrition (800-424-7887; http://www.environmentalnutrition.com)

Nutrition Action Health Letter (202-332-9110; http://www.cspinet.org/nah)

Tufts University Health & Nutrition Letter (800-274-7581; http://www.tuftshealthletter.com)

ORGANIZATIONS, HOTLINES, AND WEB SITES

American Diabetes Association. An organization with the aim of leading the fight against the deadly consequences of diabetes.
    http://www.diabetes.org/food-and-fitness
American Dietetic Association. Provides a wide variety of nutrition-related educational materials.
    http://www.eatright.org
American Heart Association: Delicious Decisions. Provides basic information about nutrition, tips for shopping and eating out, and heart-healthy recipes.
    http://www.deliciousdecisions.org
FDA Center for Food Safety and Applied Nutrition. Offers information about topics such as food labeling, food additives, dietary supplements, and foodborne illness.
    http://www.fda.gov/food
Food Safety Hotlines. Provide information on safe purchase, handling, cooking, and storage of food.
    888-SAFEFOOD (FDA)
    800-535-4555 (USDA)
Fruits & Veggies: More Matters. A nonprofit organization that encourages Americans to increase consumption of fruits and vegetables to five or more servings a day.
    http://www.fruitsandveggiesmorematters.org
Gateways to Government Nutrition Information. Provide access to government resources relating to food safety and nutrition.
    http://www.foodsafety.gov
    http://www.nutrition.gov
Harvard School of Public Health Nutrition Source. Provides recent key research findings, an overview of the Healthy Eating Pyramid, and suggestions for building a healthy diet.
    http://www.hsph.harvard.edu/nutritionsource
Mayo Clinic. Nutrition Basics. Medical, nutrition, and health information and tools for healthy living.
    http://www.mayoclinic.com/health/nutrition-and-healthy-eating/NY00431
MyPyramid.gov. Provides personalized dietary plans and interactive food and activity tracking tools.
    http://www.mypyramid.gov

National Academies' Food and Nutrition Board. Provides information about the Dietary Reference Intakes and related guidelines.

http://www.iom.edu/CMS/3788.aspx

USDA Food and Nutrition Information Center. Provides a variety of materials and extensive links relating to the Dietary Guidelines, food labels, MyPyramid, and many other topics.

http://www.nal.usda.gov/fnic

SELECTED BIBLIOGRAPHY

American Heart Association. 2010. *Diet and Lifestyle Recommendations* (http://www.americanheart.org/presenter.jhtml?identifier=851; retrieved November 5, 2010).

American Heart Association. 2010. *Fish, Levels of Mercury and Omega-3 Fatty Acids* (http://www.americanheart.org/presenter.jhtml?identifier=3013797; retrieved November 5, 2010).

American Heart Association. 2010. *Trans Fats* (http://www.americanheart.org/presenter.jhtml?identifier=3045792; retrieved November 5, 2010).

Bleich. S. N., et al. 2009. Increasing consumption of sugar-sweetened beverages among U. S. adults: 1988–1994 to 1999–2004. *American Journal of Clinical Nutrition* 89(1): 372–381.

Centers for Disease Control and Prevention. 2007. *vCJD (Variant Creutzfeldt Jakob Disease)* (http://www.cdc.gov/ncidod/dvrd/vcjd/index.htm; retrieved November 5, 2010).

Centers for Disease Control and Prevention. 2009. Application of lower sodium intake recommendations to adults–United States, 1999–2006. *Morbidity and Mortality Weekly Report* 58(11): 281–283.

Centers for Disease Control and Prevention. 2009. *Listeriosis* (http://www.cdc.gov/nczved/divisons/dfbmd; retrieved November 5, 2010).

Centers for Disease Control and Prevention. 2010. *Foodborne Illness* (http://www.cdc.gov/ncidod/dbmd/diseaseinfo/foodborneinfections_g.htm; retrieved November 5, 2010).

Council for Responsible Nutrition. 2009. *Dietary Supplements: Safe, Regulated and Beneficial* (http://www.crnusa.org/pdfs/CRN_FACT_DSSafeRegulated-Beneficial_09.pdf; retrieved November 5, 2010).

Food and Agriculture Organization of the United Nations. 2009. *1.02 Billion People Hungry* (http://www.fao.org/news/story/en/item/20568/icode/: retrieved November 5, 2010).

Harris, W. S., et al. 2009. Omega-6 fatty acids and risk for cardiovascular disease: A science advisory from the American Heart Association Nutrition Subcommittee of the Council on Nutrition, Physical Activity, and Metabolism; Council on Cardiovascular Nursing; and Council on Epidemiology and Prevention. *Circulation* 119(6): 902–907.

Harvard School of Public Health. Department of Nutrition. 2010. *The Nutrition Source: Knowledge for Healthy Eating* (http://www.hsph.harvard.edu/nutritionsource; retrieved November 5, 2010).

Hasler, C. M., et al. 2009. Position of the American Dietetic Association: Functional foods. *Journal of the American Dietetic Association* 109(4): 735–736.

Johnson, R. K., et al. 2009. Dietary sugars intake and cardiovascular health: A scientific statement from the American Heart Association. *Circulation* 120(11): 1011–1020.

Liebman, B. 2006. Whole grains: The inside story. *Nutrition Action Health Letter* 33(4): 1–5.

Maki, K. C., et al. 2010. Whole-grain ready-to-eat oat cereal, as part of a dietary program for weight loss, reduces low-density lipoprotein cholesterol in adults with overweight and obesity more than a dietary program including low-fiber control foods. *Journal of the American Dietetic Association* 110(2): 205–214.

Mayo Clinic. 2009. *Food Pyramid: An Option for Better Eating* (http://www.mayoclinic.com/health/healthy-diet/NU00190; retrieved November 5, 2010).

Nicholls, S. J., et al. 2006. Consumption of saturated fat impairs the anti-inflammatory properties of high-density lipoproteins and endothelial function. *Journal of the American College of Cardiology* 48(4): 715–720.

Siri-Tarino, P. W., et al. 2010. Meta-analysis of prospective cohort studies evaluating the association of saturated fat with cardiovascular disease. *American Journal of Clinical Nutrition* 91(3): 535–546.

Trump, D. L., et al. 2010. Vitamin D: Considerations in the continued developments as an agent for cancer prevention and therapy. *Cancer Journal* 16(1): 1–9.

Tucker, K. L., 2009. Osteoporosis prevention and nutrition. *Current Osteoporosis Reports* 7(4): 111–117.

U.S. Department of Agriculture and Centers for Disease Control and Prevention. 2009. *What We Eat in America* (http://www.ars.usda.gov/Services/docs.html?docid=15044; retrieved November 5, 2010).

U.S. Department of Health and Human Services and U.S. Department of Agriculture. 2005. *Finding Your Way to a Healthier You: Based on the Dietary Guidelines for Americans* (http://www.health.gov/dietaryguidelines/dga2005/document/html/brochure.htm; retrieved November 5, 2010).

U.S. Department of Health and Human Services and U.S. Department of Agriculture. 2009. *Dietary Guidelines for Americans 2005* (http://www.health.gov/dietaryguidelines; retrieved November 5, 2010).

U.S. Department of Health and Human Services and U.S. Department of Agriculture. 2010. *Report of the Dietary Guidelines Advisory Committee on the Dietary Guidelines for Americans, 2010* (http://www.cnpp.usda.gov/DGAs2010-DGACReport.htm; retrieved November 5, 2010).

U.S. Food and Drug Administration. 2009. *Food Allergies* (http://www.fda.gov/Food/FoodSafety/FoodAllergens/default.htm; retrieved November 5, 2010).

Varraso, R., et al. 2010. Prospective study of the dietary fiber and risk of chronic obstructive pulmonary disease among U.S. women and men. *American Journal of Epidemiology* 171(7): 776–784.

Wang, Y. C., et al. 2008. Increasing caloric contribution from sugar-sweetened beverages and 100% fruit juices among U.S. children and adolescents, 1988–2004. *Pediatrics* 121(6): e1604–e1614.

Nutrition Resources

Table 1 — Dietary Reference Intakes (DRIs): Recommended Levels for Individual Intake

LIFE STAGE	GROUP	BIOTIN (µG/DAY)	CHOLINE (MG/DAY)[a]	FOLATE (µG/DAY)[b]	NIACIN (MG/DAY)[c]	PANTOTHENIC ACID (MG/DAY)	RIBOFLAVIN (MG/DAY)
Infants	0–6 months	5	125	65	2	1.7	0.3
	7–12 months	6	150	80	4	1.8	0.4
Children	1–3 years	8	200	**150**	6	2	0.5
	4–8 years	12	250	**200**	8	3	0.6
Males	9–13 years	20	375	**300**	**12**	4	0.9
	14–18 years	25	550	**400**	**16**	5	1.3
	19–30 years	30	550	**400**	**16**	5	1.3
	31–50 years	30	550	**400**	**16**	5	1.3
	51–70 years	30	550	**400**	**16**	5	1.3
	>70 years	30	550	**400**	**16**	5	1.3
Females	9–13 years	20	375	**300**	**12**	4	0.9
	14–18 years	25	400	**400**[i]	**14**	5	1.0
	19–30 years	30	425	**400**[i]	**14**	5	1.1
	31–50 years	30	425	**400**[i]	**14**	5	1.1
	51–70 years	30	425	**400**[i]	**14**	5	1.1
	>70 years	30	425	**400**	**14**	5	1.1
Pregnancy	≤18 years	30	450	**600**[i]	**18**	6	1.4
	19–30 years	30	450	**600**[j]	**18**	6	1.4
	31–50 years	30	450	**600**[j]	**18**	6	1.4
Lactation	≤18 years	35	550	**500**	**17**	7	1.6
	19–30 years	35	550	**500**	**17**	7	1.6
	31–50 years	35	550	**500**	**17**	7	1.6
Tolerable Upper Intake Levels for Adults (19–70)			*3500*	*1000*[k]	*35*[k]		

LIFE STAGE	GROUP	THIAMIN (MG/DAY)	VITAMIN A (µG/DAY)[d]	VITAMIN B-6 (MG/DAY)	VITAMIN B-12 (µG/DAY)	VITAMIN C (MG/DAY)[e]	VITAMIN D (µG/DAY)[f]	VITAMIN E (MG/DAY)[g]
Infants	0–6 months	0.2	400	0.1	0.4	40	5	4
	7–12 months	0.3	500	0.3	0.5	50	5	5
Children	1–3 years	**0.5**	**300**	**0.5**	**0.9**	**15**	5	6
	4–8 years	**0.6**	**400**	**0.6**	**1.2**	**25**	5	7
Males	9–13 years	**0.9**	**600**	**1.0**	**1.8**	**45**	5	11
	14–18 years	**1.2**	**900**	**1.3**	**2.4**	**75**	5	15
	19–30 years	**1.2**	**900**	**1.3**	**2.4**	**90**	5	15
	31–50 years	**1.2**	**900**	**1.3**	**2.4**	**90**	5	15
	51–70 years	**1.2**	**900**	**1.7**	**2.4**[h]	**90**	10	15
	>70 years	**1.2**	**900**	**1.7**	**2.4**[h]	**90**	15	15
Females	9–13 years	**0.9**	**600**	**1.0**	**1.8**	**45**	5	11
	14–18 years	**1.0**	**700**	**1.2**	**2.4**	**65**	5	15
	19–30 years	**1.1**	**700**	**1.3**	**2.4**	**75**	5	15
	31–50 years	**1.1**	**700**	**1.3**	**2.4**	**75**	5	15
	51–70 years	**1.1**	**700**	**1.5**	**2.4**[h]	**75**	10	15
	>70 years	**1.1**	**700**	**1.5**	**2.4**[h]	**75**	15	15
Pregnancy	≤18 years	**1.4**	**750**	**1.9**	**2.6**	**80**	5	15
	19–30 years	**1.4**	**770**	**1.9**	**2.6**	**85**	5	15
	31–50 years	**1.4**	**770**	**1.9**	**2.6**	**85**	5	15
Lactation	≤18 years	**1.4**	**1200**	**2.0**	**2.8**	**115**	5	19
	19–30 years	**1.4**	**1300**	**2.0**	**2.8**	**120**	5	19
	31–50 years	**1.4**	**1300**	**2.0**	**2.8**	**120**	5	19
Tolerable Upper Intake Levels for Adults (19–70)			*3000*	*100*		*2000*	*50*	*1000*[k]

NOTE: The table includes values for the type of DRI standard—Adequate Intake (AI) or Recommended Dietary Allowance (RDA)—that has been established for that particular nutrient and life stage; RDAs are shown in **bold type**. The final row of the table shows the Tolerable Upper Intake Levels (ULs) for adults; refer to the full DRI report for information on other ages and life stages. A UL is the maximum level of daily nutrient intake that is likely to pose no risk of adverse effects. There are insufficient data to set ULs for all nutrients, but this does not mean that there is no potential for adverse effects; source of intake should be from food only to prevent high levels of intake of nutrients without established ULs. In healthy individuals, there is no established benefit from nutrient intakes above the RDA or AI.

[a]Although AIs have been set for choline, there are few data to assess whether a dietary supply of choline is needed at all stages of the life cycle, and it may be that the choline requirement can be met by endogenous synthesis at some of these stages.

[b]As dietary folate equivalents (DFE): 1 DFE = 1 µg food folate = 0.6 µg folate from fortified food or as a supplement consumed with food = 0.5 µg of a supplement taken on an empty stomach.

[c]As niacin equivalents (NE): 1 µg niacin = 60 µg tryptophan.

[d]As retinol activity equivalents (RAE s): 1 RAE = 1 µg retinol, 12 µg β-carotene, or 24 µg α-carotene or β-cryptoxanthin. Preformed vitamin A (retinol) is abundant in animal-derived foods; provitamin A carotenoids are abundant in some dark yellow, orange, red, and deep-green fruits and vegetables. For preformed vitamin A and for provitamin A carotenoids in supplements, 1RE = 1 RAE; for provitamin A carotenoids in foods, divide the REs by 2 to obtain RAEs. The UL applies only to preformed vitamin A.

LIFE STAGE	GROUP	VITAMIN K (µG/DAY)	CALCIUM (MG/DAY)	CHROMIUM (µG/DAY)	COPPER (µG/DAY)	FLUORIDE (MG/DAY)	IODINE (µG/DAY)
Infants	0–6 months	2.0	210	0.2	200	0.01	110
	7–12 months	2.5	270	5.5	220	0.5	130
Children	1–3 years	30	500	11	340	0.7	90
	4–8 years	55	800	15	440	1	90
Males	9–13 years	60	1300	25	700	2	120
	14–18 years	75	1300	35	890	3	150
	19–30 years	120	1000	35	900	4	150
	31–50 years	120	1000	35	900	4	150
	51–70 years	120	1200	30	900	4	150
	>70 years	120	1200	30	900	4	150
Females	9–13 years	60	1300	21	700	2	120
	14–18 years	75	1300	24	890	3	150
	19–30 years	90	1000	25	900	3	150
	31–50 years	90	1000	25	900	3	150
	51–70 years	90	1200	20	900	3	150
	>70 years	90	1200	20	900	3	150
Pregnancy	≤8 years	75	1300	29	1000	3	220
	19–30 years	90	1000	30	1000	3	220
	31–50 years	90	1000	30	1000	3	220
Lactation	≤18 years	75	1300	44	1300	3	290
	19–30 years	90	1000	45	1300	3	290
	31–50 years	90	1000	45	1300	3	290
Tolerable Upper Intake Levels for Adults (19–70)			2500		10,000	10	1100

LIFE STAGE	GROUP	IRON (MG/DAY)[l]	MAGNESIUM (MG/DAY)	MANGANESE (MG/DAY)	MOLYBDENUM (MG/DAY)	PHOSPHORUS (MG/DAY)	SELENIUM (MG/DAY)	ZINC (MG/DAY)[m]
Infants	0–6 months	0.27	30	0.003	2	100	15	2
	7–12 months	11	75	0.6	3	275	20	3
Children	1–3 years	7	80	1.2	17	460	20	3
	4–8 years	10	130	1.5	22	500	30	5
Males	9–13 years	8	240	1.9	34	1250	40	8
	14–18 years	11	410	2.2	43	1250	55	11
	19–30 years	8	400	2.3	45	700	55	11
	31–50 years	8	420	2.3	45	700	55	11
	51–70 years	8	420	2.3	45	700	55	11
	>70 years	8	420	2.3	45	700	55	11
Females	9–13 years	8	240	1.6	34	1250	40	8
	14–18 years	15	360	1.6	43	1250	55	9
	19–30 years	18	310	1.8	45	700	55	8
	31–50 years	18	320	1.8	45	700	55	8
	51–70 years	8	320	1.8	45	700	55	8
	>70 years	8	320	1.8	45	700	55	8
Pregnancy	≤8 years	27	400	2.0	50	1250	60	13
	19–30 years	27	350	2.0	50	700	60	11
	31–50 years	27	360	2.0	50	700	60	11
Lactation	≤18 years	10	360	2.6	50	1250	70	14
	19–30 years	9	310	2.6	50	700	70	12
	31–50 years	9	320	2.6	50	700	70	12
Tolerable Upper Intake Levels for Adults (19–70)		45	350[k]	11	2000	4000	400	40

[e]Individuals who smoke require an additional 35 mg/day of vitamin C over that needed by nonsmokers; nonsmokers regularly exposed to tobacco smoke should ensure they meet the RDA for vitamin C.

[f]As cholecalciferol: 1 µg cholecalciferol = 40 IU vitamin D. DRI values are based on the absence of adequate exposure to sunlight.

[g]As α-tocopherol. Includes naturally occurring RRR-α-tocopherol and the 2R-stereoisomeric forms from supplements; does not include the 2S-stereoisomeric forms from supplements.

[h]Because 10–30% of older people may malabsorb food-bound B-12, those over age 50 should meet their RDA mainly with supplements or foods fortified with B-12.

[i]In view of evidence linking folate intake with neural tube defects in the fetus, it is recommended that all women capable of becoming pregnant consume 400 µg from supplements or fortified foods in addition to consuming folate from a varied diet.

[j]It is assumed that women will continue consuming 400 µg from supplements or fortified food until their pregnancy is confirmed and they enter prenatal care, which ordinarily occurs after the end of the periconceptional period—the critical time for formation of the neural tube.

[k]The UL applies only to intake from supplements, fortified foods, and/or pharmacological agents and not to intake from foods.

[l]Because the absorption of iron from plant foods is low compared to that from animal foods, the RDA for strict vegetarians is approximately 1.8 times higher than the values established for omnivores (14 mg/day for adult male vegetarians; 33 mg/day for premenopausal female vegetarians). Oral contraceptives (OCs) reduce menstrual blood losses, so women taking them need less daily iron; the RDA for premenopausal women taking OCs is 10.9 mg/day. For more on iron requirements for other special situations, refer to *Dietary Reference Intakes for Vitamin A, Vitamin K, Arsenic, Boron, Chromium, Copper, Iodine, Iron, Manganese, Molybdenum, Nickel, Silicon, Vanadium, and Zinc* (visit http://www.nap.edu for the complete report).

[m]Zinc absorption is lower for those consuming vegetarian diets so the zinc requirement for vegetarians is approximately twofold greater than for those consuming a nonvegetarian diet.

LIFE STAGE	GROUP	POTASSIUM (G/DAY)	SODIUM (G/DAY)	CHLORIDE (G/DAY)	CARBOHYDRATE RDA/AI (G/DAY)	CARBOHYDRATE AMDR[o] (%)	TOTAL FIBER RDA/AI (G/DAY)	TOTAL FAT AMDR[o] (%)
Infants	0–6 months	0.4	0.12	0.18	60	ND[q]	ND	[r]
	7–12 months	0.7	0.37	0.57	95	ND[q]	ND	[r]
Children	1–3 years	3.0	1.0	1.5	130	45–65	19	30–40
	4–8 years	3.8	1.2	1.9	130	45–65	25	25–35
Males	9–13 years	4.5	1.5	2.3	130	45–65	31	25–35
	14–18 years	4.7	1.5	2.3	130	45–65	38	25–35
	19–30 years	4.7	1.5	2.3	130	45–65	38	20–35
	31–50 years	4.7	1.5	2.3	130	45–65	38	20–35
	51–70 years	4.7	1.3	2.0	130	45–65	30	20–35
	>70 years	4.7	1.2	1.8	130	45–65	30	20–35
Females	9–13 years	4.5	1.5	2.3	130	45–65	26	25–35
	14–18 years	4.7	1.5	2.3	130	45–65	26	25–35
	19–30 years	4.7	1.5	2.3	130	45–65	25	20–35
	31–50 years	4.7	1.5	2.3	130	45–65	25	20–35
	51–70 years	4.7	1.3	2.0	130	45–65	21	20–35
	>70 years	4.7	1.2	1.8	130	45–65	21	20–35
Pregnancy	≤18 years	4.7	1.5	2.3	175	45–65	28	20–35
	19–30 years	4.7	1.5	2.3	175	45–65	28	20–35
	31–50 years	4.7	1.5	2.3	175	45–65	28	20–35
Lactation	≤18 years	5.1	1.5	2.3	210	45–65	29	20–35
	19–30 years	5.1	1.5	2.3	210	45–65	29	20–35
	31–50 years	5.1	1.5	2.3	210	45–65	29	20–35
Tolerable Upper Intake Levels for Adults (19–70)			2.3	3.6				

LIFE STAGE	GROUP	LINOLEIC ACID RDA/AI (G/DAY)	LINOLEIC ACID AMDR[o] (%)	ALPHA-LINOLENIC ACID RDA/AI (G/DAY)	ALPHA-LINOLENIC ACID AMDR[o] (%)	PROTEIN[n] RDA/AI (G/DAY)	PROTEIN[n] AMDR[o] (%)	WATER[p] (L/DAY)
Infants	0–6 months	4.4	ND[q]	0.5	ND[q]	9.1	ND[q]	0.7
	7–12 months	4.6	ND[q]	0.5	ND[q]	13.5	ND[q]	0.8
Children	1–3 years	7	5–10	0.7	0.6–1.2	13	5–20	1.3
	4–8 years	10	5–10	0.9	0.6–1.2	19	10–30	1.7
Males	9–13 years	12	5–10	1.2	0.6–1.2	34	10–30	2.4
	14–18 years	16	5–10	1.6	0.6–1.2	52	10–30	3.3
	19–30 years	17	5–10	1.6	0.6–1.2	56	10–35	3.7
	31–50 years	17	5–10	1.6	0.6–1.2	56	10–35	3.7
	51–70 years	14	5–10	1.6	0.6–1.2	56	10–35	3.7
	>70 years	14	5–10	1.6	0.6–1.2	56	10–35	3.7
Females	9–13 years	10	5–10	1.0	0.6–1.2	34	10–30	2.1
	14–18 years	11	5–10	1.1	0.6–1.2	46	10–30	2.3
	19–30 years	12	5–10	1.1	0.6–1.2	46	10–35	2.7
	31–50 years	12	5–10	1.1	0.6–1.2	46	10–35	2.7
	51–70 years	11	5–10	1.1	0.6–1.2	46	10–35	2.7
	>70 years	11	5–10	1.1	0.6–1.2	46	10–35	2.7
Pregnancy	≤18 years	13	5–10	1.4	0.6–1.2	71	10–35	3.0
	19–30 years	13	5–10	1.4	0.6–1.2	71	10–35	3.0
	31–50 years	13	5–10	1.4	0.6–1.2	71	10–35	3.0
Lactation	≤18 years	13	5–10	1.3	0.6–1.2	71	10–35	3.8
	19–30 years	13	5–10	1.3	0.6–1.2	71	10–35	3.8
	31–50 years	13	5–10	1.3	0.6–1.2	71	10–35	3.8

[n] Daily protein recommendations are based on body weight for reference body weights. To calculate for a specific body weight, use the following values: 1.5 g/kg for infants, 1.1 g/kg for 1–3 years, 0.95 g/kg for 4–13 years, 0.85 g/kg for 14–18 years, 0.8 g/kg for adults, and 1.1 g/kg for pregnant (using prepregnancy weight) and lactating women.

[o] Acceptable Macronutrient Distribution Range (AMDR), expressed as a percent of total daily calories, is the range of intake for a particular energy source that is associated with reduced risk of chronic disease while providing intakes of essential nutrients. If an individual consumes in excess of the AMDR, there is a potential for increasing the risk of chronic diseases and/or insufficient intakes of essential nutrients.

[p] Total water intake from fluids and food.

[q] Not determinable due to lack of data of adverse effects in this age group and concern with regard to lack of ability to handle excess amounts. Source of intake should be from food only to prevent high levels of intake.

[r] For infants, Adequate Intake of total fat is 31 grams/day (0–6 months) and 30 grams per day (7–12 months) from breast milk and, for infants 7–12 months, complementary food and beverages.

SOURCE: Food and Nutrition Board, Institute of Medicine, National Academies. 2010. *Dietary Reference Intakes: The Essential Guide to Nutrient Requirements.* Washington, DC: National Academies Press. http://www.iom.edu/Activities/Nutrition/SummaryDRIs/DRI-Tables.aspx. Reprinted with permission from the National Academies Press, Copyright 2010, National Academy of Sciences.

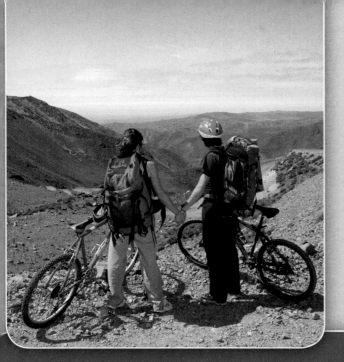

LOOKING AHEAD...

After reading this chapter, you should be able to:

- Define physical fitness, and list the health-related components of fitness

- Explain the wellness benefits of physical activity and exercise

- Describe how to develop each of the health-related components of fitness

- Discuss how to choose appropriate exercise equipment, how to eat and drink for exercise, how to assess fitness, and how to prevent and manage injuries

- Put together a personalized exercise program that you enjoy and that will enable you to achieve your fitness goals

Exercise for Health and Fitness

10

Your body is a wonderful moving machine made to work best when it is physically active. It readily adapts to practically any level of activity and exercise: The more you ask of your body, the stronger and more fit it becomes. The opposite is also true. Left unchallenged, bones lose their density, joints stiffen, muscles become weak, and cellular energy systems begin to degenerate. To be truly healthy, human beings must be active. If approached correctly, physical activity and exercise can contribute immeasurably to overall wellness, add fun and joy to life, and provide the foundation for a lifetime of fitness.

WHAT IS PHYSICAL FITNESS? ✓

Physical fitness is the body's ability to respond or adapt to the demands and stress of physical effort—that is, to perform moderate to vigorous levels of physical activity without becoming overly tired. Some components of fitness are related to specific activities or sports; others relate to general health. **Health-related fitness** includes cardiorespiratory endurance, muscular strength, muscular

endurance, flexibility, and body composition. Health-related fitness helps you withstand physical challenges and protects you from diseases.

Cardiorespiratory Endurance

Cardiorespiratory endurance is the ability to perform prolonged, large-muscle, dynamic exercise at moderate to high intensity. When cardiorespiratory fitness is low, the heart has to work hard during normal daily activities and may not be able to work hard enough to sustain high-intensity physical activity in an emergency. Poor cardiorespiratory fitness is linked with heart disease, diabetes, colon cancer, stroke, depression, anxiety, and premature death from all causes. Regular **cardiorespiratory endurance training**, however, makes the heart stronger and improves the function of the entire cardiorespiratory system. As cardiorespiratory fitness improves, related physical functions also improve. The heart pumps more blood per heartbeat, resting heart rate slows and resting blood pressure decreases, blood volume increases, blood supply to tissues improves, the body can cool itself better, and metabolic health improves, which helps the body process fuel and

QUICK STATS

Only **3.8%** of elementary schools, **7.9%** of middle schools, and **2.1%** of high schools require daily physical education.

—CDC, 2009

regulate cell function. A healthy heart can better withstand the strains of daily life, the stress of occasional emergencies, and the wear and tear of time. You can develop cardiorespiratory endurance through activities that involve continuous, rhythmic movements of large-muscle groups, such as the legs. Such activities include walking, jogging, cycling, and aerobic dancing.

Muscular Strength

Muscular strength is the amount of force a muscle can produce with a single maximum effort. It depends on such factors as the size of muscle cells and the ability of nerves to activate muscle cells. Strong muscles are important for everyday activities, such as climbing stairs, as well as for emergencies. They help keep the skeleton in proper alignment, preventing back and leg pain and providing the support necessary for good posture. Muscular strength has obvious importance in recreational activities. Strong people can hit a tennis ball harder, kick a soccer ball farther, and ride a bicycle uphill more easily.

Muscle tissue is an important element of overall body composition. Greater muscle mass makes possible a higher rate of metabolism and faster energy use, which help to maintain a healthy body weight. Strength training helps maintain muscle mass, function, and balance in older people, which greatly enhances their quality of life and prevents injuries. Strength training promotes cardiovascular health, reduces the risk of osteoporosis (bone

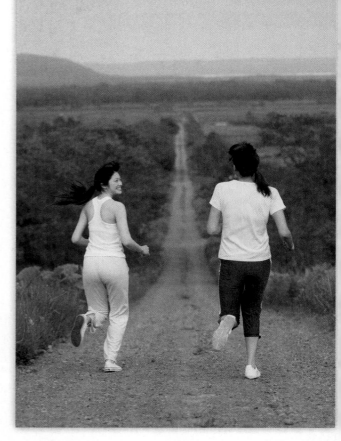

Cardiorespiratory endurance is a critical component of health-related fitness.

loss), and prevents premature death from all causes. Muscular strength can be developed by training with weights or by using the weight of the body for resistance during calisthenic exercises such as push-ups and curl-ups.

Muscular Endurance

Muscular endurance is the ability to resist fatigue and sustain a given level of muscle tension—that is, to hold a muscle contraction for a long time or to contract a muscle over and over again. It depends on such factors as the size of muscle cells, the ability of muscles to store fuel, the content of mitochondria (cell energy centers), and the blood supply to muscles. Muscular endurance is important for good posture and for injury prevention. Muscular endurance helps people cope with the physical demands of everyday life and enhances performance in sports and work. Like muscular strength, muscular endurance is developed by stressing the muscles with a greater load (weight) than they are used to. The degree to which strength or endurance develops depends on the type and amount of stress that is applied.

Flexibility

Flexibility is the ability of joints to move through their full range of motion. Flexible, pain-free joints are important

TERMS

physical fitness The body's ability to respond or adapt to the demands and stress of physical effort.

health-related fitness Physical capabilities that contribute to health, including cardiorespiratory endurance, muscular strength, muscular endurance, flexibility, and body composition.

cardiorespiratory endurance The ability of the body to perform prolonged, large-muscle, dynamic exercise at moderate to high levels of intensity.

cardiorespiratory endurance training Exercise intended to improve cardiorespiratory endurance.

muscular strength The amount of force a muscle can produce with a single maximum effort.

muscular endurance The ability of a muscle or group of muscles to remain contracted or to contract repeatedly for a long period of time.

for good health and well-being. Inactivity causes the joints to become stiffer with age. Stiffness, in turn, often causes older people to assume unnatural body postures that can stress joints and muscles. Stretching exercises can help ensure a healthy range of motion for all major joints.

Body Composition

Body composition refers to the proportion of fat and **fat-free mass** (muscle, bone, and water) in the body. Healthy body composition involves a high proportion of fat-free mass and an acceptably low level of body fat, adjusted for age and sex. A person with excessive body fat is more likely to experience health problems, including heart disease, high blood pressure, stroke, joint problems, diabetes, gallbladder disease, cancer, and back pain. The best way to lose fat is through a lifestyle that includes a sensible diet and exercise. The best way to add muscle mass is through resistance training such as weight training.

Skill-Related Components of Fitness

In addition to the five health-related components of physical fitness, the ability to perform a particular sport or activity may depend on **skill-related fitness** components such as speed, power, agility, balance, coordination, and reaction time. Skill-related fitness tends to be sport-specific and is best developed through practice. Playing a sport can be fun, can help build fitness, and may contribute to other areas of wellness.

PHYSICAL ACTIVITY AND EXERCISE FOR HEALTH AND FITNESS

Physical activity is any body movement carried out by the skeletal muscles and requiring energy. Quick, easy movements such as standing up or walking down a hallway require little energy or effort; more intense, sustained activities such as cycling 5 miles or running in a race require considerably more. **Exercise** refers to a subset of physical activity—planned, structured, repetitive movement of the body intended specifically to improve or maintain physical fitness. To develop fitness, a person must perform enough physical activity to stress the body

and cause long-term physiological changes. Physical activity is essential to health and confers wide-ranging health benefits, but exercise is necessary to significantly improve physical fitness.

The CDC reports that only about 31% of Americans participate in some leisure-time physical activity and that leisure-type physical activity decreased by nearly 6% between 2003 and 2009. Physical activity levels are higher in men than in women but decline with age in both. Levels are lower in Hispanics, American Indians, and blacks than in whites. People with higher levels of education are more active than people with lower educational attainment. For example, 54% of college graduates exercise regularly, compared to 31% of high school dropouts. Evidence is growing that for most Americans, becoming more physically active may be the single most important lifestyle change for promoting health and well-being.

In 2008 the U.S. Department of Health and Human Services issued *Physical Activity Guidelines for Americans,* making specific recommendations for promoting health. These recommendations echoed and reinforced earlier recommendations issued by the Surgeon General, the American College of Sports Medicine (ACSM), the American Heart Association, and other organizations. The 2008 guidelines stressed the importance of regular physical activity for health promotion and disease prevention and emphasized that some activity is better than none. The report included these guidelines for adults:

- For substantial health benefits, adults should do at least 150 minutes (2½ hours) a week of moderate-intensity aerobic physical activity, or 75 minutes (1¼ hours) a week of vigorous-intensity aerobic physical activity, or an equivalent combination of moderate- and vigorous-intensity activity. Preferably, activity should be spread throughout the week.

- For additional health benefits, adults should increase their activity to 300 minutes (5 hours) a week of moderate-intensity activity, or 150 minutes of vigorous-intensity activity, or an equivalent combination.

Ask Yourself

QUESTIONS FOR CRITICAL THINKING AND REFLECTION

When you think about exercise, do you think of only one or two of the five components of health-related fitness, such as muscular strength or body composition? If so, where do you think your ideas come from? What role do the media play in shaping your ideas about fitness?

- Adults should also do muscle-strengthening activities that are moderate or high intensity and involve all major muscle groups on 2 or more days a week.

- All adults should avoid inactivity.

Research shows that these levels of physical activity promote health and wellness in specific ways: by lowering the risk of high blood pressure, stroke, heart disease, type 2 diabetes, colon cancer, and osteoporosis and by reducing feelings of mild to moderate depression and anxiety. For people who need to prevent weight gain, lose weight, or maintain weight loss, 150 minutes per week of physical activity may not be enough, and 300 minutes or more are recommended.

The 2008 guidelines define moderate-intensity physical activity as activity that causes a noticeable increase in heart rate, such as a brisk walk. The report defines vigorous-intensity physical activity as activity that causes rapid breathing and a substantial increase in heart rate, as exemplified by jogging.

A daily total of physical activity can be accumulated in multiple bouts of 10 or more minutes—for example, two 10-minute bike rides to and from class and a brisk 10-minute walk to the store. More vigorous activity, as in a structured, systematic exercise program, is also needed to improve physical fitness; moderate physical activity alone is not enough. Physical fitness requires more intense movement that poses a substantially greater challenge to the body.

THE BENEFITS OF EXERCISE

The greater the demands made on the human body, the more it adjusts to meet the demands—it becomes fit. Over time, immediate, short-term adjustments translate into long-term changes and improvements (see page T1-4 of the color transparency insert "Touring Lifestyle Behaviors" in Chapter 8). The goal of regular physical activity is to bring about these kinds of long-term changes and improvements in the body's functioning.

Reduced Risk of Premature Death

Physically active people have a reduced risk of dying prematurely from all causes, with the greatest benefits found in the most active people. Physical inactivity is as important a risk factor as smoking, high blood pressure, obesity, and diabetes. Poor muscle strength also increases the risk of premature death.

Improved Cardiorespiratory Functioning

During exercise, the cardiorespiratory system (heart, lungs, and circulatory system) must work harder to meet the body's increased demand for oxygen. Regular endurance exercise improves the functioning of the heart and the ability of the cardiorespiratory system to carry oxygen to body tissues. Exercise directly affects the health of your arteries, keeping them from stiffening or clogging with plaque and reducing the risk of cardiovascular disease. Exercise also improves sexual function and general vitality.

More Efficient Metabolism and Improved Cell Health

Endurance exercise improves metabolism, the process that converts food to energy and builds tissue. This process involves oxygen, nutrients, hormones, and enzymes. A physically fit person is better able to generate energy, to use carbohydrates and fats for energy, and to regulate hormones. Exercise may also protect cells from damage from free radicals, from destructive chemicals produced during normal metabolism, and from inflammation caused by high blood pressure or cholesterol, nicotine, and overeating. Training activates antioxidant enzymes that prevent free-radical damage and maintain the health of the body's cells. Regular physical activity prevents the deterioration of telomeres, which form the protective ends of chromosomes that are vital for cell health and repair.

Improved Body Composition

Exercise can improve body composition in several ways. Endurance exercise significantly increases daily calorie expenditure; it can also slightly raise *metabolic rate,* the rate at which the body burns calories, for several hours after an exercise session. Strength training increases muscle mass, thereby tipping the body composition ratio toward fat-free mass and away from fat. It can also help with losing fat because metabolic rate is directly proportional to fat-free mass: The more muscle mass, the higher the metabolic rate.

> Only **32%** of Americans are at a healthy weight.
>
> —*The Healthy People 2010 Database,* 2010

Disease Prevention and Management

Regular physical activity lowers your risk of many chronic, disabling diseases.

Making Time for Physical Activity

"Too little time" is a common excuse for not being physically active. Learning to manage your time successfully is crucial if you are to maintain a wellness lifestyle. You can begin by keeping a record of how you are currently spending your time; in your health journal, use a grid broken into blocks of 15, 20, or 30 minutes to track your daily activities. Then analyze your record: List each type of activity and the total time you engaged in it on a given day—for example, sleeping, 7 hours; eating, 1.5 hours; studying, 3 hours; and so on. Take a close look at your list of activities, and prioritize them according to how important they are to you, from essential to somewhat important to not important at all.

Based on the priorities you set, make changes in your daily schedule by subtracting time from some activities in order to make time for physical activity. Look carefully at your leisure-time activities and your methods of transportation; these are areas where it is easy to build in physical activity. Make changes using a system of trade-offs. For example, you may choose to reduce the total amount of time you spend playing computer games to make time for an after-dinner bike ride or a walk with a friend. You may decide to watch 10 fewer minutes of television in the morning to change your 5-minute drive to class into a 15-minute walk. The following are just a few ways to become more active:

- Take the stairs instead of the elevator or escalator.
- Walk to the post office, store, bank, or library when possible.
- Park your car a mile or even just a few blocks from your destination, and walk briskly.
- Do at least one chore every day that requires physical activity: Wash the windows or your car, clean your room or house, mow the lawn, or rake the leaves.
- Take study or work breaks to avoid sitting for more than 30 minutes at a time. Get up and walk around the library, office, or your home; go up and down a flight of stairs.
- Stretch when you stand in line or watch TV.
- When you take public transportation, get off one stop early and walk to your destination.
- Take the dog for a walk (or an extra walk) every day.
- If weather or neighborhood safety rule out walking outside, look for alternative locations—an indoor track, an enclosed shopping mall, or even a long hallway.
- Seize every opportunity to get up and walk around. Move more and sit less.

Visit the U.S. Department of Health and Human Services Small Step Web site (www.smallstep.gov) for more ideas.

Cardiovascular Disease   A sedentary lifestyle is one of the six major risk factors for cardiovascular disease (CVD). Sedentary people have CVD death rates significantly higher than those of fit individuals. Physical inactivity increases the risk of CVD by 50–240%. The benefits of physical activity begin at moderate levels of activity and rise with increasing levels of activity. Exercise positively affects the risk factors for CVD, including cholesterol levels, insulin resistance, and high blood pressure. Exercise also interferes with the disease process itself, directly lowering the risk of heart disease and stroke.

Cancer   Studies have shown a relationship between increased physical activity and a reduced risk of cancer, but these findings are not conclusive. There is evidence that exercise reduces the risk of colon cancer and promising data that it reduces the risk of cancer of the breast and reproductive organs in women and prostate cancer in men.

Osteoporosis   A special benefit of exercise, especially for women, is protection against osteoporosis, a disease that results in loss of bone density and poor bone strength. Weight-bearing exercise, which includes almost everything except swimming, helps build bone during childhood and the teens and twenties. Strength training and impact exercises such as jumping rope can increase bone density throughout life. With stronger bones and muscles and better balance, fit people are less likely to experience debilitating falls and bone fractures.

Type 2 Diabetes   People with diabetes are prone to heart disease, blindness, and severe problems of the nervous and circulatory systems. Exercise prevents the development of type 2 diabetes, the most common form of the disease. Exercise burns excess sugar and makes cells more sensitive to insulin. Exercise also helps keep body fat at healthy levels. (Obesity is a key risk factor for type 2 diabetes.) For people who have diabetes, physical activity is an important part of treatment.

Improved Psychological and Emotional Wellness

People who are physically active experience many social, psychological, and emotional benefits. Numerous research studies have found evidence for the following benefits:

- *Reduced anxiety and depression.* Exercise reduces symptoms of anxiety, such as worry and self-doubt, and is associated with lowered risk for panic attacks. Exercise also relieves feelings of sadness and hopelessness, improves mood, and increases feelings of well-being in both depressed and nondepressed people.

- *Improved sleep.* Regular physical activity helps people fall asleep more easily and improves sleep quality.
- *Reduced stress.* Exercise reduces the body's overall response to stressors and helps people deal more effectively with stress.
- *Enhanced self-esteem and sense of self-efficacy.* Exercise boosts self-esteem by providing opportunities for people to succeed and excel. It also improves body image and increases people's belief in their ability to take charge of their lives.
- *Enhanced creativity and intellectual functioning.* Exercise improves alertness and memory in the short term and helps maintain reaction time, reasoning skills, and memory in the long term. Studies show that exercise can improve brain function and may delay the decline in cognitive ability that occurs for many people as they age. It may even prevent the onset of age-related brain disorders like Alzheimer's disease.
- *Improved interpersonal wellness.* Regular physical activity offers many opportunities for positive interactions with other people.

Improved Immune Function

Exercise can have either positive or negative effects on the immune system, the physiological processes that protect us from disease. Moderate endurance exercise boosts immune function, whereas excessive training depresses it. Physically fit people get fewer colds and upper respiratory tract infections than people who are not fit.

Prevention of Injuries and Low-Back Pain

Increased muscle strength provides protection against injury because it helps people maintain spinal stability, good posture, and appropriate body mechanics when carrying out everyday activities such as walking, lifting, and carrying. Good muscle endurance in the abdomen, hips, lower back, and legs supports the back in proper alignment and helps prevent low-back pain, which affects more than 85% of Americans at some time in their lives.

Improved Wellness for Life

Although people differ in the maximum levels of fitness they can achieve through exercise, the wellness benefits of exercise are available to everyone (see the box "Exercise for People with Special Health Concerns"). Exercising regularly may be the single most important thing you can do now to improve the quality of your life in the future.

DESIGNING YOUR EXERCISE PROGRAM

The best exercise program has two primary characteristics: It promotes your health, and it's fun for you to do. Exercise does not have to be a chore. On the contrary, it can provide some of the most pleasurable moments of your day, once you make it a habit.

Figure 10.1 shows a physical activity pyramid to guide you in meeting goals for physical activity. If you are sedentary, start at the bottom of the pyramid and gradually

Sedentary Activities
Do infrequently
Watching television, surfing the Internet, talking on the telephone

Strength Training
2–3 nonconsecutive days per week (all major muscle groups)
Biceps curls, push-ups, abdominal curls, bench press, calf raises

Flexibility Training
At least 2–3 days per week (all major joints)
Calf stretch, side lunge, step stretch, hurdler stretch

Cardiorespiratory Endurance Exercise
3–5 days per week (20–60 minutes per day)

Walking, jogging, bicycling, swimming, aerobic dancing, in-line skating, cross-country skiing, dancing, playing basketball

Moderate-Intensity Physical Activity
150 minutes per week; for weight loss or prevention of weight regain following weight loss, 60–90 minutes per day

Walking to the store or bank, washing windows or your car, climbing stairs, working in your yard, walking your dog, cleaning your room

FIGURE 10.1 Physical activity pyramid.

Regular, appropriate exercise is safe and beneficial for many people with chronic conditions or other special health concerns. In fact, the risks associated with inactivity are usually far greater than those associated with a program of regular moderate exercise.

If you have a special health concern and hesitate to become more active, one helpful strategy is to take a class or join an exercise group specifically designed for your condition. If you prefer to exercise at home, exercise videos are available for people with a variety of conditions.

The fitness recommendations for the general population presented in this chapter can serve as general guidelines for any exercise program. However, for people with special health concerns, certain precautions and monitoring may be required. *Anyone with special health concerns should consult a physician before beginning an exercise program.* Guidelines and cautions for some common conditions are described below:

Asthma

- Carry medication during workouts and avoid exercising alone. Use your inhaler before exercise, if recommended by your physician.

- Exercise regularly, and warm up and cool down slowly.

- When starting a fitness program, choose self-paced endurance activities, especially those involving interval training (short bouts of exercise followed by rest periods).

- When possible, avoid circumstances that may trigger an asthma attack, including cold, dry air or pollen or dust. Drink water to keep your airways moist, and in cold weather, cover your mouth with a mask or scarf to warm and humidify the air you breathe. Swimming is a good activity for people with asthma.

Diabetes

- Don't exercise alone; wear a bracelet identifying yourself as having diabetes.

- If you are taking insulin or another medication, you may need to adjust the timing and amount of each dose as you learn to balance your energy intake and output and your medication dosage.

- To prevent abnormally rapid absorption of injected insulin, inject it over a muscle that won't be exercised and wait at least an hour before exercising.

- Check blood sugar levels before, during, and after exercise, and adjust your diet or insulin dosage if needed. Avoid exercise if your blood sugar level is above 250 mg/dl, and ingest carbohydrates prior to exercise if your blood sugar level is below 100 mg/dl. Have high-carbohydrate foods available during a workout.

- Check your skin regularly for blisters and abrasions, especially on your feet.

Obesity

- For maximum benefit and minimum risk, begin with low- to moderate-intensity activities and increase intensity slowly as fitness improves.

- To lose weight or maintain lost weight, exercise moderately for 30–60 minutes or more daily and reduce food intake.

- At first choose non- or low-weight-bearing activities like swimming, water exercises, cycling, or walking.

- Stay alert for symptoms of heat-related problems during exercise.

- Try to include as much lifestyle physical activity in your daily routine as possible.

- Include strength training in your program to build muscle mass.

Heart Disease and Hypertension

- Warm-up and cool-down sessions should be gradual and last at least 10 minutes.

- Exercise at a moderate rather than a high intensity; monitor your heart rate during exercise, and stop if you experience dizziness or chest pain.

- Increase exercise frequency, intensity, and time very gradually.

- Don't hold your breath when exercising as this can cause a sudden, steep increase in blood pressure.

- Discuss the effects of your medication with your physician. If your physi-

cian has prescribed nitroglycerine, carry it with you during exercise.

Arthritis

- Begin an exercise program as early as possible in the course of the disease.

- Warm up thoroughly before each workout to loosen stiff muscles and lower the risk of injury.

- Avoid high-impact activities that may damage arthritic joints; consider swimming or water aerobics.

- In strength training, pay special attention to muscles that support and protect affected joints; add weight very gradually.

- Stretch regularly.

Osteoporosis

- If possible, choose low-impact, weight-bearing activities to help safely maintain bone density.

- To prevent fractures, avoid any activity or movement that stresses the back or carries a risk of falling.

- Weight train to improve strength and balance and to reduce the risk of falls and fractures, but avoid lifting heavy weights.

Table 10.1	ACSM Exercise Recommendations for Fitness Development in Healthy Adults

EXERCISE TO DEVELOP AND MAINTAIN CARDIORESPIRATORY ENDURANCE AND BODY COMPOSITION

Frequency of training	3–5 days per week.
Intensity of training	55/65–90% of maximum heart rate or 40/50–85% of heart rate reserve or maximum oxygen uptake reserve. The lower intensity values (55–64% of maximum heart rate and 40–49% of heart rate reserve) are most applicable to individuals who are quite unfit. For average individuals, intensities of 70–85% of maximum heart rate or 60–80% of heart rate reserve are appropriate; see page 250 for instructions for determining target heart rate.
Time (duration) of training	20–60 total minutes of continuous or intermittent (in sessions lasting 10 or more minutes) aerobic activity. Duration is dependent on the intensity of activity; thus, low-intensity activity should be conducted over a longer period of time (30 minutes or more). Low- to moderate-intensity activity of longer duration is recommended for nonathletic adults.
Type (mode) of activity	Any activity that uses large-muscle groups, can be maintained continuously, and is rhythmic and aerobic in nature—for example, walking-hiking, running-jogging, cycling-bicycling, cross-country skiing, aerobic dance, stair climbing, swimming, and skating.

EXERCISE TO DEVELOP AND MAINTAIN MUSCULAR STRENGTH AND ENDURANCE, FLEXIBILITY, AND BODY COMPOSITION

Resistance training	One set of 8–10 exercises that condition the major muscle groups should be performed at least 2 days per week. Most people should complete 8–12 repetitions of each exercise to the point of fatigue; practicing other repetition ranges (for example, 3–5 or 12–15) also builds strength and endurance; for older and frailer people (approximately 50–60 and older), 10–15 repetitions with a lighter weight may be more appropriate. Multiple-set regimens will provide greater benefits if time allows. Any mode of exercise that is comfortable throughout the full range of motion is appropriate (for example, free weights, bands, or machines).
Flexibility training	Static stretches should be performed for the major muscle groups at least 2–3 days per week, ideally 5–7 days per week. Stretch to the point of tightness, holding each stretch for 15–30 seconds; perform 2–4 repetitions of each stretch.

SOURCE: Adapted from American College of Sports Medicine. 2009. *ACSM'S Guidelines for Exercise Testing and Prescription*, 8th ed. Philadelphia: Lippincott Williams & Wilkins.

increase the moderate-intensity physical activity in your daily life. You don't have to exercise vigorously, but you should experience a moderate increase in your heart and breathing rates. If weight management is a concern for you, begin by achieving the goal of 150 minutes per week and then gradually raise your activity level to 300 minutes per week or more.

For even greater benefits, move up to the next two levels of the pyramid, which illustrate parts of a formal exercise program. The American College of Sports Medicine has established guidelines for an exercise program that includes cardiorespiratory endurance (aerobic) exercise, strength training, and flexibility training (Table 10.1). Such a program will develop all the health-related components of physical fitness. For a summary of the health and fitness benefits of different levels of physical activity, see Figure 10.2.

First Steps

Are you thinking about starting a formal exercise program? A little planning can help make it a success.

Medical Clearance Previously inactive men over 40 and women over 50 should get a medical examination before beginning an exercise program. Diabetes, asthma, heart disease, and extreme obesity are conditions that may call for a modified program. If you have an increased risk of heart disease because of smoking, high blood pressure, or obesity, get a physical checkup, including an **electrocardiogram (ECG or EKG),** before beginning an exercise program.

Basic Principles of Physical Training To put together an effective exercise program, you should first understand the basic principles of physical training.

TERMS

electrocardiogram (ECG or EKG) A recording of the changes in electrical activity of the heart.

	Lifestyle physical activity	Moderate exercise program	Vigorous exercise program
Description	Moderate physical activity (150 minutes per week; muscle-strengthening exercises 2 or more days per week)	Cardiorespiratory endurance exercise (20–60 minutes, 3–5 days per week); strength training (2–3 nonconsecutive days per week); and stretching exercises (2 or more days per week)	Cardiorespiratory endurance exercise (20–60 minutes, 3–5 days per week); interval training; strength training (3–4 nonconsecutive days per week); and stretching exercises (5–7 days per week)
Sample activities or program	• Walking to and from work, 15 minutes each way • Cycling to and from class, 10 minutes each way • Doing yard work for 30 minutes • Dancing (fast) for 30 minutes • Playing basketball for 20 minutes • Muscle exercises such as push-ups, squats, or back exercises	• Jogging for 30 minutes, 3 days per week • Weight training, 1 set of 8 exercises, 2 days per week • Stretching exercises, 3 days per week	• Running for 45 minutes, 3 days per week • Intervals, running 400 m at high effort, 4 sets, 2 days per week • Weight training, 3 sets of 10 exercises, 3 days per week • Stretching exercises, 6 days per week
Health and fitness benefits	Better blood cholesterol levels, reduced body fat, better control of blood pressure, improved metabolic health, and enhanced glucose metabolism; improved quality of life; reduced risk of some chronic diseases Greater amounts of activity can help prevent weight gain and promote weight loss	All the benefits of lifestyle physical activity, plus improved physical fitness (increased cardiorespiratory endurance, muscular strength and endurance, and flexibility) and even greater improvements in health and quality of life and reductions in chronic disease risk	All the benefits of lifestyle physical activity and a moderate exercise program, with greater increases in fitness and somewhat greater reductions in chronic disease risk Participating in a vigorous exercise program may increase risk of injury and overtraining

FIGURE 10.2   Health and fitness benefits of different amounts of physical activity and exercise.

SPECIFICITY   To develop a fitness component, you must perform exercises that are specifically designed for that component. This is the principle of **specificity.** Weight training, for example, develops muscular strength, but is less effective for developing flexibility or cardiorespiratory endurance. A well-rounded exercise program includes exercises geared to each component of fitness, to different parts of the body, and to specific activities or sports.

PROGRESSIVE OVERLOAD   When the amount of exercise, or overload, is progressively increased, fitness continues to improve. This is the principle of **progressive overload.** Too little exercise will have no effect on fitness; too much may cause injury. The appropriate amount depends on your current level of fitness, your genetic capacity to adapt to exercise, your fitness goals, and the fitness components being developed.

The amount of overload needed to maintain or improve a particular level of fitness is determined in four dimensions: Frequency, Intensity, Time, and Type. These dimensions of overload, represented by the acronym FITT, are described individually as they apply to the health-related components of fitness discussed in this chapter.

REVERSIBILITY   The body adjusts to lower levels of physical activity in the same way it adjusts to higher levels—the principle of **reversibility.** Try to exercise consistently, and don't quit if you miss a few workouts.

INDIVIDUAL DIFFERENCES   There are limits to the potential for improvement and large individual differences in our ability to improve fitness, achieve a desirable body composition, and perform and learn sports skills. But physical training improves fitness and wellness regardless of heredity.

Determining Your Target Heart Rate Range

Your target heart rate is the range of rates at which you should exercise to experience cardiorespiratory benefits. Your target heart rate range is based on your maximum heart rate, which can be estimated from your age. (If you are a serious athlete or face possible cardiovascular risks from exercise, you may want to have your maximum heart rate determined more accurately through a treadmill test in a physician's office, hospital, or sports medicine laboratory.) Your target heart rate is a range: The lower value corresponds to moderate-intensity exercise, and the higher value is associated with high-intensity exercise. Target heart rate ranges are shown in the table.

You can monitor the intensity of your workouts by measuring your pulse either at your wrist or at one of your carotid arteries, located on either side of your Adam's apple. Your pulse rate drops rapidly after exercise, so begin counting immediately after you have finished exercising. You will obtain the most accurate results by counting beats for 10 seconds and then multiplying by 6 to get your heart rate in beats per minute (bpm). The 10-second counts corresponding to each target heart rate range are also shown in the table.

AGE (YEARS)	TARGET HEART RATE RANGE (BPM)*	10-SECOND COUNT (BEATS)*
20–24	127–180	21–30
25–29	124–176	20–29
30–34	121–171	20–28
35–39	118–167	19–27
40–44	114–162	19–27
45–49	111–158	18–26
50–54	108–153	18–25
55–59	105–149	17–24
60–64	101–144	16–24
65+	97–140	16–23

*Target heart rates lower than those shown here are appropriate for individuals with a very low initial level of fitness. Ranges are based on the following formula: Target heart rate = 0.65 to 0.90 of maximum heart rate, assuming maximum heart rate = 220 – age.

Selecting Activities If you have been inactive, you should begin slowly by gradually increasing the amount of moderate physical activity in your life (the bottom of the activity pyramid). Once your body adjusts to your new level of activity, you can choose additional activities for your exercise program.

Be sure the activities you choose contribute to your overall wellness and make sense for you. Are you competitive? If so, try racquetball, basketball, or squash. Do you prefer to exercise alone? Then consider cross-country skiing or road running. Have you been sedentary? A walking program may be a good place to start. If you think you may have trouble sticking with an exercise program, find a structured activity that you can do with a friend, a personal trainer, or a group. Be realistic about the constraints presented by some sports, such as accessibility, expense, and time.

Cardiorespiratory Endurance Exercises

Exercises that condition your heart and lungs and improve metabolism should have a central role in your fitness program.

Frequency The optimal workout schedule for endurance training is 3–5 days per week. Beginners should start with 3 and work up to 5 days. Training more than 5 days a week often leads to injury for recreational athletes.

Intensity Intensity is the crucial factor in attaining a significant training effect—that is, in increasing the body's cardiorespiratory capacity. A primary purpose of endurance training is to increase **maximal oxygen consumption ($\dot{V}O_{2max}$)**. $\dot{V}O_{2max}$ represents the maximum ability of the cells to use oxygen and is considered the best measure of cardiorespiratory capacity. Intensity of training is the crucial factor in improving $\dot{V}O_{2max}$.

One of the easiest ways to determine exactly how intensely you should work involves measuring your heart rate. It is not necessary or desirable to exercise at your maximum heart rate—the fastest heart rate possible before exhaustion sets in—in order to improve your cardiorespiratory capacity. Beneficial effects occur at lower heart rates with a much lower risk of injury. **Target heart rate range** is the range of rates within which you should exercise to obtain cardiorespiratory benefits. To determine the intensity at which you should exercise, refer to the box "Determining Your Target Heart Rate Range."

Time (Duration) A total time of 20–60 minutes per workout is recommended for cardiorespiratory endurance training. Exercise can take place in a single session or several sessions lasting 10 or more minutes. The total duration of exercise depends on its intensity. To improve cardiorespiratory endurance during a moderate-intensity activity such as walking or slow swimming, exercise for 45–60 minutes. For high-intensity exercise performed at the top of your target heart rate zone, a duration of 20 minutes is sufficient. Start with less vigorous activities and gradually increase intensity.

Type The best exercises for developing cardiorespiratory endurance stress a large portion of the body's muscle mass for a prolonged period of time. These include walking, jogging, running, swimming, bicycling, and aerobic dancing. Many popular sports and recreational activities, such as racquetball, tennis, basketball, and soccer, are also good if the skill level and intensity of the game are sufficient to provide a vigorous workout.

The Warm-Up and Cool-Down It is always important to warm up before you exercise and to cool down afterward. Warming up enhances your performance and decreases your chances of injury. A warm-up session should include low-intensity movements similar to those in the activity that will follow. For example, hit forehands and backhands before a tennis game or jog slowly for 400 meters before progressing to an 8-minute mile.

Experts recommend that you stretch *after* the active part of your warm-up, when your body temperature has been elevated. Studies have found that stretching prior to exercise can temporarily decrease muscle strength and power, so if a high-performance workout is your goal, it is best to stretch after a workout.

Cooling down after exercise is important to restore the body's circulation to its normal resting condition. When you are at rest, a relatively small percentage of your total blood volume is directed to muscles, but during exercise, as much as 90% of the heart's output is directed to them. During recovery from exercise, it is important to continue exercising at a low level to provide a smooth transition to the resting state. Do not take a hot shower until after you have cooled down.

5–10 minutes
of warming up and cooling down is adequate for a 30-minute workout of brisk walking.

—CDC, 2010

Developing Muscular Strength and Endurance

Any program designed to promote health should include exercises that develop muscular strength and endurance (see the box "Gender Differences in Muscular Strength").

Types of Strength Training Exercises Muscular strength and endurance can be developed in many ways, from weight training to calisthenics. Common exercises such as curl-ups, push-ups, pull-ups, and non-weighted squats maintain the muscular strength of most people if they practice them several times a week. To condition and tone your whole body, choose exercises that work the major muscles of the shoulders, chest, back, arms, abdomen, and legs.

To increase muscular strength and endurance, you must do **resistance exercise**—exercises in which your muscles must exert force against a significant amount of resistance. Resistance can be provided by weights, exercise machines, your own body weight, or even objects such as rocks. **Isometric (static) exercises** involve applying force without movement, such as when you contract your abdominal muscles. This static type of exercise is valuable for toning and strengthening muscles. Isometrics can be practiced anywhere and do not require any equipment. For maximum strength gains, hold an isometric contraction maximally for 6 seconds; do five to ten repetitions. Don't hold your breath—that can restrict blood flow to your heart and brain. Within a few weeks, you will notice the effect of this exercise. Isometrics are particularly useful when recovering from an injury.

Isotonic (dynamic) exercises involve applying force with movement, as in weight training exercises such as the bench press. These are the most popular type of exercises for increasing muscle strength and seem to be most valuable for developing strength that can be transferred to other forms of physical activity. They include exercises using barbells, dumbbells, kettlebells, weight machines, and body weight, as in push-ups.

Choosing Equipment Weight machines are preferred by many people because they are safe, convenient, and easy to use. You just set the resistance, sit down at the machine, and start working. Machines make it easy to isolate and work specific muscles. Free weights require more care, balance, and coordination to use, but they strengthen your body in ways that are more adaptable to real life. When using free weights, you need to use a spotter, someone who stands by to assist in case you lose control over a weight.

Choosing Exercises A complete weight training program works all the major muscle groups: neck, upper back, shoulders, arms, chest, abdomen, lower back, thighs, buttocks, and calves. Different exercises work different muscles, so it usually takes about eight to ten exercises to get a complete workout for general fitness—for example, bench presses to develop the chest, shoulders, and upper arms; pull-ups to work the biceps and upper back; squats to develop the legs and buttocks; toe raises to work the calves; and so on.

Frequency For general fitness, the American College of Sports Medicine recommends a frequency of at least

Gender Differences in Muscular Strength

Men are generally stronger than women because they typically have larger bodies overall and a larger proportion of their total body mass is made up of muscle. But when strength is expressed per unit of muscle tissue, men are only 1–2% stronger than women in the upper body and about equal to women in the lower body. Individual muscle cells are larger in men, but the functioning of the cells is the same in both sexes.

Two factors that help explain these disparities are testosterone levels and the speed of nervous control of muscle. Testosterone promotes the growth of muscle tissue in both males and females, but testosterone levels are about 6–10 times higher in men than in women, so men develop larger muscles. Also, because the male nervous system can activate muscles faster, men tend to have more power.

Some women are concerned that they will develop large muscles from strength training. Because of hormonal differences, most women do not develop large muscles unless they train intensely over many years or take anabolic steroids. A study of average women who weight trained 2–3 days per week for 8 weeks found that the women gained about 1.75 pounds of muscle and lost about 3.5 pounds of fat. Another study followed women who trained with weights for 2 years. Not only did the women reduce their overall body fat levels but they ended up with less fat around their midsection.

Losing muscle over time is a much greater health concern for women than small gains in muscle weight in response to strength training, especially as any gains in muscle weight are typically more than balanced with loss of fat weight. Both men and women lose muscle mass and power as they age, but because men start out with more muscle when they are young and don't lose power as quickly as women, older women tend to have greater impairment of muscle function than older men. This may partially explain the higher incidence of life-threatening falls in older women.

Healthy People 2010 sets a national health objective of increasing to 30% the proportion of adults who perform strength training exercises on 2 or more days per week. In 2008, however, the CDC reported that only 22% of men and 17% of women met this goal, underscoring the need for additional programs and campaigns that promote resistance exercise.

SOURCES: Fahey, T. D. 2010. *Basic Weight Training for Men and Women,* 7th ed. New York: McGraw-Hill; Centers for Disease Control and Prevention. 2006. Trends in strength training— United States, 1998–2004. *Morbidity and Mortality Weekly Report* 55(28): 769–772.

---

2 nonconsecutive days per week. This allows your muscles one or more days of rest between workouts to avoid soreness and injury. If you enjoy weight training and would like to train more often, try working different muscle groups on alternate days.

Intensity and Time   The amount of weight (resistance) you lift in weight training exercises is equivalent to intensity in cardiorespiratory endurance training; the number of repetitions of each exercise is equivalent to time. In order to improve fitness, you must do enough repetitions of each exercise to temporarily fatigue your muscles. The number of repetitions needed to cause fatigue depends on the amount of resistance: the heavier the weight, the fewer repetitions to reach fatigue. In general, a heavy weight and a low number of repetitions (1–5) build strength, whereas a light weight and a high number of repetitions (10–25) build endurance. For a general fitness program to build

both strength and endurance, try to do 8–12 repetitions of each exercise. For people over 50, using a lighter weight for 10–15 repetitions is recommended.

To start, choose a weight that you can move easily through 8–12 repetitions. Add weight when you can do more than 12 repetitions of an exercise. If adding weight means you can do only 7 or 8 repetitions before your muscles fatigue, stay with that weight until you can again complete 12 repetitions. If you can do only 4–6

> **Among competitive athletes, a significant number of failed drug tests are attributable to supplement misuse.**
>
> —**World Anti-Doping Agency, 2010**

Drugs and Supplements for Improved Athletic Performance

Doping scandals have snared athletes in sports as diverse as swimming, cycling, tennis, baseball, and track and field. In 2010, 30 athletes failed drug tests at the Winter Olympics in Canada. In 2008, Martina Hingis retired from tennis after testing positive for cocaine. In 2007, Olympic sprinter Marion Jones admitted using banned substances before the 2000 Olympic games and was stripped of her five metals. And baseball legends Barry Bonds, Alex Rodriguez, and Roger Clemens have all fought allegations of steroid abuse.

Professional and Olympic athletes aren't the only ones using performance-enhancing drugs. About 2–6% of high school and college students report having used anabolic steroids, and over-the-counter dietary supplements are much more popular. Many such substances are ineffective and expensive, and many are also dangerous.

Anabolic Steroids These synthetic derivatives of testosterone are taken to increase strength, power, speed, endurance, muscle size, and aggressiveness. **Anabolic steroids** have dangerous side effects, including disruption of the body's hormone system, liver disease, acne, breast development and testicular shrinkage in males, masculinization in women and children, and increased risk of heart disease and cancer. Evidence links anabolic steroid use and risk of heart attack, stroke, and sudden death. Steroid users who inject the drugs face the same health risks as other injection drug users, including increased risk of HIV infection.

Adrenal Androgens This group of drugs, which includes dehydroepiandrosterone (DHEA) and androstenedione, are typically taken to stimulate muscle growth and aid in weight control. The few studies of these agents done on humans show that they are of little value in improving athletic performance, and they have side effects similar to those of anabolic steroids.

Stimulants These drugs may be taken to increase training intensity, to suppress hunger, to reduce fatigue, and to promote weight loss. They raise heart rate and blood pressure and, at high doses, may increase the risk of heart attack, stroke, and heat-related illness. Several stimulants, including ephedra and phenylpropanolamine, have been banned by the FDA.

Erythropoietin (EPO) A hormone that boosts the concentration of red blood cells, EPO is used by athletes to improve performance. EPO can cause blood clots and death.

Creatine Monohydrate Creatine is thought to improve performance in short-term, high-intensity, repetitive exercise and decrease the risk of injury. People vary in their responses to creatine. The long-term effects of creatine use, especially among young people, are not well established.

Protein, Amino Acid, and Polypeptide Supplements Little research supports excessive protein intake, even in athletes on extremely heavy training regimens. The protein requirements of athletes are not much higher than those of sedentary individuals, and most people take in more than enough protein in their diets. By substituting supplements for food sources of protein, people may risk deficiencies in other key nutrients typically found in such foods, including iron and B vitamins.

Chromium Picolinate Sold over the counter, chromium picolinate is a more easily digested form of the trace mineral chromium. Although it is often marketed as a means to build muscle and reduce fat, most studies have found no positive effects. Long-term use of high dosages may have serious health consequences.

---

repetitions after adding weight, or if you can't maintain good form, you've added too much and should take some off.

For developing strength and endurance for general fitness, a single set (group of repetitions) of each exercise is sufficient, provided you use enough weight to fatigue your muscles. Doing more than one set of each exercise may increase strength development, and most serious weight trainers do at least three sets of each exercise. If you do more than one set of an exercise, rest long enough between sets to allow your muscles to recover. You should warm up before every weight training session and cool down afterward.

A Caution About Supplements No nutritional supplement or drug will change a weak person into a strong person. Those changes require regular training that stresses the body and causes physiological adaptations. Supplements or drugs that promise quick, large gains in strength usually don't work and are often either dangerous, expensive, or both (see the box "Drugs and Supplements for Improved Athletic Performance"). Over-the-counter supplements are not carefully regulated, and their long-term effects have not been systematically studied.

Flexibility Exercises

Flexibility, or stretching, exercises are important for maintaining the normal range of motion in the major joints of the body. Some exercises, such as running, can decrease flexibility because they require only a partial range of motion. Like a good weight training program, a good stretching program includes exercises for all the major muscle

> **anabolic steroids** Synthetic male hormones used to increase muscle size and strength.

TERMS

Core Training

The core muscles include those in the abdomen, pelvic floor, sides of the trunk, back, buttocks, hips, and pelvis. There are 29 of these muscles, attaching to the ribs, hips, spinal column, and other bones in the trunk of the body. The core muscles stabilize the spine and help transfer force between the upper and lower body. They stabilize the midsection when you sit, stand, reach, walk, jump, twist, squat, throw, or bend. The muscles on the front, back, and sides of your trunk support your spine when you sit in a chair and fix your midsection as you use your legs to stand up. When a person hits a forehand in tennis or bats a softball, most of the force is transferred from the legs and hips, across the core muscles, to the arms. Strong core muscles make movements more forceful and help prevent back pain.

During any dynamic movement, the core muscles work together. Some shorten to cause movement, while others contract and hold to provide stability, lengthen to brake the movement, or send signals to the brain about the movements and positions of the muscles and bones (proprioception). When specific core muscles are weak or tired, the nervous system steps in and uses other muscles. This substitution causes abnormal stress on the joints, decreases power, and increases the risk of injury.

The best exercises for low-back health are whole-body exercises that force the core muscles to stabilize the spine in many different directions. Low-back exercises that focus on the core muscles include the lunge, side bridges, and spine extensions. These exercises are generally safe for beginning exercisers and, with physician approval, people with some back pain. More challenging core exercises utilize stability balls or free weights. Stability ball exercises require the core muscles to stabilize the ball and the body while performing nearly any type of exercise. Many traditional exercises with free weights can strengthen the core muscles if you do them in a standing position. Weight machines train muscles in isolation, while exercises with free weights done while standing help train the body for real-world movements—an essential principle of core training.

groups and joints of the body: neck, shoulders, back, hips, thighs, hamstrings, and calves. In tandem with core training, flexibility training is important for preventing low-back injuries and maintaining low-back health (see the box "Core Training").

Proper Stretching Technique   Stretching should be performed statically, although more advanced athletes can also include dynamic stretching (actively moving through a joint's range of motion). Ballistic stretching ("bouncing") is dangerous and counterproductive. In active stretching, a muscle is stretched under a person's own power by contracting the opposing muscles. In passive stretching, an outside force or resistance provided by yourself, a partner, gravity, or a weight helps elongate the targeted muscle. You can achieve a greater range of motion and a more intense stretch using passive stretching, but there is a greater risk of injury. The safest and most convenient technique may be active static stretching with a passive assist. For example, you might do a seated stretch of your calf muscles both by contracting the muscles on the top of your shin and by grabbing your feet and pulling them toward you.

Frequency   Do stretching exercises at least 2–3 days per week. If you stretch after cardiorespiratory endurance exercise or strength training, during your cool-down, you may develop more flexibility, because your muscles are warmer then and can be stretched farther.

Intensity and Time   For each exercise, stretch to the point of tightness in the muscle, then hold the position for 15–30 seconds. Rest for 30–60 seconds, then repeat, trying to stretch a bit farther. Relax and breathe easily as you stretch. You should feel a pleasant, mild stretch as you let the muscles relax; stretching should not be painful. Do 2–4 repetitions of each exercise. A complete flexibility workout usually takes about 20–30 minutes.

Increase your intensity gradually over time. Improved flexibility takes many months to develop. There are large individual differences in joint flexibility. Don't feel you have to compete with others during stretching workouts.

Training in Specific Skills

The final component in your fitness program is learning the skills required for the sports or activities in which you choose to participate. The first step in learning a new skill is getting help. Sports like tennis, golf, sailing, and skiing require mastery of basic movements and techniques, so instruction from a qualified teacher or coach can save you hours of frustration and increase your enjoyment of the sport. Skill is also important in conditioning activities such as jogging, swimming, and cycling. Even if you learned a sport as a child, additional instruction now can help you refine your technique.

Putting It All Together

Now that you know the basic components of a fitness program, you can put them all together in a program that works for you. Refer to Figure 10.3 for a summary of the FITT principle for the health-related fitness components.

	Cardiorespiratory endurance training	Strength training	Flexibility training
Frequency	3–5 days per week	2–3 nonconsecutive days per week	2–3 days per week (minimum); 5–7 days per week (ideal)
Intensity	55/65–90% of maximum heart rate	Sufficient resistance to fatigue muscles	Stretch to the point of tension
Time	20–60 minutes in sessions lasting 10 minutes or more	8–12 repetitions of each exercise, 1 or more sets	2–4 repetitions of each exercise, held for 15–30 seconds
Type	Continuous rhythmic activities using large muscle groups	Resistance exercises for all major muscle groups	Stretching exercises for all major joints

FIGURE 10.3   A summary of the FITT principle for the health-related components of fitness.

GETTING STARTED AND STAYING ON TRACK

Once you have a program that fulfills your basic fitness needs and suits your personal tastes, adhering to a few basic principles will help you improve at the fastest rate, have more fun, and minimize the risk of injury.

Selecting Instructors, Equipment, and Facilities

One of the best places to get help is an exercise class, where an expert instructor can help you learn the basics of training and answer your questions. A qualified personal trainer can also get you started on an exercise program or a new form of training. Make sure that your instructor or trainer has proper qualifications, such as a college degree in exercise physiology or physical education and certification by the American College of Sports Medicine (ACSM), National Strength and Conditioning Association (NSCA), or another professional organization.

Many Web sites provide fitness programs, including ongoing support and feedback via e-mail. Many of these sites charge a fee, so it is important to review the sites, decide which ones seem most appropriate, and if possible go through a free trial period before subscribing. Also remember to consider the reliability of the information at fitness Web sites, especially those that also advertise or sell products.

If you plan to purchase equipment, try to buy the best you can afford. Good equipment will enhance your enjoyment and decrease your risk of injury. Appropriate safety equipment, such as pads and helmets for in-line skating, is particularly important. Before you invest in a new piece of equipment, try it out at a local gym to make sure that you'll use it regularly. Footwear is an important piece of equipment for almost any activity (see the box "Choosing Exercise Footwear").

If you are thinking of joining a health club or fitness center, be sure to choose one that has the right programs and equipment available at the times you will use them. Also make sure the facility is certified; look for the displayed names American College of Sports Medicine (ACSM); National Strength and Conditioning Association (NSCA); American Council on Exercise (ACE); Aerobics and Fitness Association of America (AFAA); or International Health, Racquet, and Sportsclub Association (IHRSA). These trade associations have established standards to help protect consumer health, safety, and rights. Ask for a free trial workout, a 1-day pass, or an inexpensive 1- to 2-week trial membership before committing to a long-term contract. Be wary of promotional gimmicks and high-pressure sales tactics.

Eating and Drinking for Exercise

Most people do not need to change their eating habits when they begin a fitness program. In almost every case, a well-balanced diet contains all the energy and nutrients needed to sustain an exercise program. A balanced diet is also the key to improving your body composition when you begin to exercise more. One of the promises of a fitness program is a decrease in body fat and an increase in muscle mass. The best way to control body fat is to follow a reduced-calorie diet and to be physically active.

One of the most important principles to follow when exercising is to drink enough water. Sweating during exercise depletes the body's water supply and can lead to dehydration if fluids are not replaced. Serious dehydration

Choosing Exercise Footwear

Footwear is perhaps the most important item of equipment for almost any activity. Shoes protect and support your feet and improve your traction. When you jump or run, you place as much as six times more force on your feet than when you stand still. Shoes can help cushion against the stress that this additional force places on your lower legs, thereby preventing injuries. Some athletic shoes are also designed to help prevent ankle rollover, another common source of injury.

General Guidelines

When choosing athletic shoes, first consider the activity you've chosen for your exercise program. Shoes appropriate for different activities have very different characteristics.

Foot type is another important consideration. If your feet tend to roll inward excessively, you may need shoes with additional stability features on the inner side of the shoe to counteract this movement. If your feet tend to roll outward excessively, you may need highly flexible and cushioned shoes that promote foot motion. Most women will get a better fit if they choose shoes that are specifically designed for women's feet rather than downsized versions of men's shoes.

Successful Shopping

For successful shoe shopping, keep the following strategies in mind:

- Shop late in the day or, ideally, following a workout. Your foot size increases over the course of the day and after exercise.

- Wear socks like those you plan to wear during exercise.

- Try on both shoes and wear them around for 10 or more minutes. Try walking on a noncarpeted surface. Approximate the movements of your activity: walk, jog, run, jump, and so on.

- Check the fit and style carefully.

  - Is the toe box roomy enough? Your toes will spread out when your foot hits the ground or you push off. There should be at least one thumb's width of space from the longest toe to the end of the toe box.
  - Do the shoes have enough cushioning? Do your feet feel supported when you bounce up and down? Try bouncing on your toes and on your heels.
  - Do your heels fit snugly into the shoe? Do they stay put when you walk, or do they slide up?
  - Are the arches of your feet right on top of the shoe's arch supports?
  - Do the shoes feel stable when you twist and turn on the balls of your feet? Try twisting from side to side while standing on one foot.
  - Do you feel any pressure points?

- If you exercise at dawn or dusk, choose shoes with reflective sections for added visibility and safety.

- Replace athletic shoes about every 3 months or 300–500 miles of jogging or walking.

---

can cause reduced blood volume, accelerated heart rate, elevated body temperature, muscle cramps, heat stroke, and other serious problems.

During heavy or prolonged exercise or exercise in hot weather, thirst alone isn't a good indication of how much fluid you need to drink. As a rule of thumb, drink at least 2 cups (16 ounces) of fluid 2 hours before exercise and then drink enough during exercise to match fluid loss in sweat—at least 1 cup of fluid every 20–30 minutes of exercise, more in hot weather or if you sweat heavily. To determine if you're drinking the right amount of fluid, weigh yourself before and after an exercise session: Any weight loss is due to fluid loss that needs to be replaced. Any weight gain is due to over-consumption of fluid.

Bring a bottle of water when you exercise so you can replace your fluids when they're depleted (see the box "Bottled Water and the Environment"). For exercise sessions lasting less than 60–90 minutes, cool water is an excellent fluid replacement. For longer workouts, a sports drink that contains water and small amounts of electrolytes (sodium, potassium, and magnesium) and simple carbohydrates (sugar, usually in the form of sucrose or glucose) is recommended.

Managing Your Fitness Program

How can you tell when you're in shape? When do you stop improving and start maintaining? How can you stay motivated? If your program is going to become an integral part of your life, and if the principles behind it are going to serve you well in the future, these are key questions.

Start Slowly, Get in Shape Gradually An exercise program can be divided into three phases:

- *Beginning phase.* The body adjusts to the new type and level of activity.
- *Progress phase.* Fitness increases.
- *Maintenance phase.* The targeted level of fitness is sustained over the long term.

Start slowly to give your body time to adapt to the stress of exercise. Choose activities carefully, according to your fitness status.

Exercising Consistently Steady fitness improvement comes when you overload your body consistently over

Bottled Water and the Environment

Wherever you see people exercising, you will see bottled water in abundance. For several years, however, a debate has been raging about the quality and safety of commercial bottled water, as well its impact on the environment.

Evidence has emerged showing that most bottled waters are no better for you than regular tap water, and some bottled waters may actually be bad for you. In a 2008 analysis, the Environmental Working Group (EWG) found 38 different contaminants in ten popular brands of bottled water. Contaminants included heavy metals such as arsenic, pharmaceutical residues, pollutants commonly found in urban wastewater, and a variety of industrial chemicals.

Government and private agencies have also found that many commercially bottled water products are really just tap water drawn from municipal water systems. These products are priced many times higher (in some cases, 1900 times higher, according to the EWG) than water from a residential tap. They also provide no benefit over standard tap water. For the most part, the tap water supply in the United States is well regulated and very safe.

From an environmental perspective, the enormous popularity of bottled water has turned into an ecological disaster. Plastic water bottles have become a huge solid waste problem, as billions of bottles end up in landfills and the world's oceans every year. Once in a landfill, many kinds of plastic bottles will never decompose at all, although some newer types of bottles (made from corn) are biodegradable. Only 12–20% of plastic water bottles are recycled. Some bottled water producers buy land near natural springs and pump water from them, depleting underground water supplies.

According to estimates published by the Environmental Defense Fund (EDF) in 2008:

● American manufacturers produce about 30 billion plastic water bottles each year, a number that rises annually.

● The manufacturing process uses about 17 million barrels of oil each year—enough to power about a million vehicles for a year. Add the fuel required to transport all those bottles to market, and the energy requirement jumps to nearly 50 million barrels of oil annually.

● Each year, the water bottle manufacturing process releases 2.5 million tons of carbon dioxide (a greenhouse gas) into the atmosphere.

● The process of making a plastic water bottle requires three times more water than the bottle itself will hold.

Government agencies and private businesses are stepping up their efforts to reduce the use of bottled water products. Several small retail grocers, for example, have announced that they will no longer carry water bottled in plastic containers. New York City has implemented a program to place portable drinking fountains all over the city; the fountains draw their water from nearby fire hydrants.

On a larger scale, many experts and environmental advocacy groups are promoting an additional sales tax on water and sodas sold in plastic containers or a return to the old-fashioned deposit system (which allows consumers to return used containers for a refund and ensures that the containers will be recycled). Meanwhile, a national bottle bill is being considered in Congress, which would address the production and reuse of plastic beverage containers.

Consumers can take simple but concrete steps to help reduce the environmental impact of plastic containers:

● Always dispose of containers—whether plastic, glass, or metal—by recycling them.

● Buy a reusable water container (preferably made of stainless steel) that can be cleaned and sterilized after each use and fill it with tap water. If there is a problem with tap water quality or taste, the Sierra Club suggests buying a water filter for your tap water.

● If you buy water in disposable bottles, see what type of material the bottles are made of. A few beverage makers are now using bottles made from 70% traditionally produced plastics and 30% plant-based plastics. The manufacturing process for such bottles requires less petroleum and produces fewer carbon emissions, and the bottles are entirely recyclable.

For a detailed discussion of environmental health—how the environment affects you and how you affect the environment—see Chapter 14.

SOURCES: Environmental Defense Fund. 2008. *Bottles, Bottles, Everywhere . . .* (http://blogs.edf.org/climate411/2008/03/26/bottled_water/?s_src=ggad&s_subsrc=bottled&gclid=CL_Looyj5qlCFY1N2godCkCubg; retrieved July 10, 2010); Environmental Working Group. 2009. *Is Your Bottled Water Worth It?* (http://www.ewg.org/health/report/bottledwater-scorecard; retrieved July 10, 2010); Pacific Institute. 2008. *Bottled Water Fact Sheet* (http://www.pacinst.org/topics/integrity_of_science/case_studies/bottled_water_factsheet.pdf; retrieved July 10, 2010).

Table 10.2 Care of Common Exercise Injuries and Discomforts

INJURY	SYMPTOMS	TREATMENT
Blister	Accumulation of fluid in one spot under the skin	Don't pop or drain it unless it interferes too much with your daily activities. If it does pop, clean the area with antiseptic and cover with a bandage. Do not remove the skin covering the blister.
Bruise (contusion)	Pain, swelling, and discoloration	R-I-C-E: rest, ice, compression, elevation.
Fracture and/or dislocation	Pain, swelling, tenderness, loss of function, and deformity	Seek medical attention, immobilize the affected area, and apply cold.
Joint sprain	Pain, tenderness, swelling, discoloration, and loss of function	R-I-C-E. Apply heat when swelling has disappeared. Stretch and strengthen affected area.
Muscle cramp	Painful, spasmodic muscle contractions	Gently stretch for 15–30 seconds at a time and/or massage the cramped area. Drink fluids and increase dietary salt intake if exercising in hot weather.
Muscle soreness or stiffness	Pain and tenderness in the affected muscle	Stretch the affected muscle gently; exercise at a low intensity; apply heat. Nonsteroidal anti-inflammatory drugs, such as ibuprofen, help some people.
Muscle strain	Pain, tenderness, swelling, and loss of strength in the affected muscle	R-I-C-E; apply heat when swelling has disappeared. Stretch and strengthen the affected area.
Plantar fasciitis	Pain and tenderness in the connective tissue on the bottom of your feet	Apply ice, take nonsteroidal anti-inflammatory drugs, and stretch. Wear night splints when sleeping.
Shin splint	Pain and tenderness on the front of the lower leg; sometimes also pain in the calf muscle	Rest; apply ice to the affected area several times a day and before exercise; wrap with tape for support. Stretch and strengthen muscles in the lower legs. Purchase good-quality footwear and run on soft surfaces.
Side stitch	Pain on the side of the abdomen	Stretch the arm on the affected side as high as possible; if that doesn't help, try bending forward while tightening the abdominal muscles.
Tendinitis	Pain, swelling, and tenderness of the affected area	R-I-C-E; apply heat when swelling has disappeared. Stretch and strengthen the affected area.

SOURCE: Fahey, T. D., P. M. Insel, and W. T. Roth. 2011. *Fit and Well: Core Concepts and Labs in Physical Fitness and Wellness,* 9th ed. New York: McGraw-Hill. Copyright © 2011 The McGraw-Hill Companies, Inc.

time. The best way to ensure consistency is to record the details of your workouts in a journal: how far you ran, how much weight you lifted, and so on. This record will help you evaluate your progress and plan workout sessions intelligently. Don't increase your exercise volume by more than 5–10% per week.

Assessing Your Fitness   When are you in shape? It depends. One person may be out of shape running a mile in 5 minutes; another may be in shape running a mile in 12 minutes. Your ultimate level of fitness depends on your goals, your program, and your natural ability. The important thing is to set goals that make sense for you. If you are interested in finding out exactly how fit you are before you begin a program, the best approach is to get an assessment from a sports medicine laboratory.

Preventing and Managing Athletic Injuries   It is important to learn how to deal with injuries so they don't derail your fitness program or escalate into a chronic problem (Table 10.2). Some injuries require medical attention. See a physician for head and eye injuries, possible ligament injuries, broken bones, and internal disorders such as chest pain, fainting, and intolerance

to heat. Also seek medical attention for apparently minor injuries that do not get better within a reasonable amount of time.

For minor cuts and scrapes, stop the bleeding and clean the wound with soap and water. Treat soft tissue injuries (muscles and joints) with the R-I-C-E principle:

Rest: Stop using the injured area as soon as you experience pain, protect it from further injury, and avoid any activity that causes pain.

Ice: Apply ice to the injured area to reduce swelling and alleviate pain. Apply ice immediately for 10–20 minutes, and repeat every few hours until the swelling disappears. Let the injured part return to normal temperature between icings, and do not apply ice to one area for more than 20 minutes (10 minutes if you are using a cold gel pack).

Compression: Wrap the injured area with an elastic or compression bandage between icings. If the area starts throbbing or begins to change color, the bandage may be wrapped too tightly. Do not sleep with the bandage on.

Elevation: Raise the injured area above heart level to decrease the blood supply and reduce swelling.

After 36–48 hours, apply heat, if the swelling has disappeared, to relieve pain, relax muscles, and reduce stiffness. Immerse the affected area in warm water or apply warm compresses, a hot water bottle, or a heating pad.

To prevent injuries in the future, follow a few basic guidelines:

- Stay in condition; haphazard exercise programs invite injury.
- Warm up thoroughly before exercise.
- Use proper body mechanics when lifting objects or executing sports skills.
- Don't exercise when you're ill or overtrained (experiencing extreme fatigue due to overexercising).
- Use the proper equipment.
- Don't return to your normal exercise program until athletic injuries have healed.

You can minimize the risk of injury by following safety guidelines, respecting signals from your body that something may be wrong, and treating injuries promptly. Use special caution in extreme heat or humidity (over 80°F and/or 60% humidity): Exercise slowly, rest frequently in the shade, wear clothing that breathes, and drink plenty of fluids. Slow down or stop if you begin to feel uncomfortable. During hot weather, exercise in the early morning or evening, when temperatures are lowest.

Staying with Your Program Once you have attained your desired level of fitness, you can maintain it by exercising regularly at a consistent intensity, 3 to 5 days a week. In general, if you exercise at the same intensity over a long period, your fitness will level out and can be maintained easily.

Adapt your program to changes in environment or schedule. Don't use wet weather or a new job as an excuse to give up your fitness program. If you walk in the summer, dress appropriately and walk in the winter as well. If you can't go out because of darkness or an unsafe neighborhood, walk in a local shopping mall or on campus or join a gym and walk on a treadmill.

What if you run out of steam? Although good health is an important *reason* to exercise, it's a poor *motivator*. It's a good idea to have a meaningful goal, anything from fitting into the same-size jeans you used to wear to successfully skiing down a new slope.

Varying your program is another key strategy. Some people alternate two or more activities—swimming and jogging, for example—to improve a particular component of fitness. The practice, called **cross-training**, can help prevent boredom and overuse injuries. Try new activities, especially ones that you will be able to do for the rest of your life.

TIPS FOR TODAY AND THE FUTURE

Physical activity and exercise offer benefits in nearly every area of wellness. Even a low to moderate level of activity provides valuable health benefits.

RIGHT NOW YOU CAN

- Go outside and take a brisk 15-minute walk.
- Look at your calendar for the rest of the week and write in some physical activity—such as walking, running, or playing Frisbee—on as many days as you can. Schedule the activity for a specific time and stick to it.
- Call a friend and invite him or her to start planning a regular exercise program with you.

IN THE FUTURE YOU CAN

- Schedule a session with a qualified personal trainer who can evaluate your current fitness level and help you set personalized fitness goals.
- Create seasonal workout programs for the summer, spring, fall, and winter. Develop programs that are varied but consistent with your overall fitness goals.

Connect to Your Choices

Have you ever thought about how you came to have the physical activity patterns you have? Many factors can influence our physical activity and exercise choices, some not as obvious as others. Was your family physically active when you were growing up? Do you have access to a fitness center or facilities and equipment for working out? Do you hang out with people who make physical activity part of their daily lives—or with couch potatoes?

What are the external factors that influence your choices about exercise? What are your inner motivations and core values, and how do they affect your choices? Based on what you learned in this chapter, will you make some different choices in the future? If so, what will they be?

Go online to Connect to complete this activity. www.mcgraw-hillconnect.com

Ask Yourself

QUESTIONS FOR CRITICAL THINKING AND REFLECTION

Have you ever suffered an injury while exercising? If so, how did you treat the injury? Compare your treatment with the guidelines given in this chapter. Did you do the right things? What can you do to avoid such injuries in the future?

cross-training Participating in two or more activities to develop a particular component of fitness.

TERMS

Planning a Personal Exercise Program

Although most people recognize the importance of incorporating exercise into their lives, many find it difficult to do. No single strategy will work for everyone, but the general steps outlined here should help you create an exercise program that fits your goals, preferences, and lifestyle. A carefully designed contract and program plan can help you convert your vague wishes into a detailed plan of action. And the strategies for program compliance outlined here and in Chapter 1 can help you enjoy and stick with your program for the rest of your life.

Step 1: Set Goals

Setting specific goals to accomplish by exercising is an important first step in a successful fitness program because it establishes the direction you want to take. Your goals might be specifically related to health, such as lowering your blood pressure and risk of heart disease, or they might relate to other aspects of your life, such as improving your tennis game or the fit of your clothes. If you can decide why you're starting to exercise, it can help you keep going.

Step 2: Select Activities

As discussed in the chapter, the success of your fitness program depends on the consistency of your involvement. Select activities that encourage your commitment: The right program will be its own incentive to continue; poor activity choices provide obstacles and can turn exercise into a chore.

When choosing activities for your fitness program, consider the following:

- Is this activity fun? Will it hold my interest over time?
- Will this activity help me reach the goals I have set?

- Will my current fitness and skill level enable me to participate fully in this activity?
- Can I easily fit this activity into my daily schedule? Are there any special requirements (facilities, partners, equipment, etc.) that I must plan for?
- Can I afford any special costs required for equipment or facilities?
- If you have special exercise needs due to a particular health problem: Does this activity conform to those exercise needs? Will it enhance my ability to cope with my specific health problem?

Using the guidelines listed above, select a number of sports and activities.

Step 3: Make a Commitment

To affirm your commitment, sign a contract like the one shown in Chapter 1 and have a friend sign it as a witness. By completing a contract, you make a firm commitment and will be more likely to follow through until you meet your goals.

Step 4: Begin and Maintain Your Program

Start out slowly to allow your body time to adjust. Be realistic and patient—meeting your goals will take time. The following guidelines may help you start and stick with your program:

- Set aside regular periods for exercise. Choose times that fit in best with your schedule, and stick to them. Allow an adequate amount of time for warm-up, cool-down, and a shower.
- Take advantage of any opportunity for exercise that presents itself (for example,

walk to class, take the stairs instead of the elevator).
- Do what you can to avoid boredom. Do stretching exercises or jumping jacks to music, or watch the evening news while riding your stationary bicycle.
- Exercise with a group that shares your goals and general level of competence.
- Vary the program. Change your activities periodically. Alter your route or distance if biking or jogging. Change racquetball partners, or find a new volleyball court.
- Establish minigoals or a point system, and work rewards into your program. Until you reach your main goals, a series of small rewards will help you stick with your program. Rewards should be things you enjoy that are easily obtainable.

Step 5: Record and Assess Your Progress

Keeping a record that notes the daily results of your program will help remind you of your ongoing commitment to your program and give you a sense of accomplishment. Create daily and weekly program logs that you can use to track your progress. Record the activity frequency, intensity, time, and type. Keep your log handy, and fill it in immediately after each exercise session. Post it in a visible place to remind you of your activity schedule and to provide incentive for improvement.

SOURCE: Adapted from Kusinitz, I., and M. Fine. 1995. *Your Guide to Getting Fit,* 3rd ed. Mountain View, Calif.: Mayfield.

SUMMARY

- The five components of physical fitness most important to health are cardiorespiratory endurance, muscular strength, muscular endurance, flexibility, and body composition.

- Exercise improves the functioning of the heart and the ability of the cardiorespiratory system to carry oxygen to the body's

tissues. It also increases metabolic efficiency and improves body composition.

- Exercise lowers the risk of cardiovascular disease, cancer, osteoporosis, and diabetes. It improves immune function and psychological health and helps prevent injuries and low-back pain.

- Everyone should accumulate at 150 minutes per week of moderate-intensity physical activity or 75 minutes per week of vigorous-intensity physical activity. Additional health and fitness benefits can be achieved through longer or more vigorous activity.

- Cardiorespiratory endurance exercises stress a large portion of the body's muscle mass. Endurance exercise should be performed 3–5 days per week for a total of 20–60 minutes per day. Intensity can be evaluated by measuring the heart rate.

- Warming up before exercising and cooling down afterward improve your performance and decrease your chances of injury.

- Exercises that develop muscular strength and endurance involve exerting force against a significant resistance. A strength training program for general fitness typically involves one set of 8–12 repetitions of 8–10 exercises, at least 2 nonconsecutive days per week.

- A good stretching program includes exercises for all the major muscle groups and joints of the body. Do a series of active, static stretches at least 2–3 days per week. Hold each stretch for 15–30 seconds; do two to four repetitions. Stretch when muscles are warm.

- Instructors, equipment, and facilities should be chosen carefully to enhance enjoyment and prevent injuries.

- A well-balanced diet contains all the energy and nutrients needed to sustain a fitness program. When exercising, remember to drink enough fluids.

- Rest, ice, compression, and elevation (R-I-C-E) are treatments for minor muscle and joint injuries.

FOR MORE INFORMATION

BOOKS

Anderson, B. 2010. *Stretching: 30th Anniversary Edition.* Bolinas, Calif.: Shelter Publications. *An illustrated guide to stretching for the layperson, with stretches grouped by activity and sport; includes a section on office fitness.*

Fahey, T. 2011. *Basic Weight Training for Men and Women,* 7th ed. New York: McGraw-Hill. *Weight training and plyometric exercises for fitness, weight control, and improved sports performance.*

Fahey, T., P. Insel, and W. Roth. 2011. *Fit and Well: Core Concepts and Labs in Physical Fitness and Wellness,* 9th ed. New York: McGraw-Hill. *A comprehensive guide to developing a complete fitness program.*

Fenton, M. 2008. *The Complete Guide to Walking, New and Revised: For Health, Weight Loss, and Fitness.* Guildford, Conn.: Lyons Press. *Discusses walking as a fitness method and a way to avoid diseases such as diabetes.*

Gotlin, R. 2007. *Sport Injuries Guidebook.* Champaign, Ill.: Human Kinetics. *Provides information and care instructions on many types of sports-related injuries.*

Nieman, D. C. 2007. *Exercise Testing and Prescription. A Health-Related Approach,* 6th ed. New York: McGraw-Hill. *A comprehensive discussion of the effects of exercise and exercise testing and prescription.*

Woods, R., and C. Jordon. 2010. *Energy Every Day.* Champaign, Ill.: Human Kinetics. *A sensible guide to fitness and nutrition.*

ORGANIZATIONS, HOTLINES, AND WEB SITES

American Academy of Orthopaedic Surgeons. Provides fact sheets on many fitness and sports topics, including how to begin a program, how to choose equipment, and how to prevent and treat many types of injuries.

http://orthoinfo.aaos.org

American College of Sports Medicine. Provides brochures, publications, and audio- and videotapes on the positive effects of exercise.

http://www.acsm.org

American Heart Association: MyStart! Provides practical advice for people of all fitness levels plus an online fitness diary.

http://www.americanheart.org/presenter.jhtml?identifier=3040839

CDC Physical Activity Information. Provides information on the benefits of physical activity and suggestions for incorporating moderate physical activity into daily life.

http://www.cdc.gov/nccdphp/dnpa

Disabled Sports USA. Provides sport and recreation services to people with physical or mobility disorders.

http://www.dsusa.org

National Institute on Drug Abuse: Anabolic Steroid Abuse. Provides information and links about the dangers of anabolic steroids.

http://www.steroidabuse.org

President's Council on Physical Fitness and Sports (PCPFS). Provides information on PCPFS programs and publications.

http://www.fitness.gov
http://www.presidentschallenge.org

SmallStep.gov. Provides resources for increasing activity and improving diet through small changes in daily habits.

http://www.smallstep.gov

SELECTED BIBLIOGRAPHY

American College of Sports Medicine. 2009. *ACSM's Guidelines for Exercise Testing and Prescription,* 8th ed. Philadelphia: Lippincott Williams & Wilkins.

American College of Sports Medicine. 2009. *ACSM's Resource Manual for Guidelines for Exercise Testing and Prescription,* 6th ed. Philadelphia: Lippincott Williams & Wilkins.

American Heart Association. 2010. *Heart Disease and Stroke Statistics—2010 Update.* Dallas: American Heart Association.

Brooks, G. A., et al. 2005. *Exercise Physiology: Human Bioenergetics and Its Applications,* 4th ed. New York: McGraw-Hill.

Blair, S. N., and J. N. Morris. 2009. Healthy hearts—and the universal benefits of being physically active: Physical activity and health. *Annals of Epidemiology* 19(4): 253–256.

Brownson, R. C., T. K. Boehmer, and D. A. Luke. 2005. Declining rates of physical activity in the United States: What are the contributors? *Annual Review of Public Health* 26: 421–443.

Burns, R. W. 2010. Exercise guidelines for adults: Past, present & future. *Missouri Medical Journal* 107(1): 65–68.

Centers for Disease Control and Prevention. 2008. Prevalence of self-reported physically active adults—United States, 2007. *Morbidity and Mortality Weekly Report* 57(48): 1297–1300.

Fahey, T. D., P. M. Insel, and W. T. Roth. 2011. *Fit and Well: Core Concepts and Labs in Physical Fitness and Wellness,* 9th ed. New York: McGraw-Hill.

Hamer, M., and G. O'Donovan. 2010. Cardiorespiratory fitness and metabolic risk factors in obesity. *Current Opinion Lipidology* 21(1): 1–7.

Haskell, W. L., et al. 2007. Physical activity and public health: Updated recommendations for adults from the American College of Sports Medicine and the American Heart Association. *Circulation* 116(9): 1081–1093.

Janiszewski, P. M., and R. Ross. 2009. The utility of physical activity in the management of global cardiometabolic risk. *Obesity* 17(Suppl. 3): s3–s14.

Kloubec, J. A. 2010. Pilates for improvement of muscle endurance, flexibility, balance, and posture, *Journal of Strength Conditioning Research* 24(3): 661–667.

Kohler, J. M., S. P. Flanagan, and W. C. Whiting. 2010. Muscle activation patterns while lifting stable and unstable loads on stable and unstable surfaces. *Journal of Strength Conditioning Research* 24(2): 313–321.

Lanza, I. R., and K. S. Nair. 2010. Mitochondrial function as a determinant of life span. *Pflugers Archives* 459(2): 277–289.

Larson-Meyer, D. E., et al. 2010. Caloric restriction with or without exercise: The fitness versus fatness debate. *Medicine and Science in Sports Exercise* 42(1): 152–159.

Lum, D., G. Landers, and P. Peeling. 2010. Effects of a recovery swim on subsequent running performance. *International Journal of Sports Medicine* 31(1): 26–30.

McAuley, P. A., et al. 2010. Obesity paradox and cardiorespiratory fitness in 12,417 male veterans aged 40 to 70 years. *Mayo Clinic Proceedings* 85(2): 115–121.

McGill, S. M. 2010. Core training: Evidence translating to better performance and injury prevention. *Strength and Conditioning Journal* 32(3): 33–46.

McGill, S. M., and A. Karpowicz. 2009. Exercises for spine stabilization: Motion/motor patterns, stability progressions and clinical technique. *Archives of Physical Medicine and Rehabilitation* 90: 118–126.

Nelson, M. E., et al. 2007. Physical activity and public health in older adults: Recommendations from the American College of Sports Medicine and the American Heart Association. *Medicine and Science in Sports and Exercise* 39(8): 1435–1445.

Pescatello, L. S., et al. 2004. American College of Sports Medicine position stand: Exercise and hypertension. *Medicine and Science in Sports and Exercise* 36(3): 533–553.

U.S. Department of Health and Human Services. 2008. *2008 Physical Activity Guidelines for Americans.* Hyattsville, Md.: U.S. Department of Health and Human Services. ODPHP Publication U0036.

U.S. Department of Health and Human Services. 2010. *The Surgeon General's Vision for a Healthy and Fit Nation.* Rockville, Md.: U.S. Department of Health and Human Services, Office of the Surgeon General.

Warner, S. O., et al. 2010. The effects of resistance training on metabolic health with weight regain. *Journal of Clinical Hypertension* 12(1): 64–72.

Willis, F. B. 2009. Frequency of exercise for body fat loss: A controlled, cohort study. *Journal of Strength Conditioning Research* 23(8): 2377–2380.

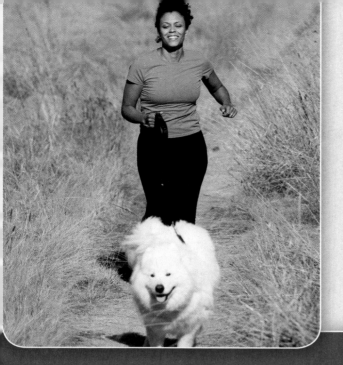

LOOKING AHEAD...

After reading this chapter, you should be [...]:

- Discuss different methods for assessing body w[...] and body composition

- Explain the health risks associated with overweight and obesity

- Explain factors that may contribute to a weight problem, including genetic, physiological, lifestyle, and psychosocial factors

- Describe lifestyle factors that contribute to weight gain and loss, including the roles of diet, exercise, and emotional factors

- Identify and describe the symptoms of eating disorders and the health risks associated with them

- Design a personal plan for successfully managing body weight

Weight Management

11

Achieving and maintaining a healthy body weight are a serious public health challenge and a source of distress for many Americans. Under standards developed by the National Institutes of Health (NIH), about 68% of American adults are overweight, including more than 33.8% who are obese (Figure 11.1). In 2007–2008, 32.2% of adult men and 35.5% of adult women were obese. And while millions struggle to lose weight, others fall into dangerous eating patterns such as binge eating or self-starvation.

Although not completely understood, managing body weight is not a mysterious process. It's basically a matter of balancing calories consumed with calories expended in daily activities—in other words, eating a moderate diet and being physically active. Successful weight management requires the long-term coordination of many aspects of a wellness lifestyle, including nutrition, physical activity, and stress management.

This chapter explores the factors that contribute to the development of overweight and to eating disorders. It also takes a closer look at weight management through lifestyle behaviors and suggests specific strategies for reaching and maintaining a healthy weight.

BASIC CONCEPTS OF WEIGHT MANAGEMENT

If you are like most people, you are concerned about your weight. But at what point does being overweight present a health risk? And how thin is too thin?

Body Composition

The human body can be divided into fat-free mass and body fat. Fat-free mass is composed of all the body's non-fat tissues: bone, water, muscle, connective tissue, organ tissues, and teeth. A certain amount of body fat is necessary for the body to function. Fat is incorporated into the nerves, brain, heart, lungs, liver, mammary glands, and other organs and tissues. It is the main source of stored energy in the body; it also cushions body organs and helps regulate body temperature. This **essential fat** makes up about 3–5% of total body weight in men and about 8–12% in women. The percentage is higher in women because of fat deposits in the breast, uterus, and other sex-specific sites.

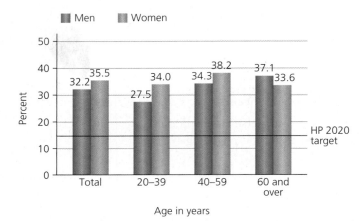

FIGURE 11.1 Obesity prevalence, by age and sex, of American adults, 2007–2008. *Healthy People 2020* sets a target obesity prevalence of not greater than 15% for all adults.

SOURCE: Flegal, K. M., et al. 2010. Prevalence and trends in obesity among U.S. adults, 1998–2008. *Journal of the American Medical Association* 303(3): 235–241.

Most of the fat in the body is stored in fat cells, or **adipose tissue,** located under the skin (**subcutaneous fat**) and around major organs (**visceral fat** or *intra-abdominal fat*). People have a genetically determined number of fat cells, but these cells can increase or decrease in size depending on several factors, including age, sex, metabolism, diet, and activity level. The primary source of excess body fat is excess calories consumed in the diet—that is, calories consumed in excess of calories expended in metabolism, physical activity, and exercise.

A pound of body fat is equal to 3500 calories. If you take in 100 calories per day in excess of the calories you expend, you will gain 10 pounds in a year.

What is most important for health is not total weight, however, but rather the proportion of the body's total weight that is fat—the **percent body fat.** For example, two women may both be 5 feet, 5 inches tall and weigh 130 pounds. But one woman, an endurance runner, may have only 15% of her body weight as fat, whereas the other woman, who is sedentary, may have 34% body fat. Although 130 pounds is not considered overweight for

ENERGY IN
Food calories

ENERGY OUT
Physical activity 20–30%
Food digestion ±10%
Resting metabolism 65–7

FIGURE 11.2 The energy balance equation.

women of this height by most standards, the sedentary woman may be overfat.

Too much body fat (not total weight) has a negative effect on health and well-being. Just as the amount of body fat is important, so is its location on your body. Visceral fat is more harmful to health than subcutaneous fat.

Overweight is usually defined as total body weight above the recommended range for good health (as determined by large-scale population surveys). **Obesity** is defined as a more serious degree of overweight. Many methods are available for measuring and evaluating body weight and percent body fat, and the cutoff points for defining overweight and obesity vary with the method chosen.

Energy Balance

The key to keeping a healthy ratio of fat to fat-free mass is maintaining an energy balance (Figure 11.2). You take in energy (calories) from the food you eat. Your body uses energy (calories) to maintain vital body functions (resting metabolism), to digest food, and to fuel physical activity. When energy in equals energy out, you maintain your current weight. To change your

In 1960, **13%** of adult Americans were obese. In 2008, nearly **34%** were obese.

—National Center for Health Statistics, 2010

weight and body composition, you must tip the energy balance equation in a particular direction. If you take in more calories daily than your body burns, the excess calories will be stored as fat and you will gain weight over

---

TERMS

essential fat   The fat incorporated in various tissues of the body; critical for normal body functioning.

adipose tissue   Connective tissue in which fat is stored.

subcutaneous fat   Fat located under the skin.

visceral fat   Fat located around major organs, also called *intra-abdominal fat.*

percent body fat   The percentage of total body weight that is composed of fat.

overweight   Body weight above the recommended range for good health.

obesity   Severe overweight, characterized by an excessive accumulation of body fat.

	<18.5 Underweight		18.5–24.9 Normal						25–29.9 Overweight					30–34.9 Obesity (Class I)					35–39.9 Obesity (Class II)					≥40 Extreme obesity
BMI	17	18	19	20	21	22	23	24	25	26	27	28	29	30	31	32	33	34	35	36	37	38	39	40
Height							Body Weight (pounds)																	
10"	81	86	91	96	101	105	110	115	120	124	129	134	139	144	148	153	158	163	168	172	177	182	187	192
11"	84	89	94	99	104	109	114	119	124	129	134	139	144	149	154	159	163	168	173	178	183	188	193	198
	87	92	97	102	108	113	118	123	128	133	138	143	149	154	159	164	169	174	179	184	190	195	200	205
1"	90	95	101	106	111	117	122	127	132	138	143	148	154	159	164	169	175	180	185	191	196	201	207	212
2"	93	98	104	109	115	120	126	131	137	142	148	153	159	164	170	175	181	186	191	197	202	208	213	219
3"	96	102	107	113	119	124	130	136	141	147	153	158	164	169	175	181	186	192	198	203	209	215	220	226
4"	99	105	111	117	122	128	134	140	146	152	157	163	169	175	181	187	192	198	204	210	216	222	227	233
5"	102	108	114	120	126	132	138	144	150	156	162	168	174	180	186	192	198	204	210	216	222	229	235	241
6"	105	112	118	124	130	136	143	149	155	161	167	174	180	186	192	198	205	211	217	223	229	236	242	248
7"	109	115	121	128	134	141	147	153	160	166	173	179	185	192	198	204	211	217	224	230	236	243	249	256
8"	112	118	125	132	138	145	151	158	165	171	178	184	191	197	204	211	217	224	230	237	244	250	257	263
9"	115	122	129	136	142	149	156	163	169	176	183	190	197	203	210	217	224	230	237	244	251	258	264	271
10"	119	126	133	139	146	153	160	167	174	181	188	195	202	209	216	223	230	237	244	251	258	265	272	279
11"	122	129	136	143	151	158	165	172	179	187	194	201	208	215	222	230	237	244	251	258	265	273	280	287
	125	133	140	148	155	162	170	177	184	192	199	207	214	221	229	236	243	251	258	266	273	280	288	295
1"	129	137	144	152	159	167	174	182	190	197	205	212	220	228	235	243	250	258	265	273	281	288	296	303
2"	132	140	148	156	164	171	179	187	195	203	210	218	226	234	242	249	257	265	273	281	288	296	304	312
3"	136	144	152	160	168	176	184	192	200	208	216	224	232	240	248	256	264	272	280	288	296	304	312	320
4"	140	148	156	164	173	181	189	197	206	214	222	230	238	247	255	263	271	280	288	296	304	312	321	329

FIGURE 11.3 Body mass index (BMI). To determine your BMI, find your height in the left column. Move across the appropriate row until you find the weight closest to your own. The number at the top of the column is the BMI at that height and weight.

SOURCE: Ratings from National Heart, Lung, and Blood Institute. 1998. *Clinical Guidelines on the Identification, Evaluation, and Treatment of Overweight and Obesity in Adults: The Evidence Report.* Bethesda, Md.: National Institutes of Health.

time. If you eat fewer calories than you burn each day, you will lose some of the stored fat and probably lose weight.

Our environment is rich in large portion sizes; high-fat, high-calorie foods; and palatable, easily available, and inexpensive foods. Unfortunately, we've decreased work-related physical activity, decreased activity associated with daily living, and increased time spent in sedentary pastimes like TV watching and computer use. The good news, however, is that you control both parts of the energy balance equation.

Evaluating Body Weight and Body Composition

Although a scale can tell your total weight, it can't differentiate between overweight and overfat. These are several simple, inexpensive ways to estimate body weight and body composition.

Body Mass Index   Body mass index (BMI) is a measure of body weight that is useful for classifying the health risks of body weight if you don't have access to more sophisticated methods. BMI is based on the concept that weight should be proportional to height. Easy to calculate and rate, BMI is a fairly accurate measure of the health risks of body weight for average people.

You can look up your BMI by using the chart in Figure 11.3, or use the following formula to calculate it more precisely.

1. Divide your body weight in pounds by 2.2 to convert the amount to kilograms.
2. Multiply your height in inches by 0.0254 to convert the amount to meters.
3. Multiply the result of step 2 by itself to get the square of the height measurement.
4. Divide the result of step 1 by the result of step 3 to determine your BMI.

Under standards issued by the National Institutes of Health, a BMI between 18.5 and 24.9 is considered healthy; a person with a BMI of 25 or above is classified as overweight, and a person with a BMI of 30 or above is classified as obese. A person with a BMI below 18.5 is classified as underweight, although low BMI values may be healthy in some cases if they are not the result of smoking, an eating disorder, or an underlying disease; a BMI of 17.5 or less is sometimes used as a diagnostic criterion for the eating disorder anorexia nervosa.

> **body mass index (BMI)**   A measure of relative body weight that takes height into account and is highly correlated with more direct measures of body fat; calculated by dividing total body weight (in kilograms) by the square of height (in meters).

TERMS

Table 11.1	Body Composition Ratings Based on Percent Body Fat	
	PERCENT BODY FAT	
CATEGORY	MALES	FEMALES
Normal	12–20%	20–30%
Borderline	21–25%	31–33%
Obese	>25%	>33%

SOURCE: Bray, G. A. 2003. *Contemporary Diagnosis and Management of Obesity and the Metabolic Syndrome*, 3rd ed. Newton, Pa.: Handbooks in Health Care.

Calipers are used to perform skinfold measurements, which is a simple and inexpensive way to determine body fat levels.

The use of BMI has some drawbacks. Because BMI does not distinguish between fat weight and fat-free weight, it can be very inaccurate for some groups, including short people (under 5 feet tall), muscular athletes, and older adults with little muscle mass. If you are in one of these groups, use one of the methods described in the next section for estimating percent body fat to assess whether your current weight and body composition are healthy. BMI is also not particularly useful for tracking changes in body composition—gains in muscle mass and losses of fat. Women are likely to have more body fat for a given BMI than men.

Body Composition Analysis The most accurate and direct way to evaluate body composition is to determine percent body fat. See Table 11.1 for body composition ratings based on percent body fat.

HYDROSTATIC WEIGHING AND BOD POD In hydrostatic (underwater) weighing, a person is submerged and weighed under water. Percent body fat can be calculated from body density. Muscle has a higher density and fat a lower density than water, so people with more fat tend to float and weigh less under water, while lean people tend to sink and weigh more under water. A specialized body composition analysis device called the Bod Pod uses air instead of water. A person sits in a chamber, and computerized pressure sensors determine the amount of air displaced by the person's body.

> *To be accurate, body composition measurements must be done by someone with appropriate training.*

SKINFOLD MEASUREMENTS The skinfold thickness technique measures the thickness of fat under the skin. Measurements are taken at several sites and plugged into formulas that calculate body fat percentages.

BIOELECTRICAL IMPEDANCE ANALYSIS (BIA) In this method, electrodes are attached to the body and a harmless electrical current is transmitted from electrode to electrode. The electrical conduction through the body favors the path of the fat-free tissues over the fat tissues. A computer can calculate fat percentages from measurements of current.

Excess Body Fat and Wellness

The amount of fat in the body—and its location—can have profound effects on health.

The Health Risks of Excess Body Fat Obesity doubles mortality rates and can reduce life expectancy by 10–20 years. If the current trends continue, scientists believe that the average American's life expectancy will soon decline by 5 years. Obesity is associated with unhealthy cholesterol and triglyceride levels, impaired heart function, and death from cardiovascular disease. Other health risks include hypertension, many kinds of cancer, impaired immune function, gallbladder and kidney diseases, skin problems, impotence, sleep and breathing disorders, back pain, arthritis, and other bone and joint disorders. Obesity is also associated with complications of pregnancy, menstrual irregularities, urine leakage (stress incontinence), and increased surgical risk.

There is a strong association between excess body fat and **diabetes mellitus**, a disease that causes a disruption of normal metabolism. The pancreas normally secretes the hormone insulin, which stimulates cells to take up blood sugar (glucose) to produce energy. In diabetes, this process is disrupted, causing a buildup of glucose in the bloodstream (see page T2-5 of the transparency insert "Touring the Cardiorespiratory System" in Chapter 12). Diabetes is associated with kidney failure; nerve damage; circulation problems and amputations; retinal damage and blindness; and increased rates of heart attack, stroke, and hypertension (see the box "Diabetes").

The risks from obesity increase with its severity, and they are much more likely to occur in people who are more than twice their desirable body weight. The NIH recommends weight loss for people whose BMI places them in the obese category and for those who are overweight *and* have two or more major risk factors for disease. If your BMI is 25 or above, consult a physician for help in determining a healthy BMI for you.

The Nurses' Health Study, in which Harvard researchers have followed more than 120,000 women since 1976,

> ## About **10%** of infants and toddlers have BMIs above the normal range, as do **18%** of teenagers.
> —CDC, 2010

has found that even mildly to moderately overweight women have an 80% increased risk of developing coronary heart disease compared to leaner women. This study also confirmed that to reduce the risk of dying prematurely of any cause, maintaining a desirable body weight is important. But it is also important to realize that small weight losses— 5–10% of total body weight—can lead to significant health improvements.

Body Fat Distribution and Health   The distribution of body fat is also an important indicator of health. Men and postmenopausal women tend to store fat in the upper regions of their bodies, particularly in the abdominal area (the apple shape). Premenopausal women usually store fat in hips, buttocks, and thighs (the pear shape). Excess fat in the abdominal area increases risk of high blood pressure, diabetes, early-onset heart disease, stroke, certain types of cancer, and mortality. It appears that abdominal fat is more easily mobilized and sent into the bloodstream, increasing disease-related blood fat levels.

> *Abdominal obesity is a primary component of metabolic syndrome and a forewarning of diabetes and heart disease.*

Ask Yourself

QUESTIONS FOR CRITICAL THINKING AND REFLECTION

Calculate or look up your BMI, then compare it with the BMIs of some classmates. Do the results surprise you? How well do you think BMI reflects body composition? Why do you think it is such a commonly used measure?

The risks from body fat distribution are usually assessed by measuring waist circumference (the distance around the abdomen at the level of the hip bone). A total waist measurement of more than 40 inches for men and 35 inches for women is associated with a significantly increased risk of disease. Large waist circumference can be a marker for increased risk of diabetes, high blood pressure, and CVD even in people with a BMI in the normal range.

Body Image   The collective picture of the body as seen through the mind's eye, **body image** consists of perceptions, images, thoughts, attitudes, and emotions. A negative body image is characterized by dissatisfaction with the body in general or some part of the body in particular. Recent surveys indicate that the majority of Americans, many of whom are not actually overweight, are unhappy with their body weight or with some aspect of their appearance.

Losing weight or getting cosmetic surgery does not necessarily improve body image. However, improvements in body image may occur in the absence of changes in weight or appearance. Many experts now believe that body image issues must be dealt with as part of treating obesity and eating disorders.

Problems Associated with Very Low Levels of Body Fat   Health experts have generally viewed very low levels of body fat—less than 8–12% for women and 3–5% for men—as a threat to wellness. Extreme leanness has been linked with reproductive, circulatory, and immune system disorders. Extremely lean people may experience muscle wasting and fatigue; they are also more likely to suffer from dangerous eating disorders.

In physically active women and girls, particularly those involved in sports where weight and appearance are important (ballet, gymnastics, skating, and distance running,

> **diabetes mellitus**   A disease that disrupts normal metabolism, interfering with cells' ability to take in glucose for energy production.
>
> **body image**   The mental representation a person holds about his or her body at any given moment in time, consisting of perceptions, images, thoughts, attitudes, and emotions about the body.

IN FOCUS

Types of Diabetes

About 24 million Americans (or 8% of the population) have one of two major forms of diabetes. About 5–10% of people with diabetes have the more serious form, known as *type 1 diabetes*. In this type of diabetes, the pancreas produces little or no insulin, so daily doses of insulin are required. Type 1 diabetes occurs when the body's immune system, triggered by a viral infection or some other environmental factor, mistakenly destroys the insulin-producing cells in the pancreas. It usually strikes before age 30.

The remaining 90–95% of Americans with diabetes have *type 2 diabetes,* and the prevalence is rising dramatically. This condition can develop slowly, and about 25% of affected individuals are unaware of their condition. In type 2 diabetes, the pancreas doesn't produce enough insulin, cells are resistant to insulin, or both. This condition is usually diagnosed in people over age 40, although there has been a tenfold increase in type 2 diabetes in children in the past two decades. About one-third of people with type 2 diabetes must take insulin; others may take medications that increase insulin production or stimulate cells to take up glucose.

A third type of diabetes occurs in about 7% of women during pregnancy. *Gestational diabetes* usually disappears after pregnancy, but more than half of women who experience it eventually develop type 2 diabetes.

The term *pre-diabetes* describes blood glucose levels that are higher than normal but not high enough for a diagnosis of full-blown diabetes. About 57 million Americans have pre-diabetes, and most people with the condition will develop type 2 diabetes unless they adopt preventive lifestyle measures. Pre-diabetes poses a risk to health beyond just the development of diabetes: Blood glucose levels in the pre-diabetes range increase the risk of heart attack or stroke by 50%. The insulin resistance and elevated glucose levels associated with pre-diabetes (and diabetes) are among the defining risk factors of metabolic syndrome.

The major factors involved in the development of diabetes are age, obesity, physical inactivity, a family history of diabetes, and lifestyle. Excess body fat reduces cell sensitivity to insulin, and insulin resistance is almost always a precursor of type 2 diabetes.

Ethnicity also plays a role. According to statistics released by the CDC, the rate of diagnosed diabetes cases is highest among Native Americans and Alaska Natives (16.5%), followed by blacks (11.8%), Hispanics (10.4%), Asian Americans (7.5%), and white Americans (6.6%). Across all races, about 25% of Americans age 60 and older have diabetes.

Prevention

It is estimated that 90% of cases of type 2 diabetes could be prevented if people adopted healthy lifestyle behaviors, including regular physical activity, a moderate diet, and modest weight loss. For people with pre-diabetes, lifestyle measures are more effective than medication for delaying or preventing the development of diabetes. Studies of people with pre-diabetes show that just a 5–7% weight loss can lower diabetes onset by nearly 60%. Exercise (endurance and/or strength training) makes cells more sensitive to insulin and helps stabilize blood glucose levels; it also helps keep body fat at healthy levels.

A moderate diet to control body fat is perhaps the most important dietary recommendation for the prevention of diabetes. However, the composition of the diet may also be important. Studies have linked diets low in fiber and high in sugar, refined carbohydrates, saturated fat, red meat, and high-fat dairy products to increased risk of diabetes; diets rich in whole grains, fruits, vegetables, legumes, fish, and poultry may be protective. Specific foods linked to higher risk of diabetes include soft drinks, white bread, white rice, french fries, processed meats, and sugary desserts.

Treatment

There is no cure for diabetes, but it can be successfully managed by keeping blood sugar levels within safe limits through diet, exercise, and, if necessary, medication. Blood sugar levels can be monitored using a home test; close monitoring and control of glucose levels can significantly reduce the rate of serious complications. New drug therapies include inhibitors known as DDP-4, which lower blood sugar levels without causing weight gain.

Nearly 90% of people with type 2 diabetes are overweight when diagnosed, including 55% who are obese. An important step in treatment is to lose weight; even a small amount of weight loss can be beneficial. People with diabetes should get their carbohydrates from whole grains, fruits, vegetables, and low-fat dairy products; carbohydrates and monounsaturated fats together should provide 60–70% of total daily calories. Regular exercise and a healthy diet are often sufficient to control type 2 diabetes.

Warning Signs and Testing

Be alert for the warning signs of diabetes:

- Frequent urination
- Extreme hunger or thirst
- Unexplained weight loss
- Extreme fatigue
- Blurred vision
- Frequent infections
- Cuts and bruises that are slow to heal
- Tingling or numbness in hands or feet
- Generalized itching with no rash

The best way to avoid complications is to recognize these symptoms and get early diagnosis and treatment. Type 2 diabetes is often asymptomatic in the early stages, however, so routine screening is recommended for people over age 45 and anyone younger who is at high risk. Screening involves a blood test to check glucose levels after either a period of fasting or the administration of a set dose of glucose. A fasting glucose level of 126 mg/dl or higher indicates diabetes; a level of 100–125 mg/dl indicates pre-diabetes.

for example), a condition called the **female athlete triad** may develop. The triad consists of three interrelated disorders: abnormal eating patterns (and excessive exercising), followed by **amenorrhea** (absence of menstruation), followed by decreased bone density (premature osteoporosis). Prolonged amenorrhea can cause bone density to erode to a point that a woman in her twenties will have the bone density of a woman in her sixties. Left untreated, the triad can lead to decreased physical performance, increased incidence of bone fractures, disturbances of heart rhythm and metabolism, and even death.

What Is the Right Weight for You?

BMI, percent body fat, and waist circumference measurement can best serve as general guides or estimates for body weight. To answer the question of what you should weigh, let your lifestyle be your guide. Don't focus on a particular weight as your goal. Instead, focus on living a lifestyle that includes eating moderate amounts of healthful foods, getting plenty of exercise, thinking positively, and learning to cope with stress. Then let the pounds fall where they may. For most people, the result will be close to the recommended weight ranges discussed earlier. For some, their weight will be somewhat higher than societal standards—but right for them. By letting a healthy lifestyle determine your weight, you can avoid developing unhealthy patterns of eating and a negative body image.

FACTORS CONTRIBUTING TO EXCESS BODY FAT

Body weight and body composition may be determined by multiple factors that may vary with each individual.

Genetic Factors

Estimates of the genetic contribution to obesity vary widely, from about 25% to 40% of an individual's body fat. Genes influence body size and shape, body fat distribution, and metabolic rate. Genetic factors also affect the ease with which weight is gained as a result of overeating and where on the body extra weight is added. If both parents are obese, their children have an 80% risk of being obese; children with only one obese parent face a 40% risk of becoming obese. In studies that compared adoptees and their biological parents, the weights of the adoptees were found to be more like those of the biological parents than those of the adoptive parents, again indicating a strong genetic link.

Hereditary influences, however, must be balanced against the contribution of environmental factors. Not all children of obese parents become obese, and normal-weight parents may have overweight children. The *tendency* to develop obesity may be inherited, but the expression of this tendency is affected by environmental influences.

The message you should take from this research is that genes are not destiny. It is true that some people have a harder time losing weight and maintaining weight loss than others. However, with increased exercise and attention to diet, even those with a genetic tendency toward obesity can maintain a healthy body weight.

Physiological Factors

Metabolism is the sum of all the vital processes by which food energy and nutrients are made available to and used by the body. The largest component of metabolism, **resting metabolic rate (RMR)**, is the energy required to maintain vital body functions, including respiration, heart rate, body temperature, and blood pressure, while the body is at rest. As shown in Figure 11.2, RMR accounts for about 65–70% of daily energy expenditure. The energy required to digest food accounts for an additional ±10% of daily energy expenditure. The remaining 20–30% is expended during physical activity.

Both heredity and behavior affect metabolic rate. Men, who have a higher proportion of muscle mass than women, have a higher RMR because muscle tissue is more metabolically active than fat. Also, some individuals inherit a higher or lower RMR than others. A higher RMR means that a person burns more calories while at rest and can therefore take in more calories without gaining weight.

Weight loss or gain also affects metabolic rate. When a person loses weight, both RMR and the energy required to perform physical tasks decrease. The reverse occurs when weight is gained. Exercise has a positive effect on metabolism. When people exercise, they slightly increase their RMR—the number of calories their bodies burn at rest. They also increase their muscle mass, which is associated with a higher metabolic rate. The exercise itself also burns calories, raising total energy expenditure. The higher the energy expenditure, the more the person can eat without gaining weight.

Lifestyle Factors

Although genetic and physiological factors may increase risk for excess body fat, they are not sufficient to explain the increasingly high rate of obesity seen in the United

---

female athlete triad   A condition consisting of three interrelated disorders: abnormal eating patterns (and excessive exercising) followed by lack of menstrual periods (amenorrhea) and decreased bone density (premature osteoporosis).

amenorrhea   The absence of menstruation.

resting metabolic rate (RMR)   The energy required to maintain vital body functions, including respiration, heart rate, body temperature, and blood pressure, while the body is at rest.

TERMS

Are Diet Sodas Bad for You?

Consumption of sodas has grown significantly in the past 30 years across all segments of the population. Regular soft drinks are now the leading source of calories in the American diet.

A can of regular soda contains about 150 calories. High consumption of sugary soda has been linked with obesity and diabetes in children and adolescents and with high blood pressure in adults. Some studies have shown that the added sweeteners in soft drinks are linked to increased triglycerides in the blood, leading to a greater risk of heart disease.

Many weight-conscious people have changed to diet soda in the hope that this is a healthier alternative to regular soda. But recent research indicates that drinking more than one soft drink a day, even if it is diet soda, may be associated with an increased incidence of metabolic syndrome, a cluster of risk factors linked to the development of diabetes, heart disease, and stroke. The syndrome includes high blood pressure, elevated triglyceride levels, low levels of HDL ("good" cholesterol), high fasting blood sugar levels, and excessive waist circumference.

Compared to people who did not drink soda, researchers found that people who consumed more than one soft drink per day—regular or diet—were associated with the following:

- 44% more likely to develop metabolic syndrome

- 31% more likely to be obese

- 25% more likely to have higher-than-average blood pressure

- 18% more likely to have high blood pressure

Some research has suggested that the artificial sweeteners in diet drinks make a person more prone to eat sweet, higher-calorie foods. Another theory is that the caramel content in both regular and diet sodas may play a role in insulin resistance.

On the other hand, some contradictory studies show the benefit of diet soda consumption in overweight individuals and suggest that other factors could explain the development of risk factors for heart disease. Regardless, everyone agrees that more research should be done before a final verdict on diet soda consumption is reached.

States. The gene pool has not changed in the past 40 years, but the rate of obesity among Americans has more than doubled. Clearly, other factors are at work—particularly lifestyle factors such as increased eating and decreased physical activity.

Eating Americans have access to plenty of calorie-dense foods, and many have eating habits that contribute to weight gain. (See the box "Are Diet Sodas Bad for You?.") Most overweight adults admit to eating more than they should of high-fat, high-sugar, high-calorie foods. Americans eat out more frequently now than in the past, and we rely more heavily on fast food and packaged convenience foods. Restaurant and convenience food portion sizes tend to be large, and the foods themselves are likely to be high in fat, sugar, and calories and low in nutrients. Studies have consistently found that people underestimate portion sizes by as much as 25%.

Physical Activity Activity levels among Americans are declining, beginning in childhood and continuing throughout life. Many schools have cut back on physical education classes and recess. Most adults drive to work, sit all day, and then relax in front of the TV at night. Modern conveniences such as remote controls, elevators, and power mowers have also reduced daily physical activity.

Psychosocial Factors

Many people have learned to use food as a means of coping with stress and negative emotions. Eating can provide a powerful distraction from difficult feelings—loneliness, anger, boredom, anxiety, shame, sadness, inadequacy. It can be used to combat low moods, low energy levels, and low self-esteem. When food and eating become the primary means of regulating emotions, binge eating or other disturbed eating patterns can develop.

Obesity is strongly associated with socioeconomic status. The prevalence of obesity goes down as income level goes up. More women than men are obese at lower income levels, but men are somewhat more obese at higher levels. These differences may reflect the greater sensitivity and concern for a slim physical appearance among upper-income women, as well as greater access to information about nutrition, to low-fat and low-calorie foods, and to opportunities for physical activity. It may also reflect the greater acceptance of obesity among certain ethnic groups, as well as different cultural values related to food choices.

In some families and cultures, food is used as a symbol of love and caring. It is an integral part of social gatherings and celebrations. In such cases, it may be difficult to change established eating patterns because they are linked to cultural and family values.

ADOPTING A HEALTHY LIFESTYLE FOR SUCCESSFUL WEIGHT MANAGEMENT

Permanent weight loss is not something you start and stop. You need to adopt healthy behaviors that you can maintain throughout your life.

Diet and Eating Habits

In contrast to dieting, which involves some form of food restriction, the term *diet* refers to your daily food choices. Everyone has a diet, but not everyone is dieting. You need to develop a diet that you enjoy and that enables you to maintain a healthy body composition. Use MyPyramid as the basis for a healthy diet (see Chapter 9). For weight management, pay special attention to total calories, portion sizes, energy density, fat and carbohydrate intake, and eating habits.

Total Calories   MyPyramid suggests approximate daily energy intakes based on gender, age, and activity level. However, energy balance may be a more important consideration for weight management than total calories consumed (refer back to Figure 11.2). To maintain your current weight, the total number of calories you eat must equal the number you burn. To lose weight, you must decrease your calorie intake and/or increase the number of calories you burn; to gain weight, the reverse is true. (One pound of body fat represents 3500 calories.)

The best approach for weight loss is combining an increase in physical activity with moderate calorie restriction. Don't go on a crash diet. To maintain weight loss, you many need to maintain some degree of the calorie restriction you used to lose the weight. Therefore, you need to adopt a level of food intake that provides all the essential nutrients that you can live with over the long term. For most people, maintaining weight loss is more difficult than losing the weight in the first place.

Portion Sizes   Overconsumption of total calories is closely tied to portion sizes. Many Americans are unaware that the portions of packaged foods and of foods served at restaurants have increased in size, and most of us significantly underestimate the amount of food we eat. Limiting portion sizes is critical for maintaining good health. Check the serving sizes listed on packaged foods, and order the smallest-sized items on the menu when you eat out. Don't supersize your meals and snacks; although huge servings may seem like the best deal, it is more important to order just what you need.

Energy (Calorie) Density   To cut back on calories and still feel full, you should favor foods that are low in energy density, foods that have more volume and bulk—that is, they are relatively heavy but have few calories. For example, for the same 100 calories, you could eat 21 baby carrots or 4 pretzel twists; you are more likely to feel full after eating

the serving of carrots because it weighs 10 times as much as the serving of pretzels (10 ounces versus 1 ounce).

Fresh fruits and vegetables, with their high water and fiber content, are low in energy density, as are whole-grain foods. Fresh fruits contain fewer calories and more fiber than fruit juices or drinks. Meat, ice cream, potato chips, croissants, crackers, and cakes and cookies are examples of foods high in energy density. Strategies for lowering the energy density of your diet include the following:

- Eat fruit with breakfast and for dessert.
- Add extra vegetables to sandwiches, casseroles, stir-fry dishes, pizza, pasta dishes, and fajitas.
- Start meals with a bowl of broth-based soup; include a green salad or fruit salad.
- Snack on fresh fruits and vegetables rather than crackers, chips, or other energy-dense snack foods.

Limit serving sizes of energy-dense foods such as butter, mayonnaise, cheese, chocolate, fatty meats, croissants, and snack foods that are fried, are high in added sugars (including reduced-fat products), or contain trans fats.

It is also important to watch out for processed foods, which can be high in fat and sodium. Even processed foods labeled "fat-free" or "reduced fat" may be high in calories; such products may contain sugar and fat substitutes.

Eating Habits   Equally important to weight management is the habit of eating small, frequent meals—four to five meals per day, including breakfast and snacks—on a regular schedule. Skipping meals leads to excessive hunger, feelings of deprivation, and increased vulnerability to binge eating or snacking. For weight management, it's better to consume the majority of calories during the day rather than in the evening.

In addition to establishing a regular pattern of eating, set some rules to govern your food choices. Rules for breakfast might be these, for example: Choose a sugar-free, high-fiber cereal with fat-free milk on most days; have a hard-boiled egg (no more than 3 per week); save pancakes and waffles for special occasions, unless they are whole-grain. The ultimate goal is to eat in moderation; no foods need to be entirely off-limits, though some should be eaten judiciously.

Physical Activity and Exercise

Physical activity and exercise burn calories and keep the metabolism geared to using food for energy instead of storing it as fat. Making significant cuts in food intake in order to lose weight is a difficult strategy to maintain; increasing your physical

> For weight management, *it's better to consume the majority of calories during the day* rather than in the evening.

activity is a much better approach. Regular physical activity protects against weight gain, is essential for maintaining weight loss, and improves quality of life. The sooner you establish good habits, the better.

Thinking and Emotions

The way you think about yourself and the world influences, and is influenced by, how you feel and how you act. Often, people with low self-esteem mentally compare the actual self to an internally held picture of an "ideal self," an image based on perfectionistic goals and beliefs about how they and others should be. The more these two pictures differ, the larger the impact on self-esteem and the more likely the presence of negative emotions.

Besides the internal picture we carry of ourselves, all of us carry on an internal dialogue about events happening to us and around us. This *self-talk* can be either self-deprecating or positively motivating, depending on our beliefs and attitudes. Having realistic beliefs and goals, and practicing positive self-talk and problem solving support a healthy lifestyle.

Coping Strategies

Appropriate coping strategies help you deal with the stresses of life; they are also an important lifestyle factor in weight management. Those who overeat might use food to alleviate loneliness or to serve as a pickup for fatigue, as an antidote to boredom, or as a distraction from problems. Some people even overeat to punish themselves for real or imagined transgressions. Those who recognize that they are misusing food can consciously attempt to find new coping strategies and begin to use food appropriately—to fuel life's activities, to foster growth, and to bring pleasure, but *not* as a way to manage stress.

APPROACHES TO OVERCOMING A WEIGHT PROBLEM

Each year, Americans spend more than $40 billion on weight-loss plans and products. If you are overweight, you may already be creating a plan to lose weight and keep it off. You have many options.

Ask Yourself

QUESTIONS FOR CRITICAL THINKING AND REFLECTION
Have you ever used food as an escape when you were stressed out? Were you aware of what you were doing at the time? How can you avoid using food as a coping mechanism in the future?

Doing It Yourself

If you need to lose weight, focus on adopting the healthy lifestyle described throughout this book. The right weight for you will naturally evolve. Combine modest cuts in energy intake with exercise, and avoid very-low-calorie diets. (In general, a low-calorie diet should provide 1200–1500 calories per day.) By producing a negative energy balance of 250–1000 calories per day, you will produce the recommended weight loss of 0.5–2.0 pounds per week. Realize that most low-calorie diets cause a rapid loss of body water at first. When this phase passes, weight loss declines, and dieters are often misled into believing that their efforts are not working. They then give up, not realizing that smaller, mostly fat, losses later in the diet are actually better than the initial larger, mostly fluid losses. Reasonable weight loss is 8–10% of body weight over 6 months. A registered dietitian or nutritionist can recommend an appropriate plan for you when you want to lose weight on your own.

> A 16-ounce whole-milk latte has **265 calories,** and a 20-ounce bottle of regular soda has **227 calories.** Beverages have a huge impact on calorie intake.
>
> —CDC, 2010

Dietary Supplements and Diet Aids

Dietary supplements marketed for weight loss are subject to fewer regulations than OTC medications. The Federal Trade Commission reports that more than half of advertisements for weight-loss products made representations that are likely to be false.

In 2008, the FDA alerted consumers not to use or purchase more than 25 weight-loss products and ordered the products recalled from stores. Such recalls are becoming more common. Some of recalled supplements contained pharmaceuticals in amounts far exceeding FDA-recommended levels, and some contained substances not approved for sale in the United States. The use of these drugs could lead to complications such as heart attack, stroke, cancer, and suicide.

Formula Drinks and Food Bars Canned diet drinks, powders used to make shakes, and diet food bars and snacks are designed to achieve weight loss by substituting for some or all of a person's daily food intake. However, most people find it difficult to use these products for long periods, and muscle loss and other serious health problems may result if they are used as the sole source of nutrition for an extended period. Use of such products sometimes

Is Any Diet Best for Weight Loss?

Many popular weight-loss plans promote specific food choices and macronutrient (protein, fat, carbohydrate) combinations as best for weight loss. Research findings have been mixed, but two points are clear. Total calorie intake matters, and the best diet is probably the one you can stick with.

Low-Carbohydrate Diets

Some low-carb diets advocate fewer than 10% of total calories from carbohydrates, compared to the 45–65% recommended by the Food and Nutrition Board. Some suggest daily carbohydrate intake below the 130 grams needed to provide essential carbohydrates in the diet. Small studies have found that low-carbohydrate diets can help with short-term weight loss and be safe for relatively short periods of time—although unpleasant effects such as bad breath, constipation, and headache are fairly common.

Some low-carb diets tend to be very high in protein and saturated fat and low in fiber, whole grains, vegetables, and fruits (and thus lack some essential nutrients). Such diets have been linked to an increased risk of heart disease, high blood pressure, and cancer. Other low-carb diets, though still emphasizing protein, limit saturated fats, allow most vegetables after an initial period, and advocate switching to "healthy carbs." These diets are healthier than the more extreme versions.

Low-Fat Diets

Many experts advocate diets that are relatively low in fat, high in carbohydrates, and moderate in protein. Critics of these diets blame them for rising rates of obesity. However, low-fat diets combined with physical activity can be safe and effective for many people.

The debate has highlighted the importance of total calorie intake and the quality of carbohydrate choices. A low-fat diet is not a license to consume excess calories, even in low-fat foods.

How Do Popular Diets Measure Up?

One study followed participants in four popular diets that emphasize different strategies—Weight Watchers (restricted portion sizes and calories), Atkins (low-carbohydrate, high-fat), Zone (relatively high protein, moderate fat and carbohydrate), and Ornish (very low fat). Each of these diets modestly reduced body weight and heart disease risk factors. There was no significant difference in weight loss at 1 year among the diets, and the more closely people adhered to each diet, the more weight they lost. Dropout rates were high—about 50% for Atkins and Ornish and 35% for Weight Watchers and Zone.

Energy Balance Counts: The National Weight Control Registry

Important lessons about energy balance can be drawn from the National Weight Control Registry, an ongoing study of people who have lost significant amounts of weight and kept it off. The average participant in the registry has lost 71 pounds and kept the weight off for more than 5 years. Nearly all participants use a combination of diet and exercise to manage their weight. Most consume diets moderate in calories and relatively low in fat and fried foods; they monitor their body weight and their food intake frequently. Participants engage in an average of 60 minutes of moderate physical activity daily. The National Weight Control Registry study illustrates that to lose weight and keep it off, you must decrease daily calorie intake and/or increase daily physical activity—and continue to do so over your lifetime.

SOURCES: Sacks, F. M., et al. 2009. Comparison of weight-loss diets with different compositions of fat, protein, and carbohydrates. *New England Journal of Medicine* 360(9): 859–873. Battle of the diet books II. 2006. *Nutrition Action Healthletter,* July/August; Dansinger, M. L., et al. 2005. Comparison of the Atkins, Ornish, Weight Watchers, and Zone diets for weight loss and heart disease risk reduction. *Journal of the American Medical Association* 293(1): 43–53; Hill, J., and R. Wing. 2003. The National Weight Control Registry. *Permanente Journal* 7(3): 34–37.

results in rapid short-term weight loss, but the weight is typically regained because users don't learn to change their eating and lifestyle behaviors.

Herbal Supplements   Herbs are marketed as dietary supplements, so there is little information about effectiveness, proper dosage, drug interactions, and side effects. The FDA has banned the sale of ephedra (*ma huang*), stating that it presented a significant and unreasonable risk to human health. Ephedrine, the active ingredient in ephedra, is structurally similar to amphetamine and was widely used in weight-loss supplements. It may suppress appetite, but adverse effects have included elevated blood pressure, panic attacks, seizures, insomnia, and increased risk of heart attack or stroke, particularly when combined with another stimulant, such as caffeine. The FDA banned the synthetic stimulant phenylpropanolamine for similar reasons.

Other Supplements   Fiber is another common ingredient in OTC diet aids, promoted for appetite control. However, dietary fiber acts as a bulking agent in the large intestine, not the stomach, so it doesn't have a pronounced effect on appetite. Other popular dietary supplements include conjugated linoleic acid, carnitine, chromium, pyruvate, calcium, B vitamins, chitosan, and a number of products labeled "fat absorbers," "fat blockers," and "starch blockers." Research has not found these products to be effective, and many have potentially adverse side effects.

Weight-Loss Programs

Weight-loss programs come in a variety of types, including noncommercial support organizations, commercial programs, Web sites, and clinical programs.

Noncommercial Weight-Loss Programs Noncommercial programs such as TOPS (Take Off Pounds Sensibly) and Overeaters Anonymous (OA) mainly provide group support. They do not advocate any particular diet but do recommend seeking professional advice for creating an individualized plan. These types of programs are generally free. Your physician or a registered dietitian can also provide information and support for weight loss.

Commercial Weight-Loss Programs Commercial weight-loss programs typically provide group support, nutrition education, physical activity recommendations, and behavior modification advice. Some also make available packaged foods to assist in following dietary advice.

A responsible and safe weight-loss program should have the following features:

- The recommended diet should be safe and balanced, include all the food groups, and meet the DRIs for all nutrients. Physical activity and exercise should be strongly encouraged.

- The program should promote slow, steady weight loss averaging 0.5–2.0 pounds per week.

- If a participant plans to lose more than 20 pounds, has any health problems, or is taking medication on a regular basis, physician evaluation and monitoring should be recommended. The staff of the program should include qualified counselors and health professionals.

- The program should include plans for weight maintenance after the weight-loss phase is over.

- The program should provide information on all fees and costs, including those of supplements and prepackaged foods, as well as data on risks and expected outcomes of participating in the program.

A strong commitment and a plan for maintenance are especially important because only about 10–15% of program participants maintain their weight loss—the rest gain back all or more than they had lost. One study of participants found that regular exercise was the best predictor of maintaining weight loss, whereas frequent television viewing was the best predictor of weight gain.

Clinical Weight-Loss Programs Medically supervised clinical programs are usually located in a hospital or other medical setting. Designed to help those who are severely obese, these programs typically involve a closely monitored very-low-calorie diet. The cost of a clinical program is usually high, but insurance will often cover part of the fee.

Prescription Drugs

The medications most often prescribed for weight loss are appetite suppressants that reduce feelings of hunger or increase feelings of fullness. Appetite suppressants usually

Ask Yourself

QUESTIONS FOR CRITICAL THINKING AND REFLECTION

Why do you think people continue to buy into fad diets and weight-loss gimmicks, even though they are constantly reminded that the key to weight management is lifestyle change? Have you ever tried a fad diet or weight-loss supplement? If so, what were your reasons for trying it? What were the results?

work by increasing levels of brain chemicals that affect mood and appetite. All prescription weight-loss drugs have potential side effects, including sleeplessness, nervousness, and euphoria. Sibutramine (Meridia) may trigger increases in blood pressure and heart rate. Headaches, constipation or diarrhea, dry mouth, and insomnia are other side effects.

Orlistat (Xenical), an appetite suppressant with FDA approval for long-term use, blocks fat absorption in the intestines, preventing about 30% of the fat in food from being digested. Orlistat also reduces the absorption of fat-soluble vitamins and antioxidants, so a vitamin supplement is highly recommended for those taking the drug. Side effects include diarrhea, cramping, and other gastrointestinal problems if users do not follow a low-fat diet. The OTC drug Alli is a lower-dose version of Orlistat.

These medications work best in conjunction with behavior modification. Studies have generally found that appetite suppressants produce modest weight loss—about 5–22 pounds above the loss expected with nondrug obesity treatments. Individuals respond very differently, however, and some experience more weight loss than others. Unfortunately, weight loss tends to level off or reverse after 4–6 months on a medication, and many people regain the weight they've lost when they stop taking the drug.

> **Most bariatric surgery patients can expect to lose 50–60% of their excess weight within 2 years of the procedure.**
>
> —Mayo Clinic, 2010

Prescription drugs are recommended only for people who have been unable to lose weight with nondrug options and who have a BMI over 30 (or over 27 if two or more additional risk factors such as diabetes and high blood pressure are present).

Surgery

It is estimated that 5.7% of adult Americans have a BMI greater than 40, qualifying them as severely, or "morbidly," obese. Severe obesity is a serious medical condition that is often complicated by other health problems such as diabetes, sleep disorders, heart disease, and arthritis. Surgical intervention may be necessary as a treatment of last resort. According to the NIH, weight-loss (bariatric) surgery is recommended for patients with a BMI greater than 40, or greater than 35 with obesity-related illnesses.

Bariatric surgery modifies the gastrointestinal tract by changing either the size of the stomach or how the intestine drains, thereby reducing food intake. The keys to success with surgical weight-loss procedures are adequate follow-up and continued motivation so that eating patterns and lifestyle behaviors are permanently changed.

BODY IMAGE

Developing a positive body image is an important aspect of psychological wellness and an important component of successful weight management.

Severe Body Image Problems

A person can become preoccupied with a perceived defect in appearance, thereby damaging self-esteem and interfering with relationships. Adolescents and adults who have a negative body image are more likely to diet restrictively, eat compulsively, or develop some other form of disordered eating.

When dissatisfaction becomes extreme, the condition is called *body dysmorphic disorder (BDD).* BDD affects about 2% of Americans, males and females in equal numbers; BDD usually begins before age 18 but can begin in adulthood. Sufferers are overly concerned with physical appearance, often focusing on slight flaws that are not obvious to others. Low self-esteem is common. Individuals with BDD may spend hours every day thinking about their flaws and looking at themselves in mirrors; they may desire and seek repeated cosmetic surgeries. BDD is related to obsessive-compulsive disorder and can lead to depression, social phobia, and suicide if left untreated. An individual with BDD needs to get professional evaluation and treatment; medication and therapy can help people with BDD.

In some cases, body image may bear little resemblance to fact. A person suffering from the eating disorder anorexia nervosa typically has a severely distorted body image—she believes herself to be fat even when she has become emaciated. Distorted body image is also a hallmark of *muscle dysmorphia,* a disorder experienced by some bodybuilders and other active people who see themselves as small and out of shape despite being very muscular. Those who suffer from muscle dysmorphia may let obsessive exercise interfere with their work and relationships. They may also use steroids and other potentially dangerous muscle-building drugs.

Acceptance and Change

There are limits to the changes that can be made to body weight and body shape, both of which are influenced by heredity. The changes that can and should be made are lifestyle changes.

Knowing when you've reached the limits of healthy change—and accepting those limits—are crucial for overall wellness. Obesity is a serious health risk, but weight management needs to take place in a positive and realistic atmosphere. For an obese person, losing as few as 10 pounds can reduce blood pressure and improve mood. The hazards of excessive dieting and overconcern about body weight need to be countered by a change in attitude. A reasonable weight must take into account a person's weight history, social circumstances, metabolic profile, and psychological well-being.

EATING DISORDERS

Problems with body weight and weight control are not limited to excessive body fat. A growing number of people, especially adolescent girls and young women, experience **eating disorders,** characterized by severe disturbances in body image, eating patterns, and eating-related behaviors. The major eating disorders are anorexia nervosa, bulimia nervosa, and binge-eating disorder. Disordered eating affects an estimated 10 million American females and 1 million males. About 90% of eating disorders begin during adolescence. In recent years, however, cases of eating disorders have increased among children as young as 8.

> *Knowing when you've **reached the limits of healthy change**—and accepting those limits—are crucial for overall wellness.*

eating disorder   A serious disturbance in eating patterns or eating-related behavior, characterized by a negative body image and concerns about body weight or body fat.

Exercise is a healthy practice, but people with eating disorders sometimes exercise compulsively, building their lives around their workouts. Compulsive exercise can lead to injuries, low body fat, and other health problems.

Anorexia Nervosa

A person with **anorexia nervosa** does not eat enough food to maintain a reasonable body weight. Anorexia affects about 3 million people, 95% of them female. Although it can occur later, anorexia typically develops between the ages of 12 and 18.

Characteristics of Anorexia Nervosa People with anorexia have an intense fear of gaining weight or becoming fat. Their body image is so distorted that even when emaciated they think they are fat. People with anorexia may engage in compulsive behaviors or rituals that help keep them from eating, though some may also binge and **purge.** They often use vigorous and prolonged exercise to reduce body weight as well. Although they may express a great interest in food, even taking over the cooking responsibilities for the rest of the family, their own diet becomes more and more extreme. People with anorexia often hide or hoard food without eating it.

Anorexic people are typically introverted, emotionally reserved, and socially insecure. They are often model children who rarely complain and are anxious to please others and win their approval. Although school performance is typically above average, they are often critical of themselves and not satisfied with their accomplishments. For people with anorexia nervosa, their entire sense of self-esteem may be tied up in their evaluation of their body shape and weight.

Health Risks of Anorexia Nervosa Because of extreme weight loss, females with anorexia often stop menstruating, become intolerant of cold, and develop low blood pressure and heart rate. They develop dry skin that is often covered by fine body hair like that of an infant. Their hands and feet may swell and take on a blue tinge.

Anorexia nervosa has been linked to a variety of medical complications, including disorders of the cardiovascular, gastrointestinal, endocrine, and skeletal systems. When body fat is virtually gone and muscles are severely wasted, the body turns to its own organs in a desperate search for protein. Death can occur from heart failure caused by electrolyte imbalances. About one in ten women with anorexia dies of starvation, cardiac arrest, or other medical complications—the highest death rate for any psychiatric disorder. Depression is also a serious risk, and about half the fatalities related to anorexia are suicides.

Bulimia Nervosa

A person suffering from **bulimia nervosa** engages in recurrent episodes of binge eating followed by purging. Bulimia is often difficult to recognize because sufferers conceal their eating habits and usually maintain a normal weight, although they may experience weight fluctuations of 10–15 pounds. Although bulimia usually begins in adolescence or young adulthood, it has begun to emerge at increasingly younger (11–12 years) and older (40–60 years) ages.

Characteristics of Bulimia Nervosa During a binge, a bulimic person may rapidly consume thousands of calories. This is followed by an attempt to get rid of the food by purging, usually by vomiting or using laxatives or diuretics. During a binge, bulimics feel as though they

Gender, Ethnicity, and Body Image

Body Image and Gender

Women are more likely than men to be dissatisfied with their bodies, often wanting to be thinner than they are. In one study, only 30% of eighth-grade girls reported being content with their bodies, while 70% of their male classmates expressed satisfaction with their looks. Girls and women are more likely than boys and men to diet, develop eating disorders, and be obese.

The image of the ideal woman presented in the media is often unrealistic and even unhealthy. In a review of BMI data for Miss America pageant winners since 1922, researchers noted a significant decline in BMI over time, with an increasing number of recent winners having BMIs in the "underweight" category.

Our culture may be promoting an unattainable masculine ideal as well. Researchers studying male action figures such as GI Joe from the past 40 years noted that they have become increasingly muscular. A recent Batman action figure, if projected onto a man of average height, would result in someone with a 30-inch waist, 57-inch chest, and 27-inch biceps.

Body Image and Ethnicity

Although some groups espouse thinness as an ideal body type, others do not. In many traditional African societies, for example, full-figured women are seen as symbols of health, prosperity, and fertility. African American teenage girls have a more positive body image than do white girls; in one survey, two-thirds of them defined beauty as "the right attitude," whereas white girls were more preoccupied with weight and body shape.

Nevertheless, recent evidence indicates that African American women are as likely to engage in disordered eating behavior, especially binge eating and vomiting, as their Latina, American Indian, and white counterparts.

Avoiding Body Image Problems

To minimize your risk of developing a body image problem, keep the following strategies in mind:

- Focus on healthy habits and good physical health.

- Focus on good psychological health and put concerns about physical appearance in perspective.

- Practice body acceptance. You can influence your body size and type to some degree through lifestyle, but the basic fact is that some people are genetically designed to be bigger or heavier than others.

- Find things to appreciate in yourself besides an idealized body image. What you can do is more important than how you look.

- See the beauty and fitness industries for what they are. One of their goals is to prompt dissatisfaction with yourself so that you will buy their products.

---

have lost control and cannot stop or limit how much they eat. Some binge and purge only occasionally; others do so many times every day.

People with bulimia may appear to eat normally, but they are rarely comfortable around food. Binges usually occur in secret and can become nightmarish—raiding the kitchen for food, going from one grocery store to another to buy food, or even stealing food. During the binge, food acts as an anesthetic, and all feelings are blocked out. Afterward, bulimics feel physically drained and emotionally spent. They usually feel deeply ashamed and disgusted with both themselves and their behavior and terrified that they will gain weight from the binge.

Major life changes such as leaving for college, getting married, having a baby, or losing a job can trigger a binge-purge cycle. At such times, stress is high and the person may have no good outlet for emotional conflict or tension. As with anorexia, bulimia sufferers are often insecure and depend on others for approval and self-esteem. They may hide difficult emotions such as anger and disappointment from themselves and others. Binge eating and purging become a way of dealing with feelings.

Health Risks of Bulimia Nervosa The binge-purge cycle of bulimia places a tremendous strain on the body. Contact with vomited stomach acids erodes tooth enamel. Repeated vomiting or the use of laxatives, in combination with deficient calorie intake, can damage the liver and kidneys and cause cardiac arrhythmia. Chronic hoarseness and esophageal tearing with bleeding may also result from vomiting. More rarely, binge eating can lead to rupture of the stomach. Although less often associated with suicide or premature death than anorexia, bulimia is associated with increased depression, excessive preoccupation with food and body image, and sometimes disturbances in cognitive functioning.

Binge-Eating Disorder

Binge-eating disorder affects about 2% of American adults. It is characterized by uncontrollable eating, usually followed by feelings of guilt and shame with weight gain. Common eating patterns are eating more rapidly than normal, eating until uncomfortably full, eating when not hungry, and preferring to eat alone. Binge eaters may eat large amounts of food throughout the day, with no planned mealtimes. Many people with binge-eating disorder mistakenly see rigid dieting as the only solution to their problem. However, rigid dieting usually causes feelings of deprivation and a return to overeating.

Compulsive overeaters rarely eat because of hunger. Instead, food is used as a means of coping with stress, conflict, and other difficult emotions or to provide solace and entertainment. People who do not have the resources to deal effectively with stress may be more vulnerable to binge-eating disorder. Inappropriate overeating often begins during childhood. In some families, eating may be used as an activity to fill otherwise empty time. Parents may reward children with food for good behavior or withhold food as a means of punishment, thereby creating distorted feelings about the use of food.

Binge eaters are almost always obese, so they face all the health risks associated with obesity. In addition, binge eaters may have higher rates of depression and anxiety.

Borderline Disordered Eating

Eating habits and body image run along a continuum from healthy to seriously disordered. Where each of us falls along that continuum can change depending on life stresses, illnesses, and many other factors. People with borderline disordered eating have some symptoms of eating disorders but do not meet the full diagnostic criteria for anorexia, bulimia, or binge-eating disorder. Behaviors such as excessive dieting, occasional bingeing or purging, or the inability to control eating turn food into the enemy and create havoc in the lives of millions of Americans.

How do you know if you have disordered eating habits? When thoughts about food and weight dominate your life, you have a problem. If you're convinced that your worth as a person hinges on how you look and how much you weigh, it's time to get help. Other danger signs include frequent feelings of guilt after a meal or snack, any use of vomiting or laxatives after meals, or overexercising or severely restricting your food intake to compensate for what you've already eaten.

If you suspect you have an eating problem, don't go it alone or delay getting help, as disordered eating habits can develop into a full-blown eating disorder. Check with your student health or counseling center—nearly all colleges have counselors and medical personnel who can help you or refer you to a specialist if needed.

Treating Eating Disorders

The treatment of eating disorders must address both problematic eating behaviors and the misuse of food to manage stress and emotions. Anorexia nervosa treatment first involves averting a medical crisis by restoring adequate body weight; then the psychological aspects of the disorder can be addressed. The treatment of bulimia nervosa or binge-eating disorder involves first stabilizing the eating patterns, then identifying and changing the patterns of thinking that led to disordered eating, and then improving coping skills. Concurrent problems, such as depression or anxiety, must also be addressed. Antidepressants like Prozac have been used in the treatment of anorexia but with mixed results.

Treatment of eating disorders usually involves a combination of psychotherapy and medical management. The therapy may be carried out individually or in a group; sessions involving the entire family may be recommended. A support or self-help group can be a useful adjunct to such treatment.

> **About 30%** of people with anorexia receive treatment; only **6%** of bulimics receive treatment.
>
> —National Eating Disorders Association, 2005

TERMS

binge-eating disorder An eating disorder characterized by binge eating and a lack of control over eating behavior in general.

Ask Yourself

QUESTIONS FOR CRITICAL THINKING AND REFLECTION

Do you know someone you suspect may suffer from an eating disorder? Does the advice in this chapter seem helpful to you? Do you think you could follow it? Why or why not? Have you ever experienced a disordered eating pattern yourself? If so, can you identify the reasons for it?

Creating a Personal Weight-Management Plan

The behavior management plan described in Chapter 1 provides an excellent framework for a weight-management program. Following are some suggestions about specific ways you can adapt that general plan to controlling your weight.

Motivation and Commitment

Make sure you are motivated and committed before you begin. Failure at weight loss is a frustrating experience that can make it more difficult to lose weight in the future. Think about why you want to lose weight. Self-focused reasons, such as to feel good about yourself or to have a greater sense of well-being, are often associated with success. Trying to lose weight for others or out of concern for how others view you is a poor foundation for a weight-loss program. Make a list of your reasons for wanting to lose weight, and post it in a prominent place.

Setting Goals

Choose a reasonable weight you think you would like to reach over the long term, and be willing to renegotiate it as you get further along. Break down your long-term weight and behavioral goals into a series of short-term goals. Develop a new way of behaving by designing small, manageable steps that will get you to where you want to go.

Creating a Negative Energy Balance

When your weight is constant, you are burning approximately the same number of calories as you are taking in. To tip the energy balance toward weight loss, you must either consume fewer calories, or burn more calories through physical activity, or both. One pound of body fat represents 3500 calories. To lose weight at the recommended rate of 0.5–2.0 pounds per week, you must create a negative energy balance of 1750–7000 calories per week or 250–1000 calories per day. To generate a negative energy balance, it's usually best to begin by increasing activity level rather than decreasing your calorie consumption.

Physical Activity

Consider how you can increase your energy output simply by increasing routine physical activity, such as walking or taking the stairs. If you are not already involved in a regular exercise routine aimed at increasing endurance and building or maintaining muscle mass, seek help from someone who is competent to help you plan and start an appropriate exercise routine. If you are already doing regular physical exercise, evaluate your program according to the guidelines in Chapter 10.

Don't try to use exercise to spot reduce. Leg lifts, for example, contribute to fat loss only to the extent that they burn calories; they don't burn fat just from your legs. You can make parts of your body appear more fit by exercising them, but the only way you can reduce fat in any specific part of your body is to create an overall negative energy balance.

Diet and Eating Habits

If you can't generate a large enough negative energy balance solely by increasing physical activity, you may want to supplement exercise with modest cuts in your calorie intake. Don't think of this as going on a diet; your goal is to make small changes in your diet that you can maintain for a lifetime. Focus on cutting your intake of saturated and trans fats and added sugars and on eating a variety of nutritious foods in moderation. Don't skip meals, fast, or go on a very-low-calorie diet or a diet that is unbalanced.

Making changes in eating habits is another important strategy for weight management. If your program centers on a conscious restriction of certain food items, you're likely to spend all your time thinking about the forbidden foods. Focus on *how* to eat rather than *what* to eat.

Self-Monitoring

Keep a record of your weight and behavior change progress. Try keeping a record of everything you eat. Write down what you plan to eat, in what quantity, *before* you eat. You'll find that just having to record something that is not OK to eat is likely to stop you from eating it. If you also note what seems to be triggering your urges to eat (for example, you feel bored, or someone offered you something), you'll become more aware of your weak spots and be better able to take corrective action. Also, keep track of your daily activities and your formal exercise program so you can monitor increases in physical activity.

Putting Your Plan into Action

- Examine the environmental cues that trigger poor eating and exercise habits, and devise strategies for dealing with them. For example, you may need to remove problem foods from your house temporarily or put a sign on the refrigerator reminding you to go for a walk instead of having a snack. Anticipate problem situations, and plan ways to handle them more effectively.

- Create new environmental cues that will support your new healthy behaviors. Put your walking shoes by the front door. Move fruits and vegetables to the front of the refrigerator.

- Get others to help. Talk to friends and family members about what they can do to support your efforts. Find a buddy to join you in your exercise program.

- Give yourself lots of praise and rewards. Think about your accomplishments and achievements and congratulate yourself. Plan special nonfood treats for yourself, such as a walk or a movie. Reward yourself often and for anything that counts toward success.

- If you slip, tell yourself to get back on track immediately, and don't waste time on self-criticism. Think positively instead of getting into a cycle of guilt and self-blame. Don't demand too much of yourself.

- Don't get discouraged. Be aware that although weight loss is bound to slow down after the first loss of body fluid, the weight loss at this slower rate is more permanent than earlier, more dramatic, losses.

- Remember that weight management is a lifelong project. You need to adopt reasonable goals and strategies that you can maintain over the long term.

TIPS FOR TODAY AND THE FUTURE

Many approaches work, but the simplest formula for weight management is moderate food intake coupled with regular exercise.

RIGHT NOW YOU CAN

- Assess your weight-management needs. Do you need to gain weight, lose weight, or stay at your current weight?
- List five things you can do to add more physical activity (not exercise) to your daily routine.
- Identify the foods you regularly eat that may be sabotaging your ability to manage your weight.

IN THE FUTURE YOU CAN

- Make an honest assessment of your current body image. Is it accurate and fair, or is it unduly negative and unhealthy? If your body image presents a problem, consider getting professional advice on how to view yourself realistically.
- Keep track of your energy needs to determine whether your energy balance equation is correct. Use this information as part of your long-term weight-management efforts.

Connect to Your Choices

Have you ever thought about how you came to have the body weight and body composition you have? Many factors can influence our weight-management choices, some not as obvious as others. Do you have easy access to high-calorie, high-fat snacks in your dorm or dining hall? Does your school provide transportation around campus, making it less appealing to walk to class? Does your TV or computer lure you into hours of sedentary entertainment?

What are the external factors that influence your choices about weight management? What are your inner motivations and core values, and how do they affect your choices? Based on what you learned in this chapter, will you make some different choices in the future? If so, what will they be?

Go online to Connect to complete this activity. www.mcgraw-hillconnect.com

SUMMARY

- Body composition is the relative amounts of fat-free mass and fat in the body. *Overweight* and *obesity* refer to body weight or the percentage of body fat that exceeds what is associated with good health.

- The key to weight management is maintaining a balance of calories in (food) and calories out (resting metabolism, food digestion, and physical activity).

- Standards for assessing body weight and body composition include body mass index (BMI) and percent body fat.

- Too much or too little body fat is linked to health problems; the distribution of body fat can also be a significant risk factor for many health problems.

- An inaccurate or negative body image is common and can lead to psychological distress.

- Factors involved in the regulation of body weight and body fat include heredity and metabolic rate.

- Nutritional guidelines for weight management include consuming a moderate number of calories; limiting portion sizes, energy density, and the intake of fat, simple sugars, refined carbohydrates, and protein to recommended levels; and developing an eating schedule and rules for food choices.

- Activity guidelines for weight management emphasize daily physical activity and regular sessions of cardiorespiratory endurance exercise and strength training.

- Weight management requires developing positive, realistic self-talk and self-esteem and a repertoire of appropriate techniques for handling stress and other emotional and physical challenges.

- People can be successful at long-term weight loss on their own, by combining diet and exercise.

- OTC diet aids and supplements and formal weight-loss programs should be assessed for safety and efficacy.

- Professional help is needed in cases of severe obesity; medical treatments include prescription drugs, surgery, and psychological therapy.

- Dissatisfaction with weight and shape is common to all eating disorders. Anorexia nervosa is characterized by self-starvation, distorted body image, and an intense fear of gaining weight. Bulimia nervosa is characterized by recurrent episodes of uncontrolled binge eating and frequent purging. Binge-eating disorder involves binge eating without regular use of compensatory purging.

FOR MORE INFORMATION

BOOKS

American Heart Association. 2011. *American Heart Association No-Fad Diet, 2nd Edition: A Personal Plan for Healthy Weight Loss.* New York: Clarkson Potter. *Provides guidelines for successful weight management.*

Dillon, E. 2009. *Issues That Concern You: Obesity.* New York: Greenhaven Press. *A collection of perspectives on the causes of obesity, its management, and its impact on individuals and society.*

Hochstrasser, A. 2009. *The Patient's Guide to Weight Loss Surgery*, rev. ed. New York: Hatherleigh. *An easy-to-read guide to the benefits and risks of weight-loss surgery.*

Mayo Clinic. 2009. *Mayo Clinic's Essential Diabetes Book*. Rochester, Minn.: Mayo Clinic. *A user-friendly guide to diabetes.*

Smolin, K., and M. B. Grosvenor. 2010. *Nutrition and Eating Disorders*. New York: Chelsea House Publications. *An easy-to-understand guide to eating disorders.*

ORGANIZATIONS, HOTLINES, AND WEB SITES

American Diabetes Association. Provides information, a free newsletter, and referrals to local support groups; the Web site includes an online diabetes risk assessment.

  http://www.diabetes.org

FDA Center for Food Safety and Applied Nutrition: Dietary Supplements. Provides background facts and information on the current regulatory status of dietary supplements, including compounds marketed for weight loss.

  http://www.cfsan.fda.gov/Food/DietarySupplements/default.htm

National Heart, Lung, and Blood Institute (NHLBI): Aim for a Healthy Weight. Provides information and tips on diet and physical activity, as well as a BMI calculator.

  http://www.nhlbi.nih.gov/health/public/heart/obesity/lose_wt

National Institute of Diabetes and Digestive and Kidney Diseases (NIDDK): Weight-Control Information Network. Provides information and referrals for problems related to obesity, weight control, and nutritional disorders.

  http://win.niddk.nih.gov/

SmallStep.gov. Provides resources for increasing activity and improving diet through small changes in daily habits.

  http://www.smallstep.gov

USDA Food and Nutrition Information Center: Weight and Obesity. Reports and studies on the issue of obesity among Americans.

  http://www.nal.usda.gov/fnic/reports/obesity.html

Resources for people concerned about eating disorders:

Eating Disorder Referral and Information Center
  http://www.edreferral.com

MedlinePlus: Eating Disorders
  http://www.nlm.nih.gov/medlineplus/eatingdisorders.html

National Association of Anorexia Nervosa and Associated Eating Disorders
  630-571-1330 (help line)
  http://www.anad.org

National Eating Disorders Association
  800-931-2237
  http://www.nationaleatingdisorders.org

SELECTED BIBLIOGRAPHY

Adams, K. F., et al. 2006. Overweight, obesity, and mortality in a large prospective cohort of persons 50 to 71 years old. *New England Journal of Medicine* 355(8): 763–778.

Baker, B. 2006. Weight loss and diet plans. *American Journal of Nursing* 106(6): 52–59.

Behn, A., and E. Ur. 2006. The obesity epidemic and its cardiovascular consequences. *Current Opinions in Cardiology* 21(4): 353–360.

Centers for Disease Control and Prevention. 2007. *Take Charge of Your Diabetes*, 4th ed. Atlanta, Ga.: U.S. Department of Health and Human Services, Centers for Disease Control and Prevention.

Centers for Disease Control and Prevention. 2008. *National Diabetes Fact Sheet: General Information and National Estimates on Diabetes in the United States, 2007.* Atlanta, Ga: U.S. Department of Health and Human Services, Centers for Disease Control and Prevention.

Dhingra, R., et al. 2007. Soft drink consumption and risk of developing cardiometabolic risk factors and the metabolic syndrome in middle-aged adults in the community. *Circulation* 116(5): 480–488.

Drewnowski, A., and P. Eichelsdoerfer. 2010. Can low-income Americans afford a healthy diet? *Nutrition Today* 44(6): 246–249.

Flegal, K. M., et al. 2010. Prevalence and trends in obesity among US adults, 1999–2008. *Journal of the American Medical Association* 303(3): 235–241.

Hamilton, M., et al. 2007. Role of low energy expenditure and sitting in obesity, metabolic syndrome, type 2 diabetes, and cardiovascular disease. *Diabetes* 56(11): 2655–2667.

Karlamangla, A. S., et al. 2010. Socioeconomic and ethnic disparities in cardiovascular risk in the United States, 2001–2006. *Annals of Epidemiology* 20(8): 617–628.

Mata, J., et al. 2010. When weight management lasts: Lower perceived rule complexity increases adherence. *Appetite* 54(1): 37–43.

McCullough, P. A., et al. 2006. Cardiorespiratory fitness and short-term complications after bariatric surgery. *CHEST* 130: 517–525.

National Center for Health Statistics. 2010. *Prevalence of Overweight, Obesity, and Extreme Obesity Among Adults: United States, Trends 1976–1980 Through 2007–2008* (http://www.cdc.gov/NCHS/data/hestat/obesity_adult_07_08/obesity_adult_07_08.pdf; retrieved July 8, 2010).

O'Brien, P., et al. 2006. Treatment of mild to moderate obesity with laparoscopic adjustable gastric banding or an intensive medical program. *Annals of Internal Medicine* 144(9): 625–633.

Ogden, C. L., et al. 2010. Prevalence of high body mass index in US children and adolescents, 2007–2008. *Journal of the American Medical Association* 303(3): 242–249.

Olshansky, S. J., et al. 2005. A potential decline in life expectancy in the United States in the 21st century. *New England Journal of Medicine* 352(11): 1138–1145.

van Dam, R. M., et al. 2006. The relationship between overweight in adolescence and premature death in women. *Annals of Internal Medicine* 145(2): 91–97.

Vorona, R. D., et al. 2005. Overweight and obese patients in a primary care population report less sleep than patients with a normal body mass index. *Archives of Internal Medicine* 165: 25–30.

Wang, Y., and M. A. Beydoun. 2007. The obesity epidemic in the United States—gender, age, socioeconomic, racial/ethnic and geographical characteristics: A systematic review and meta-regression analysis. *Epidemiologic Reviews* 29: 6–28.

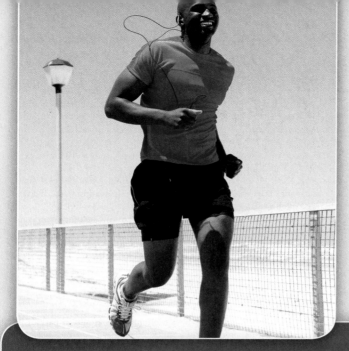

LOOKING AHEAD...

After reading this chapter, you should be able to:

- List the major components of the cardiovascular system and describe how blood is pumped and circulated throughout the body

- Describe the controllable and uncontrollable risk factors associated with cardiovascular disease

- Discuss the major forms of cardiovascular disease and how they develop

- Explain what cancer is and how it spreads

- List and describe common cancers—their risk factors, signs and symptoms, and treatments, as well as approaches to prevention

- List the steps you can take to lower your personal risk of cardiovascular disease and cancer

Cardiovascular Disease and Cancer

12

Cardiovascular disease (CVD) affects more than 81 million Americans and is the leading cause of death in the United States, claiming one life every 38 seconds—nearly 2300 Americans every day. Heart attacks and strokes are the number-one and number-three causes of death, respectively, making them the most common life-threatening manifestations of CVD. Cancer is the second leading cause of death in the United States, claiming nearly 70,000 lives annually—more than 1500 each day. Although age, genetics, and the environment play roles in the development of CVD and cancers, these diseases are primarily lifestyle diseases, linked to many controllable lifestyle factors. This chapter describes the forms and causes of these two diseases and provides information about how you can reduce your risk of developing and dying from CVD or cancer.

THE CARDIOVASCULAR SYSTEM

The **cardiovascular system** consists of the heart and blood vessels; together, they move blood throughout the body. When the lungs are included, the system is known as the cardiorespiratory system (see page T2-2 of the color transparency insert "Touring the Cardiorespiratory System" in this chapter).

The heart is a four-chambered, fist-sized muscle located just beneath the sternum (breastbone). It pumps deoxygenated (oxygen-poor) blood to the lungs and delivers oxygenated (oxygen-rich) blood to the rest of the body. Blood actually travels through two separate circulatory systems. The right side of the heart pumps blood to the lungs in what is called **pulmonary circulation**, and the left side pumps blood through the rest of the body in **systemic circulation** (see page T2-3 of the color transparency insert "Touring the Cardiorespiratory System" in this chapter).

Waste-laden, oxygen-poor blood travels the **venae cavae** into the heart's right upper chamber, or **atrium.** After the right atrium fills, it contracts and pumps blood into the heart's right lower chamber, or **ventricle.** When the right ventricle is full, it contracts and pumps blood through the pulmonary artery into the lungs. There, blood picks up oxygen and discards carbon dioxide. Cleaned, oxygenated blood then flows from the lungs through the pulmonary veins into the left atrium. After this chamber fills, it contracts and pumps blood into the left ventricle, which then pumps blood through the **aorta**—the body's largest artery—for distribution to the rest of the body's blood vessels. The period of the heart's contraction is called **systole;** the period of relaxation is called **diastole.**

Hypertension isn't just a risk factor for CVD; it is a type of CVD in itself.

Blood vessels are classified by size and function. **Veins** carry blood to the heart. **Arteries** carry blood away from the heart. Veins have thin walls, but arteries have thick elastic walls that enable them to expand and relax with the volume of blood being pumped through them. After leaving the heart, the aorta branches into smaller and smaller vessels. The smallest arteries branch still further into **capillaries,** tiny vessels only one cell thick. The capillaries deliver oxygen and nutrient-rich blood to the tissues and pick up oxygen-poor, waste-laden blood. From the capillaries, this blood empties into small veins and then into larger veins that return it to the heart to repeat the cycle. Two large vessels, the right and left **coronary arteries,** branch off the aorta and supply the heart muscle with oxygenated blood (see page T2-3 of the color transparency insert "Touring the Cardiorespiratory System" in this chapter). Blockage of a coronary artery is a leading cause of heart attacks.

RISK FACTORS FOR CARDIOVASCULAR DISEASE

Researchers have identified a variety of factors associated with an increased risk of developing CVD. They are grouped into two categories: major risk factors and contributing risk factors. Some risk factors are linked to controllable aspects of lifestyle and can therefore be changed. Others are beyond your control.

Major Risk Factors That Can Be Changed

The American Heart Association (AHA) has identified six major risk factors for CVD that can be changed: tobacco use, high blood pressure, unhealthy blood cholesterol levels, physical inactivity, overweight and obesity, and diabetes.

Ask Yourself

QUESTIONS FOR CRITICAL THINKING AND REFLECTION
How often do you think about the health of your heart? Are there certain situations, for example, that make you aware of your heart rate or make you wonder how strong your heart is?

Tobacco Use   About one in five deaths is attributable to smoking. People who smoke a pack of cigarettes a day have twice the risk of heart attack as nonsmokers; smoking two or more packs a day triples the risk. When smokers have heart attacks, they are two to three times more likely than nonsmokers to die from them. Cigarette smoking also doubles the risk of stroke.

Smoking harms the cardiovascular system in several ways. It damages the lining of arteries. It reduces the level of high-density lipoproteins (HDL), or "good" cholesterol, and raises the levels of triglycerides and low-density lipoproteins (LDL), or "bad" cholesterol. Nicotine increases blood pressure and heart rate. The carbon monoxide in cigarette smoke displaces oxygen in the blood, reducing the amount of oxygen available to the body. Smoking causes **platelets** to stick together in the bloodstream, leading to clotting, and it also speeds the development of fatty deposits in the arteries.

You don't have to smoke to be affected. The risk of developing heart disease increases up to 30% among those exposed to environmental tobacco smoke (ETS) at home or at work. Researchers estimate that about 35,000 nonsmokers die from heart disease each year as a result of exposure to ETS.

TERMS

cardiovascular disease (CVD)   The collective term for various diseases of the heart and blood vessels.

cardiovascular system   The system that circulates blood through the body; consists of the heart and blood vessels.

pulmonary circulation   The part of the circulatory system governed by the right side of the heart; the circulation of blood between the heart and the lungs.

systemic circulation   The part of the circulatory system governed by the left side of the heart; the circulation of blood between the heart and the rest of the body.

vena cava   Either of two large veins through which blood is returned to the right atrium of the heart; plural, *venae cavae.*

atrium   Either of the two upper chambers of the heart in which blood collects before passing to the ventricles; plural, *atria.*

ventricle   Either of the two lower chambers of the heart that pump blood to the lungs and other parts of the body.

aorta   The large artery that receives blood from the left ventricle and distributes it to the body.

systole   The contraction phase of the heart.

diastole   The relaxation phase of the heart.

vein   A vessel that carries blood to the heart.

artery   A vessel that carries blood away from the heart.

capillary   A very small blood vessel that serves to exchange oxygen and nutrients between the blood and tissues.

coronary artery   One of the system of arteries branching from the aorta that provides blood to the heart muscle.

platelets   Cell fragments in the blood that are necessary for the formation of blood clots.

Exam ✕

Table 12.1	Blood Pressure Classification for Healthy Adults		
CATEGORY[a]	SYSTOLIC (MM HG)		DIASTOLIC (MM HG)
Normal[b]	below 120	and	below 80
Prehypertension	120–139	or	80–89
Hypertension[c]			
Stage 1	140–159	or	90–99
Stage 2	160 and above	or	100 and above

[a]When systolic and diastolic pressure fall into different categories, the higher category should be used to classify blood pressure status.
[b]The risk of death from heart attack and stroke begins to rise when blood pressure is above 115/75.
[c]Based on the average of two or more readings taken at different physician visits. In persons over 50, systolic blood pressure greater than 140 is a much more significant CVD risk factor than diastolic blood pressure.

SOURCE: *The Seventh Report of the Joint National Committee on Prevention, Detection, Evaluation, and Treatment of High Blood Pressure.* 2003. Bethesda, Md.: National Heart, Lung, and Blood Institute. National Institutes of Health (NIH Publication No. 03-5233).

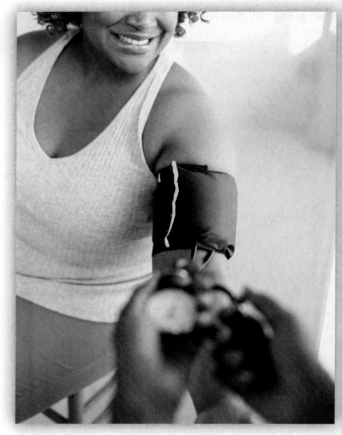

Monitoring blood pressure is a key strategy for the prevention of CVD. Blood pressure can be measured by a health care professional during a health care visit or at home with a home blood pressure monitor.

High Blood Pressure   High blood pressure, or **hypertension,** is a risk factor for many forms of cardiovascular disease, including heart attacks and strokes, and is itself considered a form of CVD.

Blood pressure, the force exerted by the blood on the vessel walls, is created by the pumping action of the heart. High blood pressure occurs when too much force is exerted against the walls of the arteries. Many factors affect blood pressure, such as exercise or excitement. Short periods of high blood pressure are normal, but chronic high blood pressure is a health risk.

Blood pressure is measured with a stethoscope and an instrument called a *sphygmomanometer.* It is expressed as two numbers—for example, 120 over 80—and measured in millimeters of mercury (mm Hg). The first number is the systolic blood pressure; the second is the diastolic blood pressure. A normal blood pressure reading for a healthy adult is below 120 systolic and below 80 diastolic; CVD risk increases when blood pressure rises above 120 over 80. High blood pressure in adults is defined as equal to or greater than 140 over 90 (Table 12.1).

High blood pressure results from an increased output of blood by the heart or from increased resistance to blood flow in the arteries. The latter condition can be caused by constriction of smooth muscle surrounding the arteries or by **atherosclerosis,** a disease process that causes arteries to become clogged and narrowed. High blood pressure also scars and hardens arteries, making them less elastic and further increasing blood pressure. When a person has high blood pressure, the heart must work harder than normal to force blood through the narrowed and stiffened arteries, straining both the heart and the arteries. High blood pressure is often called a silent killer, because it usually has no symptoms. A person may have high blood pressure for years without realizing it. But during that time, it damages vital organs and increases the risk of heart attack, congestive heart failure, stroke, kidney failure, and blindness.

Recent research has shed new light on the importance of lowering blood pressure to improve cardiovascular health. Death rates from CVD begin to rise when blood pressure is above 115 over 75, well below the traditional 140 over 90 cutoff for a diagnosis of hypertension. People with blood pressure in the prehypertension range are at an increased risk of heart attack and stroke as well as at significant risk of developing full-blown hypertension.

PREVALENCE   Hypertension is common, and its incidence increases with age. The rate of hypertension is highest in African Americans (41%), in whom, compared with other groups, the disorder is often more severe, more resistant to treatment, and more likely to be fatal at an early age.

TERMS

hypertension   Sustained abnormally high blood pressure.

atherosclerosis   A form of CVD in which the inner layers of artery walls are made thick and irregular by plaque deposits; arteries become narrow, and blood supply is reduced.

Primary hypertension cannot be cured, but it can be controlled. Because hypertension has no early warning signs, it's crucial to have your blood pressure tested at least once every 2 years (more often if you have other CVD risk factors). Lifestyle changes are recommended for everyone with prehypertension and hypertension. These changes include weight reduction, regular exercise, a healthy diet, and moderation of alcohol use. The DASH diet is recommended; it emphasizes eating more fruits, vegetables, and whole grains and increasing potassium and fiber intake. Even small increases in fruit and vegetable intake can create measurable drops in blood pressure.

Sodium restriction is also helpful for most people with hypertension. The American Heart Association and the 2010 Dietary Guidelines Advisory Committee recommend restricting sodium consumption to no more than 1500 mg per day. For people whose blood pressure isn't adequately controlled with lifestyle changes, medication is prescribed.

> **33%** of Americans have high blood pressure; **22%** of them aren't aware of their condition.
>
> —American Heart Association, 2010

High Cholesterol Cholesterol is a fatty, waxlike substance that circulates through the bloodstream and is an important component of cell membranes, sex hormones, vitamin D, the fluid that coats the lungs, and the protective sheaths around nerves. Adequate cholesterol is essential for the proper functioning of the body. Excess cholesterol, however, can clog arteries and increase the risk of CVD. Your liver manufactures cholesterol; you also get cholesterol from the foods you eat.

GOOD VERSUS BAD CHOLESTEROL Cholesterol is carried in the blood in protein-lipid packages called **lipoproteins**. **Low-density lipoproteins (LDLs)** shuttle cholesterol from the liver to the organs and tissues that require it. LDL is known as "bad" cholesterol because if there is more than the body can use, the excess is deposited in the blood vessels. If coronary arteries are blocked, the result may be a heart attack; if an artery carrying blood to the brain is blocked, a stroke may occur. **High-density lipoproteins (HDLs),** or "good" cholesterol, shuttle unused cholesterol back to the liver for recycling. By removing cholesterol from blood vessels, HDL helps protect against atherosclerosis.

RECOMMENDED BLOOD CHOLESTEROL LEVELS The risk for cardiovascular disease increases with higher blood cholesterol levels, especially LDL. The National Cholesterol Education Program (NCEP) recommends lipoprotein testing at least once every 5 years for all adults, beginning at age 20. The recommended test measures total cholesterol, LDL cholesterol, HDL cholesterol, and triglycerides (another blood fat). In general, high LDL, total cholesterol,

Table 12.2 Cholesterol Guidelines

TOTAL CHOLESTEROL (MG/DL)	
Less than 200	Desirable
200–239	Borderline high
240 or more	High
LDL CHOLESTEROL (MG/DL)	
Less than 100	Optimal
100–129	Near optimal/above optimal
130–159	Borderline high
160–189	High
190 or more	Very high
HDL CHOLESTEROL (MG/DL)	
Less than 40	Low (undesirable)
60 or more	High (desirable)
TRIGLYCERIDES (MG/DL)	
Less than 150	Normal
150–199	Borderline high
200–499	High
500 or more	Very high

SOURCE: Expert Panel on Detection, Evaluation, and Treatment of High Blood Cholesterol in Adults. 2001. Executive Summary of the Third Report of the National Cholesterol Education Program (NCEP) Expert Panel on Detection, Evaluation, and Treatment of High Blood Cholesterol in Adults (Adult Treatment Panel III). *Journal of the American Medical Association* 285(19).

and triglyceride levels combined with low HDL levels are associated with a higher risk for CVD. You can reduce this risk by lowering LDL, total cholesterol, and triglycerides. Raising HDL is important because a high HDL level seems to offer protection from CVD even in cases where total cholesterol is high. This seems to be especially true for women.

As shown in Table 12.2, LDL levels below 100 mg/dl (milligrams per deciliter) and total cholesterol levels below 200 mg/dl are desirable. An estimated 102 million American adults have total cholesterol levels of 200 mg/dl or higher. The CVD risk associated with elevated cholesterol levels also depends on other factors. For example, an above-optimal level of LDL would be of more concern for someone who also smokes and has high blood pressure than for someone without these additional CVD risk factors, and it is especially a concern for diabetics.

> **lipoproteins** Protein-and-lipid substances in the blood that carry fats and cholesterol; classified according to size, density, and chemical composition.
>
> **low-density lipoprotein (LDL)** A lipoprotein containing a moderate amount of protein and a large amount of cholesterol; "bad" cholesterol.
>
> **high-density lipoprotein (HDL)** A lipoprotein containing relatively little cholesterol that helps transport cholesterol out of the arteries and thus protects against heart diseases; "good" cholesterol.

BENEFITS OF CONTROLLING CHOLESTEROL Important dietary changes for reducing LDL levels include increasing fiber intake and substituting unsaturated for saturated and trans fats. Decreasing saturated and trans fats is particularly important because they promote the production of cholesterol by the liver. Exercising regularly and eating more fruits, vegetables, fish, and whole grains also help. You can raise your HDL levels by exercising regularly, losing weight if you are overweight, quitting smoking, and altering the amount and type of fat you consume.

> *Exercise is thought to be **the closest thing we have to a magic bullet** against heart disease.*

Physical Inactivity An estimated 40–60 million Americans are so sedentary that they are at high risk for developing CVD. Exercise is thought to be the closest thing we have to a magic bullet against heart disease. It lowers CVD risk by helping to decrease blood pressure and resting heart rate, increase HDL levels, maintain desirable weight, improve the condition of blood vessels, and prevent or control diabetes. One study found that women who accumulated at least 3 hours of brisk walking each week cut their risk of heart attack and stroke by more than 50%.

Obesity Death from CVD is two to three times more likely in obese people (BMI ≥ 30) than it is in lean people (BMI 18.5–24.9), and for every 5-unit increment of BMI, a person's risk of death from coronary heart disease increases by 30%. Excess body fat is strongly associated with hypertension, high cholesterol levels, insulin resistance, diabetes, physical inactivity, and increasing age. With excess weight, there is also more blood to pump and the heart has to work harder. This causes chronically elevated pressures within the heart chambers that can lead to ventricular **hypertrophy** (enlargement), and eventually the heart muscle can start to fail.

Physical activity and physical fitness have a strong positive influence on cardiovascular health in those who are overweight and obese. People who are obese but have at least moderate cardiorespiratory fitness may have lower rates of cardiovascular disease than their normal-weight but unfit peers. For someone who is overweight, even modest weight reduction—5–10% of body weight—can reduce CVD risk.

Overweight and obesity are major risk factors for cardiovascular disease, but physical activity, including walking, can lower that risk. Modest weight loss can also reduce CVD risk.

Diabetes Diabetes is a disorder characterized by elevated blood glucose levels due to an insufficient supply or inadequate action of insulin (see page T2-5 of the color transparency insert "Touring the Cardiorespiratory System" in this chapter). Diabetes doubles the risk of CVD for men and triples the risk for women. Diabetics tend to have higher rates of other CVD risk factors, including hypertension, obesity, and unhealthy blood lipid levels (typically, high triglyceride levels and low HDL levels). The elevated blood glucose and insulin levels that occur in diabetes can damage the endothelial cells that line the arteries, making them more vulnerable to atherosclerosis; diabetics also often have platelet and blood coagulation abnormalities that increase the risk of heart attacks and strokes. People with pre-diabetes also face a significantly increased risk of CVD.

> **65%** of people with diabetes die from CVD.
>
> —**American Heart Association, 2010**

In people with pre-diabetes, a healthy diet and exercise [ar]e more effective than medication at preventing diabetes. [F]or people with diabetes, a healthy diet, exercise, and [ca]reful control of glucose levels are recommended to de-[cr]ease chances of developing complications. Even people [w]hose diabetes is under control face a high risk of CVD, [s]o control of other risk factors is critical.

Contributing Risk Factors That Can Be Changed

Other factors that can be changed have been identified as contributing to CVD risk, including triglyceride levels and psychological and social factors.

High Triglyceride Levels Like cholesterol, **triglycerides** are blood fats that are obtained from food and manufactured by the body. High triglyceride levels are a reliable predictor of heart disease, especially if associated with other risk factors. Factors contributing to elevated triglyceride levels include excess body fat, physical inactivity, cigarette smoking, type 2 diabetes, excess alcohol intake, very high carbohydrate diets, and certain diseases and medications.

A full lipid profile should include testing and evaluation of triglyceride levels (see Table 12.2). For people with borderline high triglyceride levels, increased physical activity, reduced intake of added sugars, and weight reduction can help bring levels down into the healthy range; for people with high triglyceride levels, drug therapy may be recommended. Being moderate in the use of alcohol and quitting smoking are also important.

Psychological and Social Factors Many of the psychological and social factors that influence other areas of wellness are also important risk factors for CVD.

STRESS Excessive stress can strain the heart and blood vessels over time and contribute to CVD. When you experience stress, stress hormones activate the sympathetic nervous system, which causes the fight-or-flight response and increases heart rate and blood pressure in anticipation of physical activity. If you are healthy, you can tolerate the cardiovascular responses that take place during stress, but if you already have CVD, stress can lead to abnormal heart rhythms (arrhythmias), heart attacks, and sudden cardiac death.

CHRONIC HOSTILITY AND ANGER Certain traits in the hard-driving Type A personality—hostility, cynicism, and anger—are associated with increased risk of heart disease. Men prone to anger have two to three times the heart attack risk of calmer men and are much more likely to develop CVD at young ages (see the box "Anger, Hostility, and Heart Disease").

SUPPRESSING PSYCHOLOGICAL DISTRESS Suppressing anger and other negative emotions may also be hazardous to a healthy heart. People who hide psychological distress appear to have higher rates of heart disease than people who experience similar distress but share it with others. People with such "Type D" personalities tend to be pessimistic, negative, and unhappy and to suppress these feelings.

DEPRESSION Depression appears to increase the risk of CVD in healthy people and the risk of adverse cardiac events in those who already have heart disease. Depression also causes physiological changes; for example, it elevates basal levels of stress hormones, which induce a variety of stress-related responses.

ANXIETY Chronic anxiety and anxiety disorders (such as phobias and panic disorder) are associated with up to a threefold increased risk of coronary heart disease, heart attack, and sudden cardiac death. People with anxiety are more likely to have a subsequent adverse cardiac event after having a heart attack.

SOCIAL ISOLATION Social isolation and low social support (living alone, or having few friends or family members) are associated with an increased incidence of coronary heart disease (CHD) and poorer outcomes after the first diagnosis of CHD. A strong social support network is a major antidote to stress. Friends and family members can also promote and support a healthy lifestyle.

LOW SOCIOECONOMIC STATUS Low socioeconomic status and low educational attainment also increase risk for CVD. These associations are probably due to a variety of factors, including lifestyle and access to health care.

Alcohol and Drugs Although moderate drinking may have health benefits for some people, drinking too much alcohol raises blood pressure and can increase the risk of stroke and heart failure. Stimulant drugs, particularly cocaine, can also cause serious cardiac problems, including heart attack, stroke, and sudden cardiac death. Injection drug use can cause infection of the heart and stroke.

Major Risk Factors That Can't Be Changed

A number of major risk factors for CVD cannot be changed. They include heredity, aging, being male, and ethnicity.

Heredity Multiple genes contribute to the development of CVD and its associated risk factors, such as high cholesterol, hypertension, diabetes, and obesity. Having a favorable set of genes decreases your risk of developing

---

triglyceride A type of blood fat that can be a predictor of heart disease.

TERMS

Anger, Hostility, and Heart Disease

People with a quick temper, a persistently hostile outlook, and a cynical, mistrusting attitude toward life are more likely to develop heart disease than those with a calmer, more trusting attitude. People who are angry frequently, intensely, and for long periods experience the stress response much more often than more relaxed individuals. Over the long term, the effects of stress may damage arteries and promote CVD.

Are You Too Hostile?

To help answer that question, Duke University researcher Redford Williams, M.D., has devised a short self-test. It's not a scientific evaluation, but it does offer a rough measure of hostility. Are the following statements true or false for you?

1. I often get annoyed at checkout cashiers or the people in front of me when I'm waiting in line.
2. I usually keep an eye on the people I work or live with to make sure they do what they should.
3. I often wonder how homeless people can have so little respect for themselves.

4. I believe that most people will take advantage of you if you let them.
5. The habits of friends or family members often annoy me.
6. When I'm stuck in traffic, I often start breathing faster and my heart pounds.
7. When I'm annoyed with people, I really want to let them know it.
8. If someone does me wrong, I want to get even.
9. I'd like to have the last word in any argument.
10. At least once a week, I have the urge to yell at or even hit someone.

According to Williams, five or more "true" statements suggest that you're excessively hostile and should consider taking steps to mellow out.

Managing Your Anger

Begin by monitoring your angry responses and looking for triggers—people or situations that typically make you angry. Familiarize yourself with the patterns of thinking that lead to angry or hostile feelings, and then try to head them off before they develop into full-blown

anger. If you feel your anger starting to build, try reasoning with yourself by asking the following questions:

1. *Is this really important enough to get angry about?*
2. *Am I really justified in getting angry?*
3. *Is getting angry going to make a real and positive difference in this situation?*

If you answer yes to all three questions, then calm but assertive communication may be an appropriate response. If your anger isn't reasonable, try distracting yourself or removing yourself from the situation. Exercise, humor, social support, and other stress-management techniques can also help (see Chapter 3 for additional anger-management tips). Your heart—and the people around you—will benefit from your calmer, more positive outlook.

SOURCE: Virginia Williams and Redford Williams, 1999, *Lifeskills: 8 Simple Ways to Build Stronger Relationships, Communicate More Clearly, and Improve Your Health,* New York: Times Books.

CVD; having an unfavorable set of genes increases your risk. Risk, however, is modifiable by lifestyle factors.

Aging About 70% of all heart attack victims are age 65 or older, and about 75% who suffer fatal heart attacks are over 65. For people over 55, the incidence of stroke more than doubles in each successive decade. However, even people in their thirties and forties, especially men, can have heart attacks.

Being Male Although CVD is the leading killer of both men and women in the United States, men face a greater risk of heart attack than women, especially earlier in life. Until age 55, men also have a greater risk of hypertension. By age 75, the gender gap nearly disappears (see the box "Women and CVD").

Ethnicity Rates of heart disease vary among ethnic groups in the United States, with African Americans having much higher rates of hypertension, heart disease, and stroke than other groups (see the box "Ethnicity and CVD"). Puerto Rican Americans, Cuban Americans, and Mexican Americans are also more likely to suffer from

high blood pressure and angina (a warning sign of heart disease) than non-Hispanic white Americans. Asian Americans historically have had far lower rates of CVD than white Americans.

Inflammation and C-Reactive Protein Inflammation plays a key role in the development of CVD. When an artery is injured by smoking, cholesterol, hypertension, or other factors, the body's response is to produce inflammation. A substance called *C-reactive protein (CRP)* is released into the bloodstream during the inflammatory response, and high levels of CRP indicate a substantially elevated risk of heart attack and stroke. CRP may also be harmful to the coronary arteries themselves.

> In general, **men face a greater risk of heart attack, hypertension, and stroke than women.**

Lifestyle changes and certain drugs can reduce CRP levels. Statin drugs, widely prescribed to lower cholesterol,

On average, women live 10–15 more years free of coronary heart disease than men do. But heart disease is the leading cause of death among women, and it has killed more women than men every year since 1984.

Polls indicate that women vastly underestimate their risk of dying of a heart attack and, in turn, overestimate their risk of dying of breast cancer. In reality, nearly 1 in 3 women dies of CVD, whereas 1 in 30 dies of breast cancer. Minority women face the highest risk of developing CVD, but their awareness of heart disease as a killer of women is lower than that of white women.

Risk factors for CVD are similar for men and women and include age, family history, smoking, hypertension, high cholesterol, and diabetes. But there are gender differences. HDL appears to be an even more powerful predictor of CVD risk in women than it is in men. Also, women with diabetes have a greater risk of having CVD events like heart attack and stroke than men with diabetes.

Estrogen: A Heart Protector?

The hormone estrogen, produced naturally by a woman's ovaries until menopause, improves blood lipid concentrations and other CVD risk factors. For the past several decades, many physicians encouraged menopausal women to take hormone replacement therapy (HT) to relieve menopause symptoms and pre-sumably reduce the risk of CVD. However, studies found that HT may actually *increase* a woman's risk for heart disease and certain other health problems, including breast cancer. Some newer studies have found that the increased risk of CVD in women who start HT may be age dependent; women in the early stages of menopause (usually ages 40–49) or ages 50–59 did not appear to have excess risk. This suggests that outcomes may depend on several factors, including the timing of hormone use. The U.S. Preventive Services Task Force and the American Heart Association recommend that HT not be used to protect against CVD.

For younger women, the most common form of hormonal medication is oral contraceptives (OCs). Typical OCs contain estrogen and progestin in relatively low doses and are generally considered safe for most nonsmoking women. But women who smoke and use OCs are up to 32 times more likely to have a heart attack than nonsmoking OC users.

Postmenopausal Women: At Risk

Women who have heart attacks are more likely than men to die within a year. One reason is that because women develop heart disease at older ages, they are more likely to have other health problems that complicate treatment. Women have smaller hearts and arteries than men, possibly making diagnosis and treatment more difficult. There may also be biological or psychosocial risk factors contributing to women's mortality.

Also, medical personnel appear to evaluate and treat women less aggressively than men. Women with positive stress tests and those whose evaluation raises concern about a heart attack are less likely to be referred to further testing than are men. In addition, studies of heart attack patients have found that women usually have to wait longer than men to receive clot-dissolving drugs in an emergency room.

Women presenting with CHD are just as likely as men to report chest pain, but are also likely to report non-chest-pain symptoms, which may obscure their diagnosis. These additional symptoms include fatigue, weakness, shortness of breath, nausea, vomiting, and pain in the abdomen, neck, jaw, and back. Women are also more likely to have pain at rest, during sleep, or with mental stress.

Careful diagnosis of symptoms is also key in cases of stress-induced cardiomyopathy ("broken heart syndrome"), which occurs much more often in women. In this condition, a severe stress response stuns the heart, producing heart-attack-like symptoms and decreased pumping function of the heart, but no damage to the heart muscle. Typically, the condition reverses quickly, and correct diagnosis is important to avoid unnecessary invasive procedures.

---

also decrease inflammation and reduce CRP levels; this may be one reason that statin drugs seem to lower CVD risk even in people with normal blood lipid levels.

Possible Risk Factors Currently Being Studied

2.9 million
American teenagers have metabolic syndrome.

—American Heart Association, 2010

In recent years, other possible risk factors for cardiovascular disease have been identified.

Insulin Resistance and Metabolic Syndrome As people gain weight and engage in less physical activity, their muscles, fat, and liver become less sensitive to the effect of insulin—a condition known as insulin resistance (or pre-diabetes). As the body becomes increasingly insulin resistant, the pancreas must secrete more and more insulin to keep glucose levels within a normal range. Eventually, however, even high levels of insulin may become insufficient, and blood glucose levels will also start to rise (hyperglycemia), resulting in type 2 diabetes.

Those who have insulin resistance tend to have several other related risk factors; as a group, this cluster of abnormalities is called metabolic syndrome or insulin resistance syndrome (Table 12.3). Metabolic syndrome significantly increases the risk of CVD—more so in women than in men. It is estimated that about 34% of the adult U.S. population has metabolic syndrome.

To reduce your risk for metabolic syndrome, choose a healthy diet and get plenty of exercise. The amount and

African Americans are at substantially higher risk for death from CVD than other groups. The rate of hypertension among African Americans is among the highest of any group in the world. Blacks tend to develop hypertension at an earlier age than whites, and their average blood pressures are much higher. African Americans have a higher risk of stroke, have strokes at younger ages, and, if they survive, have more significant stroke-related disabilities. Some experts recommend that blacks be treated with antihypertensive drugs at an earlier stage—when blood pressure reaches 130/80 rather than the typical 140/90 cutoff for hypertension.

A number of genetic and biological factors may contribute to CVD in African Americans. They may be more sensitive to dietary sodium, leading to greater blood pressure elevation in response to a given amount of sodium. African Americans may also experience less dilation of blood vessels in response to stress, an attribute that also raises blood pressure.

Heredity also plays a large role in the tendency to develop diabetes, another important CVD risk factor that is more common in blacks than whites. However, Latinos are even more likely to develop diabetes and insulin resistance, and at a younger age, than African Americans. There is variation within the Latino population, however, with a higher prevalence of diabetes occurring among Mexican Americans and Puerto Ricans and a relatively lower prevalence among Cuban Americans.

Another factor that likely contributes to the high incidence of CVD among ethnic minority groups is low income. Economic deprivation usually means reduced access to adequate health care and health insurance. Also associated with low income is low educational attainment, which often means less information about preventive health measures, such as diet and stress management. And people with low incomes tend to smoke more, use more salt, and exercise less than those with higher incomes.

Discrimination may also play a role in CVD. Physicians and hospitals may treat the medical problems of ethnic minorities differently than those of whites. Discrimination, along with low income and other forms of deprivation, may also increase stress, which is linked with hypertension and CVD. In terms of access to care, factors such as insurance coverage and availability of high-tech cardiac equipment in hospitals used most often by minorities may also play a role.

CVD risk in ethnic groups is further affected by immigration and one's place of birth. Upon immigration to the United States, an Asian's risk for CVD tends to increase and reflect that of a typical American more than a typical Asian, perhaps in part because Asian immigrants often abandon their traditional (and healthier) diets.

However, birthplace (and its associated lifestyle factors) also seems to be a strong determinant of risk. One study found that among New Yorkers born in the Northeast, blacks and whites have nearly identical risk of CVD. But black New Yorkers who were born in the South have a sharply higher risk, and black New Yorkers born in the Caribbean have a significantly lower risk. Researchers speculate that instead of abandoning their traditional diets and lifestyles, blacks from the South bring these traditions with them. Some risk factors for CVD, including smoking and a high-fat diet, are more common in the South. Combined with urban stress, these factors create a lifestyle that is far from heart-healthy.

All Americans are advised to have their blood pressure checked regularly, exercise, eat a healthy diet, manage stress, and avoid smoking. These general preventive strategies may be particularly helpful for ethnic minorities. Tailoring your lifestyle to your particular ethnic risk may also be helpful in some cases. Discuss your particular risk profile with your physician to help identify lifestyle changes most appropriate for you.

Table 12.3	Defining Characteristics of Metabolic Syndrome*	
Abdominal obesity (waist circumference)		
Men	>40 in (>102 cm)	
Women	>35 in (>88 cm)	
Triglycerides	≥150 mg/dl	
HDL cholesterol		
Men	<40 mg/dl or drug-treated	
Women	<50 mg/dl or drug-treated	
Blood pressure	≥130/≥85 mm Hg or drug-treated	
Fasting glucose	≥100 mg/dl or drug-treated	

*A person is diagnosed with metabolic syndrome if she or he has three or more of the risk factors listed here.

SOURCE: Grundy, S. M., et al. 2005. Diagnosis and management of the metabolic syndrome: An American Heart Association/National Heart, Lung, and Blood Institute Scientific Statement. *Circulation* 112: 2735.

type of carbohydrate intake is also important: Diets high in carbohydrates, especially high-glycemic-index foods, can raise levels of glucose and triglycerides and lower HDL, thus contributing to the development or worsening of metabolic syndrome and CVD, particularly in people who are already sedentary and overweight. For people prone to insulin resistance, eating more unsaturated fats, protein, vegetables, and fiber while limiting added sugars and starches may be beneficial.

Homocysteine Elevated levels of homocysteine, an amino acid circulating in the blood, are associated with an increased risk of CVD. Homocysteine appears to damage the lining of blood vessels, resulting in inflammation and the development of fatty deposits in artery walls. These changes can lead to the formation of clots and blockages in arteries, which in turn can cause heart attacks and strokes. High homocysteine levels are also associated with cognitive impairment, such as memory loss. Men generally have higher homocysteine levels than women, as do individuals with diets low in folic acid, vitamin B-12, and vitamin B-6. If your homocysteine level is high, it may be helpful to follow a diet rich in fruits, vegetables, and whole grains.

MAJOR FORMS OF CARDIOVASCULAR DISEASE

According to the CDC, heart diseases killed nearly 632,000 Americans in 2006. Figure 12.1 shows the death rates among various ethnic groups due to heart disease in 2006, the most recent year for which data are available. The main forms of CVD are atherosclerosis, heart disease and heart attack, stroke, peripheral arterial disease (PAD), congestive heart failure, congenital heart disease, rheumatic heart disease, and heart valve problems. Many forms are interrelated and have elements in common; we treat them separately here for the sake of clarity. Hypertension, which is both a major risk factor and a form of CVD, was described earlier in the chapter.

> The estimated annual financial burden of CVD is **$475.3 billion.**
>
> —American Heart Association, 2009

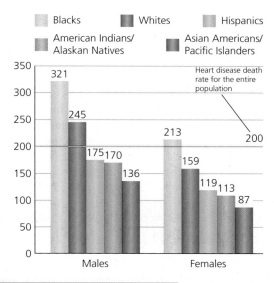

Blacks · Whites · Hispanics · American Indians/Alaskan Natives · Asian Americans/Pacific Islanders

Heart disease death rate for the entire population — 200

Males: 321, 245, 175, 170, 136
Females: 213, 159, 119, 113, 87

VITAL STATISTICS

FIGURE 12.1 Heart disease death rates of Americans, 2006. Deaths due to various forms of heart disease per 100,000 people.

SOURCE: National Center for Health Statistics. 2010. *Health, United States, 2009.* Hyattsville, Md.: National Center for Health Statistics.

Ask Yourself

QUESTIONS FOR CRITICAL THINKING AND REFLECTION

What risk factors do you have for cardiovascular disease? Which ones are factors you have control over, and which are factors you can't change? If you have risk factors you cannot change (such as a family history of CVD), were you aware that you can make lifestyle adjustments to reduce your risk? Do you think you will make them?

Atherosclerosis *Exam* ✳

Atherosclerosis is a form of arteriosclerosis, or thickening and hardening of the arteries. In atherosclerosis, arteries become narrowed by deposits of fat, cholesterol, and other substances (see page T2-4 of the color transparency insert "Touring the Cardiorespiratory System" in this chapter). The process begins when the endothelial cells (cells that line the arteries) become damaged, most likely through a combination of factors such as smoking, high blood pressure, high insulin or glucose levels, and deposits of oxidized LDL particles. The body's response to this damage results in inflammation and changes in the artery lining that create a sort of magnet for LDL, platelets, and other cells; these cells build up and cause a bulge in the wall of the artery. As these deposits, called **plaques,** accumulate on artery walls, the arteries lose their elasticity and their ability to expand and contract, restricting blood flow. Once narrowed by a plaque, an artery is vulnerable to blockage by blood clots.

If the heart, brain, and/or other organs are deprived of blood and the oxygen it carries, the effects of atherosclerosis can be deadly. Coronary arteries, which supply the heart with blood, are particularly susceptible to plaque buildup, a condition called **coronary heart disease (CHD),** or *coronary artery disease (CAD).* The blockage of a coronary artery causes a heart attack. If a cerebral artery (leading to the brain) is blocked, the result is a stroke. If an artery in a limb becomes narrowed or blocked, it causes *peripheral arterial disease,* a condition that causes pain and sometimes loss of the affected limb.

The main risk factors for atherosclerosis are cigarette smoking, physical inactivity, high levels of blood cholesterol, high blood pressure, and diabetes. Atherosclerosis often begins in childhood.

plaque A deposit of fatty (and other) substances on the inner wall of an artery.

coronary heart disease (CHD) Heart disease caused by atherosclerosis in the arteries that supply blood to the heart muscle; also called *coronary artery disease.*

TERMS

Heart Disease and Heart Attack

When one of the coronary arteries becomes blocked, a **heart attack,** or *myocardial infarction (MI),* results. Although a heart attack may come without warning, it is usually the end result of a long-term disease process. Heart attack symptoms may include chest pain or pressure, arm, neck, or jaw pain, difficulty breathing, excessive sweating, nausea and vomiting, and loss of consciousness. Most people having a heart attack suffer chest pain, but about one-third of heart attack victims do not. Women, ethnic minorities, older adults, and people with diabetes are the most likely groups to experience heart attack without chest pain.

Angina Arteries narrowed by disease may still be open enough to deliver blood to the heart. At times, however—during stress or exertion, for example—the heart needs more oxygen than can flow through narrowed arteries. When the need for oxygen exceeds the supply, chest pain, called **angina pectoris,** may occur. Angina pain is usually felt as an extreme tightness in the chest and heavy pressure behind the breastbone or in the shoulder, neck, arm, hand, or back. Angina may be controlled in a number of ways (with drugs and surgical or nonsurgical procedures), but its course is unpredictable. Over a period ranging from hours to years, the narrowing may go on to full blockage and a heart attack.

Arrhythmias and Sudden Cardiac Death The pumping of the heart is controlled by electrical impulses from the sinus node, located in the right atrium, that maintain a regular heartbeat of 60–100 beats per minute. If this electrical conduction system is disrupted, the heart may beat too quickly, too slowly, or in an irregular fashion, a condition known as **arrhythmia.** Arrhythmia can cause symptoms ranging from imperceptible to severe and even fatal.

Sudden cardiac death, also called *cardiac arrest,* is most often caused by an arrhythmia called *ventricular fibrillation,* a kind of quivering of the ventricle that makes it ineffective in pumping blood. If ventricular fibrillation continues for more than a few minutes, it is generally fatal. Cardiac defibrillation, in which an electrical shock is delivered to the heart, can be effective in jolting the heart into a more efficient rhythm. Automated external defibrillators (AEDs) are becoming increasingly available in public places for use by the general public. (Training in the use of AEDs is available from organizations such as the American Red Cross and the American Heart Association.) Some arrhythmias cause no problems and resolve without treatment; more serious arrhythmias are usually treated with medication or a surgically implanted pacemaker or defibrillator that delivers electrical stimulation to the heart to create a more normal rhythm.

Helping a Heart Attack Victim Most people who die from a heart attack expire within 2 hours from the time they experience the first symptoms. If you or someone you are with has any of the warning signs of heart attack listed in the box "What to Do in Case of a Heart Attack, Stroke, or Cardiac Arrest," take immediate action. Many experts also suggest that the heart attack victim chew and swallow one adult aspirin tablet (325 mg) as soon as possible after symptoms begin; aspirin has an immediate anticlotting effect.

If the victim loses consciousness, a qualified person should immediately start administering emergency **cardiopulmonary resuscitation (CPR).** Damage to the heart muscle increases with time. If the person receives emergency care quickly enough, a clot-dissolving agent can be injected to break up a clot in the coronary artery.

Detecting and Treating Heart Disease Currently, the most common initial screening tool for CAD is the stress, or exercise, test, in which a patient runs or walks on a treadmill or pedals a stationary cycle while being monitored for abnormalities with an **electrocardiogram (ECG** or **EKG).** Certain characteristic changes in the heart's electrical activity while under stress can reveal particular heart problems, such as restricted blood flow. Exercise testing can also be performed in conjunction with imaging techniques such as nuclear medicine or echocardiography that provide pictures of the heart, which can help pinpoint problems.

TERMS

heart attack Damage to, or death of, heart muscle, resulting from a failure of the coronary arteries to deliver enough blood to the heart; also known as *myocardial infarction (MI).*

angina pectoris Pain in the chest, and often in the left arm and shoulder, caused by the heart muscle not receiving enough blood.

arrhythmia A change in the normal pattern of the heartbeat.

sudden cardiac death A nontraumatic, unexpected death from sudden cardiac arrest, most often due to arrhythmia; in most instances, victims have underlying heart disease.

cardiopulmonary resuscitation (CPR) A technique involving mouth-to-mouth breathing and/or chest compression to keep oxygen flowing to the brain.

electrocardiogram (ECG or EKG) A test to detect abnormalities by evaluating the electrical activity in the heart.

Ask Yourself

QUESTIONS FOR CRITICAL THINKING AND REFLECTION

Has anyone you know ever had a heart attack? If so, was the onset gradual or sudden? Were appropriate steps taken to help the person (for example, did anyone call 911, give CPR, or use an AED)? Do you feel comfortable dealing with a cardiac emergency? If not, what can you do to improve your readiness?

What to Do in Case of a Heart Attack, Stroke, or Cardiac Arrest

Warning Signs of Heart Attack

Some heart attacks are sudden and intense—the "movie heart attack," where no one doubts what's happening. But most heart attacks start slowly, with mild pain or discomfort. Often people affected aren't sure what's wrong and wait too long before getting help. Here are signs that can mean a heart attack is happening:

- **Chest discomfort.** Heart attacks often involve discomfort in the chest that lasts more than a few minutes, or that goes away and comes back. It can feel like uncomfortable pressure, squeezing, fullness, or pain.

- **Discomfort in other areas of the upper body.** Symptoms can include pain or discomfort in one or both arms, the back, neck, jaw, or stomach.

- **Shortness of breath.** This may occur with or without chest discomfort.

- **Other signs.** Signs may include breaking out in a cold sweat, nausea, vomiting, or lightheadedness.

Not all the signs occur in every heart attack. As with men, women's most common heart attack symptom is chest pain or discomfort, but women are somewhat more likely than men to experience some of the other symptoms, particularly shortness of breath, nausea/vomiting, and back or jaw pain.

If you or someone you're with has chest discomfort, especially with one or more of the other signs, don't wait longer than a few minutes (no more than 5) before calling for help.

Calling 9-1-1 is almost always the fastest way to get life-saving treatment. Emergency medical services staff can begin treatment when they arrive—up to an hour sooner than if someone gets to the hospital by car. Patients with chest pain who arrive by ambulance usually receive faster treatment at the hospital, too. Today, medications and treatments are available that weren't available in the past, but they must be given relatively quickly after the heart attack to be effective.

If you can't access the emergency medical services (EMS), have someone drive you to the hospital right away. If you're the one having symptoms, don't drive yourself, unless you have absolutely no other option.

Warning Signs of Stroke

The American Stroke Association says these are the warning signs of stroke:

- Sudden numbness or weakness of the face, arm, or leg, especially on one side of the body

- Sudden confusion, trouble speaking or understanding

- Sudden trouble seeing in one or both eyes

- Sudden trouble walking, dizziness, or loss of balance or coordination

- Sudden, severe headache with no known cause

If you or someone with you has one or more of these signs, call 9-1-1 immediately. If given within 3 hours of the start of symptoms, a clot-busting drug called tissue plasminogen activator (tPA) can reduce long-term disability for the most common type of stroke. tPA is the only FDA-approved medication for the treatment of stroke within 3 hours of symptom onset.

Signs of Cardiac Arrest

Cardiac arrest strikes immediately and without warning. Here are the signs:

- Sudden loss of responsiveness. No response to tapping on shoulders.

- No normal breathing. The victim does not take a normal breath when you tilt the head up and check for at least 5 seconds.

If these signs of cardiac arrest are present, tell someone to call 9-1-1 and to get an automated external defibrillator (AED) if one is available before you begin CPR. Use the AED as soon as it arrives.

For more on emergency care for cardiac arrest, see the inside back cover.

SOURCE: Adapted from American Heart Association. 2005. *Heart Attack, Stroke, and Cardiac Arrest Warning Signs.* www.americanheart.org—OID=3053. Copyright © 2007 American Heart Association.

If symptoms or noninvasive tests such as **magnetic resonance imaging (MRI)** or positron emission tomography (PET) suggest coronary artery disease, the next step is usually a coronary **angiogram,** performed in a cardiac catheterization lab. In this test, a catheter (a small plastic tube) is threaded into an artery, usually in the groin, and advanced through the aorta to the coronary arteries. The catheter is then placed into the opening of the coronary artery and a special dye is injected. The dye can be seen moving through the arteries under moving X ray, and any narrowings or blockages can be identified. If a problem is found, it is commonly treated with **balloon angioplasty,** which involves placing a small wire in the artery and feeding a deflated balloon over it. The balloon is advanced to the site of the narrowing and then inflated, flattening the fatty plaque and widening the arterial opening. This is generally followed by placement of a stent, a small metal tube that helps keep the artery open.

Other treatments, ranging from medication to major surgery, are also available. Along with a low-fat diet, regular exercise, and smoking cessation, one frequent recommendation for people at high risk for CVD is to take a low-dose aspirin tablet every day. Aspirin has an anticlotting effect, discouraging platelets in the blood from sticking to arterial plaques and forming clots; it also reduces inflammation.

In cases of a more severe blockage, **coronary bypass surgery** may be performed. Cardiothoracic surgeons remove a healthy blood vessel, usually a vein from one of the patient's legs, and graft it from the aorta to one or more coronary arteries to bypass a blockage.

Stroke

A **stroke,** also called a *cerebrovascular accident (CVA),* occurs when the blood supply to the brain is cut off.

> **795,000**
> Americans suffer strokes each year.
> —American Heart Association, 2010

Types of Strokes   There are two major types of strokes (Figure 12.2).

ISCHEMIC STROKE   An **ischemic stroke** is caused by a blockage in a blood vessel. There are two types of ischemic strokes: A *thrombotic stroke* is caused by a **thrombus,** a blood clot that forms in a cerebral artery that has been narrowed or damaged by atherosclerosis; an *embolic stroke* is caused by an **embolus,** a wandering blood clot that is carried in the bloodstream and may become wedged in a cerebral artery. Many embolic strokes are linked to a type of abnormal heart rhythm called *atrial fibrillation.* Ischemic strokes account for 87% of all strokes.

HEMORRHAGIC STROKE   A **hemorrhagic stroke** occurs when a blood vessel in the brain bursts, spilling blood into the surrounding tissue. Cells normally nourished by the artery are deprived of blood and cannot function. In addition, accumulated blood from the burst vessel may put pressure on surrounding brain tissue, causing damage and even death. There are two types of hemorrhagic strokes: An *intracerebral hemorrhage* occurs when a blood vessel ruptures within the brain; a *subarachnoid hemorrhage* occurs when a blood vessel on the brain's surface ruptures and bleeds into the space between the brain and the skull. Hemorrhages can be caused by head injuries or the bursting of a malformed blood vessel or an **aneurysm,** a blood-filled pocket that bulges out from a weak spot in an artery wall. Aneurysms in the brain may remain stable and never break. But when they do, the result is a stroke. Aneurysms may be caused or worsened by hypertension.

The Effects of a Stroke   The interruption of the blood supply to any area of the brain prevents the nerve cells there from functioning—in some cases causing death. Stroke survivors usually have some lasting disability. A stroke may cause paralysis, walking disability, speech impairment, memory loss, and changes in behavior. The severity of the stroke and its long-term effects depend on which brain cells have been injured, how widespread the damage is, how effectively the body can restore the blood supply, and how rapidly other areas of the brain can take over the functions of the damaged areas.

HEMORRHAGIC STROKE

- 13% of strokes
- Caused by ruptured blood vessels followed by blood leaking into tissue
- Usually more serious than ischemic stroke

Subarachnoid hemorrhage
- A bleed into the space between the brain and the skull
- Develops most often from an *aneurysm*, a weakened, ballooned area in the wall of an artery

Intracerebral hemorrhage
- A bleed from a blood vessel inside the brain
- Often caused by high blood pressure and the damage it does to arteries

ISCHEMIC STROKE

- 87% of strokes
- Caused by blockages in brain blood vessels; potentially treatable with clot-busting drugs
- Brain tissue dies when blood flow is blocked

Embolic stroke
- Caused by *emboli*, blood clots that travel from elsewhere in the body to the brain blood vessels
- 25% of embolic strokes are related to atrial fibrillation

Thrombotic stroke
- Caused by *thrombi*, blood clots that form where an artery has been narrowed by atherosclerosis
- Most often develops when part of a thrombus breaks away and causes a blockage in a downstream artery

FIGURE 12.2   Types of stroke.

SOURCE: Excerpted from *Harvard Health Letter,* April 2000. © 2000, Harvard University. Reprinted with permission. For more information visit: http://www.health.harvard.edu/newsletters/Harvard_Health_Letter.

> *Full-blown strokes are **sometimes** preceded by **symptomless "silent" strokes** or by ministrokes.*

Detecting and Treating Stroke   Effective treatment requires the prompt recognition of symptoms and correct diagnosis of the type of stroke. Many people have strokes without knowing it. These "silent strokes" do not cause any noticeable symptoms while they are occurring. Although they may be mild, silent strokes leave their victims at a higher risk for subsequent and more serious strokes later in life. They also contribute to loss of mental and cognitive skills.

Some stroke victims have a **transient ischemic attack (TIA),** or ministroke, days, weeks, or months before they have a full-blown stroke. A TIA produces temporary stroke-like symptoms, such as weakness or numbness in an arm or a leg, speech difficulty, or dizziness. These symptoms are brief, often lasting just a few minutes, and do not cause permanent damage. TIAs should be taken as warning signs of a stroke, however, and anyone with a suspected TIA should get immediate medical help.

A person with stroke symptoms should be rushed to the hospital. A **computed tomography (CT)** scan, which uses a computer to construct an image of the brain from X rays, can assess brain damage and determine the type of stroke. Newer techniques using MRI and ultrasound are becoming increasingly available and should improve the speed and accuracy of stroke diagnosis.

If tests reveal that a stroke is caused by a blood clot—and if help is sought within a few hours of the onset of symptoms—the person can be treated with the same kind of clot-dissolving drugs that are used to treat coronary artery blockages. If the clot is dissolved quickly enough, brain damage is minimized and symptoms may disappear.

If tests reveal that a stroke was caused by a cerebral hemorrhage, drugs may be prescribed to lower the blood pressure, which will usually be high. Careful diagnosis is crucial, because administering clot-dissolving drugs to a person suffering a hemorrhagic stroke would cause more bleeding and potentially more brain damage.

If detection and treatment of stroke come too late, rehabilitation is the only treatment. Although damaged or destroyed brain tissue does not normally regenerate, nerve cells in the brain can make new pathways, and some functions can be taken over by other parts of the

transient ischemic attack (TIA)   A small stroke; usually a temporary interruption of blood supply to the brain, causing numbness or difficulty with speech.

computed tomography (CT)   The use of computerized X ray images to create a cross-sectional depiction (scan) of tissue density.

TERMS

brain. Some people recover completely in a matter of days or weeks, but most stroke victims who survive must adapt to some disability.

Congestive Heart Failure

When the heart has been damaged by high blood pressure or other disease conditions and cannot maintain its regular pumping rate and force, fluids begin to back up into body tissue. When extra fluid seeps through capillary walls, edema (swelling) results, usually in the legs and ankles, but sometimes in other parts of the body as well. Fluid can collect in the lungs and interfere with breathing, particularly when a person is lying down. This condition is called **pulmonary edema,** and the entire process is known as **congestive heart failure.** Treatment includes reducing the workload on the heart, modifying salt intake, and using drugs that help the body eliminate excess fluid. When medical therapy is ineffective, heart transplant is a solution for some patients with severe heart failure, but the need greatly exceeds the number of hearts available.

Other Forms of Heart Disease

Other, less common, disorders and diseases also affect the heart.

Congenital Heart Defects About 36,000 children born each year in the United States have a malformation of the heart or major blood vessels. These conditions are collectively referred to as **congenital heart defects,** and they cause about 3600 deaths a year. The most common congenital defects are holes in the wall that divides the chambers of the heart and *coarctation of the aorta,* a narrowing, or constriction, of the aorta. Most of the common congenital defects can now be accurately diagnosed and treated with medication or surgery.

Hypertrophic cardiomyopathy (HCM) occurs in 1 out of every 500 people and is the most common cause of sudden death among athletes younger than age 35. The disease causes the heart muscle to become hypertrophic (enlarged). People with hypertrophic cardiomyopathy are at high risk for sudden death, mainly due to serious arrhythmias. Hypertrophic cardiomyopathy may be identified by a **murmur,** then diagnosed using echocardiography. Possible treatments include medication and a pacemaker or internal defibrillator.

Rheumatic Heart Disease **Rheumatic fever,** a consequence of certain types of untreated streptococcal throat infections, is a leading cause of heart disease worldwide. Rheumatic fever can permanently damage the heart muscle and heart valves, a condition called *rheumatic heart disease (RHD).* Symptoms of strep throat include the sudden onset of a sore throat, painful swallowing, fever, swollen glands, headache, nausea, and vomiting. If left untreated, up to 3% of strep infections progress into rheumatic fever.

Heart Valve Disorders Congenital defects and certain types of infections can cause abnormalities in the valves between the chambers of the heart. The most common heart valve disorder is **mitral valve prolapse (MVP),** which occurs in about 3% of the population. Most people with MVP have no symptoms; they have the same ability to exercise and live as long as people without MVP. Treatment for MVP is usually unnecessary, although surgery may be needed in the rare cases where leakage through the faulty valve is severe.

PROTECTING YOURSELF AGAINST CARDIOVASCULAR DISEASE

CVD can begin very early in life. For example, fatty streaks (very early atherosclerosis) can be seen on the aorta in children younger than age 10. Reducing CVD risk factors when you are young can pay off with many extra years of life and health.

Eat Heart-Healthy

For most Americans, eating a heart-healthy diet involves cutting total fat intake, substituting unsaturated fats for saturated and trans fats, and increasing intake of whole grains and fiber. Several other dietary factors also affect CVD risk.

- *Fat and cholesterol.* The National Cholesterol Education Program (NCEP) recommends that all Americans over age 2 adopt a diet in which total fat

TERMS

pulmonary edema The accumulation of fluid in the lungs.

congestive heart failure A condition resulting from the heart's inability to pump out all the blood that returns to it; blood backs up in the veins leading to the heart, causing an accumulation of fluid in various parts of the body.

congenital heart defect A defect or malformation of the heart or its major blood vessels, present at birth.

hypertrophic cardiomyopathy (HCM) An inherited condition in which there is an enlargement of the heart muscle, especially between the two ventricles.

murmur An abnormal heart sound indicating turbulent blood flow through a valve or hole in the heart.

rheumatic fever A disease, mainly of children, characterized by fever, inflammation, and pain in the joints; often damages the heart valves and muscle, a condition called *rheumatic heart disease.*

mitral valve prolapse (MVP) A condition in which the mitral valve billows out during ventricular contraction, possibly allowing leakage of blood from the left ventricle into the left atrium.

consumption is no more than 30% of total daily calories, with no more than one-third of total fat calories (10% of total daily calories) coming from saturated fat. The American Heart Association and the 2010 Dietary Guidelines Advisory Committee recommend that no more than 7% of daily calories come from saturated fat. The NCEP recommends that most Americans limit dietary cholesterol intake to no more than 300 mg per day; for people with heart disease or high LDL levels, the suggested daily limit is 200 mg. Animal products contain cholesterol as well as saturated fat; vegetable products do not contain cholesterol.

- *Fiber.* Studies have shown that a high-fiber diet is associated with a 40–50% reduction in the risk of heart attack and stroke. To get the recommended 25–38 grams of dietary fiber per day, eat whole grains, fruits, and vegetables. Good sources of fiber include oatmeal, some breakfast cereals, barley, legumes, and most fruits and vegetables.

- *Sodium and potassium.* Reducing sodium intake to recommended levels, while also increasing potassium intake, can help reduce blood pressure for many people. The American Heart Association and the 2010 Dietary Guidelines Advisory Committee recommend that sodium intake be reduced to no more than 1500 mg per day for all Americans.

- *Alcohol.* Moderate alcohol use may increase HDL cholesterol; it may also reduce stroke risk, possibly by dampening the inflammatory response or by affecting blood clotting. For most people under age 45, however, the risks of alcohol use probably outweigh any health benefit. Excessive alchohol consumption increases the risk of a variety of serious health problems, including hypertension, stroke, some cancers, liver disease, alcohol dependence, and injuries.

- *Omega-3 fatty acids.* Found in fish, shellfish, and some plant foods (nuts and canola, soybean, and flaxseed oils), omega-3 fatty acids may reduce clotting, abnormal heart rhythms, and inflammation and have other heart-healthy effects, such as lowering triglycerides. The American Heart Association recommends eating fish two or more times a week.

- *Plant stanols and sterols.* Plant stanols and sterols, found in some types of trans fat-free margarines and other products, reduce the absorption of cholesterol in the body and help lower LDL levels.

- *Folic acid, vitamin B-6, and vitamin B-12.* These vitamins lower homocysteine levels, and folic acid has also been found to reduce the risk of hypertension.

- *Calcium.* Diets rich in calcium may help prevent hypertension and possibly stroke by reducing insulin resistance and platelet aggegration.

Ask Yourself

QUESTIONS FOR CRITICAL THINKING AND REFLECTION

Do you know what your blood pressure and cholesterol levels are? If not, is there a reason you don't know? Is there something preventing you from getting this information about yourself? How can you motivate yourself to have these easy but important health checks?

- *Soy protein.* Replacing some animal proteins with soy protein may help lower LDL cholesterol.

- *Healthy carbohydrates.* Healthier carbohydrate choices, including whole grains, fruits, and non-starchy vegetables, typically provide more nutrients than refined grains and starchy foods. Healthy carbohydrates are important for people with insulin resistance, pre-diabetes, or diabetes.

- *Total calories.* Reducing energy intake can improve cholesterol and triglyceride levels as much as reducing fat intake does. Reduced calorie intake also helps control body weight.

A diet plan that reflects many of these recommendations is the DASH diet (Dietary Approaches to Stop Hypertension). The DASH study found that a diet low in fat and high in fruits, vegetables, and low-fat dairy products reduces blood pressure. The DASH diet is one of the recommended eating patterns in the report of the 2010 Dietary Guidelines Advisory Committee.

Exercise Regularly

You can significantly reduce your risk of CVD with a moderate amount of physical activity (see the box "Exercise and CVD Risk"). The American Heart Association recommends strength training in addition to aerobic exercise for building and maintaining cardiovascular health. Strength training helps reduce body fat and improve lipid levels and glucose metabolism.

Avoid Tobacco

The number-one risk factor for CVD that you can control is smoking. If you smoke, quit. If you don't, don't start. If you find yourself breathing in ETS, take steps to prevent or stop the exposure.

Know and Manage Your Blood Pressure

If you have no CVD risk factors, have your blood pressure measured by a trained professional

QUICK STATS

Only **19%** of Americans with hypertension follow the DASH diet.

—**American Heart Association, 2010**

at least once every 2 years; yearly tests are recommended if you have other risk factors. If your blood pressure is high, follow your physician's advice on how to lower it.

Know and Manage Your Cholesterol Levels

All people age 20 and over should have their cholesterol checked at least once every 5 years. The NCEP recommends a fasting lipoprotein profile that measures total cholesterol, HDL, LDL, and triglyceride levels. Once you know your baseline numbers, you and your physician can develop an LDL goal and lifestyle plan.

Develop Effective Ways to Handle Stress and Anger

To reduce the psychological and social risk factors for CVD, develop effective strategies for handling the stress in your life. Shore up your social support network, and try some of the techniques described in Chapter 2 for managing stress.

WHAT IS CANCER?

Cancer is the abnormal, uncontrolled multiplication of cells, which can ultimately cause death if left untreated.

Tumors

Most cancers take the form of tumors, although not all tumors are cancerous. A **tumor** (or *neoplasm*) is a mass of tissue that serves no physiological purpose. **Benign** (noncancerous) **tumors** are made up of cells similar to the

surrounding normal cells and are enclosed in a membrane that prevents them from penetrating neighboring tissues. They are dangerous only if their physical presence interferes with body functions. A benign brain tumor, for example, can cause death if it blocks the blood supply to the brain.

The term **malignant tumor** is synonymous with cancer. A malignant tumor can invade surrounding structures, including blood vessels, the **lymphatic system,** and nerves. It can also spread to distant sites via the blood and lymphatic circulation, producing invasive tumors in almost any part of the body. A few cancers, like leukemia (cancer of the blood), do not produce a mass but still have the fundamental property of rapid, uncontrolled cell multiplication; for this reason, such diseases are considered to be a form of cancer.

Every case of cancer begins as a change in a cell that allows the cell to grow and divide when it should not. Normally (in adults), cells multiply at a rate just sufficient to replace dying cells. In contrast, a malignant cell divides without regard for normal control mechanisms and gradually produces a mass of abnormal cells, or a tumor. It takes about a billion cells to make a mass the size of a pea, so a single tumor cell must go through many divisions, often taking years, before the tumor grows to a noticeable size.

Eventually a tumor produces a sign or symptom. In the breast, for example, a tumor may be felt as a lump or diagnosed as cancer by an X ray or **biopsy.** In less accessible locations, like the lung, a tumor may be noticed only after it has grown considerably and may then be detected only by an indirect symptom, such as a persistent cough or unexplained bleeding. In the case of leukemia, changes in the blood are eventually noticed as increasing fatigue, infection, or abnormal bleeding.

Metastasis

Metastasis, the spreading of cancer cells, occurs because cancer cells do not stick to each other as strongly as normal cells do and therefore may not remain at the site of the *primary tumor* (the original location). They break away and can pass through the lining of lymph or blood vessels to invade nearby tissue. They can also travel to different parts of the body where they establish new cancer cells. This traveling and seeding process is called *metastasizing,* and the new tumors are called *secondary tumors,* or *metastases.* The ability of cancer cells to metastasize makes early cancer detection critical. To control the cancer, every cancerous cell must be removed. Once cancer cells enter either the lymphatic system or the bloodstream, it is extremely difficult to stop their spread to other organs of the body.

A significant number of cancer cases go into **remission,** which in some cases lasts for years. In remission, signs and symptoms of cancer disappear, and the disease is considered to be under control Remission typically results from treatment, but some patients have entered remission for no apparent reason.

TERMS

cancer The abnormal, uncontrolled multiplication of cells.

tumor A mass of tissue that serves no physiological purpose; also called a *neoplasm.*

benign tumor A tumor that is not cancerous.

malignant tumor A tumor that is capable of spreading and, thus, is cancerous.

lymphatic system A system of vessels that returns proteins, lipids, and other substances from fluid in the tissues to the circulatory system.

biopsy The removal and examination of a small piece of body tissue; a needle biopsy uses a needle to remove a small sample, but some biopsies require surgery.

metastasis The spread of cancer cells from one part of the body to another.

remission A period during the course of cancer in which there are no symptoms or other evidence of disease.

Exercise and CVD Risk

Regular exercise directly and indirectly benefits your cardiovascular health and can actually help you avoid having a heart attack or stroke. The evidence comes from dozens of large-scale, population-based studies conducted over the past several decades. There is so much evidence about the cardiovascular health benefits of exercise, in fact, that physicians regard physical activity as a magic bullet against heart disease.

Physical activity has an inverse relationship with cardiovascular health, meaning that the more exercise you get, the less likely you are to develop or die from CVD. Compared to sedentary individuals, people who engage in regular, moderate physical activity lower their risk of CVD by 20% or more. People who get regular, vigorous exercise reduce their risk of CVD by 30% or more. This positive benefit applies regardless of gender, age, race, or ethnicity.

Most studies focus on various aerobic endurance exercises, such as walking, running on a treadmill, or biking. The type of exercise performed is less important than the amount of energy expended during the activity. The greater the energy expenditure, the greater the health benefits. Exercise affects heart health via many mechanisms, all of which are being studied. For example, exercise helps people lose weight and improve body composition. Weight loss can improve heart health by reducing the amount of stress on the heart. Changing body composition to a more positive ratio of fat-free mass to fat boosts resting metabolic rate. Exercise can also prevent metabolic syndrome and reverse many of its negative effects on the body. Exercise directly strengthens the heart muscle itself, and it improves the balance of fats in the blood by boosting HDL and reducing LDL and triglyceride levels.

One of the clearest positive effects of exercise is on hypertension. Many studies, involving thousands of people, have shown that physical activity reduces both systolic and diastolic blood pressure. These studies showed that people who did regular aerobic exercise lowered their resting blood pressure by 2–4% on average. Lowered blood pressure itself reduces the risk of other kinds of cardiovascular disease.

Fewer studies have been conducted on exercise and risk of stroke. Even with limited evidence, however, there appears to be a similar inverse relationship between physical activity and stroke. According to a handful of studies, the most physically active people reduced their risk of both ischemic and hemorrhagic strokes by up to 30%. Although this benefit appears to apply equally to men and women, there is not sufficient evidence that it applies equally across races or ethnicities.

Of course, exercise isn't possible for everyone and may actually be dangerous for some people. Anyone who has CVD or serious risk factors for heart disease should work with their physician to determine whether or how to exercise.

SOURCES: Physical Activity Guidelines Advisory Committee. 2008. *Physical Activity Guidelines Advisory Committee Report*, 2008. Washington, D.C.: U.S. Department of Health and Human Services; Williams, M. A., et al. 2007. Resistance exercise in individuals with and without cardiovascular disease: 2007 update: A scientific statement from the American Heart Association Council on Clinical Cardiology and Council on Nutrition, Physical Activity, and Metabolism. *Circulation* 116(5): 572–584.

Types of Cancer

The behavior of tumors arising in different body organs is characteristic of the tissue of origin. (Figure 12.3 shows the major cancer sites and the incidence of each type.) Malignant tumors are classified according to the types of cells that give rise to them:

- **Carcinomas** arise from **epithelia,** tissues that cover external body surfaces, line internal tubes and cavities, and form the secreting portion of glands. They are the most common type of cancers; major sites include the skin, breast, uterus, prostate, lungs, and gastrointestinal tract.

- **Sarcomas** arise from connective and fibrous tissues such as muscle, bone, cartilage, and the membranes covering muscles and fat.

- **Lymphomas** are cancers of the lymph nodes, part of the body's infection-fighting system.

- **Leukemias** are cancers of the blood-forming cells, which reside chiefly in the **bone marrow.**

Cancers vary greatly in how easily they can be detected and how well they respond to treatment. For example, certain types of skin cancer are easily detected, grow slowly, and are very easy to remove; virtually all of these cancers are cured. Cancer of the pancreas, on the other hand, is very difficult to detect or treat, and very few patients survive the disease.

The Incidence of Cancer

Each year, more than 1.5 million people in the United States are diagnosed with cancer. Most will be cured, or be able to live years longer. In fact, the American Cancer

TERMS

carcinoma Cancer that originates in epithelial tissue (skin, glands, and lining of internal organs).

epithelia Tissue that covers a surface or lines a tube or cavity of the body, enclosing and protecting other parts of the body.

sarcoma Cancer arising from bone, cartilage, or striated muscle.

lymphoma A tumor originating from lymphatic tissue.

leukemia Cancer of the blood or the blood-forming cells.

bone marrow Soft vascular tissue in the interior cavities of bones that produces blood cells.

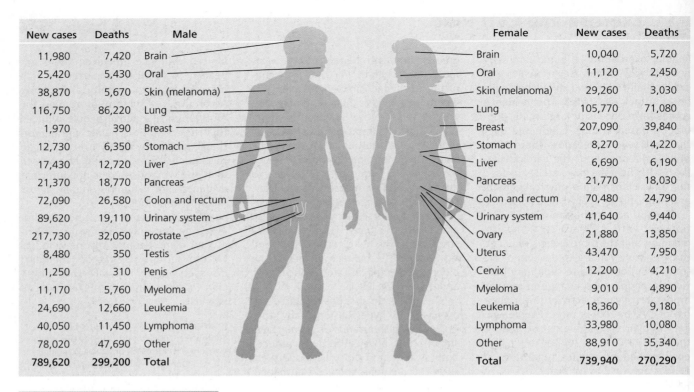

New cases	Deaths	Male			Female	New cases	Deaths
11,980	7,420	Brain			Brain	10,040	5,720
25,420	5,430	Oral			Oral	11,120	2,450
38,870	5,670	Skin (melanoma)			Skin (melanoma)	29,260	3,030
116,750	86,220	Lung			Lung	105,770	71,080
1,970	390	Breast			Breast	207,090	39,840
12,730	6,350	Stomach			Stomach	8,270	4,220
17,430	12,720	Liver			Liver	6,690	6,190
21,370	18,770	Pancreas			Pancreas	21,770	18,030
72,090	26,580	Colon and rectum			Colon and rectum	70,480	24,790
89,620	19,110	Urinary system			Urinary system	41,640	9,440
217,730	32,050	Prostate			Ovary	21,880	13,850
8,480	350	Testis			Uterus	43,470	7,950
1,250	310	Penis			Cervix	12,200	4,210
11,170	5,760	Myeloma			Myeloma	9,010	4,890
24,690	12,660	Leukemia			Leukemia	18,360	9,180
40,050	11,450	Lymphoma			Lymphoma	33,980	10,080
78,020	47,690	Other			Other	88,910	35,340
789,620	**299,200**	**Total**			**Total**	**739,940**	**270,290**

VITAL STATISTICS

FIGURE 12.3   Cancer cases and deaths by site and sex. The *New Cases* column indicates the number of cancers that occur annually in each site; the *Deaths* column indicates the number of cancer deaths that are annually attributed to each type.

SOURCE: American Cancer Society. 2010. *Cancer Facts and Figures, 2010.* Atlanta: American Cancer Society.

Society (ACS) estimates that the 5-year survival rate for all cancers diagnosed between 1995 and 2005 is 68%. These statistics exclude more than 1 million cases of the curable types of skin cancer. At current U.S. rates, however, nearly 1 in 2 men and more than 1 in 3 women will develop cancer at some point in their lives.

Death rates from cancer are not declining as fast as those from heart disease, in large part because of the differing effects that quitting smoking has on disease risk. Heart-related damage of smoking reverses more quickly and more significantly than the cancer-related damage from smoking. Smoking-related gene mutations cannot be reversed, although other mechanisms can sometimes control cellular changes. If heart disease death rates continue to decline faster than cancer death rates, cancer may overtake heart disease as the leading cause of death among Americans of all ages.

The American Cancer Society estimates that 90% of skin cancer could be prevented by protecting the skin from the rays of the sun and 87% of lung cancer could be prevented by avoiding exposure to tobacco smoke. Thousands of cases of colon, breast, and uterine cancer could be prevented by improving the diet and controlling body weight. Regular screenings and self-examinations have the potential to save an additional 100,000 lives per year.

COMMON CANCERS

In this section we look at some of the most common cancers and their causes, prevention, and treatment.

Lung Cancer

Lung cancer is the most common cause of cancer death in the United States, responsible for about 157,000 deaths each year. Since 1987 lung cancer has surpassed breast cancer as the leading cause of cancer death in women.

Risk Factors   The chief risk factor for lung cancer is tobacco smoke, which currently accounts for 30% of all

Ask Yourself

QUESTIONS FOR CRITICAL THINKING AND REFLECTION

Most people think of cancer as a death sentence, but is that necessarily true? Have you or has anyone you know had an experience with cancer? If so, what was the outcome? Have you ever considered whether you might be at risk for some type of cancer? Have you taken any steps to reduce your risk?

cancer deaths and 90% of lung cancer deaths. When smoking is combined with exposure to other carcinogens, such as asbestos particles or certain pollutants, the risk of cancer can be multiplied by a factor of 10 or more. Environmental tobacco smoke (ETS) is a human carcinogen; even brief exposure can cause serious harm. ETS causes about 3400 lung cancer deaths each year in nonsmokers.

Detection and Treatment   Lung cancer is difficult to detect at an early stage and hard to cure even when detected early. Symptoms of lung cancer do not usually appear until the disease has advanced to the invasive stage. Signals such as a persistent cough, chest pain, or recurring bronchitis may be the first indication of a tumor's presence. A diagnosis can usually be made by CT scanning, chest X rays, or analysis of the cells in sputum. If caught early, localized cancers can be treated with surgery. But because only about 15% of lung cancers are detected before they spread, radiation and **chemotherapy** are often used in addition to surgery. For cases detected early, 53% of patients are alive 5 years after diagnosis; but overall, the 5-year survival rate is only 15%.

Colon and Rectal Cancer   ✳ Exam

Although there are effective screening methods for colorectal cancer, it is the third most common type of cancer.

Risk Factors   Age is a key risk factor for colon and rectal cancer, with more than 91% of cases diagnosed in people age 50 and older. Heredity also plays a role. Many cancers arise from preexisting **polyps,** small growths on the wall of the colon that may gradually develop into malignancies. The tendency to form colon polyps appears to be determined by specific genes, so many colon cancers may be due to inherited gene mutations.

Excessive alcohol use and smoking may increase the risk of colorectal cancer. Regular physical activity appears to reduce a person's risk, whereas obesity increases risk. A diet rich in red and processed meats increases risk, whereas eating fruits, vegetables, and whole grains is associated with lower risk. However, research findings on whether dietary fiber prevents colon cancer have been mixed. Studies have suggested a protective role for folic acid, magnesium, vitamin D, and calcium; in contrast, high intake of refined carbohydrates, simple sugars, and smoked meats and fish may increase risk.

Use of oral contraceptives or hormone replacement therapy may reduce risk in women. Regular use of nonsteroidal anti-inflammatory drugs such as aspirin and ibuprofen may decrease the risk of colon cancer and other cancers of the digestive tract. However, these agents are not recommended for colorectal cancer prevention, given that they can have other, negative health effects.

Detection and Treatment   If identified early, precancerous polyps and early-stage cancers can be removed before they become malignant or spread. Because polyps may bleed as they progress, the standard warning signs of colon cancer are bleeding from the rectum and a change in bowel habits. Regular screening tests are recommended beginning at age 50 (earlier for people with a family history of the disease). A yearly stool blood test can detect small amounts of blood in the stool long before obvious bleeding would be noticed. More involved screening tests are recommended at 5- or 10-year intervals.

Surgery is the primary treatment for colon and rectal cancer. Radiation and chemotherapy may be used before surgery to shrink a tumor or after surgery to destroy any remaining cancerous cells. The survival rate is 91% for colon and rectal cancers detected early and 65% overall.

Breast Cancer

Breast cancer is the most common cancer in women. In the United States, about 1 woman in 8 will develop breast cancer during her lifetime, and 1 woman in 30 will die from the disease. About 207,000 American women are diagnosed with breast cancer each year, and about 40,000 women die from it each year.

Less than 2% of breast cancer cases occur in women under age 35, but incidence increases quickly with age. About 50% of cases are diagnosed in women age 45–65. Rates decrease slightly for women in their seventies and eighties, although this could reflect a decrease in screening for this age population.

Risk Factors   There is a strong genetic factor in breast cancer. A woman who has two close relatives with breast cancer is more than four times more likely to develop the disease than a woman who has no close relatives with it. However, even though genetic factors are important, only about 15% of cancers occur in women with a family history of breast cancer.

Other risk factors include early onset of menstruation, late onset of menopause, having no children or having a first child after age 30, current use of hormone replacement therapy (HT), obesity, and alcohol use. Estrogen may be a unifying element for many of these risk factors. Estrogen circulates in a woman's body in high concentrations between puberty and menopause. Fat cells also produce

chemotherapy   The treatment of cancer with chemicals that selectively destroy cancerous cells.

polyp   A small, usually harmless, mass of tissue that projects from the inner surface of the colon or rectum.

TERMS

estrogen, and estrogen levels are higher in obese women. Alcohol can interfere with estrogen metabolism in the liver and increase estrogen levels in the blood. Estrogen promotes the growth of cells in responsive sites, including the breast and the uterus, so any factor that increases estrogen exposure may raise breast cancer risk. A dramatic drop in rates of breast cancer from 2001 to 2004 was attributed in part to reduced use of HT by women over age 50 beginning in July 2002. Millions of women stopped taking the hormones after research linked HT with an increased risk of breast cancer and heart disease.

Eating a low-fat, vegetable-rich diet, exercising regularly, limiting alcohol intake, and maintaining a healthy body weight can minimize the chance of developing breast cancer. Despite some popular myths, studies have shown that breast cancer incidence is not increased by underwire bras, antiperspirants, breast implants, or abortions.

Early Detection   A cure is most likely if breast cancer is detected early, so regular screening is a good investment, even for younger women. The ACS advises a three-part personal program for the early detection of breast cancer:

- The ACS recommends a **mammogram** (low-dose breast X ray) every year for women over 40. Some groups have argued that women should not begin receiving mammograms until age 50 because of the number of false positive results between 40 and 50, but most organizations still recommend beginning mammograms at 40. Studies show that magnetic resonance imaging (MRI) may be better than mammography at detecting breast abnormalities in some women.

- Women between ages 20 and 39 should have a clinical breast exam every 3 years, and women age 40 and older should have one every year before their scheduled mammogram.

- Breast self-exam (BSE) allows a woman to become familiar with her breasts, so she can alert her health care provider to any changes. Women who choose to do breast self-exams should begin at age 20 (see the box "How to Perform a Breast Self-Exam").

Breast pain or tenderness is usually associated with benign conditions such as menstruation rather than breast cancer. The first physical signs of breast cancer are more likely to be a lump, swelling, or thickening; skin irritation or dimpling; or nipple pain, scaliness, or retraction. Although most breast lumps are benign, any breast lump should be brought to the attention of a health care provider.

Treatment   If a lump is detected, it may be scanned by **ultrasonography** and biopsied to see if it is cancerous. In most cases, the lump is found to be a cyst or other harmless growth, and no further treatment is needed. If the lump contains cancer cells, a variety of surgeries may be called for, ranging from a lumpectomy (removal of the lump and surrounding tissue) to a mastectomy (removal of the breast).

If the tumor is discovered before it has spread to the adjacent lymph nodes, the patient has about a 98% chance of surviving more than 5 years. The survival rate for all stages is 90% at 5 years.

New Strategies for Treatment and Prevention   A number of drugs have been developed for the treatment or prevention of breast cancer. A family of drugs called selective estrogen-receptor modulators, or SERMs, act like estrogen in some tissues of the body but block estrogen's effects in others. One SERM, tamoxifen, has long been used in breast cancer treatment because it blocks the action of estrogen in breast tissue. In 1998, the FDA approved the use of tamoxifen to reduce the risk of breast cancer in healthy women who are at high risk for the disease. Another SERM, named raloxifene, was approved in 2007 for the reduction of invasive breast cancer risk in postmenopausal women at high risk for breast cancer. Compared to tamoxifen, raloxifene has been shown to pose a slightly lower risk of blood clots, but the risk is still higher than that of a placebo. Raloxifene has also been shown to improve bone mineral density.

For advanced cancer, treatment with trastuzumab, a **monoclonal antibody,** is an option for some women. Monoclonal antibodies are a special type of antibody that is produced in the laboratory and designed to bind to a specific cancer-related target. Many other monoclonal antibodies are currently in development for breast cancer.

Prostate Cancer

The prostate gland is situated at the base of the bladder in men, and completely surrounds the male's urethra. It produces seminal fluid; if enlarged, it can block the flow of urine. Prostate cancer is the most common cancer in men and the second leading cause of cancer death in men. Nearly 218,000 new cases are diagnosed each year, and more than 32,000 American men die from the disease each year.

TERMS

mammogram   Low-dose X ray of the breasts used to check for early signs of breast cancer.

ultrasonography   An imaging method in which sound waves are bounced off body structures to create an image on a TV monitor; also called *ultrasound.*

monoclonal antibody   An antibody designed to bind to a specific cancer-related target.

How to Perform a Breast Self-Exam

The best time for a woman to examine her breasts is when the breasts are not tender or swollen. Women who examine their breasts should have their technique reviewed during their periodic health exams by their health care professional.

Women with breast implants can do BSE. It may be helpful to have the surgeon help identify the edges of the implant so that you know what you are feeling. There is some thought that the implants push out the breast tissue and may actually make it easier to examine. Women who are pregnant or breast-feeding can also choose to examine their breasts regularly.

It is acceptable for women to choose not to do BSE or to do BSE once in a while. Women who choose not to do BSE should still be aware of the normal look and feel of their breasts and report any changes to their doctor right away.

How to Examine Your Breasts

- Lie down and place your right arm behind your head. The exam is done while lying down, not standing up. This is because when you are lying down, the breast tissue spreads evenly over the chest wall and is as thin as possible, making it much easier to feel all the breast tissue.

- Use the finger pads of the three middle fingers on your left hand to feel for lumps in the right breast. Use overlapping dime-sized circular motions of the finger pads to feel the breast tissue.

- Use three different levels of pressure to feel all the breast tissue. Light pressure is needed to feel the tissue closest to the

skin; medium pressure to feel a little deeper; and firm pressure to feel the tissue closest to the chest and ribs. A firm ridge in the lower curve of each breast is normal, but you should tell your doctor if you feel anything else out of the ordinary. If you're not sure how hard to press, talk with your doctor or nurse. Use each pressure level to feel the breast tissue before moving on to the next spot.

- Move around the breast in an up-and-down pattern starting at an imaginary line drawn straight down your side from the underarm and moving across the breast to the middle of the chest bone (sternum or breastbone). Be sure to check the entire breast area going down until you feel only ribs and up to the neck or collar bone (clavicle).

- There is some evidence to suggest that the up-and-down pattern (sometimes called the vertical pattern) is the most effective pattern for covering the entire breast, without missing any breast tissue.

- Repeat the exam on your left breast, using the finger pads of the right hand.

- While standing in front of a mirror with your hands pressing firmly down on your hips, look at your breasts for any changes of size, shape, contour, or dimpling, or redness or scaliness of the nipple or breast skin. (The pressing down on the hips position contracts the chest wall muscles and enhances any breast changes.)

- Examine each underarm while sitting up or standing and with your arm only slightly raised so you can easily feel in this area. Raising your arm straight up tightens the tissue in this area and makes it harder to examine.

This procedure for doing breast self-exam is different than in previous recommendations. These changes represent an extensive review of the medical literature and input from an expert advisory group. These is evidence that this position (lying down), area felt, pattern of coverage of the breast, and use of different amounts of pressure increase a woman's ability to find abnormal areas.

Risk Factors   Age is the strongest predictor of the risk, with more than 60% of cases of prostate cancer diagnosed in men over age 65. Inherited genetic predisposition may be responsible for 5–10% of cases, and men with a family history of the disease should be particularly vigilant about screening. African American men and Jamaican men of African descent have the highest rates of prostate cancer of any groups in the world; both genetic and lifestyle factors may be involved. Diets high in calories, dairy products, and animal fats and low in plant foods have also been

implicated as possible culprits, as have obesity, inactivity, and a history of sexually transmitted diseases. Type 2 diabetes and insulin resistance are also associated with prostate cancer. Soy foods, tomatoes, and cruciferous vegetables are being investigated for their possible protective effects.

Detection   Warning signs of prostate cancer can include changes in urinary frequency, weak or interrupted urine flow, painful urination, and blood in the urine. Techniques for early detection include a digital rectal examination and the **prostate-specific antigen (PSA) blood test.** Annual screening tests for early detection are recommended, beginning at age 50, for men who are at average risk of prostate cancer, do not have any major medical problems, and have a life expectancy of at least 10 years. Men at high risk, including African Americans and those with a family history of the disease, should consider beginning screening at age 45. Men with multiple family members who have been diagnosed with the disease should begin screening at age 40.

PSA testing has been a subject of controversy among experts for several years because of its tendency to yield misleading results, leading to further testing that can potentially cause harm. This is especially a concern for older men (over 75), who are more likely to die of other causes even if they have slow-growing prostate cancer. The American Cancer Society recommends that physicians discuss PSA and other prostate-cancer tests with their male patients and offer the tests to any man over age 50 (or younger if the patient is at high risk for the disease).

Treatment　Treatments vary based on the stage of the cancer and the age of the patient. A small, slow-growing tumor in an older man may be treated with watchful waiting, because he is more likely to die from another cause before his cancer becomes life threatening. More aggressive treatment would be indicated for younger men or those with more advanced cancers. Treatment involves radical prostatectomy, in which the prostate is removed surgically. Although radical surgery has an excellent cure rate, it is major surgery and often results in **incontinence** and/or erectile dysfunction. Minimally invasive surgery, which utilizes a laparoscopic or robotic approach, is being offered at many centers throughout the world and can sometimes offer fewer complications and quicker recovery. A less invasive alternative involves surgical implantation of radioactive seeds that destroy the tumor and much of the normal prostate tissue but leave surrounding tissue relatively untouched. Survival rates for all stages of this cancer have improved steadily since 1940; the 5-year survival rate is now nearly 100%.

Cancers of the Female Reproductive Tract

Several types of cancer can affect the female reproductive tract, and a few of these cancers are relatively common.

Cervical Cancer　Cancer of the cervix occurs frequently in women in their thirties or even twenties. Virtually all cases of cervical cancer stem from infection by the human papillomavirus (HPV), a group of about 100 related viruses that also cause common warts and genital warts. When certain types of HPV are introduced into the cervix, usually by an infected sex partner, the virus infects cervical cells, causing the cells to divide and grow. If unchecked, this growth can develop into cervical cancer.

Cervical cancer is associated with multiple sex partners. Smoking, immunosuppression, and prolonged use of oral contraceptives have also been associated with increased risk. The regular use of condoms can reduce the risk of transmitting HPV. Studies also suggest that women whose sexual partners are circumcised may be at reduced risk because circumcised men are less likely to harbor a chronic HPV infection and pass it to their partners.

Screening for the changes in cervical cells that precede cancer is done chiefly by means of the **Pap test.** During a pelvic exam, loose cells are scraped from the cervix and examined under a microscope to see whether they are normal. If cells are abnormal but not yet cancerous, a condition commonly referred to as *cervical dysplasia,* the Pap test is repeated at intervals. Sometimes cervical cells spontaneously return to normal, but in about one-third of cases, the cellular changes progress toward malignancy. If this happens, the abnormal cells must be removed, either surgically or by destroying them with a cryoscopic (ultracold) probe or localized laser treatment. Without timely surgery, the malignant patch of cells goes on to invade the wall of the cervix and spreads to the uterus and adjacent lymph nodes. At this stage, chemotherapy may be used with radiation to kill the fast-growing cancer cells, but chances for a complete cure are lower.

55 million
Pap tests are performed each year in the United States; about **6%** are abnormal and require medical follow-up.

—National Cancer Institute, 2009

Because the Pap test is highly effective, all sexually active women and women between ages 18 and 65 should be tested. The recommended schedule for testing depends on risk factors, the type of Pap test performed, and whether the Pap test is combined with HPV testing. Two HPV vaccines have been approved by the FDA for the prevention of cervical cancer. Women who receive one of the vaccines should continue to receive routine Pap tests, since the vaccines do not protect against all genotypes of the virus (see the box "HPV and Cancer").

TERMS

prostate-specific antigen (PSA) blood test　A diagnostic test for prostate cancer that measures blood levels of prostate-specific antigen (PSA).

incontinence　The inability to control the flow of urine.

Pap test　A scraping of cells from the cervix for examination under a microscope to detect cancer.

HPV (human papillomavirus), the most commonly diagnosed sexually transmitted disease in the United States, has been linked to several serious cancers, including cervical cancer, oropharyngeal cancer (cancers of the oropharynx, the back of the mouth and opening of the throat), and cancers of the male and female genitals.

About 75–80% of sexually active adults will acquire HPV before the age of 50. There are more than 100 types of HPV, but only a few are responsible for the majority of infections that lead to potentially deadly illnesses. Much of the time, the infection clears and the person may never know that he or she was infected. People with persistent HPV infection are at the highest risk for precancerous or cancerous lesions, a process that can take months to years.

HPV may be best known for causing genital warts, which usually appear as pink- or gray-colored protuberances of the skin on the penis, vulva, cervix, vagina, or anal region. Two types of HPV (genotypes 6 and 11) cause approximately 90% of all cases of genital warts. For some people, infections are asymptomatic, but others require treatment with chemical agents, immunotherapy, or surgery.

Cancers linked to HPV infection include the following:

- Cervical cancer. HPV is thought to be responsible for more than 99% of all cervical cancers. Each year in the United States, approximately 11,000 women develop cervical cancer, and nearly 4,000 die from it. In developing countries, cervical cancer is the second most common cause of cancer-related deaths. On average, it takes about 15 years from the time of initial HPV infection for invasive cervical cancer to develop.

- Oropharyngeal cancer. Close to 50% of all cancers of the oropharynx—in particular, the tonsils and base of the tongue—are related to HPV infection. Patients require aggressive therapy with combined chemotherapy and radiation, which have severe side effects of their own.

- Other cancers. Between 40 and 70% of cancers of the vulva, vagina, and penis, and up to 93% of anal cancers have been linked to HPV infection. Even when they can be treated locally, such cancers can cause significant compromise of sexual function and lead to long-term illness.

Currently, two commercially available HPV vaccines are approved by the FDA. Gardasil™, approved in 2006, targets four types of HPV (genotypes 16, 18, 6, 11). It is administered in three doses. Cervarix, approved in 2009, targets genotypes 16 and 18 only. It is also administered in three doses. In 2007, the Advisory Committee on Immunization Practices recommended that all females be vaccinated at age 11–12 with Gardasil and that females age 13–26 who had not been previously vaccinated receive catch-up vaccinations. In 2009, the committee added Cervarix to the list of approved vaccines for the prevention of cervical cancer, and an FDA panel expanded the recommendation for Gardasil vaccination to males age 9–26 for the prevention of genital warts.

Young girls are targeted for vaccination because the greatest benefits are experienced by those who are not yet sexually active. However, it is also likely that young sexually active individuals will not have been exposed to all HPV genotypes targeted by the vaccines. Thus, individuals who have already been infected with one or more HPV types will still derive protection from the vaccine types they have not acquired. Women who are vaccinated still need to receive regular Pap tests for cervical cancer screening, since 30% of the HPV genotypes responsible for cervical cancer are not covered by the vaccine.

Although studies suggest that vaccination of the entire U.S. population of 12-year-old girls would prevent more than 200,000 HPV infections and 3300 cases of cervical cancer, so far the actual vaccination rates have been much lower than were initially predicted. One study reported at the CDC's 2010 STD conference found that only 15% of 11–12-year-olds and 25% of 13–17-year-olds had received at least one dose of HPV vaccine. The most common barriers to vaccination were the belief that the child did not need the vaccine or was not sexually active and lack of knowledge about the vaccines. As more educational programs are launched, it is hoped that vaccination rates will increase, leading to associated declines in cancer incidence.

SOURCES: Broomall, E. M., et al. 2010. Epidemiology, clinical manifestations, and recent advances in vaccination against human papillomavirus. *Postgraduate Medicine* 122(2): 121–129; Ryerson, A. B., et al. 2008. Burden of potentially human papillomavirus-associated cancers of the oropharynx and oral cavity in the U.S., 1998–2003. *Cancer* 113(10 Suppl.): 2901–2909; Slade, B. A., et al. 2009. Postlicensure safety surveillance for quadrivalent human papillomavirus recombinant vaccine. *Journal of the American Medical Association* 302(7): 750–757; Wong, C., et al. 2010. *National HPV Vaccine Uptake and Vaccination Predictors and Barriers for Girls 8–17 Years Old.* Oral Presentation at the National STD Prevention Conference, March 8–11, 2010. Atlanta, Ga.

Uterine, or Endometrial, Cancer   Cancer of the lining of the uterus, or endometrium, most often occurs after the age of 55. The risk factors are similar to those for breast cancer, including prolonged exposure to estrogen, early onset of menstruation, late menopause, never having been pregnant, and obesity. Type 2 diabetes is also associated with increased risk. The use of oral contraceptives, which combine estrogen and progestin, appears to provide protection.

Endometrial cancer often presents with abnormal vaginal bleeding in a postmenopausal woman. It is treated surgically, commonly by hysterectomy, or removal of the uterus. Radiation treatment, hormones, and chemotherapy may be used in addition to surgery. When the tumor is detected at an early stage, about 96% of patients are alive and disease-free 5 years later. When the disease has spread beyond the uterus, the 5-year survival rate is less than 68%.

Ovarian Cancer   Although ovarian cancer is rare compared with cervical or uterine cancer, it causes more deaths than the other two combined. There are often no warning signs of developing ovarian cancer. Early clues may include increased abdominal size and bloating, urinary urgency, and pelvic pain. It cannot be detected by Pap tests or any other simple screening method and is often diagnosed only late in its development, when surgery and other therapies are unlikely to be successful.

The risk factors are similar to those for breast and endometrial cancer: increasing age (most ovarian cancer occurs after age 60), never having been pregnant, a family history of breast or ovarian cancer, obesity, and specific genetic mutations. A high number of ovulations appears to increase the chance that a cancer-causing genetic mutation will occur, so anything that lowers the number of lifetime ovulation cycles—pregnancy, breastfeeding, or use of oral contraceptives—reduces a woman's risk of ovarian cancer.

Women with symptoms or who are at high risk because of family history or because they harbor a mutant gene should have thorough pelvic exams at regular intervals. Ovarian cancer is treated by surgical removal of both ovaries, the fallopian tubes, and the uterus. Radiation and chemotherapy are sometimes used in addition to surgery.

Skin Cancer

Skin cancer is the most common cancer of all when cases of the highly curable forms are included in the

Tanning, either under direct sunlight or in a tanning bed, is a known cause of skin cancer.

count. (Usually these forms are not included, precisely because they are easily treated.) Of the more than 1 million cases of skin cancer diagnosed each year, about 68,000 are of the most serious type, **melanoma.** Treatments are usually simple and successful when the cancers are caught early.

Risk Factors   Almost all cases of skin cancer can be traced to excessive exposure to **ultraviolet (UV) radiation** from the sun, including longer-wavelength ultraviolet A (UVA) and shorter-wavelength ultraviolet B (UVB) radiation. UVB radiation causes sunburns and can damage the eyes and the immune system. UVA is less likely to cause an immediate sunburn, but by damaging connective tissue it leads to premature aging of the skin. (Tanning lamps and tanning-salon beds emit mostly UVA radiation.) Both UVA and UVB radiation have been linked to the development of skin cancer, and the National Toxicology Program has declared both solar and artificial sources of UV radiation, including sunlamps and tanning beds, to be known human carcinogens.

Both severe, acute sun reactions (sunburns) and chronic low-level sun reactions (suntans) can lead to skin cancer. People with fair skin have less natural protection against skin damage from the sun and a higher risk of developing skin cancer; people with naturally dark skin have a considerable degree of protection. Caucasians are about 10 times more likely than African Americans to develop melanoma, but African Americans and Latinos are still at risk.

Severe sunburns in childhood have been linked to a greatly increased risk of skin cancer in later life, so

TERMS

melanoma   A malignant tumor of the skin that arises from pigmented cells, usually a mole.

ultraviolet (UV) radiation   Light rays of a specific wavelength emitted by the sun; most UV rays are blocked by the ozone layer in the upper atmosphere.

children in particular should be protected. According to the Skin Cancer Foundation, the risk of skin cancer doubles in people who have had five or more sunburns in their lifetime. Because of damage to the ozone layer of the atmosphere, there is a chance that we may all be exposed to increasing amounts of UV radiation in the future.

Other risk factors for skin cancer include having many moles, particularly large ones; spending time at high altitudes; and a family history of the disease.

Types of Skin Cancer   There are three main types of skin cancer, named for the types of skin cells from which they develop. **Basal cell** and **squamous cell carcinomas** together account for about 95% of the skin cancers diagnosed each year. They are usually found in chronically sun-exposed areas, such as the face, neck, hands, and arms. They usually appear as pale, waxlike, pearly nodules or red, scaly, sharply outlined patches. These cancers are often painless, although they may bleed, crust, and form an open sore on the skin.

Melanoma is by far the most dangerous skin cancer because it spreads so rapidly. It can occur anywhere on the body, but the most common sites are the back, chest, abdomen, and lower legs. A melanoma usually appears at the site of a preexisting mole. The mole may begin to enlarge, become mottled or varied in color (colors can include blue, pink, and white), or develop an irregular surface or irregular borders. Tissue invaded by melanoma may also itch, burn, or bleed easily.

Prevention   One of the major steps you can take to protect yourself against all forms of skin cancer is to avoid lifelong overexposure to sunlight. Blistering, peeling sunburns from unprotected sun exposure are particularly dangerous, but suntans—whether from sunlight or from tanning lamps—also increase your risk of developing skin cancer later in life. People of every age, especially babies and children, need to be protected from the sun with sunscreens and protective clothing (see the box "Choosing and Using Sunscreens and Sun-Protective Clothing").

Detection and Treatment   Make it a habit to examine your skin regularly. Most of the spots, freckles, moles, and blemishes on your body are normal; you were born with some of them, and others appear and disappear throughout your life. But if you notice an unusual growth, discoloration, sore that does not heal, or mole that undergoes a sudden or progressive change, see your physician or a dermatologist immediately.

> *Most cases of skin cancer are **so easily detected and treated** that they aren't even included in cancer surveillances.*

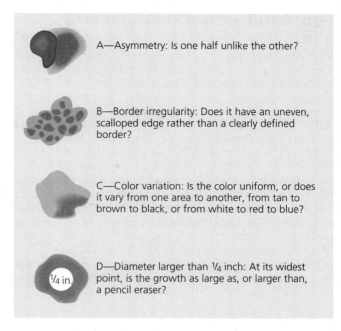

A—Asymmetry: Is one half unlike the other?

B—Border irregularity: Does it have an uneven, scalloped edge rather than a clearly defined border?

C—Color variation: Is the color uniform, or does it vary from one area to another, from tan to brown to black, or from white to red to blue?

D—Diameter larger than ¼ inch: At its widest point, is the growth as large as, or larger than, a pencil eraser?

FIGURE 12.4   The ABCD test for melanoma. To see a variety of photos of melanoma and benign moles, visit the National Cancer Institute's Visuals Online site (http://visualsonline.cancer.gov).

The characteristics that may signal that a skin lesion is a melanoma—asymmetry, border irregularity, color change, and a diameter greater than ¼ inch—are illustrated in Figure 12.4. If you have an unusual skin lesion, your physician will examine it and possibly perform a biopsy. If the lesion is cancerous, it is usually removed surgically, a procedure that can almost always be performed in the physician's office using a local anesthetic.

Head and Neck Cancers

Head and neck cancers—cancers of the oral cavity, pharynx, larynx, and nasal cavity—can be traced principally to cigarette, cigar, or pipe smoking, the use of spit tobacco, and the excessive consumption of alcohol. The incidence of head and neck cancer is twice as great in men as in women and most frequent in men over 40.

Chemotherapy, radiation, and surgery are the primary methods of treatment for head and neck cancers. Often patients endure intense mouth and throat inflammation and some require disfiguring surgeries, but many can be cured. Among those who survive, a significant number will develop another primary cancer of the head and neck. The 5-year survival rate is about 61%.

basal cell carcinoma   Cancer of the deepest layers of the skin.

squamous cell carcinoma   Cancer of the surface layers of the skin.

TERMS

Choosing and Using Sunscreens and Sun-Protective Clothing

With consistent use of the proper clothing, sunscreens, and common sense, you can lead an active outdoor life *and* protect your skin against most sun-induced damage.

Clothing

- Wear long-sleeved shirts and long pants. Dark-colored, tightly woven fabrics provide reasonable protection from the sun. Another good choice is clothing made from special sun-protective fabrics; these garments have an ultraviolet protection factor (UPF) rating, similar to the SPF for sunscreens. For example, a fabric with a UPF rating of 20 allows only one-twentieth of the sun's UV radiation to pass through. There are three categories of UPF protection: A UPF of 15–24 provides "good" UV protection; a UPF of 25–39 provides "very good" protection; and a UPF of 40–50 provides "excellent" protection. By comparison, typical shirts provide a UPF of only 5–9, a value that drops when clothing is wet.

- Wear a hat. A good choice is a broad-brimmed hat or a legionnaire-style cap that covers the ears and neck. Wear sunscreen on your face even if you are wearing a hat.

- Wear sunglasses. Exposure to UV rays can damage the eyes and cause cataracts.

Sunscreen

- Use a sunscreen and lip balm with a sun protection factor (SPF) of 15 or higher. An SPF rating refers to the amount of time you can stay out in the sun before you burn, compared with not using sunscreen. For example, a product with an SPF of 15 would allow you to remain in the sun without burning 15 times longer, on average, than if you didn't apply sunscreen. If you're fair-skinned, have a family history of skin cancer, are at high altitude, or will be outdoors for many hours, use a sunscreen with a high SPF (30+).

- Choose a broad-spectrum sunscreen that protects against both UVA and UVB radiation. The SPF rating of a sunscreen currently applies only to UVB, but a number of ingredients, especially titanium dioxide and zinc oxide, are effective at blocking most UVA radiation. In 2006, the FDA approved a product called Anthelios SX that protects against both UVA and UVB radiation. Use a water-resistant sunscreen if you

swim or sweat a great deal. If you have acne, look for a sunscreen that is labeled "noncomedogenic," which means that it will not cause pimples.

- Shake sunscreen before applying. Apply it 30 minutes before exposure to allow it time to bond to the skin. Reapply sunscreen frequently and generously to all sun-exposed areas (many people overlook their temples, ears, and sides and backs of their necks). Most people use less than half as much as they need to attain the full SPF rating. One ounce of sunscreen is enough to cover an average-size adult in a swimsuit. Reapply sunscreen 15–30 minutes after sun exposure begins and then every 2 hours after that and/or following activities, such as swimming, that could remove sunscreen.

- If you're taking medications, ask your physician or pharmacist about possible reactions to sunlight or interactions with sunscreens. Medications for acne, allergies, and diabetes are just a few of the products that can trigger reactions. If you're using sunscreen and an insect repellent containing DEET, use extra sunscreen (DEET may decrease sunscreen effectiveness).

Time of Day and Location

- Avoid sun exposure between 10 A.M. and 4 P.M., when the sun's rays are most intense. Clouds allow as much as 80% of UV rays to reach your skin. Stay in the shade when you can.

- Consult the day's UV Index, which predicts UV levels on a 0–10+ scale, to get a sense of the amount of sun protection you'll need; take special care on days with a rating of 5 or above. UV Index ratings are available in local newspapers, from the weather bureau, or from certain Web sites.

- Be aware that UV rays can penetrate at least 3 feet in water. Thus swimmers should wear water-resistant sunscreens. Snow, sand, water, concrete, and white-painted surfaces are also highly reflective.

Tanning Salons

- Stay away from tanning salons! Despite advertising claims to the contrary, the lights used in tanning parlors are damaging to your skin. Tanning beds and lamps emit mostly UVA radiation, increasing your risk of premature skin aging (such as wrinkles) and skin cancer.

Testicular Cancer

Testicular cancer is relatively rare, accounting for only 1% of cancer in men (about 8500 cases per year), but it is the most common cancer in men age 20–35. It is much more common among white Americans than among Latinos, Asian Americans, or African Americans and among men whose fathers had testicular cancer. Men with undescended testicles are at increased risk for testicular cancer, and for this reason the condition should be corrected in early childhood. Self-examination may help in the early detection of testicular cancer (see the box "Testicle Self-Examination"). Tumors are treated

by surgical removal of the testicle and, if the tumor has spread, by chemotherapy; radiation treatment is used only rarely.

Ask Yourself

QUESTIONS FOR CRITICAL THINKING AND REFLECTION

Has anyone you know had cancer? If so, what type of cancer was it? What were its symptoms? Based on the information presented so far in this chapter, did the person have any of the known risk factors for the disease?

Testicle Self-Examination

The best time to perform a testicular self-exam is after a warm shower or bath, when the scrotum is relaxed.

First, stand in front of a mirror and look for any swelling of the scrotum. Then examine each testicle with both hands. Place the index and middle fingers under the testicle and the thumbs on top; roll the testicle gently between the fingers and thumbs. Don't worry if one testicle seems slightly larger than the other—that's common. Also, expect to feel the epididymis, the soft, sperm-carrying tube at the rear of the testicle.

Perform the self-exam each month. If you find a lump, swelling, or nodule, consult a physician right away. The abnormality may not be cancer, but only a physician can make a diagnosis.

Other possible signs of testicular cancer include a change in the way a testicle feels, a sudden collection of fluid in the scrotum, a dull ache in the lower abdomen or groin, a feeling of heaviness in the scrotum, or pain in a testicle or the scrotum.

SOURCES: Testicular Cancer Resource Center. 2009. *How to Do a Testicular Self Examination* (http://www.tcrc.acor.org/tcexam.html; retrieved November 18, 2010); National Cancer Institute. 2005. *Questions and Answers About Testicular Cancer* (http://www.cancer.gov/cancertips/factsheet/sites-types/testicular; retrieved November 18, 2010).

THE CAUSES OF CANCER

Although scientists do not know everything about what causes cancer, they have identified genetic, environmental, and lifestyle factors.

> **The overall cost of cancer in the U.S. is $264 billion annually.**
>
> —National Institutes of Health, 2010

The Role of DNA

Heredity and genetics are important factors in a person's risk of cancer. Certain genes may predispose some people to cancer, and specific genetic mutations— changes in the normal makeup of a gene—have been associated with cancer.

Some mutations are inherited, and others are caused by environmental agents, including radiation, certain viruses, and chemical substances in the air we breathe. An example of an inherited mutation is *BRCA1* (breast cancer gene 1): Women who inherit a damaged copy of this gene face a significantly increased risk of breast and ovarian cancer. Testing and identification of hereditary cancer risks can be helpful for some people, especially if it leads to increased attention to controllable risk factors and better medical screening.

Tobacco Use

Smoking is responsible for 80–90% of lung cancers and for about 30% of all cancer deaths. Overall, tobacco use is responsible for nearly 1 in 5 American deaths—nearly 444,000 premature deaths each year. The U.S. Surgeon General has reported that tobacco use is a direct cause of several types of cancer besides lung and bronchial cancer, including cancer of the larynx, mouth, pharynx, esophagus, stomach, pancreas, kidneys, bladder, and cervix.

Dietary Factors

The foods you eat contain many biologically active compounds, and your food choices affect your cancer risk by both exposing you to potentially dangerous compounds and depriving you of potentially protective ones.

Dietary Fat and Meat Diets high in fat and meat appear to contribute to certain cancers, including colon, stomach, and prostate. Certain types of fats may be riskier than others. Omega-6 polyunsaturated fats are associated with a higher risk of certain cancers; omega-3 fats are not.

Alcohol Alcohol is associated with an increased incidence of several cancers. Women who have 2 to 5 drinks daily have about 1.5 times the risk of women who drink no alcohol. Alcohol and tobacco interact as risk factors for oral cancer.

Fried Foods Scientists have found high levels of the chemical acrylamide (a probable human carcinogen) in starch-based foods that had been fried or baked at high temperatures, especially french fries and certain types of snack chips and crackers. Acrylamide is also found in high concentrations in tobacco.

Fruits and Vegetables Researchers have identified many mechanisms by which food components may act against cancer. Some may prevent carcinogens from forming in the first place or block them from reaching or acting on target cells. Others boost enzymes that detoxify carcinogens and render them harmless. Some essential nutrients act as **anticarcinogens**. For example, vitamin C, vitamin E, selenium, and the **carotenoids** (vitamin A precursors) may help block cancer by acting as antioxidants.

Many other anti-cancer agents in the diet fall under the broader heading of **phytochemicals**, substances in plants that help protect against chronic diseases. One of the first to be identified was sulforaphane, a potent anticarcinogen found in broccoli. Researchers are now beginning to identify the many beneficial phytochemicals contained in many fruits and vegetables.

Inactivity and Obesity

The American Cancer Society recommends maintaining a healthy weight throughout life by balancing caloric intake with physical activity, and by achieving and maintaining a healthy weight if you are currently overweight or obese. Being overweight or obese is linked with increased risk of several kinds of cancer, including breast and colon cancer.

Carcinogens in the Environment

Some carcinogens occur naturally in the environment, like viruses and the sun's UV rays. Others are manufactured or synthetic substances that show up occasionally in the general environment but more often in the work environments of specific industries.

Ingested Chemicals   The food industry uses preservatives and other additives to prevent food from becoming spoiled or stale. Some of these compounds are antioxidants and may actually decrease any cancer-causing properties the food might have. Other compounds, like the nitrates and nitrites found in processed meat, are potentially more dangerous. While nitrates and nitrites are not themselves carcinogenic, they can combine with dietary substances in the stomach and be converted to nitrosamines, which are highly potent carcinogens. Foods cured with nitrites, as well as those cured by salt or smoke, have been linked to esophageal and stomach cancer, and they should be eaten only in modest amounts.

Environmental and Industrial Pollution   Pollutants in urban air have long been suspected of contributing to the incidence of lung cancer. The best available data indicate that less than 2% of cancer deaths are caused by general environmental pollution, such as substances in our air and water, but exposure to carcinogenic materials in the workplace is a more serious problem. Occupational exposure to specific carcinogens may account for about 4% of cancer deaths. With increasing industry and government regulation, we can anticipate that the industrial sources of cancer risk will continue to diminish, at least in the United States (see the box "Cancer and the Environment").

> Worldwide, **7.6 million** people died of cancer in 2008.
>
> —World Health Organization, 2010

Radiation   All sources of radiation are potentially carcinogenic, including medical X rays, radioactive substances (radioisotopes), and UV rays from the sun. Successful efforts have been made to reduce the amount of radiation needed for mammograms, dental X rays, and other necessary medical X rays. UV radiation from the sun is also a potential carcinogen, and care should be taken to avoid excessive exposure.

DETECTING, DIAGNOSING, AND TREATING CANCER

Early cancer detection often depends on our willingness to be aware of changes in our own body and to make sure we keep up with recommended diagnostic tests.

Detecting Cancer

By being aware of the risk factors in your own life, your immediate family's cancer history, and your own history, you may bring a problem to the attention of a physician long before it would have been detected at a routine physical. In addition to self-monitoring, the ACS recommends routine cancer checkups as well as specific screening tests for certain cancers (Table 12.4).

Cancer and the Environment

The American Cancer Society estimates that about 6% of cancer deaths stem from exposure to carcinogens in the environment—about 4% from occupational exposure and about 2% from exposure to naturally occurring or human-made pollutants in the larger environment.

These cancer-inducing or cancer-promoting agents come from a wide variety of sources. Radon, for example, is a highly radioactive element that rises into the atmosphere from the ground in some regions of the country. A colorless, odorless, tasteless gas, radon is a by-product of the breakdown of uranium and radium within the earth. Exposure to radon is known to cause lung cancer and in fact is the second-leading cause of lung cancer in the United States, second only to tobacco use. The EPA estimates that radon is responsible for about 21,000 lung cancer deaths every year.

Radon is present in many buildings and residences, especially in attics, basements, crawlspaces, and other underground areas, accumulating in such areas if they are not adequately ventilated. Radon poses a special threat to people who work underground, such as miners and construction workers who work on multiple-level basements and tunnels. Homeowners can easily have their homes tested for radon with home-use test kits, but professional inspectors may offer more accurate detection. If radon is present and exceeds minimum safety levels, the homeowner may need to make modifications, such as increased ventilation, to reduce the amount of inhalable radon.

Asbestos is another substance that has long been known to cause cancer and other lung diseases. Asbestos was used for many years in home and building construction because of its fire-resistant properties. For decades, asbestos-containing insulation, tiles, and exterior sheathing were used in homes and commercial buildings. Asbestos was even used in special flame-retardant clothing for firefighters and factory workers.

Asbestos use has been banned entirely in the European Union and is now highly restricted in the United States. When asbestos is uncovered in buildings, special abatement procedures must be taken to remove the material while protecting workers and surrounding areas. The human body is so sensitive to asbestos that inhaling even a few small asbestos fibers can result in lung damage, mesothelioma (a rare form of cancer caused almost exclusively by asbestos exposure), and lung cancer.

The EPA identifies many other environmental hazards as "known human carcinogens," including the following:

- Benzene, a powerful solvent used in many industrial processes and contained in thousands of products

- Heavy metals, such as cadmium, which is commonly found in computers and other electronic devices

- X rays, which occur naturally but are used daily in health care work

- Ultraviolet light, whether from the sun or tanning beds

- Environmental tobacco smoke

Carcinogens are encountered much more often in workplaces than in the home. Many of the chemicals, metals, and plastics used in industry are known or suspected carcinogens or cancer pro-

moters. Ironically, many of the drugs used to treat cancer are known or suspected carcinogens, posing a risk of leukemia and other cancers to health care workers. Chemotherapy drugs can also cause skin rashes, infertility, miscarriage, and birth defects in people who work with or near these highly toxic substances. The National Institute for Occupational Safety and Health (NIOSH) publishes guidelines detailing proper procedures and equipment for handling these hazardous drugs. For all hazardous and potentially carcinogenic agents used throughout industry, more research is needed to determine which agents actually cause cancer and what level of exposure is dangerous.

SOURCES: American Cancer Society. 2010. *Cancer Facts and Figures 2010*. Atlanta: American Cancer Society; U.S. Department of Health and Human Services, Public Health Service, National Toxicology Program. 2005. *Report on Carcinogens*, 11th ed. Washington, D.C.: U.S. Department of Health and Human Services; U.S. Environmental Protection Agency. 2010. *Radon* (http://www.epa.gov/radon/; retrieved November 18, 2010).

Diagnosing and Treating Cancer

Methods for determining the exact location, type, and degree of malignancy of a cancer continue to improve. A biopsy may be performed to confirm the type of tumor. Several diagnostic imaging techniques have replaced exploratory surgery for some patients. They include MRIs, CT scanning, and ultrasonography.

For most cancers, surgery is the most useful treatment. Chemotherapy, or the use of cell-killing drugs to destroy rapidly growing cancer cells, works by interfering with DNA synthesis and replication in rapidly dividing cells. Chemotherapy drugs are often used in combinations or with surgery. In cancer radiation therapy, a beam of X rays or gamma rays is directed at the tumor, and the tumor cells are killed. Occasionally, when an organ is small enough, radioactive seeds are surgically placed inside the cancerous organ to destroy the tumor and then removed later if necessary. Radiation destroys both normal and cancerous cells, but because it can be precisely directed at the tumor it is usually less toxic for the patient than either surgery or chemotherapy.

CANCER SITE	POPULATION	TEST OR PROCEDURE	FREQUENCY
Breast	Women, age 20+	Breast self-examination	Beginning in their early 20s, women should be told about the benefits and limitations of breast self-examination (BSE). The importance of prompt reporting of any new breast symptoms to a health professional should be emphasized. Women who choose to do BSE should receive instruction and have their technique reviewed on the occasion of a periodic health examination. It is acceptable for women to choose not to do BSE or to do BSE irregularly.
		Clinical breast examination	For women in their 20s and 30s, it is recommended that clinical breast examination (CBE) be part of a periodic health examination, preferably at least every three years. Asymptomatic women aged 40 and over should continue to receive a clinical breast examination as part of a periodic health examination, preferably annually.
		Mammography	Begin annual mammography at age 40.*
Colorectal[†]	Men and women, age 50+	Tests that find polyps and cancer:	
		Flexible sigmoidoscopy[†], or	Every five years, starting at age 50
		Colonoscopy	Every 10 years, starting at age 50
		Double-contrast barium enema (DCBE)[†], or	Every five years, starting at age 50
		CT colonography (virtual colonoscopy)[†]	Every five years, starting at age 50
		Tests that mainly find cancer:	
		Fecal occult blood test (FOBT) with at least 50% test sensitivity for cancer, or fecal immunochemical test (FIT) with at least 50% test sensitivity for cancer[†§] or	Annual, starting at age 50
		Stool DNA test (sDNA)[†]	Interval uncertain, starting at age 50
Prostate	Men, age 50+	Prostate-specific antigen test (PSA) with or without digital rectal examination (DRE)	Asymptomatic men who have at least a 10-year life expectancy should have an opportunity to make an informed decision with their health care provider about screening for prostate cancer after receiving information about the uncertainties, risks, and potential benefits associated with screening. Men at average risk should receive this information beginning at age 50. Men at higher risk, including African American men and men with a first degree relative (father or brother) diagnosed with prostate cancer before age 65, should receive this information beginning at age 45. Men at appreciably higher risk (multiple family members diagnosed with prostate cancer before age 65) should receive this information beginning at age 40.
Cervix	Women, age 18+	Pap test	Cervical cancer screening should begin approximately three years after a woman begins having vaginal intercourse, but no later than 21 years of age. Screening should be done every year with conventional Pap tests or every two years using liquid-based Pap tests. At or after age 30, women who have had three normal test results in a row may get screened every two to three years with cervical cytology (either conventional or liquid-based Pap test) alone, or every three years with an HPV DNA test plus cervical cytology. Women 70 years of age and older who have had three or more normal Pap tests and no abnormal Pap tests in the past 10 years and women who have had a total hysterectomy may choose to stop cervical cancer screening.
Endometrial	Women, at menopause		At the time of menopause, women at average risk should be informed about risks and symptoms of endometrial cancer and strongly encouraged to report any unexpected bleeding or spotting to their physicians.
Cancer-related checkup	Men and women, age 20+		On the occasion of a periodic health examination, the cancer-related checkup should include examination for cancers of the thyroid, testicles, ovaries, lymph nodes, oral cavity, and skin, as well as health counseling about tobacco, sun exposure, diet and nutrition, risk factors, sexual practices, and environmental and occupational exposures.

*Beginning at age 40, annual clinical breast examination should be performed prior to mammography.

[†]Individuals with a personal or family history of colorectal cancer or adenomas, inflammatory bowel disease, or high-risk genetic syndromes should continue to follow the most recent recommendations for individuals at increased or high risk.

[‡]Colonoscopy should be done if test results are positive.

[§]For FOBT or FIT used as a screening test, the take-home multiple sample method should be used. A FOBT or FIT done during a digital rectal exam in the doctor's office is not adequate for screening.

SOURCE: American Cancer Society. *Cancer Facts and Figures, 2008.* Atlanta: American Cancer Society, Inc.

Connect to Your Choices

Have you ever thought about where you get your behaviors and habits related to CVD and cancer? Many factors can influence our behaviors and habits, some not as obvious as others. When you were growing up, did your family avoid risk-increasing behaviors like smoking and being physically inactive? Currently, do you live on a campus or in a community where smoking is discouraged and physical activity is encouraged? Does your health clinic offer programs to help smokers quit or to promote and facilitate physical activity? Does your clinic discourage tanning and offer free blood pressure and cholesterol checks?

What are the external factors that influence your choices about CVD and cancer? What are your inner motivations and core values, and how do they affect your choices? Based on what you learned in this chapter, will you make some different choices in the future? If so, what will they be?

Go online to Connect to complete this activity.
www.mcgraw-hillconnect.com

TIPS FOR TODAY AND THE FUTURE

A growing body of research suggests that we can take an active role in preventing CVD and many cancers by adopting a wellness lifestyle.

RIGHT NOW YOU CAN

- Plan to replace one high-fat item in your diet with one that is high in fiber. For example, replace a doughnut with a bowl of whole-grain cereal.
- Check the cancer screening guidelines in this chapter and make sure you are up-to-date on your screenings.

IN THE FUTURE YOU CAN

- Take a class in cardiopulmonary resuscitation (CPR). A CPR certification equips you to help someone who is having a heart attack or experiencing cardiac arrest.
- Learn where to find information about daily UV radiation levels in your area, and learn how to interpret the information. Many local newspapers and television stations (and their Web sites) report current UV levels every day.
- Gradually add foods with abundant phytochemicals to your diet.

New and Experimental Techniques Many new and exciting possibilities for cancer therapy are on the horizon. Although it is impossible to predict which of these new approaches will be most successful, researchers hope that cancer therapy overall will become increasingly safer and more effective. When existing treatments are not successful at curbing cancer, patients often turn to complementary and alternative medicine, and experts caution them to be wary of fraudulent approaches.

SUMMARY

- The cardiovascular system circulates blood throughout the body. The heart pumps blood to the lungs via the pulmonary artery and to the body via the aorta.

- The six major risk factors for CVD that can be changed are smoking, high blood pressure, unhealthy cholesterol levels, inactivity, overweight and obesity, and diabetes.

- Hypertension occurs when blood pressure exceeds normal limits most of the time. It weakens the heart, scars and hardens arteries, and can damage the eyes and kidneys.

- Physical inactivity, obesity, and diabetes are interrelated and are associated with high blood pressure and unhealthy cholesterol levels.

- Contributing risk factors that can be changed include high triglyceride levels and psychological and social factors.

- Risk factors for CVD that can't be changed include being over 65, being male, being African American, and having a family history of CVD.

- Atherosclerosis is a progressive hardening and narrowing of arteries that can lead to restricted blood flow and even complete blockage.

- Heart attacks are usually the result of a long-term disease process.

- A stroke occurs when the blood supply to the brain is cut off by a blood clot or hemorrhage.

- Congestive heart failure occurs when the heart's pumping action becomes less efficient and fluid collects in the lungs or in other parts of the body.

- CVD risk can be reduced by engaging in regular exercise, avoiding tobacco and environmental tobacco smoke, knowing and managing your blood pressure and cholesterol levels, and developing effective ways of handling stress and anger.

- A malignant tumor can invade surrounding structures and spread to distant sites via the blood and lymphatic system, producing additional tumors.

- Lung cancer kills more people than any other type of cancer. Tobacco smoke is the primary cause.

- Colon and rectal cancer is linked to age, heredity, obesity, and a diet rich in red meat and low in fruits and vegetables. Most colon cancers arise from preexisting polyps.

Modifying Your Diet for Heart Health and Cancer Prevention

Gradually modifying your diet to include less saturated and trans fat and more fruits and vegetables can help you avoid both CVD and cancer in the future. Begin by assessing your current diet: Keep a record in your health journal of everything you eat for a week. At the end of the week, you can evaluate your diet and start taking steps to modify it.

Reducing Saturated and Trans Fat in Your Diet

The American Heart Association recommends that no more than 10% of the calories in your diet come from saturated and trans fat. Foods high in these fats include meat, poultry skin, full-fat dairy products, coconut and palm oils, and products made with hydrogenated vegetable oils, such as deep-fried fast food and packaged baked goods. To find out if your diet is within the 10% recommendation, at the end of the week, record the grams of saturated and trans fat next to the foods you've listed in your health journal. This information is available on many food labels, in books, and on the Internet. For fast foods, use the appendix. Trans fat content can be more difficult to determine. Here are the average values per serving for a few trans fat–rich foods: french fries (large), 5 g; pound cake, 5 g; doughnut, 4 g; fried breaded chicken, 3 g; Danish pastry, 3 g; vegetable shortening, 3 g; sandwich cookies, 2 g; crackers, 2 g; margarine (stick), 2 g; margarine (tub), 1 g.

Once you have the grams of fat listed, add up what you consumed each day. For a 2000-calorie diet, the 10% limit corresponds to about 22 grams of saturated and trans fat (2000 × 10% = 200 calories; 200 divided by 9 calories per gram of fat = 22 grams). If you're not able to get all the data you need, estimate by looking at the number of servings of food high in saturated or trans fat you consume in a day.

If your diet is higher in these fats than it should be, look at your food record to see if you are choosing high-fat foods more often than you should. To reduce your intake of saturated and trans fats, try making healthy substitutions:

- Vegetable oils or trans fat–free tub margarine rather than butter, stick margarine, or vegetable shortening
- Fruits, vegetables, rice cakes, unbuttered popcorn, or pretzels instead of chips, crackers, or cheese puffs
- Low-fat or fat-free milk, cheese, yogurt, or mayonnaise instead of the full-fat versions
- Fruit or a low-fat sweet (angel food cake, frozen yogurt, sorbet) instead of cakes, cookies, pastries, or regular ice cream
- Whole-grain breads and rolls, English muffins, or bagels instead of croissants, muffins, or coffee cake
- Lean meat, skinless poultry, or a veggie burger instead of ground beef, fried chicken, or lunch meats
- Baked potato or rice instead of french fries or onion rings
- Vegetarian chili or pasta with vegetables instead of pizza or macaroni and cheese

When you do eat high-fat foods, eat smaller portions, and balance your higher-fat choices with low-fat choices over the course of the day.

Increasing Fruits and Vegetables in Your Diet

Many fruits and vegetables contain phytochemicals, compounds that help slow, stop, or even reverse the process of cancer. For this reason, the National Cancer Institute (NCI) has developed the "Fruits and Veggies Matter" program to help Americans increase their consumption of fruits and vegetables to health-promoting levels. Take a look at the foods you've listed in your health journal for a week. Have you included five or more fruits and vegetables each day? If not, here are some tips from the NCI:

- Drink 100% juice every morning.
- Add raisins, berries, or sliced fruit to cereal; top bagels with tomato slices.
- Make a fruit smoothie from fresh or frozen fruit and orange juice or low-fat yogurt.
- Have vegetable soup or a salad with your lunch.
- Replace french fries or potato chips with cut-up vegetables.
- Try adding vegetables such as roasted peppers, cucumber slices, shredded carrots, avocado, or salsa to sandwiches.
- Drink tomato or vegetable juice instead of soda (monitor the sodium content of vegetable juices).
- At the salad bar, pile your plate with healthy fruits and vegetables and use low-fat or fat-free dressing.
- At dinner, choose a vegetarian main dish, such as stir-fry, or include two servings of vegetables.
- Substitute vegetables for meat in pasta, chili, and casseroles.
- Keep raw fruits and vegetables (apples, plums, carrots) on hand for snacks.

Some fruits and vegetables are particularly rich in phytochemicals; choose them as often as you can. They include cruciferous vegetables (e.g., broccoli, cauliflower, cabbage, bok choy, brussels sprouts); citrus fruits (e.g., oranges, lemons, grapefruit); berries (e.g., strawberries, raspberries); dark-green leafy vegetables (e.g., spinach, chard, romaine lettuce); and deep-yellow, orange, and red fruits and vegetables (e.g., carrots, red and yellow bell peppers, winter squash, cantaloupe, apricots).

SOURCES: American Heart Association, 2008. *Following a Healthy Eating Plan* (http://www.americanheart.org; retrieved September 22, 2010); National Cancer Institute. 2010. *Fruits and Veggies Matter* (http://www.fruitsandveggiesmatter.gov; retrieved September 22, 2010).

- Breast cancer affects about one in eight women in the United States. Although there is a genetic component to breast cancer, diet and hormones are also risk factors.

- Prostate cancer is chiefly a disease of aging; diet and lifestyle probably are factors in its occurrence.

- Cancers of the female reproductive tract include cervical, uterine, and ovarian cancer. The Pap test is an effective screening test for cervical cancer.

- Skin cancers occur as basal cell carcinoma, squamous cell carcinoma, and melanoma.

- Head and neck cancers are caused primarily by smoking, excessive alcohol consumption, and use of spit tobacco.

- Testicular cancer can be detected early through self-examination.

- Some cancers are caused by inherited genetic mutations, but most mutations are the result of environmental and lifestyle factors, such as radiation, a poor diet, or smoking.

- Self-monitoring and regular screening tests are essential to early cancer detection.

- Methods of cancer diagnosis include magnetic resonance imaging, computed tomography, and ultrasound. Treatment methods usually consist of some combination of surgery, chemotherapy, and radiation.

FOR MORE INFORMATION

BOOKS

American Cancer Society. 2009. *The American Cancer Society Complete Guide to Complementary & Alternative Cancer Therapies.* Atlanta: American Cancer Society. *Provides in-depth information about cancer therapies being used alongside traditional Western medicine in treating cancer.*

Heller, M. 2005. *The DASH Diet Action Plan, Based on the National Institutes of Health Research: Dietary Approaches to Stop Hypertension.* Northbrook, Ill.: Amidon Press. *Provides background information and guidelines for adopting the DASH diet; also includes meal plans to suit differing caloric needs and recipes.*

Lipsky, M. S., et al. 2008. *American Medical Association Guide to Preventing and Treating Heart Disease.* New York: Wiley. *A team of doctors provides advice for heart health to consumers.*

McKinnell, R. G., et al. 2006. *The Biological Basis of Cancer,* 2nd ed. Boston: Cambridge University Press. *Examines the underlying causes of cancer and discusses actual cases of the disease and its impact on patients and families.*

Rosenbaum, E., et al. 2008. *Everyone's Guide to Cancer Therapy,* rev. 5th ed. Riverside, N.J.: Andrews McMeel. *Reviewed by a panel of more than 100 oncologists; provides articles on the known causes, diagnoses, and treatments for many types of cancer.*

ORGANIZATIONS AND WEB SITES

American Academy of Dermatology. Provides information on skin cancer prevention.
http://www.aad.org

American Cancer Society. Provides a wide range of free materials on the prevention and treatment of cancer.
http://www.cancer.org

American Heart Association. Provides information on hundreds of topics relating to cardiovascular disease: the AHA's Web site links to several sites focusing on specific heart-related topics.
http://www.heart.org (general information)

Clinical Trials. Information about clinical trials for new cancer treatments can be accessed at the following sites:
http://www.cancer.gov/clinicaltrials
http://www.centerwatch.com

Dietary Approaches to Stop Hypertension (DASH). Provides information about the design, diets, and results of the DASH study, including tips on how to follow the DASH diet at home.
http://www.nhlbi.nih.gov/health/public/heart/hbp/dash

EPA/Sunwise. Information about the UV Index and the effects of sun exposure, with links to sites with daily UV Index ratings for cities in the United States and other countries.
http://www.epa.gov/sunwise/uvindex.html

Food and Drug Administration, Center for Drug Evaluation and Research: Oncology Tools. Provides information about types of cancer, treatments, and clinical trials.
http://www.fda.gov/cder/cancer

Harvard School of Public Health: Disease Risk Index. Includes interactive risk assessments as well as tips for preventing common cancers.
http://www.diseaseriskindex.harvard.edu/update

The Human Heart: An On-Line Exploration. An online museum exhibit containing information on the structure and function of the heart, how to monitor your heart's health, and how to maintain a healthy heart.
http://www.fi.edu/learn/heart/index.html

National Cancer Institute. Provides information on treatment options, screening, and clinical trials.
http://www.cancer.gov

National Heart, Lung, and Blood Institute. Provides information on and interactive applications for a variety of topics relating to cardiovascular health and disease, including cholesterol, smoking, obesity, hypertension, and the DASH diet.
http://www.nhlbi.nih.gov

National Stroke Association. Provides information and referrals for stroke victims and their families; the Web site has a stroke risk assessment.
http://www.stroke.org

SELECTED BIBLIOGRAPHY

American Cancer Society. 2006. *Few Americans Know Connection Between Excess Weight and Cancer Risk, Survey Finds* (http://www.cancer.org/docroot/MED/content/MED_2_1x_Few_Americans_Know_Connection_Between_Excess_Weight_and_Cancer_Risk_Survey_Finds.asp; retrieved February 15, 2009).

American Cancer Society. 2009. *Cancer Prevention and Early Detection Facts and Figures 2009.* Atlanta: American Cancer Society.

American Cancer Society. 2010. *Cancer Facts and Figures, 2010.* Atlanta, Ga.: American Cancer Society.

American Heart Association. 2010. *Heart Disease and Stroke Statistics—2010 Update.* Dallas: American Heart Association.

Baker, S., and J. Kaprio. 2006. Common susceptibility genes for cancer: Search for the end of the rainbow. *British Medical Journal* 332(7550): 1150–1152.

Bibbins-Doming, K., et al. 2010. Projected effect of dietary salt reductions of future cardiovascular disease. *New England Journal of Medicine* 362(7): 590–599.

Centers for Disease Control and Prevention. 2008. Awareness of stroke warning symptoms—13 states and the District of Columbia, 2005. *Morbidity and Mortality Weekly Report* 57(18): 481–485.

Centers for Disease Control and Prevention. 2008. Surveillance for cancers associated with tobacco use—United States, 1999–2004. *Morbidity and Mortality Weekly Report Surveillance Summaries* 57(SS-08): 1–33.

Centers for Disease Control and Prevention. 2009. Application of lower sodium intake recommendations to adults—United States, 1999–2006. *Morbidity and Mortality Weekly Report* 58(11): 281–283.

Chao, A., et al. 2005. Meat consumption and risk of colorectal cancer. *Journal of the American Medical Association* 293(2): 172–182.

de Torbal, A., et al. 2006. Incidence of recognized and unrecognized myocardial infarction in men and women aged 55 and older: The Rotterdam Study. *European Heart Journal* 27(6): 729–736.

Garland, S. 2006. Efficacy of a quadrivalent HPV (types 6, 11, 16, 18) L1 VLP vaccine against external genital disease: Future 1 analysis. *European Journal of Obstetrics, Gynecology, and Reproductive Biology,* August 16.

Genetics and breast cancer. 2004. *Journal of the American Medical Association* 292(4): 522.

Giovannucci, E., et al. 2008. 25-hydroxyvitamin D and risk of myocardial infarction in men; a prospective study. *Archives of Internal Medicine* 168(11): 1174–1180.

Gommans, J., et al. 2009. Preventing strokes: The assessment and management of people with transient ischemic attack. *New Zealand Medical Journal* 122(1293): 50–60.

Harvard Medical School. 2008. The status of statins. *Harvard Women's Health Watch* 15(6): 1–3.

Kauff, N. D., et al. 2008. Risk-reducing salpingo-oophorectomy for the prevention of BRCA1- and BRCA2-associated breast and gynecologic cancer: A multicenter, prospective study. *Journal of Clinical Oncology* 26(8): 1331–1337.

Kidambi, S., et al. 2009. Hypertension, insulin resistance, and aldosterone: Sex-specific relationships. *Journal of Clinical Hypertension* 11(3): 130–137.

Kroenke, C. H., et al. 2005. Weight, weight gain, and survival after breast cancer diagnosis. *Journal of Clinical Oncology* 23(7): 1370–1378.

Ma, X., et al. 2010. Diet, lifestyle, and acute myeloid leukemia in the NIH-AARP cohort. *American Journal of Epidemiology* 171(3): 312–322.

Martinez, M. E. 2005. Primary prevention of colorectal cancer: Lifestyle, nutrition, exercise. *Recent Results in Cancer Research* 166: 177–211.

Marshall, D. A., et al. 2009. Achievement of heart health characteristics through participation in an intensive lifestyle change program (Coronary Artery Disease Reversal Study). *Journal of Cardiopulmonary Rehabilitation and Prevention* 29(2): 84–94.

Mayo Clinic. 2006. Skin cancer epidemic. Take steps to avoid sun damage. *Mayo Clinic Health Letter* 24(4): 1–3.

Mayo Clinic. 2008. Breast imaging: Advances in earlier cancer detection. *Mayo Clinic Health Letter* 26(2): 1–3.

Mirmiran, P., et al. 2009. Fruit and vegetable consumption and risk factors for cardiovascular disease. *Metabolism* 58(4): 460–468.

Müller, D., et al. 2006. How sudden is sudden cardiac death? *Circulation* 114(11): 1146–1150.

National Center for Health Statistics. 2010. Deaths: Final data for 2007. *National Vital Statistics Reports* 58(19): 1–73.

National Toxicology Program. 2005. *Report on Carcinogens,* Eleventh Edition. Research Triangle Park, N.C.: National Toxicology Program.

Nita, C., et al. 2008. Hypertensive waist: First step of the screening for metabolic syndrome. *Metabolic Syndrome and Related Disorders* 7(2): 105–110.

Ostrom, M. P., et al. 2008. Mortality incidence and the severity of coronary atherosclerosis assessed by computed tomography angiography. *Journal of the American College of Cardiology* 52(16): 1335–1343.

Raggi, P., et al. 2008. Coronary artery calcium to predict all-cause mortality in elderly men and women. *Journal of the American College of Cardiology* 52(1): 17–23.

Rho, R. W., and R. L. Page. 2007. The automated external defibrillator. *Journal of Cardiovascular Electrophysiology* 18: 1–4.

Ridker, P. M., et al. 2008. Rosuvastatin to prevent vascular events in men and women with elevated C-reactive protein. *New England Journal of Medicine* 359(21): 2195–2207.

Sesso, H. D., et al. 2008. Vitamins E and C in the prevention of cardiovascular disease in men: Physician's Health Study II randomized controlled trial. *Journal of the American Medical Association* 300(18): 2123–2133.

Sui, X., et al. 2007. Cardiorespiratory fitness and the risk of nonfatal cardiovascular disease in women and men with hypertension. *American Journal of Hypertension* 20(6): 608–615.

Terry, M. B., et al. 2004. Association of frequency and duration of aspirin use and hormone receptor status with breast cancer risk. *Journal of the American Medical Association* 291(20): 2433–2440.

Trimble, C. L., et al. 2005. Active and passive cigarette smoking and the risk of cervical neoplasia. *Obstetrics and Gynecology* 105(1): 174–181.

University of California, Berkeley. 2008. Heart tests: low- to high-tech. *University of California, Berkeley, Wellness Letter,* August, 5.

U.S. Preventive Services Task Force. 2008. Screening for prostate cancer: U.S. Preventive Services Task Force recommendation statement. *Annals of Internal Medicine* 149(3): 185–191.

Van Gils, C. H., et al. 2005. Consumption of vegetables and fruits and risk of breast cancer. *Journal of the American Medical Association* 293(3): 183–193.

Wang, X., et al. 2007. Efficacy of folic acid supplementation in stroke prevention: A meta-analysis. *Lancet* 369(9576): 1876–1882.

World Health Organization. 2005. *Cancer: Diet and Physical Activity's Impact* (http://www.who.int/dietphysicalactivity/publications/facts/cancer/en/; retrieved Feburary 15, 2009).

Touring the Cardiorespiratory System

The Cardiorespiratory System

The Heart and Lungs

Atherosclerosis: The Process of Cardiovascular Disease

Diabetes: A Disorder of Metabolism

GOALS OF THE TOUR

1. **The Cardiorespiratory System.** Identify the parts of the cardiorespiratory system and the pattern of blood flow through the body.

2. **The Heart and Lungs.** Identify the chambers of the heart and describe the flow of blood through the right side of the heart to the lungs (pulmonary circulation) and through the left side of the heart to the body (systemic circulation).

3. **Atherosclerosis.** Explain the process of cardiovascular disease and compare and contrast the outcomes affecting the heart and the brain.

4. **Diabetes.** Describe how the body uses digested food for energy and growth and how this process is disrupted when a person has diabetes.

The Cardiorespiratory System

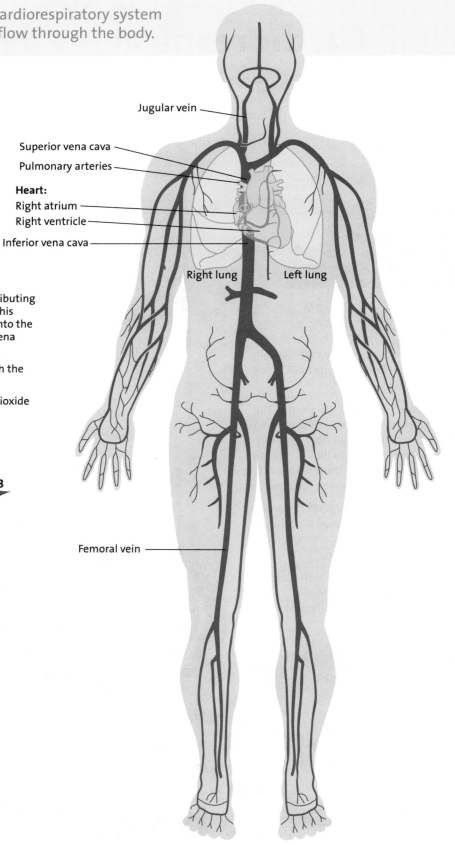

Jugular vein

Superior vena cava

Pulmonary arteries

Heart:

Right atrium

Right ventricle

Inferior vena cava

Right lung   Left lung

Femoral vein

Return of deoxygenated blood to the heart

1. Blood travels through the body, distributing oxygen and picking up carbon dioxide. This waste-laden, oxygen-poor blood flows into the right side of the heart via the superior vena cava and the inferior vena cava.

2. From there, blood is pumped through the pulmonary arteries into the lungs.

3. In the lungs, blood discards carbon dioxide and picks up oxygen.

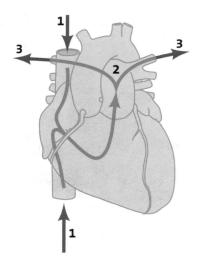

The Heart and Lungs

Identify the chambers of the heart and describe the flow of blood through the right side of the heart to the lungs (pulmonary circulation) and through the left side of the heart to the body (systemic circulation).

2

Blood is supplied to the heart muscle by the right and left coronary arteries, which branch off the aorta.

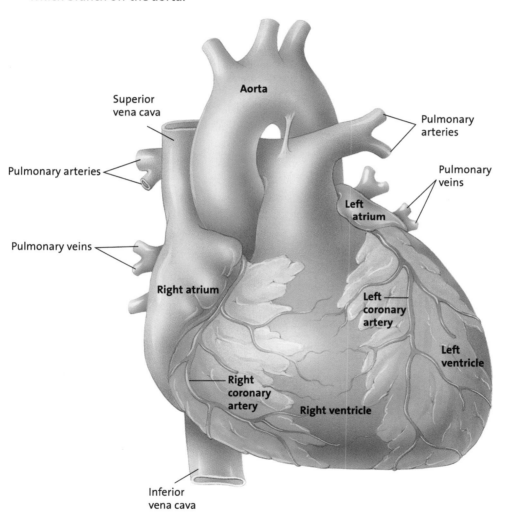

Aorta

Superior
vena cava

Pulmonary
arteries

Pulmonary arteries

Pulmonary
veins

Left
atrium

Pulmonary veins

Right atrium

Left
coronary
artery

Left
ventricle

Right
coronary
artery

Right ventricle

Inferior
vena cava

Atherosclerosis: The Process of Cardiovascular Disease

3 Explain the process of cardiovascular disease and compare and contrast the outcomes affecting the heart and the brain.

1. A healthy artery allows blood to flow through freely.

2. Plaque buildup begins when endothelial cells lining the arteries are damaged by smoking, high blood pressure, oxidized LDL cholesterol, and other causes. Excess cholesterol particles collect beneath these cells.

Coronary arteries

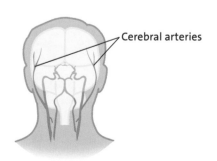

Cerebral arteries

Diabetes: A Disorder of Metabolism

Describe how the body uses digested food for energy and growth and how this process is disrupted when a person has diabetes.

Normal metabolism

1. When a meal is consumed, food is broken down into nutrients that the body can use to produce energy and build and nourish cells. Carbohydrates are broken down into glucose, which is the body's primary source of energy.

2. When glucose enters the bloodstream, the pancreas secretes the hormone insulin, which allows glucose to enter body cells.

Glucose

Bloodstream

Insulin

Body cells

Liver

Pancreas

Stomach

Kidney

LOOKING AHEAD...

After reading this chapter, you should be able to:

- Describe the step-by-step process by which infectious diseases are transmitted
- Explain how the immune system responds to an invading microorganism
- Identify the major types of pathogens and describe the common diseases they cause
- Explain how HIV infection affects the body and how it is transmitted, diagnosed, and treated
- Discuss the symptoms, risks, and treatments for the other major STDs
- Discuss steps you can take to prevent infections, including STDs, and strengthen your immune system

13

Immunity and Infection

The immune system works to keep the body from being overwhelmed, not just by external invaders that cause **infections,** but also by internal changes such as cancer. Most people don't notice these internal skirmishes unless they become sick. But people today are more knowledgeable about the complexities of immunity because they have heard about or had experience with HIV infection, which directly attacks the immune system. This chapter introduces you to the mechanisms of immunity and infection, and shows how to keep yourself well in a world of disease-causing microorganisms.

THE CHAIN OF INFECTION

Infectious diseases are transmitted from one person to another through a series of steps—a chain of infection. The infectious disease cycle begins with a **pathogen,** a microorganism that causes disease. HIV (the virus that causes AIDS) and the tuberculosis bacterium are examples of pathogens. The pathogen has a natural environment—called a **reservoir**—in which it typically lives. This reservoir can be a person, an animal, or an environmental component like soil or water. To transmit infection, the pathogen must leave the reservoir through some portal of exit. In the case of a human reservoir, portals of exit include saliva (for mumps, for example), the mucous membranes (for many sexually transmitted diseases), blood (for HIV and hepatitis), feces (for intestinal infections), and nose and throat discharges (for colds and influenza).

Transmission can occur directly or indirectly. In direct transmission, the pathogen is passed from one person to another without an intermediary; this usually requires fairly close association with an infected host, but not necessarily physical contact. For example, sneezing and coughing can discharge infectious particles into the air, where they can be inhaled by someone nearby. Most common respiratory infections and many intestinal infections are passed directly. Other means of direct transmission include sexual contact and contact with blood.

In indirect transmission, animals or insects such as rats, ticks, and mosquitoes can serve as *vectors,* carrying the pathogen from one host to another. Pathogens can also be transmitted via contaminated soil, food, or water or from inanimate objects, such as eating utensils.

To infect a new host, a pathogen must have a portal of entry into the body. Pathogens can enter in one of three general ways: direct contact with or penetration of the skin, inhalation through the mouth or nose, or ingestion of contaminated food or water. Pathogens that enter the skin or mucous membranes can cause a local infection of the tissue, or they may penetrate into the bloodstream or lymphatic system, thereby causing a more extensive **systemic infection.** Agents that cause sexually transmitted diseases (STDs) usually enter the body through the mucous membranes lining the urethra (in males) or the cervix (in females). Organisms that are transmitted via respiratory secretions may cause upper respiratory infections or pneumonia, or they may enter the bloodstream and cause systemic infection. Foodborne and waterborne organisms enter the mouth and may attack the cells of the small intestine or the colon, causing diarrhea, or they may enter the bloodstream via the digestive system and travel to other parts of the body.

Once in the new host, a variety of factors determine whether the pathogen will be able to establish itself and cause infection. People with a strong immune system or resistance to a particular pathogen are less likely to become ill than people with poor immunity. If conditions are right, the pathogen will multiply and produce disease in the new host. In such a case, the new host may become a reservoir from which a new chain of infection can be started.

Interrupting the chain of infection at any point can prevent disease. Strategies for breaking the chain include both public health measures and individual action. For example, a pathogen's reservoir can be isolated or destroyed, as when a sick individual is placed under quarantine or when insects or animals carrying pathogens are killed. Public sanitation practices, such as sewage treatment and the chlorination of drinking water, can also kill pathogens. Transmission can be disrupted through strategies like hand washing and the

use of face masks. Immunization and the treatment of infected hosts can stop the pathogen from multiplying, producing a serious disease, and being passed on to a new host.

THE BODY'S DEFENSE SYSTEM

Our bodies have very effective ways of protecting themselves against invasion by pathogens. The body's first line of defense is a formidable array of physical and chemical barriers. When these barriers are breached, the body's **immune system** comes into play.

Physical and Chemical Barriers

The skin, the body's largest organ, prevents many microorganisms from entering the body. Although many bacterial and fungal organisms live on the surface of the skin, very few can penetrate it except through a cut or break.

Wherever there is an opening in the body, or an area without skin, other barriers exist. The mouth is lined with mucous membranes, which contain cells designed to prevent the passage of unwanted organisms and particles. Body openings and the fluids that cover them (for example, tears, saliva, and vaginal secretions) are rich in antibodies and in enzymes that break down and destroy many microorganisms.

The respiratory tract is lined not only with mucous membranes but also with cells having hairlike protrusions called *cilia*. The cilia sweep foreign matter up and out of the respiratory tract. Particles that are not caught by this mechanism may be expelled from the system by a cough.

The Immune System

Once the body has been invaded by a foreign organism, an elaborate system of responses is activated. Two of these responses are the inflammatory response and the immune response.

Immunological Defenders   The immune response is carried out by different types of white blood cells, which are continuously being produced in the bone marrow.

Neutrophils, one type of white blood cell, travel in the bloodstream to areas of invasion, attacking and ingesting pathogens. Macrophages, or "big eaters," take up stations in tissues and act as scavengers, devouring pathogens and worn-out cells. Natural killer cells directly destroy virus-infected cells and cells that have turned cancerous. Dendritic cells, which reside in tissues, eat pathogens and activate lymphocytes. Lymphocytes, of which there are several types, are white blood cells that travel in both the bloodstream and the lymphatic system. At various places in the lymphatic system there are lymph nodes (or glands), where macrophages and dendritic cells congregate and filter bacteria and other substances from the lymph. When these nodes are actively involved in fighting an invasion of microorganisms, they fill with cells; physicians use the location of swollen lymph nodes as a clue to the location and cause of an infection.

The two main types of lymphocytes are T cells and B cells. T cells are further differentiated into helper T cells, killer T cells, and suppressor T cells. B cells are lymphocytes that produce **antibodies.** The first time T cells and B cells encounter a specific invader, some of them are reserved as memory T and B cells, enabling the body to mount a rapid response should the same invader appear again in the future.

The immune system is built on a remarkable feature of these defenders: the ability to distinguish foreign cells from the body's own cells. Because lymphocytes are capable of great destruction, it is essential that they not attack the body itself. When they do, they cause **autoimmune diseases,** such as lupus and rheumatoid arthritis.

All the cells in your body display markers on their surfaces—tiny molecular shapes—that identify them as "self" to lymphocytes that encounter them. Invading microorganisms also display markers on their surface; lymphocytes identify these as foreign, or "nonself." Nonself markers that trigger the immune response are known as **antigens.** Antibodies have complementary surface markers that work with antigens like a lock and key. When an antigen appears in the body, it eventually encounters an antibody with a complementary pattern. The antibody locks onto the antigen, triggering a series of events designed to destroy the invading pathogen.

> The immune system has a remarkable ability: It can distinguish foreign cells from the body's own cells.

The Inflammatory Response

When injured or infected, your body reacts by producing an inflammatory response. Special cells in the area of invasion or injury release **histamine** and other substances that cause blood vessels to dilate and fluid to flow out of capillaries into the injured tissue. This produces increased heat, swelling, and redness in the affected area. White blood cells are drawn to the area and attack the invaders—in many cases, destroying them.

The Immune Response

The immune system has two types of responses to invading pathogens: natural (innate) and acquired (adaptive). In the natural immune response, immune system cells recognize pathogens as "foreign" and respond the same way no matter how many times a pathogen invades, essentially eating the invaders. In the acquired immune response, immune system cells develop a memory for the antigen. If the body is invaded again, they recognize the pathogen and mount a much more potent response. The immune response can be thought of as having four phases, as depicted in Figure 13.1.

Immunity

After an infection, survival often confers **immunity;** that is, an infected person will never get the same illness again because some of the lymphocytes created during the second phase of the immune response are reserved as memory T and B cells. If the same antigen enters the body again, the memory T and B cells recognize and destroy it before it can cause illness. The ability of memory lymphocytes to remember previous infections is known as **acquired immunity.**

Symptoms and Contagion

The immune system is operating at the cellular level at all times, maintaining its vigilance when you're well and fighting invaders when you're sick. During **incubation,** when viruses are multiplying in the body or when bacteria are actively multiplying before the immune system has gathered momentum, you may not have any symptoms of the illness, but you may be contagious. During the second and third phases of the immune response, you may still be

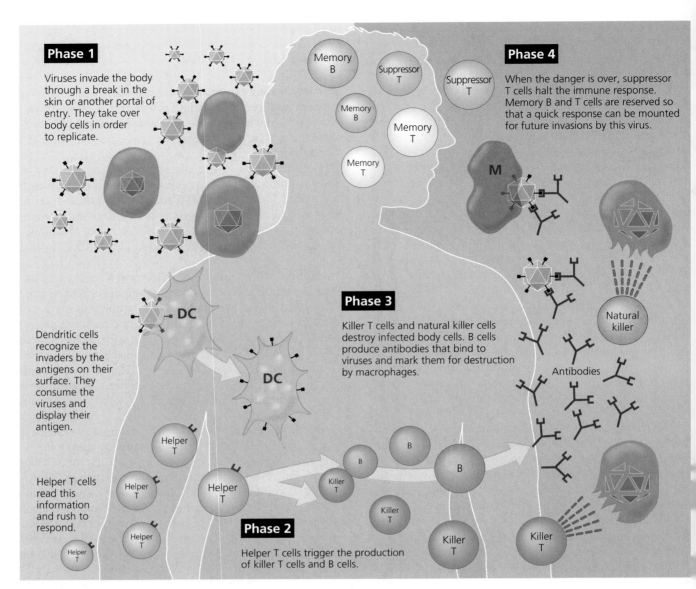

FIGURE 13.1 **The immune response.** Once invaded by a pathogen, the body mounts a complex series of reactions to eliminate the invader. Pictured here are the principal elements of the immune response to a virus.

unaware of the infection, or you may "feel a cold coming on." Symptoms first appear during the *prodromal period,* which follows incubation. If the infected host has acquired immunity, the infection may be eradicated during the *incubation period* or the prodromal period. In this case, although you may have felt you were coming down with a cold, for example, it does not develop into a full-blown illness.

Many symptoms of an illness are actually due to the immune response of the body rather than to the actions or products of the invading organism. For example, fever is caused by the release and activation of certain **cytokines** in macrophages and other cells during the immune response. These cytokines travel in the bloodstream to the brain and cause the body's thermostat to be reset to a higher level. The resulting elevated temperature helps the body in its fight against pathogens by enhancing immune responses.

> **27 common diseases can be prevented by vaccines.**
>
> —CDC, 2010

cytokine A chemical messenger produced by a variety of cell types that helps regulate many cell functions; immune system cells release cytokines that help amplify and coordinate the immune response.

Epidemics and Pandemics

The term **epidemic** refers to a rapidly spreading disease, whether caused by an infectious agent or some other factor (for example, the current "obesity epidemic"). In an epidemic, the occurrence of the disease is greater than what is expected normally.

The term **pandemic** refers to a widespread epidemic, one that has spread across a large area, such as an entire nation, continent, or even the world. Human history has been punctuated by numerous pandemics of various diseases, including bubonic plague, smallpox, and more recently HIV and the 2009 HINI influenza pandemic.

Epidemics and pandemics of influenza A are due to viral evolution. Small changes in the influenza virus proteins hemagglutinin (H) and neuraminidase (N), referred to as *antigenic drift,* arise through mutations during viral replication. The antibodies that a person's immune system produced during a prior influenza infection may no longer be able to bind to the new H and N variants or may bind weakly, and thus they may confer only partial protection from infection with the new strain of influenza.

Less frequently, an influenza A virus can undergo a dramatic change due to the exchange of genetic material with another influenza virus. For example, if a pig is infected simultaneously with both swine and human influenza A strains, there can be a more drastic change in the H and N antigens, resulting in *antigenic shift.* The novel influenza A virus may now be able to infect humans. The antibodies that an individual had produced during infection with standard human strains of influenza A will provide no protection from infection, and the new influenza A strain can spread across the human population. Luckily, antigenic shift occurs less frequently than antigenic drift. A pandemic results if three criteria are met: there is little or no preexisting immunity to the new virus, there is efficient human-to-human transmission of the virus, and the new virus can cause illness. For more information, see the box "The 2009 H1N1 Flu Pandemic."

Immunization

The ability of the immune system to remember previously encountered organisms and retain its strength against them is the basis for **immunization.** When a person is immunized, the immune system is primed with an antigen similar to the pathogenic organism but not as dangerous. The body responds by producing antibodies, which prevent serious infection if the person is exposed to the disease organism itself. The preparations used to manipulate the immune system are known as **vaccines.** Most vaccines are made from microbes that have been weakened or killed in the laboratory but still retain their ability to stimulate the production of antibodies.

Vaccines confer what is known as *active immunity*— that is, the vaccinated person produces his or her own antibodies to the microorganism. Another type of injection confers *passive immunity.* In this case, a person exposed to a disease is injected with the antibodies, which have been produced by other human beings or animals who have recovered from the disease. Injections of *gamma globulin*—a product made from the blood plasma of many individuals containing all the antibodies they have ever made—are sometimes given to people to create a rapid but temporary immunity to a particular disease.

Allergy: The Body's Defense System Gone Haywire

Allergies result from a hypersensitive and overactive immune system. In someone with an allergy, the immune system mounts a response to a harmless substance such as pollen or animal dander. Allergy symptoms—stuffy nose, sneezing, wheezing, skin rashes, and so on—result primarily from the immune response rather than from **allergens,** the substances that provoke the response.

The Allergic Response   Most allergic reactions are due to the production of a special type of antibody known as immunoglobulin E (IgE). Initial exposure to a particular allergen may cause little response, but it sensitizes the immune system. When the body is subsequently exposed to the allergen, the allergen binds to IgE, causing *mast cells* (another type of immune cell) to release large amounts of histamine and other compounds into surrounding tissues. Histamine has many effects, including increasing the inflammatory response and stimulating mucus production. In the nose, histamine may cause congestion and sneezing; in the eyes, itchiness and tearing; in the skin, redness, swelling, and itching; in the intestines, bloating and cramping; and in the

TERMS

epidemic   A rapidly spreading disease or health-related concern.

pandemic   A widespread epidemic.

immunization   The process of conferring immunity to a pathogen by administering a vaccine.

vaccine   A preparation of killed or weakened microorganisms, inactivated toxins, or components of microorganisms that is administered to stimulate an immune response; a vaccine protects against future infection by the pathogen.

allergy   A disorder caused by the body's exaggerated response to foreign chemicals and proteins; also called *hypersensitivity.*

allergen   A substance that triggers an allergic reaction.

The 2009 H1N1 Flu Pandemic

In 2009, an outbreak of influenza caused by a new virus never before identified as a cause of human illness led to fears of a disastrous worldwide pandemic. Health officials were alarmed because most people had no immunity to this new H1N1 strain, initially called swine flu, and because, like all forms of flu, it could easily spread from one person to another. History has shown that such outbreaks can spread rapidly around the world, killing millions. In addition, there was no H1N1 vaccine available at the outset.

The outbreaks began in North America in April, and within 2 months, 74 countries were reporting cases of the illness. In June, the World Health Organization decleared that a pandemic was under way. The CDC began tracking laboratory-confirmed cases in the United States, including those requiring hospitalization and those resulting in death. Between April and October of 2009, the CDC estimated that there were between 14 million and 34 million cases of H1N1 influenza infection, resulting in between 63,000 and 153,000 hospitalizations and between 2500 and 6000 deaths. By February 2010, the total number of cases had increased to between 42 million and 86 million, with a total of between 188,000 and 389,000 hospitalizations and between 8520 and 17,620 deaths. These estimates include corrections for under-reporting, given that many people with the flu do not seek medical care and an even smaller number of infected people are tested properly.

The CDC issued guidelines on good health habits to prevent the flu, including washing your hands frequently, staying home if you are sick with flulike

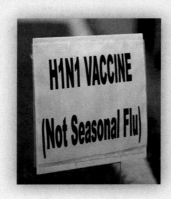

symptoms, and avoiding people who are sick. The Department of Homeland Security issued guidelines for employers, schools, and state and local public health departments, and even President Obama addressed the American public about the pandemic. Early supplies of the H1N1 vaccine were limited, so vaccination was at first available only to high-risk groups. Ultimately, the H1N1 flu did not prove as virulent as feared, so mortality in the millions was avoided.

The H1N1 influenza A virus is a remarkable recombinant influenza virus. The genetic evolution of H1N1 indicates a reassortment of four different influenza A virus genomes: two derived from swine flu (H1N1) virus, one from avian (bird) flu virus, and one from human flu virus. The swine flu components are from viruses found in Europe, North America, and Asia. Contrary to the popular perception that this evolution was a very recent development, the data indicate that it began as long ago as 1918. However, the final steps involve a recent reassortment between two swine flu viruses, which contained both avian flu and human flu virus genes.

The 2009 H1N1 pandemic had two notable characteristics that distinguished it from seasonal flu. First, it was a summer flu. It started in the spring and peaked in the second week of October. In contrast, seasonal flu outbreaks generally begin in the fall and peak in January, February, or March. Second, 90% of the hospitalizations and 87% of the deaths caused by the 2009 H1N1 pandemic occurred in persons younger than 65 years of age. In contrast, 60% of hospitalizations and 90% of flu-related deaths caused by seasonal flu occur in persons 65 years of age of older.

The CDC recommends H1N1 immunization for all persons 6 months of age or older. Vaccination is particularly important for pregnant women; for people who have asthma, chronic obstructive pulmonary disease (COPD), diabetes, or coronary artery disease; and for people who are morbidly obese.

Although the number of cases of H1N1 influenza has tapered off, the CDC continues to collect data weekly from the National Influenza Surveillance System to track trends throughout the nation. The virus's spread is also being tracked globally by the World Health Organization and other agencies.

SOURCES: Centers for Disease Control and Prevention. 2010. *Updated CDC Estimates of 2009 H1N1 Influenza Cases, Hospitalizations and Deaths in the United States, April 2009– April 10, 2010* (http://www.cdc.gov/h1n1flu/ estimates_2009_h1n1.htm; retrieved July 23, 2010); Fisher, M. C. 2009. Novel H1N1 pandemic. When pigs fly. *The Pediatric Infectious Disease Journal* 29(10): 911–914; Zimmer, S. M., and S. D. Burke. 2009. Historical perspective– Emergence of influenza A (H1N1) viruses. *New England Journal of Medicine* 361(3): 279–285.

---

lungs, coughing, wheezing, and shortness of breath. In some people, an allergen can trigger an **asthma** attack.

The most serious, but rare, kind of allergic reaction is **anaphylaxis,** which results from a release of histamine throughout the body. Anaphylactic reactions can be life-threatening because symptoms may include swelling of the throat, extremely low blood pressure, fainting, heart arrhythmia, and seizures. Anaphylaxis is a medical emergency, and treatment requires immediate injection of epinephrine.

Dealing with Allergies If you suspect you might have an allergy, visit your physician or an allergy specialist. You may be able to avoid or minimize exposure to allergens by mak-

ing changes in your environment or behavior. For example, removing carpets from the bedroom and using special bedding can reduce dust mite contact. There are also medications available for allergy sufferers. Many over-the-counter

asthma A disease that affects the lungs; characterized by wheezing, shortness of breath, a sensation of tightness in the chest, and coughing, which may be more prevalent at night or in the early morning.

anaphylaxis A severe systemic hypersensitive reaction to an allergen characterized by difficulty breathing, low blood pressure, heart arrhythmia, seizure, and sometimes death.

Type of Organism	Selected Pathogens	Associated Diseases
Bacteria Microscopic single-celled organisms	*Bordetella pertussis* *Borrelia burgdorferi* *Chlamydia* *Clostridium tetani* *Helicobacter pylori* *Legionella pneumophila* *Mycobacterium tuberculosis* Mycoplasma *Neisseria* Rickettsia Staphylococcus Streptococcus	Pertussis (whooping cough) Lyme disease Pneumonia (*C. pneumoniae*), chlamydia (*C. trachomatis*) Tetanus Peptic ulcers Legionnaire's disease Tuberculosis Pneumonia, ear infections, sore throat, urethritis Gonorrhea (*N. gonorrhoeae*), meningitis (*N. meningitidis*) Rocky Mountain spotted fever, typhus Boils and other skin infections, toxic shock syndrome Strep throat, skin infections, pneumonia, rheumatic fever and rheumatic heart disease, necrotizing fascitis
Viruses Infectious agents consisting of a protein shell enclosing DNA or RNA	Coronavirus, rhinovirus Epstein-Barr virus Hepatitis viruses Herpes simplex 1 and 2 Human immunodeficiency virus Human papillomaviruses Influenza viruses A and B Paramyxovirus Rhabdovirus Togavirus Varicella-zoster	Severe acute respiratory syndrome (SARS), common cold Infectious mononucleosis Hepatitis (inflammation of the liver) Cold sores, genital herpes HIV/AIDS Warts, cervical cancer Flu Measles, mumps Rabies Rubella Chicken pox, shingles
Fungi Single- or multicelled organisms (e.g., yeasts, molds)	*Candida albicans* *Cryptococcus neoformans* Dermatophyte fungi *Histoplasma capsulatum* *Coccidioides immitis*	Yeast infections, thrush Pneumonia, meningitis Athlete's foot, jock itch, ringworm, nail infections Histoplasmosis Coccidioidomycosis
Protozoa Single-celled organisms	*Entamoeba histolytica* *Giardia lamblia* *Plasmodia* *Trichomonas vaginalis* *Trypanosoma brucei*	Amoebic dysentery Giardiasis Malaria Trichomoniasis African sleeping sickness
Parasitic worms Worms that feed and live on or in a host	*Ancylostoma duodenale* *Ascaris lumbricoides* Beef, pork, or fish tapeworms *Enterobius vermicularis* *Necator americanus* Schistosoma	Ancylostomiasis (hookworm infection) Ascariasis (roundworm infection) Tapeworm infection Pinworm infection Hookworm infection Cercarial dermatitis (swimmer's itch), schistosomiasis
Prions Proteinaceous infectious particles	PrP^{Sc}	Creutzfeldt-Jakob disease (CJD)

FIGURE 13.2 Pathogens and associated infectious diseases.

antihistamines are effective at controlling symptoms, and prescription corticosteroids delivered by aerosol markedly reduce allergy symptoms. A third approach is immunotherapy, in which a person is desensitized to a particular allergen through the administration of gradually increasing doses of the allergen over a period of months or years.

PATHOGENS AND DISEASE

When pathogens enter body tissue, they can cause illness and sometimes death to the host. Pathogens include bacteria, viruses, fungi, protozoa, parasitic worms, and prions (Figure 13.2).

Bacteria

The most abundant living things on earth are **bacteria,** single-celled organisms that usually reproduce by splitting in two to create a pair of identical cells. We harbor both helpful and harmful bacteria on our skin and in our gastrointestinal and reproductive tracts. The human colon contains helpful bacteria that produce certain vitamins

> **bacterium (plural, bacteria)** A microscopic single-celled organism; about 100 bacterial species can cause disease in humans.

and help digest nutrients. Friendly bacteria also keep harmful bacteria in check by competing for food and resources and secreting substances toxic to pathogenic bacteria. Not all bacteria found in the body are beneficial, however.

Pneumonia   Inflammation of the lungs, called *pneumonia,* may be caused by infection with bacteria, viruses, or fungi or by contact with chemical toxins or irritants. Pneumonia often follows another illness, such as a cold or the flu, but the symptoms are typically more severe—fever, chills, shortness of breath, increased mucus production, and cough. Pneumonia is the leading infectious cause of death worldwide and one of the ten leading causes of death for Americans.

Pneumococcus bacteria are the most common cause of bacterial pneumonia; a vaccine is available and recommended for all adults age 65 and older and others at risk. Other bacteria that may cause pneumonia include *Streptococcus pneumoniae, Chlamydia pneumoniae,* and mycoplasmas. Outbreaks of infection with mycoplasmas are relatively common among young adults, especially in crowded settings such as dormitories. Bacterial pneumonia can be treated with antibiotics.

Meningitis   Infection of the *meninges,* the membranes covering the brain and spinal cord, is called *meningitis.* Viral meningitis is usually mild and goes away on its own; bacterial meningitis, however, can be life-threatening and requires immediate treatment with antibiotics. Symptoms of meningitis include fever, a severe headache, stiff neck, sensitivity to light, and confusion. The disease is fatal in 10% of cases, and about 10–20% of people who recover have permanent hearing loss or other serious effects. A vaccine is available, but it is not effective against all strains of meningitis-causing bacteria. The CDC recommends routine vaccination of children 11–18 years old, previously unvaccinated adolescents at high school entry, and first-year college students who live in dormitories.

TERMS

streptococcus   Any of a genus (*Streptococcus*) of spherical bacteria; streptococcal species can cause skin infections, strep throat, rheumatic fever, pneumonia, scarlet fever, and other diseases.

staphylococcus   Any of a genus (*Staphylococcus*) of spherical, clustered bacteria commonly found on the skin or in the nasal passages; staphylococcal species may enter the body and cause conditions such as boils, pneumonia, and toxic shock syndrome.

tuberculosis (TB)   A chronic bacterial infection that usually affects the lungs.

Strep Throat and Other Streptococcal Infections
The **streptococcus** bacterium can cause streptococcal pharyngitis, or strep throat, characterized by a red, sore throat with white patches on the tonsils, swollen lymph nodes, fever, and headache. It is typically spread through close contact with an infected person via sneezing or coughing. If left untreated, strep throat can develop into the more serious rheumatic fever. A particularly virulent type of streptococcus can invade the bloodstream, spread to other parts of the body, and produce dangerous systemic illness. It can also cause a serious but rare infection of the deeper layers of the skin, a condition called necrotizing fascitis, or "flesh-eating strep."

Toxic Shock Syndrome and Other Staphylococcal Infections   The spherical-shaped **staphylococcus** bacterium can cause infections ranging from minor skin infections to very serious conditions such as blood infections and pneumonia. The strain known as methicillin-resistant *Staphylococcus aureus* (MRSA) has become the most common cause of skin infections treated in emergency rooms *Staphylococcus aureus* is also responsible for many cases of toxic shock syndrome (TSS). The bacteria produce a toxin that causes the massive proliferation of T cells that can bind to it. The staphylococcus toxins are referred to as "super antigens" because the massive proliferation of T cells results in excessive production of proinflammatory cytokines. This "cytokine storm" causes tissue damage, widespread coagulation of blood in the blood vessels, and ultimately organ failure.

Tuberculosis   Caused by the bacterium *Mycobacterium tuberculosis,* **tuberculosis (TB)** is a chronic bacterial infection that usually affects the lungs. TB is spread via the respiratory route. Symptoms include coughing, fatigue, night sweats, weight loss, and fever. Ten to 15 million Americans have been infected with, and therefore continue to carry, *M. tuberculosis.* Only about 10% of people with latent TB infections actually develop an active case of the disease. In the United States, active TB is most common among people infected with HIV, recent immigrants from countries where TB is endemic, and those who live in the inner cities. Many strains of tuberculosis respond to antibiotics, but only over a course of treatment lasting 6–12 months. Failure to complete treatment can lead to relapse and the development of strains of antibiotic-resistant bacteria.

Tickborne Infections Lyme disease is spread by the bite of a tick of the genus *Ixodes* that is infected with the spiral-shaped bacterium *Borrelia burgdorferi.* Symptoms of Lyme disease vary but typically occur in three stages. In the first stage, about 80% of victims develop a bull's-eye-shaped red rash expanding from the area of the bite, usually about 2 weeks after the bite occurs. The second stage occurs weeks to months later in 10–20% of untreated patients; symptoms may involve the nervous and cardiovascular systems and can include impaired coordination, partial facial paralysis, and heart rhythm abnormalities. Months or years after the tick bite some untreated people may develop chronic or recurring arthritis. Lyme disease is preventable by avoiding contact with ticks or by removing a tick before it has had the chance to transmit the infection. Rocky Mountain spotted fever is also transmitted via tick bites and is characterized by sudden onset of fever, headache, and muscle pain, followed by development of a spotted rash.

Ulcers About 25 million Americans suffer from ulcers, sores in the lining of the stomach or the first part of the small intestine (duodenum). Ulcer symptoms include gnawing or burning pain in the abdomen, nausea, and loss of appetite. Up to 90% of ulcers are caused by infection with the bacterium *Helicobacter pylori.* If tests show the presence of *H. pylori,* antibiotics often cure the infection and the ulcers. Persons who take NSAIDs and contract ulcers should be tested for *H. pylori,* because it is likely that they are infected and withdrawing of NSAIDs alone will not cure them.

Antibiotic Treatments **Antibiotics** are both naturally occurring and synthetic substances that can kill bacteria. Most antibiotics work in a similar fashion: They interrupt the production of new bacteria by damaging some part of their reproductive cycle or by causing faulty parts of new bacteria to be made. Antibiotics are among the most widely prescribed and effective drugs.

When antibiotics are misused or overused, the pathogens they are designed to treat can become resistant to their effects. When exposed to antibiotics, resistant bacteria can grow and flourish, while the antibiotic-sensitive bacteria die off. Antibiotic-resistant strains of many common bacteria have developed, including strains of gonorrhea (an STD) and salmonellosis (a foodborne illness). One strain of tuberculosis is resistant to seven different antibiotics. Antibiotic resistance is a major factor contributing to the rise in problematic infectious diseases.

Resistance is promoted when people fail to take the full course of an antibiotic or when they inappropriately take antibiotics for viral infections. Another source of resistance is the use of antibiotics in agriculture, which is estimated to account for 50–80% of the 25,000 tons of antibiotics used annually in the United States.

You can help prevent the development of antibiotic-resistant strains of bacteria by using antibiotics properly:

- Don't take an antibiotic every time you get sick. They are mainly helpful for bacterial infections; they are ineffective against viruses.
- Use antibiotics as directed, and finish the full course of medication even if you begin to feel better. This helps ensure that all targeted bacteria are killed off.
- Never take an antibiotic without a prescription.

Viruses

Viruses lack all the enzymes essential to energy production and protein synthesis in normal animal cells, and they cannot grow or reproduce by themselves; they are parasites, taking what they need for growth and reproduction from the cells they invade. Once a virus is inside the host cell, it sheds its protein covering, and its genetic material takes control of the cell and manufactures more viruses like itself. Illnesses caused by viruses are the most common forms of contagious disease.

The Common Cold Although generally brief, lasting only 1–2 weeks, colds are nonetheless irritating and often interfere with one's normal activities. A cold may be caused by any of more than 200 different viruses that attack the lining of the nasal passages. Cold viruses are almost always transmitted by hand-to-hand contact. To lessen your risk of contracting a cold, wash your hands frequently; if you touch someone else, avoid touching your face until after you've washed your hands. If you catch a cold, over-the-counter cold remedies may help treat your symptoms but do not directly attack the viral cause. Avoid multisymptom cold remedies. Because these products include drugs to treat symptoms you may not even have, you risk suffering from side effects from medications you don't need. It's better to treat each symptom separately:

Antibiotics will not help a cold unless a bacterial infection such as strep throat is also present, and overuse of antibiotics leads to the development of drug resistance. The jury is still out on whether other remedies, including

> *Antibiotics are not effective against viral illnesses. It's important to talk to your doctor before taking antibiotics.*

---

antibiotics Synthetic or naturally occurring substances used as drugs to kill bacteria.

virus A very small infectious agent composed of nucleic acid (DNA or RNA) surrounded by a protein coat; lacks an independent metabolism and reproduces only within a host cell.

zinc gluconate lozenges, echinacea, and vitamin C, will relieve symptoms or shorten the duration of a cold.

Influenza   Commonly called the flu, **influenza** is an infection of the respiratory tract caused by the influenza virus. Compared to the common cold, influenza is a more serious illness, usually including a fever and extreme fatigue. Most people who get the flu recover within 1–2 weeks, but some develop potentially life-threatening complications, such as pneumonia. The highest rates of infection occur in children. Influenza is highly contagious and is spread via respiratory droplets.

Vaccination can be appropriate for anyone age 6 months or older who wants to reduce his or her risk of the flu.

Chicken Pox, Cold Sores, and Other Herpesvirus Infections   The **herpesviruses** are a large group of viruses. Once infected, the host is never free of the virus. The virus lies latent within certain cells and becomes active periodically, producing symptoms. The family of herpesviruses includes varicella-zoster virus, which causes chicken pox and shingles; herpes simplex virus (HSV) types 1 and 2, which cause cold sores and the STD herpes; and Epstein-Barr virus (EBV), which causes infectious mononucleosis. Two herpesviruses that can cause severe infections in people with a suppressed immune system are cytomegalovirus (CMV), which infects the lungs, brain, colon, and eyes, and human herpesvirus 8 (HHV-8), which has been linked to Kaposi's sarcoma.

Viral Hepatitis   Viral **hepatitis** is a term used to describe several different infections that cause inflammation of the liver. Hepatitis is usually caused by one of the three most common hepatitis viruses. Hepatitis A virus (HAV) causes the mildest form of the disease and is usually transmitted by food or water contaminated by sewage or an infected person. Hepatitis B virus (HBV) is usually transmitted sexually. Hepatitis C virus (HCV) can also be transmitted sexually, but it is much more commonly passed through direct contact with infected blood via injection drug use or, prior to the development of screening tests, blood transfusions. HBV and, to a lesser extent, HCV can also be passed from a pregnant woman to her child. There are effective vaccines for hepatitis A and B.

Symptoms of acute hepatitis infection can include fatigue, **jaundice**, abdominal pain, loss of appetite, nausea, and diarrhea. Most people recover from hepatitis A within a month or so. However, 5–10% of people infected with HBV and 85–90% of people infected with HCV become chronic carriers of the virus, capable of infecting others for the rest of their lives. Some chronic carriers remain asymptomatic, while others slowly develop chronic liver disease, cirrhosis, or liver cancer. An estimated 4 million Americans and 500 million people worldwide may be chronic carriers of hepatitis.

The extent of HCV infection has only recently been recognized, and most infected people are unaware of their condition. To ensure proper treatment and prevention, testing for HCV may be recommended for people at risk, including people who have ever injected drugs (even once), who received a blood transfusion or a donated organ prior to July 1992, who have engaged in high-risk sexual behavior, or who have had body piercing, tattoos, or acupuncture involving unsterile equipment. If you are considering getting a tattoo or body piercing, choose the artist carefully and follow aftercare directions.

Human Papillomavirus (HPV)   The more than 100 different types of HPV cause a variety of warts, including common warts on the hands, plantar warts on the soles of the feet, and genital warts. Depending on their location, warts may be removed using over-the-counter preparations or professional methods such as laser surgery or cryosurgery. Because HPV infection is chronic, warts can reappear despite treatment. HPV causes the majority of cases of cervical cancer; a vaccine is available and recommended for girls and women age 9–26. Experts now advise that boys receive HPV vaccine to protect them against genital warts and to prevent certain cancer later in life.

Treating Viral Illnesses   Antiviral drugs typically work by interfering with some part of the viral life cycle; for example, they may prevent a virus from entering body cells or from successfully reproducing within cells. Antivirals are currently available to fight infections caused by HIV, influenza, herpes simplex, varicella-zoster, HBV, and HCV. Most other viral diseases must simply run their course.

Fungi

A **fungus** is an organism that absorbs food from organic matter. Only about 50 fungi out of many thousands of species cause disease in humans, and these diseases are usually restricted to the skin, mucous membranes, and lungs.

TERMS

influenza   Infection of the respiratory tract by the influenza virus, which is highly infectious and adaptable; the form changes so easily that every year new strains arise, making treatment difficult; commonly known as the flu.

herpesvirus   A family of viruses responsible for cold sores, mononucleosis, chicken pox, and the STD known as herpes; frequently causes latent infections.

hepatitis   Inflammation of the liver, which can be caused by infection, drugs, or toxins.

jaundice   Increased bile pigment levels in the blood, characterized by yellowing of the skin and the whites of the eyes.

fungus   A single-celled or multicelled organism that absorbs food from living or dead organic matter; examples include molds, mushrooms, and yeasts. Fungal diseases include yeast infections, athlete's foot, and ringworm.

Candida albicans is a common fungus found naturally in the vagina of most women. When excessive growth occurs, the result is itching and discomfort, commonly known as a yeast infection. Other common fungal conditions, including athlete's foot, jock itch, and ringworm, affect the skin. Fungi can also cause systemic diseases that are severe, life-threatening, and extremely difficult to treat. Fungal infections can be especially deadly in people with an impaired immune system.

Protozoa

Another group of pathogens is single-celled organisms known as **protozoa.** Millions of people in developing countries suffer from protozoal infections.

> **Polio remains endemic in only 4 countries: Afghanistan, India, Nigeria, and Pakistan.**
>
> —World Health Organization, 2010

Malaria, caused by a protozoan of the genus *Plasmodium,* is a major killer worldwide; each year, there are 350–500 million new cases of malaria and more than 1 million deaths, mostly among infants and children, and drug-resistant strains of malaria have emerged, requiring new medicines.

Other protozoal diseases include **giardiasis,** caused by a single-celled parasite that lives in the intestines of humans and animals and characterized by nausea, diarrhea, bloating, and abdominal cramps; *trichomoniasis,* a common, treatable, vaginal infection; *trypanosomiasis,* known as African sleeping sickness; and *amoebic dysentery.*

Parasitic Worms

The **parasitic worms** are the largest organisms that can enter the body to cause infection. The tapeworm, for example, can grow to a length of many feet. Worms cause a variety of relatively mild infections. Pinworm, the most common worm infection in the United States, primarily affects young children. Worm infections generally originate from contaminated food or drink and can be controlled by careful attention to hygiene.

Prions

In recent years, several fatal degenerative disorders of the central nervous system have been linked to **prions,** or *proteinaceous infectious particles.* Unlike all other infectious agents, prions appear to lack DNA or RNA and to consist only of protein; their presence in the body does not trigger an immune response. Prions have an abnormal shape and form deposits in the brain. Prions are associated with a

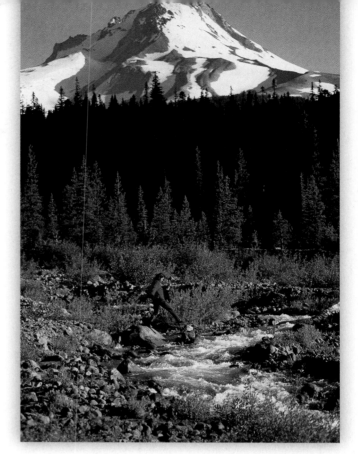

Even seemingly pristine mountain streams can be contaminated with the protozoan *Giardia lamblia,* as many unwary hikers and campers have discovered. Symptoms of giardiasis include abdominal pain, bloating, and diarrhea.

class of diseases known as *transmissible spongiform encephalopathies (TSEs),* which are characterized by spongelike holes in the brain; symptoms of TSEs include loss of coordination, weakness, dementia, and death. Known prion diseases include Creutzfeldt-Jakob disease (CJD) in humans; bovine spongiform encephalopathy (BSE), or mad cow disease, in cattle; and scrapie in sheep. Some prion diseases are inherited or the result of spontaneous genetic

TERMS

protozoan (plural, protozoa) A microscopic single-celled organism that often produces recurrent, cyclical attacks of disease.

malaria A severe, recurrent, mosquito-borne infection caused by the protozoan *Plasmodium.*

giardiasis An intestinal disease caused by the protozoan *Giardia lamblia.*

parasitic worm A pathogen that causes intestinal and other infections; includes tapeworms, hookworms, pinworms, and flukes.

prions Proteinaceous infectious particles thought to be responsible for a class of neurodegenerative diseases known as transmissible spongiform encephalopathies; Creutzfeldt-Jakob disease (CJD) in humans and bovine spongiform encephalopathy (BSE, or mad cow disease) are prion diseases.

mutations, whereas others are the result of eating infected tissue or being exposed to prions during medical procedures such as organ transplants.

Emerging Infectious Diseases

Emerging infectious diseases are those infections whose incidence in humans has increased or threatens to increase in the near future. They include both known diseases that have experienced a resurgence, such as tuberculosis and cholera, and diseases that were previously unknown or confined to specific areas, such as the Ebola and West Nile viruses.

Selected Infections of Concern   Although the chances of the average American contracting an exotic infection are very low, emerging infections represent a challenge to all nations in the future.

WEST NILE VIRUS   A mini-outbreak of encephalitis in New York in 1999 led to identification of this virus, which had previously been restricted to Africa, the Middle East, and parts of Europe. Between 1999 and 2007, the virus spread across the United States and caused more than 27,605 illnesses and 1086 deaths. West Nile virus is carried by birds and then passed to humans when mosquitoes bite first an infected bird and then a person. Most people who are bitten have few or no symptoms, but the virus can cause permanent brain damage or death in some.

SEVERE ACUTE RESPIRATORY SYNDROME (SARS)   In February 2003, SARS appeared in southern China and quickly spread to more than 15 countries; it is a form of pneumonia that is fatal in about 5–15% of cases. SARS is caused by a new type of coronavirus found in wildlife that may have crossed the species barrier. It has reemerged several times since 2003, and by 2004 had been responsible for more than 8000 illnesses and 800 deaths.

ROTAVIRUS   The leading viral cause of gastroenteritis, an intestinal inflammation that results in vomiting and diarrhea, rotavirus infects almost every child at one time or another and kills about 600,000 children each year, mostly in developing countries. Left untreated, rotavirus-induced diarrhea can become severe and lead to dehydration, which can be fatal. Rotavirus spreads through poor hygiene and sanitation practices.

ESCHERICHIA COLI O157:H7   This potentially deadly strain of *E. coli*, transmitted in contaminated food, can cause bloody diarrhea and kidney damage. Outbreaks have been linked to contaminated spinach, lettuce, alfalfa sprouts, unpasteurized juice, petting zoos, and public swimming pools. An estimated 70,000 cases and 61 deaths occur in the United States each year.

HANTAVIRUS   Since first being recognized in 1993, over 300 cases of hantavirus pulmonary syndrome (HPS) have

been reported in the United States. HPS is caused by the rodentborne Sin Nombre virus (SNV) and is spread primarily through airborne viral particles from rodent urine, droppings, or saliva. It is characterized by a dangerous fluid buildup in the lungs and is fatal in about 45% of cases.

EBOLA   Human outbreaks of the often fatal Ebola hemorrhagic fever (EHF) have occurred only in Africa. The Ebola virus is transmitted by contact with infected blood or other body secretions. Because symptoms appear quickly and 70% of victims die, usually within a few days, the virus tends not to spread widely.

Factors Contributing to Emerging Infections   What's behind this rising tide of infectious diseases? One factor is drug resistance. New or increasing drug resistance has been found in organisms that cause malaria, tuberculosis, gonorrhea, influenza, AIDS, and pneumococcal and staphylococcal infections. Some bacterial strains now appear to be resistant to all available antibiotics.

Another factor is poverty. More than 1 billion people live in extreme poverty, and half the world's population have no regular access to essential drugs. Population growth, urbanization, overcrowding, and migration (including the movement of refugees) also spread infectious diseases.

> *Some bacterial strains now appear to be **resistant to all available antibiotics.***

A poor public health infrastructure is often associated with poverty and social upheaval, but problems such as contaminated water supplies can occur even in industrial countries. Natural disasters such as hurricanes also disrupt the public health infrastructure, leaving survivors with contaminated water and food supplies and no shelter from disease-carrying insects.

Travel, commerce, and food production and distribution practices also contribute, as do human behaviors. More than 500 million travelers cross national borders each year, and international tourism and trade open the world to infectious agents. SARS was quickly spread throughout the world by infected air travelers. Food now travels long distances to our table, and microbes are transmitted along with it. Mass production of food increases the likelihood that a chance contamination can lead to mass illness. The widespread use of injectable drugs rapidly transmits HIV infection and hepatitis. Changes in sexual behavior over the past 30 years have led to a proliferation of old and new STDs. The use of day-care facilities for children has led to increases in the incidence of several infections that cause diarrhea.

Finally, the deliberate release of deadly infectious agents is an ongoing concern. In 2001, infectious anthrax spores sent through the mail sickened 11 and killed 5 people in the United States. Potential bioterrorism agents that the CDC categorizes as a highest concern are those that can be easily disseminated or transmitted from person to person and that have a high mortality rate and the potential for a major public health impact; these include anthrax, smallpox, plague, botulism, and viral hemorrhagic fevers such as Ebola.

Other Immune Disorders: Cancer and Autoimmune Diseases

Sometimes, as in the case of cancer, the body comes under attack by its own cells. The immune system can often detect cells that have recently become cancerous and then destroy them just as it would a foreign microorganism. But if the immune system breaks down, the cancer cells may multiply out of control before the immune system recognizes the danger.

Another immune disorder occurs when the body confuses its own cells with foreign organisms. This is what happens in autoimmune diseases such as rheumatoid arthritis and systemic lupus erythematosus. In this type of malady, the immune system seems to be too sensitive and begins to misapprehend itself as nonself. For reasons not well understood, these conditions are much more common in women than in men.

SUPPORTING YOUR IMMUNE SYSTEM

Pathogens threaten everyone's wellness, but you can take steps to prevent them from compromising your health. Here are some general guidelines for keeping pathogens at bay:

- Eat a balanced diet and maintain a healthy weight.
- Get enough sleep. Most people need 6–8 hours every night.
- Exercise, but not when you're sick.
- Don't smoke.
- If you drink alcohol, do so only in moderation.
- Wash your hands frequently. Use hand sanitizer when soap and water aren't available.
- Avoid contact with people who are contagious with an infectious disease.
- Practice safer sex and don't inject drugs.
- Make sure you have received all your recommended vaccinations.

Ask Yourself

QUESTIONS FOR CRITICAL THINKING AND REFLECTION

Have you ever had any of the illnesses described in the preceding section? How were you exposed to the disease? Could you have taken any precautions to avoid it?

THE MAJOR STDS

Sexually transmitted diseases (STDs) are infectious diseases that are spread from person to person mainly through sexual activity. STDs are a particularly insidious group of illnesses because a person can be infected and able to transmit the disease, yet not look or feel sick; this is why the term *sexually transmitted infection (STI)* is often used synonymously with STD. The following seven STDs pose a major health threat:

- HIV/AIDS
- Gonorrhea
- Hepatitis
- Herpes
- Syphilis
- Human papillomavirus (HPV)
- Chlamydia

These diseases are considered major threats because they are serious in themselves, cause serious complications if left untreated, and pose risks to a fetus or newborn. STDs often result in long-term consequences, including chronic pain, infertility, stillbirths, genital cancers, and death.

The United States has the highest rate of STDs of any developed nation; at current rates, half of all young people will acquire an STD by age 25. A 2007 report from the Centers for Disease Control and Prevention (CDC) showed that many of the most common STDs are on the rise in the United States. In 2008, the CDC estimated that 65 million Americans were infected with an STD, and about 19 million Americans become newly infected with an STD each year.

HIV Infection and AIDS

The **human immunodeficiency virus (HIV)** causes **acquired immunodeficiency syndrome (AIDS),** a disease that without treatment ultimately kills nearly all of its victims. An estimated total of 65 million people have been infected since the HIV/AIDS epidemic began— nearly 1% of the world's population—and tens of millions of those people have died (see the box "HIV/AIDS Around the World"). Currently, about 33 million people are infected with HIV worldwide.

Many experts believe that the global HIV epidemic peaked in the late 1990s, at about 3.5 million new infections per year, compared with an estimated 2.7 million new infections in 2008. Despite a slowing of the

DIMENSIONS OF DIVERSITY

In 2011, the world marks the thirtieth year since AIDS was diagnosed in five young men in Los Angeles. HIV/AIDS is now a worldwide scourge, with 65 million people infected and more than 25 million deaths since the epidemic began.

The vast majority of cases–95%–have occurred in developing countries, where heterosexual contact is the primary means of transmission, responsible for 85% of all adult infections. In the developed world, HIV is increasingly becoming a disease that disproportionately affects the poor and ethnic minorities. Worldwide, women are the fastest-growing group of newly infected people; half of adults living with HIV in 2008 were women. Some 2.1 million children now live with HIV infection, and about 15 million children are AIDS orphans.

Despite the ongoing tragedy of the HIV epidemic, strides have been made in treatment and prevention measures. In 2003, only 7% of infected individuals were receiving antiretroviral treatment; by 2008, 42% of HIV-positive people received treatment. In 2008, 45% of pregnant women received treatment to prevent transmission of HIV to their babies, up from just 10% in 2004. Treating HIV with effective drugs not only prolongs life and decreases suffering but also has a major impact in reducing the spread of the virus, since treated individuals are generally much less infectious than untreated people.

The HIV epidemic seems to have stabilized in many parts of the world. Rates of new infections have remained steady or have even dropped in a few regions. Sub-Saharan Africa remains the hardest-hit area of the world, but even there the number of new infections dropped from 2.3 million in 2001 to 1.9 million in 2008. Despite gradual improvement, two-thirds of all HIV-infected people in the world live in Sub-Saharan Africa, and nearly three-quarters of all deaths due to AIDS in 2008 occurred there. However, treatment rates are up to 48% in eastern and southern Africa.

Eastern Europe and parts of Asia have also been hit hard by HIV. For example, former Soviet countries have seen a 50-fold increase in HIV infection in the last decade. In many of these areas, HIV infection was initially seen primarily in intravenous drug users, but in recent year sexual transmission has become much more common.

Efforts to combat AIDS are complicated by political, economic, and cultural barriers. Education and prevention programs are often hampered by resistance from social and religious institutions and by the taboo on openly discussing sexual issues. Condoms are not commonly used in many countries, and women in many societies do not have sufficient control over their lives to demand that men use condoms. Successful prevention approaches include STD treatment and education, public education campaigns about safer sex, and syringe exchange programs for injection drug users.

Empowering women is a crucial priority in reducing the spread of HIV. In particular, reducing sexual violence against women, allowing women property rights, and increasing women's access to education and employment are essential.

International efforts are under way to make condoms more available by lowering their price and to develop effective antiviral creams that women can use without the knowledge of their partners. Other potential strategies for fighting the spread of HIV include the widespread use of drugs to suppress genital herpes simplex, an extremely common STD that can dramatically increase transmission of HIV. Also, the practice of male circumcision might be useful in reducing the spread of HIV (and chlamydia, discussed later in this chapter). Recent research has shown a 60% reduction in HIV transmission among circumcised men compared with uncircumcised men, even when controlling for other factors.

In developed nations such as the United States, new drugs are easing AIDS symptoms and lowering viral levels

---

QUICK STATS

Worldwide, about
1 million
people acquire an STD (including HIV) every day.

—World Health Organization (WHO), 2008

TERMS

HIV infection   A chronic, progressive viral infection that damages the immune system.

CD4 T cell   A type of white blood cell that helps coordinate the activity of the immune system; the primary target for HIV infection.

epidemic, however, AIDS remains a primary cause of death in Africa and continues to be a major cause of mortality around the world. In the United States, about 1.1 million people have been infected with HIV and about 56,000 new HIV infections were reported in 2006. Nearly 560,000 Americans have died from AIDS since the start of the epidemic in 1981. Today, about 21% of HIV-infected Americans are unaware of their condition.

What Is HIV Infection?   **HIV infection** is a chronic disease that progressively damages the body's immune system, making an otherwise healthy person less able to resist a variety of infections and disorders. Normally, when a virus or other pathogen enters the body, it is targeted and destroyed by the immune system. But HIV attacks the immune system itself, invading and taking over **CD4 T cells** and other essential elements of the immune system. HIV enters a human cell and converts its own genetic material, RNA, into DNA. It then inserts this DNA into the chromosomes of the host cell. The viral DNA takes over the CD4 cell, causing it to produce new copies of HIV; it also makes the CD4 cell incapable of performing its immune functions.

dramatically for some patients. In the past few years, a growing number of people in poor countries have gained access to antiviral drugs because of the introduction of inexpensive generic drugs and increased international funding for HIV treatment. Still, far too many people with HIV remain untreated, and far too many new infections are occurring. As of 2008, for every two people starting treatment, another five people became newly infected with the virus.

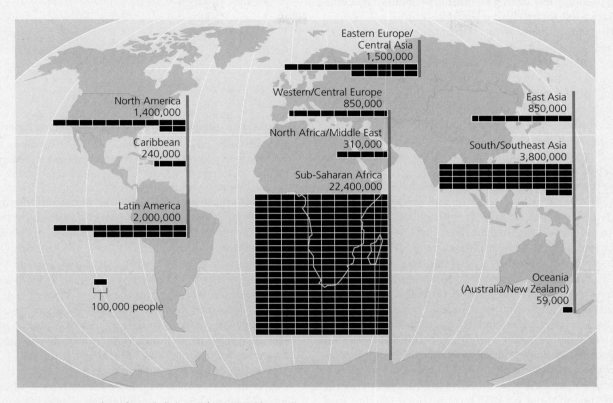

Approximate number of people living with HIV/AIDS in 2008.

SOURCE: Joint United Nations Programme on HIV/AIDS (UNAIDS). 2009. *AIDS Epidemic Update 2009*. Geneva: UNAIDS.

Immediately following infection with HIV, billions of infectious particles are produced every day. For a time, the immune system keeps pace, also producing billions of new cells. Unlike the virus, however, the immune system cannot make new cells indefinitely; as long as the virus keeps replicating, it wins in the end. The destruction of the immune system is signaled by the loss of CD4 T cells. As CD4 cells decline, an infected person may begin to experience mild to moderately severe symptoms. A person is diagnosed with full-blown AIDS when he or she develops one of the conditions defined as a marker for AIDS or when the number of CD4 cells in the blood drops below a certain level (200/µl). People with AIDS are vulnerable to a number of serious **opportunistic (secondary) infections.**

The first weeks after being infected with HIV are called the *primary infection* phase. People have large amounts of HIV in the bloodstream, making them much more infectious than they will be several months later when they enter the chronic infection stage.

The next phase of HIV infection is the chronic **asymptomatic** (symptom-free) stage, also called the *latency phase*. This period can last from 2 to 20 years, averaging 11 years in untreated adults. During this time, the virus progressively infects and destroys the cells of the immune system. People infected with HIV can transmit the disease to others, even if they are symptom-free.

Transmitting the Virus   HIV lives only within cells and body fluids, not outside the body. It is transmitted by blood and blood products, semen, vaginal and cervical secretions, and breast milk. It cannot live in air, in water, or on objects or surfaces such as toilet seats, eating utensils, or telephones. The three main routes of HIV transmission are (1) from specific kinds of sexual contact, (2) from direct exposure to infected blood, and (3) from an HIV-infected woman to her fetus during pregnancy or childbirth or to her infant during breastfeeding.

HIV is more likely to be transmitted by unprotected anal or vaginal intercourse than by other sexual activities. During vaginal intercourse, male-to-female transmission is more likely to occur than female-to-male transmission. HIV has been found in preejaculatory fluid, so transmission can occur before ejaculation. Being the receptive partner during unprotected anal intercourse is the riskiest of all sexual activities. Oral-genital contact carries some risk of transmission, although less than anal or vaginal intercourse.

The presence of lesions, blisters, or inflammation from other STDs in the genital, anal, or oral areas makes it two to nine times easier for the virus to be passed. Spermicides may also cause irritation and increase the risk of HIV transmission. Recent studies of the widely used spermicide nonoxynol-9 (N-9) found that frequent use may cause vaginal and rectal irritation, increasing the risk of transmission of HIV and other STDs. The risk of HIV transmission during oral sex increases if a person has poor oral hygiene, has oral sores, or has brushed or flossed just before or after oral sex. Studies have found that circumcised males have a lower risk of HIV infection than uncircumcised males.

Direct contact with the blood of an infected person is another major route of HIV transmission. Needles and syringes used to inject drugs (including heroin, cocaine, and anabolic steroids) are routinely contaminated by the blood of the user. Nearly 20% of all new U.S. cases of HIV are caused, directly or indirectly, by sharing drug injection equipment contaminated with HIV. HIV has also been transmitted in blood and blood products used in the medical treatment of injuries and illnesses, resulting in about 14,000 cases of AIDS in the United States. Nearly all of these cases occurred in the early days of the AIDS epidemic, before effective screening tests were available. All blood in licensed U.S. blood banks and plasma centers is now thoroughly screened for HIV.

The final major route of HIV transmission is mother-to-child, also called *vertical,* or *perinatal, transmission,* which can occur during pregnancy, childbirth, or breastfeeding. About 30–35% of infants born to untreated HIV-infected mothers are also infected with the virus; testing and treatment can dramatically lower this infection rate.

Populations of Special Concern for HIV Infection
Among Americans with AIDS, the most common means of HIV exposure is sexual activity between men; heterosexual contact and injection drug use (IDU) are the next most common (Figure 13.3). Although HIV transmission

* MSM = Men who have sex with men
IDU = Injection drug users

FIGURE 13.3 **Routes of HIV transmission among Americans.**

SOURCE: Centers for Disease Control and Prevention. 2009. *HIV/AIDS in the United States* (http://www.cdc.gov/hiv/resources/factsheets/us.htm; retrieved November 21, 2010).

occurs through specific individual behaviors, disproportionately high rates of infection in certain groups are tied to social, cultural, and economic factors. In 2008, the CDC estimated that 76% of HIV-positive Americans were men; the remaining 24% were women. HIV in the United States is increasingly becoming a disease that affects ethnic minorities, women, and the poor. Women, especially African American women and Latinas, make up an increasingly large proportion of all U.S. AIDS cases. Overall, African American men and women are vastly overrepresented among people newly diagnosed with AIDS.

Another group of people at increased risk for HIV infection are young men who have sex with men. There are probably several factors underlying this trend. Young gay men are less likely than older men to have experienced watching friends die from AIDS and thus are more removed from the reality of the disease. They may be less afraid of acquiring HIV because of advances in treatment and a false belief that a cure is just around the corner.

Another population of concern is men who

> Although **circumcision offers some protection against HIV in developing countries,** that is not the case in the United States.

have sex with men but still identify themselves as heterosexual. They are just as likely to be infected with HIV as are openly gay and bisexual men, but they are much less likely to know their HIV status and so may be more likely to transmit HIV to a male or female partner.

Symptoms of HIV Infection Within a few days or weeks (on average, 2 to 4 weeks after exposure to the virus) of infection with HIV, most people will develop symptoms of primary (also called acute) HIV infection. People who have engaged in behavior that places them at risk for HIV infection and who then experience such symptoms should immediately inform their physician of their risk status, so the proper tests can be performed. Standard tests for HIV will usually be negative in the very early stages of infection, so specialized blood tests such as the **HIV RNA assay,** which directly measures the amount of virus in the body, must be used. Immediate treatment is sometimes given to help preserve immune function, slow the progress of the disease, and reduce transmission of HIV to others.

Other than the initial flulike symptoms, most people in the first months or years of HIV infection have few if any symptoms. As the immune system weakens, however, a variety of symptoms can develop—persistent swollen lymph nodes; lumps, rashes, sores, or other growths on or under the skin or on the mucous membranes of the eyes, mouth, anus, or nasal passages; persistent yeast infections; unexplained weight loss; fever and drenching night sweats; dry cough and shortness of breath; persistent diarrhea; easy bruising and unexplained bleeding; profound fatigue; memory loss; difficulty with balance; tremors or seizures; changes in vision, hearing, taste, or smell; difficulty in swallowing; changes in mood and other psychological symptoms; and persistent or recurrent pain. Obviously, many of these symptoms can also occur with a variety of other illnesses.

People with HIV infection are highly susceptible to infections. The most common one in the United States is *Pneumocystis* pneumonia, a fungal infection. **Kaposi's sarcoma,** a previously rare form of cancer, is common in HIV-infected men. Women with HIV infection often have frequent and difficult-to-treat vaginal yeast infections. Cases of tuberculosis (TB) are increasingly being reported in people with HIV.

treatment. The immune system's status can be gauged by measuring CD4 T cells every few months. The infection itself can be monitored by tracking the amount of virus in the body through an HIV RNA assay. A new diagnostic test that may help guide treatment decisions is called HIV Replication Capacity. This test shows how fast HIV from a patient's blood sample can reproduce itself.

The CDC currently recommends universal HIV testing at least once as part of routine medical care for everyone age 13–64. People at greater risk should be tested periodically (see the box "Getting an HIV Test").

A diagnosis of AIDS is made if a person is HIV-positive and either has developed an infection defined as an AIDS indicator or has a severely damaged immune system (as measured by CD4 T-cell counts).

> *In many people, combination therapies can **reduce HIV in the blood to undetectable levels**.*

Treatment   Although there is no known cure for HIV infection, medications can significantly alter the course of the disease and extend life. The drop in the number of U.S. AIDS deaths that has occurred since 1996 is in large part due to the increasing use of combinations of new drugs.

ANTIVIRAL DRUGS   Antiviral drugs in current use to combat HIV fall into several categories based on how they block HIV replication. **Reverse transcriptase inhibitors,** including the widely used drug zidovudine (AZT), work

---

47% of Americans have been tested for HIV at least once in their life.

—Kaiser Family Foundation, 2009

Diagnosing HIV Infection   The most common HIV tests check for antibodies to the virus. **HIV antibody tests** are used because they are accurate and relatively inexpensive. Standard testing involves an initial test called an **ELISA;** if it is positive, a second test—either a **Western blot** or immunofluorescence assay—is done to confirm the results.

Babies born to HIV-infected mothers may carry HIV antibodies, passed from their mother, without being infected with HIV. Antibodies can pass through the placenta to a fetus, but in the majority of cases, even without treatment, an infant does not acquire HIV. Thus, an infant may test positive on an HIV antibody test but actually be uninfected. Further tests such as the HIV RNA assay must be done to determine if an infant is actually infected.

If a person is diagnosed as **HIV-positive,** the next step is to determine the disease's severity to plan appropriate

---

TERMS

HIV RNA assay   A test used to determine the viral load (the amount of HIV in the blood).

Pneumocystis **pneumonia**   A fungal infection common in people infected with HIV.

Kaposi's sarcoma   A form of cancer characterized by purple or brownish lesions that are generally painless and occur anywhere on the skin; usually appears in men infected with HIV.

HIV antibody test   A blood test to determine whether a person has been infected by HIV; becomes positive within weeks or months of exposure.

ELISA (enzyme-linked immunosorbent assay)   A blood test that detects the presence of antibodies to HIV.

Western blot   A blood test that detects the presence of HIV antibodies; a more accurate and more expensive test used to confirm positive results from an ELISA test.

HIV-positive   A diagnosis resulting from the presence of HIV in the bloodstream; also referred to as *seropositive*.

reverse transcriptase inhibitor   An antiviral drug used to treat HIV infection that works by inhibiting reverse transcriptase, the enzyme that converts viral RNA to DNA.

Getting an HIV Test

CRITICAL CONSUMER

You should strongly consider being tested if any of the following apply to you or any past or current sexual partners: You have had unprotected sex (vaginal, anal, or oral) with more than one partner or with a partner who was not in a mutually monogamous relationship with you; you have used or shared needles, syringes, or other paraphernalia for injecting drugs (including steroids); you received a transfusion of blood or blood products between 1978 and 1985; or you have ever been diagnosed with an STD.

You can either visit a physician or health clinic or take a home test. If the test is performed by a physician or clinician, you will get one-on-one counseling about the test and your results. The home test is a good alternative for people at low risk who just want to be sure.

Physician or Clinic Testing

Your physician, student health clinic, Planned Parenthood, public health department, or local AIDS association can arrange your HIV test. It usually costs $50–$100, but public clinics often charge little or nothing. The standard test involves drawing a sample of blood that is sent to a laboratory for analysis for the presence of antibodies; if the first stage of testing is positive, a confirmatory test is done. This standard test takes 1–2 weeks, and you'll be asked to phone or come in personally to obtain your results, which should also include appropriate counseling.

Alternative tests are available at some clinics. The Orasure test uses oral fluid, collected by placing a treated cotton pad in the mouth; urine tests are also available. New rapid tests are also available at some locations. These tests use blood or oral fluid and can provide results in as little as 20 minutes. If a rapid test is positive for HIV infection, a confirmatory test will be performed.

Before you get an HIV test, be sure you understand what will be done with the results. Results from confidential tests may still become part of your medical record and/or be

reported to state and federal public health agencies. If you decide you want to be tested anonymously, check with your physician or counselor about how to obtain an anonymous test or use a home test.

Home Testing

Home test kits for HIV are available; they cost about $40–$70. (Avoid testing kits that are not FDA-approved; unapproved kits are sold over the Internet. The only home test kit for HIV currently approved by the FDA is manufactured by Home Access.) To use a home test, you prick a finger with a supplied lancet, blot a few drops of blood onto blotting paper, and mail it to the company's laboratory. Anyone testing positive is routed to a trained counselor, who can provide emotional and medical support. The results of home test kits are anonymous.

Understanding the Results

A negative test result means that no antibodies were found in your sample. However, it usually takes at least a month after exposure to HIV (and possibly as long as 6 months in some people) for antibodies to appear. Therefore, an infected person may get a false-negative result. If you test negative but your risk of infection is high, ask about obtaining an HIV RNA assay, which allows very early diagnosis, and about the appropriateness of retesting in a few months.

A positive result means that you are infected. It is important to seek medical care and counseling immediately. You need to know more about your medical options; the possible psychological, social, and financial repercussions; and how to avoid spreading the disease. Rapid progress is being made in treating HIV, and treatments are potentially much more successful when begun early.

For more information about HIV testing and a national directory of testing sites, visit the CDC National HIV Testing Resources site (www.hivtest.org).

---

by inhibiting the enzyme reverse transcriptase, which HIV uses to integrate its genetic material into human cells. **Protease inhibitors** target the enzyme HIV protease, which the virus uses to create a protein coat for each

new copy of itself. **Entry inhibitors** block HIV from entering and infecting cells.

Treatment with combinations of drugs, referred to as *highly active antiretroviral therapy,* or *HAART,* can reduce HIV in the blood to undetectable levels in many people. However, latent virus is still present in the body, and HIV-infected people on HAART carry potentially transmissible HIV in their body fluids.

Antiviral medications are sometimes used to prevent infection in people who have been exposed to HIV, a practice called Postexposure Prophylaxis (PEP). PEP is recommended for health care workers with exposure to blood, victims of sexual assault, and people who are at

TERMS

protease inhibitor   A drug that inhibits the action of any of the protein-splitting enzymes known as proteases. Protease inhibitors have been developed to block the action of HIV protease and thus prevent the replication of HIV.

entry inhibitor   An antiviral drug that blocks the entry of HIV into cells by inhibiting the fusion of viral and cell membranes.

risk from recent unprotected sex or contact with a contaminated needle.

TREATMENTS FOR OPPORTUNISTIC INFECTIONS In addition to antiviral drugs, most patients with low CD4 T-cell counts also take a variety of antibiotics to help prevent opportunistic infections such as pneumonia and tuberculosis. A person with advanced HIV infection may need to take 20 or more pills daily.

HIV AND PREGNANCY Early-stage HIV infection does not appear to significantly affect a woman's chance of becoming pregnant. Without treatment, about one-third of infants born to HIV-infected women are themselves infected with the virus. The risk of an infected mother transmitting HIV to her baby can be reduced to less than 2% by treating the mother during her pregnancy and labor, giving the baby antiretroviral drugs during the first weeks of life, avoiding breastfeeding, and delivering the baby by cesarean section if necessary.

TREATMENT CHALLENGES The average cost of treatment for an HIV-infected person in the United States is $2100–$4000 per month. The 2010 U.S. federal budget included $26 billion in funding for HIV/AIDS. These costs are tremendous even for relatively wealthy countries, but 95% of people with HIV infection live in developing countries, where these treatments are unlikely to be available to anyone except the wealthiest few. Pharmaceutical companies and the World Bank are working to develop combination pills and to lower drug costs in developing regions. International aid is gradually increasing, but much more is needed.

Besides financial cost, receiving HIV treatment is challenging in many other ways. Common short-term side effects include nausea, vomiting, diarrhea, and fatigue. People on HIV drugs must take their medicines on time, every time, because drug resistance develops quickly if the medicines are taken inconsistently.

Patients who take antiretroviral medications for an extended period sometimes develop serious problems including abnormal blood lipids, heart disease, liver problems, bone loss, kidney disease, and cancers. Changes in body shape and facial appearance due to alterations in fat distribution are a common and troubling side effect of long-term antiretroviral drug use. Generally, people with HIV who have no symptoms and have relatively high CD4 counts may opt to delay treatment; however, immediate treatment is still recommended for anyone who is experiencing symptoms and for all pregnant women.

How Can You Protect Yourself?
Although AIDS is currently incurable, it is preventable. You can protect yourself by avoiding behaviors that may bring you into contact with HIV.

In a sexual relationship, the current and past behaviors of you and your partner determine the amount of risk

involved (Figure 13.4). If you are uninfected and in a mutually monogamous relationship with another uninfected person, you are not at risk for HIV.

People who inject drugs should avoid sharing needles, syringes, filters, or anything that might have blood on it. Any injectable drug, legal or illegal, can be associated with HIV transmission. Needles can be decontaminated with a solution of bleach and water, but it is not a foolproof procedure, and HIV can survive in a syringe for a month or longer. (Boiling needles and syringes does not necessarily destroy HIV either.) For more guidelines and tips, see the box "Preventing STD Infection."

High Risk

Unprotected anal sex is the riskiest sexual behavior, especially for the receptive partner.

Unprotected vaginal intercourse is the next riskiest, especially for women, who are much more likely to be infected by an infected male partner than vice versa.

Oral sex is probably considerably less risky than anal and vaginal intercourse but can still result in HIV transmission.

Sharing of sex toys can be risky because they can carry blood, semen, or vaginal fluid.

Use of a condom reduces risk considerably but not completely for any type of intercourse. Anal sex with a condom is riskier than vaginal sex with a condom; oral sex with a condom is less risky, especially if the man does not ejaculate.

Hand-genital contact and deep kissing are less risky but could still theoretically transmit HIV; the presence of cuts or sores increases risk.

Sex with only one uninfected and totally faithful partner is without risk, but effective only if both partners are uninfected and completely monogamous.

Activities that don't involve the exchange of body fluids carry no risk: hugging, massage, closed-mouth kissing, masturbation, phone sex, and fantasy.

Abstinence is completely without risk. For many people, it can be an effective and reasonable method of avoiding HIV infection and other STDs during certain periods of life.

No Risk

FIGURE 13.4 What's risky and what's not: The approximate relative risk of HIV transmission of various sexual activities.

One-third of surveyed HIV-positive people said they did not reveal their infection to their sexual partners.

—CDC, 2006

QUICK STATS

Preventing STD Infection

For those who aren't in a long-term monogamous relationship with an uninfected partner, abstinence is the only truly safe option for avoiding STDs.

If you are sexually active, talk with potential partners about HIV, safer sex, and condom use before you begin a sexual relationship. The following guidelines can also help you avoid infection:

● Don't drink alcohol or use drugs in sexual situations. Mood-altering drugs can affect your judgment and make you more likely to take risks.

● Limit the number of partners. Avoid sexual contact with people who have HIV or an STD or who have engaged in risky behaviors.

● Use condoms during every act of intercourse and oral sex. Condoms do not provide perfect protection, but they provide a high level of protection against HIV and greatly reduce your risk of contracting most STDs.

● Use condoms properly to obtain maximum protection.

● Use latex squares or dental dams during oral-genital or oral-anal contact.

● Avoid sexual contact that could cause cuts or tears in the skin or tissue.

● Get periodic screening tests for STDs and HIV. Sexually active young women need yearly pelvic exams and chlamydia screening. A Pap test should be done on all young women at age 21 and then every two years after that.

● Get vaccinated for hepatitis B. Young women should consider getting vaccinated against HPV.

● Get prompt treatment for any STDs you contract. Make sure your partner gets treated, too. Don't have sex until both of you have completed your treatment.

If you inject drugs of any kind, don't share needles, syringes, or anything that might have blood on it. If your community has a syringe exchange program, use it. Seek treatment.

If you are at risk for HIV infection, don't donate blood, sperm, or body organs. Get tested for HIV soon, and get treated. HIV-infected people who get early treatment generally feel better and live longer than those who delay.

Condom use reduces the risk of transmitting HIV during all forms of intercourse.

Chlamydia

Chlamydia trachomatis causes **chlamydia,** the most prevalent bacterial STD in the United States. The highest rates of infection occur in single people between ages 15 and 24. Both men and women are susceptible to chlamydia, but, as with most STDs, women bear the greater burden because of possible complications and consequences of the disease (see the box "Women Are Hit Hard by STDs"). *C. trachomatis* can be transmitted by oral and anal sex as well as by other forms of sexual intercourse. Having a chlamydia infection increases the risk of HIV transmission. In most women, chlamydia produces no early symptoms. If left untreated, it can lead to pelvic inflammatory disease (PID), which is discussed later in this chapter. Chlamydia also greatly increases a woman's risk for infertility and ectopic (tubal) pregnancy. The U.S. Preventive Services Task Force currently recommends annual chlamydia testing for all sexually active women age

25 or younger and for older women who are at increased risk (such as those who have multiple sex partners). Women who have a new sexual partner should consider being tested more often than once a year.

Chlamydia can also lead to infertility in men, although not as often as in women. In men under age 35, chlamydia is the most common cause of epididymitis, inflammation of the sperm-carrying ducts. And up to half of all cases of **urethritis,** inflammation of the urethra, in men are caused by chlamydia. Despite these statistics, many infected men have no symptoms.

Infants of infected mothers can acquire the infection through contact with the pathogen in the birth canal during delivery. Every year, over 150,000 newborns suffer from eye infections and pneumonia as a result of untreated maternal chlamydial infections.

Symptoms In men, chlamydia symptoms include painful urination, a slight watery discharge from the penis, and sometimes pain around the testicles. Although most women with chlamydia are asymptomatic, some notice increased vaginal discharge, burning with urination, pain or bleeding with intercourse, and lower abdominal pain. Symptoms in both men and women can begin within 5 days of infection. However, most people experience few or no symptoms, increasing the likelihood that they will inadvertently spread the infection to their partners.

Diagnosis and Treatment Chlamydia is typically diagnosed through laboratory tests on a urine sample or a

---

chlamydia An STD transmitted by the pathogenic bacterium *Chlamydia trachomatis.*

urethritis Inflammation of the tube that carries urine from the bladder to the outside opening.

Women Are Hit Hard by STDs

Sexually transmitted diseases cause suffering for all who are infected, but in many ways, women and girls are the hardest hit, for both biological and social reasons. Among Americans, 62% of all cases of adverse health problems from STDs occur in women. Worldwide, as many women as men now die from AIDS each year.

Male-to-female transmission of many infections is more likely to occur than female-to-male transmission. This is particularly true of HIV: Studies show that it is three to eight times easier for an HIV-positive man to transmit the virus to a woman than it is for an HIV-positive woman to infect a man.

Teenagers have been hit especially hard, and 26% of American girls age 14–19 are infected with at least one of the most common STDs. Young women are also more vulnerable to STDs for social and emotional reasons: Lack of control in relationships, fear of discussing condom use, and having an older sex partner are all linked to increased STD risk. In some cases, women who refuse sex or demand condom use become the victims of physical and sexual assault.

Once infected, women tend to suffer more consequences of STDs than men. For example, gonorrhea and chlamydia can cause PID and permanent damage to the oviducts in women, but these infections tend to have less serious effects in men. HPV infection causes nearly all cases of cervical cancer. HPV infection is also associated with penile cancer, which is much less common than cervical cancer. Women also have the added concern of the potential effects of STDs during pregnancy.

Between 1985 and 2005, the proportion of new U.S. AIDS cases in women increased from 5% to 27%. Women may become sicker at lower viral loads compared with men. Women and men with HIV do about equally well if they have similar access to treatment, but in many cases women are diagnosed later in the course of HIV infection, receive less treatment, and die sooner.

Worldwide, social and economic factors play a large role in the transmission and consequences of AIDS and other STDs for women. Sexual violence against women is spreading AIDS, as are such practices as very early marriage for girls, often to much older men who have had many sexual partners. Cultural gender norms that promote premarital and extramarital relationships for men, combined with women's lack of power to negotiate safer sex, make HIV a risk even for women who are married and monogamous. In addition, lack of education and economic opportunities can force women into commercial sex work, placing them at high risk for all STDs.

SOURCES: AVERT. 2010. *Women, HIV, and AIDS* (http://www.avert.org/women-hiv-aids.htm; retrieved June 9, 2010); Dunkle, K. M., et al. 2004. Gender-based violence, relationship power, and risk of HIV infection in women attending antenatal clinics in South Africa. *Lancet* 363(9419): 1415–1421; Ebrahim, S. H., M. T. McKenna, and J. S. Marks. 2005. Sexual behaviour: Related adverse health burden in the United States. *Sexually Transmitted Infection* 81(1): 38–40; World Health Organization. 2003. *Gender and HIV/AIDS.* Geneva: World Health Organization.

---

small amount of fluid from the urethra or cervix. Once chlamydia has been diagnosed, the infected person and his or her partner(s) are given antibiotics. Studies show that younger women were more likely than older women to be reinfected by an untreated, infected partner.

When it is unlikely that a partner of someone being treated for chlamydia will also be treated, the CDC recommends that an extra prescription for antibiotics be given to the patient to give to his or her partner. This strategy, called *expedited partner therapy,* is legal and encouraged when sexual partners are unlikely to seek medical help on their own.

Gonorrhea

More than 330,000 cases of **gonorrhea** were reported to the CDC in 2008. The highest incidence is among 15–24-year-olds. Like chlamydia, untreated gonorrhea can cause PID in women and urethritis and epididymitis in men. It can also cause arthritis, rashes, and eye infections, and it occasionally involves internal organs. A woman who is infected during pregnancy is at risk for preterm delivery and for having a baby with life-threatening gonorrheal infection of the blood or joints. An infant passing through the birth canal of an infected mother may contract **gonococcal conjunctivitis,** an infection in the eyes that can cause blindness if not treated.

Symptoms In males, the incubation period for gonorrhea is brief, generally 2–7 days. The first symptoms are due to urethritis, which causes urinary discomfort and a thick, yellowish white or yellowish green discharge from the penis. The lips of the urethral opening may become inflamed and swollen. In some cases, the lymph glands in the groin become enlarged and swollen. Up to half of males have very minor symptoms or none at all.

Most females with gonorrhea are asymptomatic. Those who do have symptoms often experience pain with urination, increased vaginal discharge, and severe menstrual cramps. Up to 40% of women with untreated gonorrhea

> **QUICK STATS**
>
> In the United States, rates of gonorrhea dropped **5.4%** from 2007 to 2008.
>
> —CDC, 2009

gonorrhea A sexually transmitted bacterial infection that usually affects mucous membranes.

gonococcal conjunctivitis An inflammation of the mucous membrane lining of the eyelids, caused by the gonococcus bacterium.

TERMS

develop PID. Gonorrhea can also infect the throat or rectum of people who engage in oral or anal sex.

Diagnosis and Treatment   Gonorrhea is detectable through several tests; depending on the test, samples of urine or cervical, urethral, throat, or rectal fluids may be collected. Gonorrhea is curable with antibiotics, but increasing drug resistance is a major concern. Today only one class of antibiotics, the cephalosporins, remains consistently effective against gonorrhea.

Pelvic Inflammatory Disease

Pelvic inflammatory disease (PID) is a major complication in 10–40% of women who have been infected with either gonorrhea or chlamydia and have not received adequate treatment. PID occurs when the initial infection with gonorrhea and/or chlamydia travels upward into the uterus, oviducts, ovaries, and pelvic cavity. PID is occasionally caused by non-sexually transmitted bacteria, but in most cases is related to a sexually transmitted infection. PID is often serious enough to require hospitalization and sometimes surgery. Even if the disease is treated successfully, about 25% of affected women will have long-term problems such as a continuing susceptibility to infection, ectopic pregnancy, infertility, and chronic pelvic pain. PID is the leading cause of infertility in young women.

Women under age 25 are much more likely to develop PID than are older women. As with all STDs, the more sex partners a woman has had, the greater her risk of PID. Smokers have twice the risk of PID as nonsmokers. Using IUDs for contraception also increases the risk of PID, although this risk is greatly reduced for women with only one uninfected sexual partner.

Symptoms   Some women, especially those with chlamydia, may be asymptomatic; others may feel very ill with abdominal pain, fever, chills, nausea, and vomiting. Early symptoms are essentially the same as those described earlier for chlamydia and gonorrhea. Symptoms often begin or worsen during or soon after a woman's menstrual period. Many women have abnormal vaginal bleeding—either bleeding between periods or heavy and painful menstrual bleeding.

Diagnosis and Treatment   Diagnosis of PID is made on the basis of symptoms, physical examination, ultrasound, and laboratory tests. Laparoscopy may be used to confirm the diagnosis and obtain material for cultures. Antibiotics are usually started immediately; in severe cases, the woman may be hospitalized and antibiotics given intravenously. It is especially important that an infected woman's partners be treated. As many as 60% of the male contacts of women with PID are infected but asymptomatic.

Human Papillomavirus

Human papillomavirus (HPV) infection is the most common STD in the United States. HPV infection causes a variety of human diseases, including common warts, **genital warts,** and genital cancers. HPV is the cause of virtually all cervical cancer, but HPV also causes penile cancer and some forms of anal and oropharyngeal cancers (the oropharynx includes the back of the mouth and the throat). Genital HPV is usually spread from one person to another through sexual activity, including oral sex. HPV is especially common in young people, with some of the highest rates of infection among college students. Many young women contract HPV infection within 3 months of becoming sexually active.

*Although **80% of sexually active people become infected with HPV by age 50,** most show no symptoms at all.*

Genital HPV infection is quite contagious. Condoms and other barrier methods can help prevent the transmission of HPV, but HPV infection frequently occurs in areas where condoms are not fully protective. These areas are the labia in women, the base of the penis and the scrotum in men, and around the anus in both men and women.

Two vaccines for HPV have FDA approval: Gardasil and Cervarix. Gardasil protects against four types of HPV virus that together account for 90% of genital warts and 70% of cervical cancers; the drug has also been shown to prevent cancers of the vagina and vulva. Cervarix does not protect against genital warts but may be more effective in protecting against cervical cancer. Vaccination is available for girls and women age 9–26. The CDC recommends the vaccine for all girls between the ages of 11 and 12 because the vaccine is most effective before the onset of sexual activity. Gardasil is also approved for boys and men. For more on HPV, see Chapter 12.

QUICK STATS

The annual direct medical cost of STDs is $15.9 billion.

—CDC, 2009

TERMS

pelvic inflammatory disease (PID)   An infection that progresses from the vagina and cervix to the uterus, oviducts, and pelvic cavity.

human papillomavirus (HPV)   The pathogen that causes human warts, including genital warts.

genital warts   A sexually transmitted viral infection characterized by growths on the genitals; also called *genital HPV infection* or *condyloma.*

Symptoms HPV-infected tissue often appears normal; it may also look like anything from a small bump on the skin to a large, warty growth. Depending on location and size, genital warts are sometimes painful. Untreated warts can grow together to form a cauliflower-like mass. In males, they appear on the penis and often involve the urethra, appearing first at the opening and then spreading inside. The growths may cause irritation and bleeding, leading to painful urination and a urethral discharge. Warts may also appear around the anus or within the rectum. In women, warts may appear on the labia or vulva and may spread to the perineum, the area between the vagina and the rectum, and on the cervix.

The incubation period ranges from 1 month to 2 years from the time of contact. People can be infected with the virus and be capable of transmitting it to their sex partners without having any symptoms at all. The vast majority of people with HPV infection have no visible warts or symptoms of any kind.

Diagnosis and Treatment Genital warts are usually diagnosed based on the appearance of the lesions. HPV infection of the cervix is often detected on routine Pap tests. Special tests are now available to detect the presence of HPV infection and to distinguish among the more common strains of HPV, including those that cause most cases of cervical cancer.

Treatment focuses on reducing the number and size of warts. The currently available treatments do not eradicate HPV infection. Warts may be removed by cryosurgery (freezing), electrocautery (burning), or laser surgery. Direct applications of podophyllin or other cytotoxic acids may be used, and there are treatments that patients can use at home. Warts are more likely to persist and become severe in people with an impaired immune system.

Even after treatment and the disappearance of visible warts, the individual may continue to carry HPV in healthy-looking tissue and can probably still infect others. Cervical HPV infection will often clear on its own, but women need to follow their health practitioners' advice on repeat testing, examination, and treatment. Cervical abnormalities that are cancerous or precancerous are treated surgically or with other techniques such as electrical excision, freezing, and laser, Oropharyngeal cancers are treated with surgery, radiation, and other methods. Anyone who has ever had HPV infection should inform all partners and use condoms, even though they do not provide total protection. Whether or not they have had the vaccine, all women should have regular pelvic exams and Pap tests.

Genital Herpes

About one in five adults in the United States has **genital herpes.** Worldwide, genital herpes is extremely common and is a major factor in the transmission of HIV. Two types of herpes simplex viruses, HSV 1 and HSV 2, cause genital

herpes and oral-labial herpes (cold sores). Genital herpes is usually caused by HSV 2, and oral-labial herpes is caused by HSV 2 or HSV 1, although both virus types can cause either genital or oral-labial lesions. Many people wrongly assume that they are unlikely to pick up an STD if they limit their sexual activity to oral sex, but this is not true, particularly in the case of genital herpes. Oral sex is a very common way of acquiring herpes infection, particularly among young people. HSV can also cause rectal lesions, usually transmitted through anal sex. Infection with HSV is generally lifelong; after infection, the virus lies dormant in nerve cells and can reactivate at any time.

HSV 1 infection is so common that 50–80% of U.S. adults have antibodies to HSV 1 (indicating previous exposure to the virus); most were exposed to HSV 1 during childhood. HSV 2 infection usually occurs during adolescence and early adulthood.

HSV 2 is almost always sexually transmitted. The infection is more easily transmitted when people have active sores, but HSV 2 can be transmitted to a sex partner even when no obvious lesions are present. Because HSV is asymptomatic in 80–90% of people, the infection is often acquired from a person who does not know that he or she is infected. If you have ever had an outbreak of genital herpes, you should consider yourself always contagious and inform your partners. Avoid intimate contact when any sores are present, and use condoms during all sexual contact. A recent study showed that using condoms for every act of intercourse results in a 30% decrease in the transmission of herpes compared with no condom use. Condoms are more effective in preventing the transmission of other STDs than for herpes, but this study shows that they can make a significant difference in preventing the spread of genital herpes.

Newborns can occasionally be infected with HSV, usually during passage through the birth canal of an infected mother or due to HSV infection acquired by the mother during the third trimester of pregnancy. Without treatment, 65% of newborns with HSV will die, and most who survive will have some degree of brain damage. The risk is low (less than 1%) in women with long-standing herpes infection.

Symptoms Up to 90% of people who are infected with HSV have no symptoms. Those who do develop symptoms

genital herpes A sexually transmitted infection caused by the herpes simplex virus.

TERMS

Stress and Genital Herpes

Patients and health care workers alike have long suspected that stress and genital herpes outbreaks are related. A recent study of women with genital herpes found that persistent stressors (those lasting more than a week) and persistent high levels of anxiety were associated with increased outbreaks. Short-term stress, mood changes, and brief negative life experiences did not influence the rate of herpes outbreaks.

Experts suspect that stress has a negative impact on the immune system.

Studies have shown that immune function and antibody levels may drop in response to psychological stress. Perhaps herpes viruses that are usually dormant in nervous system tissue become activated when immune function declines due to stress.

The next step is to investigate whether stress-reduction techniques such as meditation or exercise result in reduced rates of herpes outbreaks. Until such research becomes available, it makes sense for people who suffer recurrent genital

herpes outbreaks to do what they can to reduce stress, especially long-term stress and anxiety. If you have herpes, joining a support group may help reduce your stress and improve your ability to cope with this chronic disease. Keep in mind that regardless of stress level, genital herpes outbreaks naturally tend to become less and less frequent over time. Knowing that your outbreaks are likely to diminish can, in and of itself, help reduce your feelings of stress.

---

often first notice them within 2–20 days of having sex with an infected partner. (However, it is not unusual for the first outbreak to occur months or even years after initial exposure.) The first episode of genital herpes frequently causes flulike symptoms in addition to genital lesions. The lesions tend to be painful or itchy and can occur anywhere on the genitals, inner thighs, or anal area. Depending on their location, they can cause considerable pain with urination. Lymph nodes in the groin may become swollen and tender. The sores usually heal within 3 weeks. On average, newly diagnosed people will experience five to eight outbreaks per year, with a decrease in the frequency of outbreaks over time. Genital herpes due to HSV 2 tends to recur more frequently and have more severe symptoms than infection due to HSV 1. Recurrent episodes are usually less severe than the initial one, with fewer and less painful sores that heal more quickly. Outbreaks can be triggered by stress, illness, fatigue, sun exposure, sexual intercourse, and menstruation (see the box "Stress and Genital Herpes").

Diagnosis and Treatment Genital herpes is sometimes diagnosed on the basis of symptoms and physical examination, but laboratory testing is helpful if there is any question about the diagnosis. There are also several blood tests that can detect the presence of HSV antibodies.

There is no cure for herpes. Once infected, a person carries the virus for life. Antiviral drugs such as acyclovir can be taken at the beginning of an outbreak to shorten the severity and duration of symptoms. People who have frequent outbreaks can take acyclovir or similar drugs daily to suppress outbreaks and decrease viral shedding between outbreaks. A person on suppressive therapy can

still transmit HSV to an uninfected partner, but the risk is probably reduced by about half. Using condoms consistently and taking suppressive medication are reasonable ways to reduce the risk of passing herpes to an uninfected sexual partner. It is always important to inform a sexual partner if you have genital herpes. Herpes vaccines are in development.

Hepatitis B

Hepatitis (inflammation of the liver) can cause serious and sometimes permanent damage to the liver. One of the many types of hepatitis is caused by hepatitis B virus (HBV). HBV is somewhat similar to HIV; it is found in most body fluids of an infected person, and it can be transmitted sexually, by injection drug use, and during pregnancy and delivery. However, HBV is much more contagious than HIV, and it can also be spread through nonsexual close contact. Hepatitis B is a potentially fatal disease with no cure, but fortunately there is an effective vaccine. Vaccination is recommended for everyone under age 19 and for all adults at increased risk for hepatitis B, including people who have more than one sex partner in 6 months, men who have sex with other men, those who inject illegal drugs, and health care workers who are exposed to blood and body fluids.

Other forms of viral hepatitis can also be sexually transmitted. Hepatitis A is of particular concern for people who engage in anal sex; a vaccine is available and is recommended for all people at risk. Less commonly, hepatitis C can be transmitted sexually. Experts believe that traumatic sexual activity that causes tissue damage is most likely to transmit HCV.

Transmission HBV is easily transmitted through any sexual activity that involves the exchange of body fluids, the use of contaminated needles, and any blood-to-blood contact, including the use of contaminated razor blades, toothbrushes, and eating utensils. The primary risk factors for acquiring HBV are sexual exposure and injection drug

TERMS **hepatitis** Inflammation of the liver, which can be caused by infection, drugs, or toxins; some forms of infectious hepatitis can be transmitted sexually.

use; having multiple partners greatly increases risk. A pregnant woman can transmit HBV to her unborn child.

Symptoms Many people infected with HBV never develop symptoms; they have what are known as silent infections. Mild cases of hepatitis can cause flulike symptoms such as fever, body aches, chills, and loss of appetite. As the illness progresses, there may be nausea, vomiting, dark-colored urine, abdominal pain, and jaundice.

Most adults who have acute hepatitis B recover completely, but they can become chronic carriers of the virus, capable of infecting others for the rest of their life. Some chronic carriers remain asymptomatic, while others develop chronic liver disease. Chronic hepatitis can cause cirrhosis of the liver, liver failure, and a deadly form of liver cancer.

Diagnosis and Treatment Blood tests can diagnose hepatitis by analyzing liver function, detecting the infecting organism, and detecting antibodies to the virus. There is no cure for hepatitis B and no specific treatment for acute infections; antiviral drugs and immune system modulators may be used for cases of chronic HBV infection.

Syphilis

Syphilis, a disease that once caused death and disability for millions, can now be effectively treated with antibiotics. The number of new cases in the United States hit an all-time low in 2000 but has been on the rise since then. Studies have found an association between syphilis infection and the use of the Internet as a means to meet sex partners among men who have sex with men. Another recent trend is an increase in the proportion of cases of syphilis from oral sex.

Syphilis is caused by a spirochete called *Treponema pallidum,* a thin, corkscrew-shaped bacterium. The disease is usually acquired through sexual contact, although infected pregnant women can transmit it to the fetus. The pathogen passes through any break or opening in the skin or mucous membranes and can be transmitted by kissing, vaginal or anal intercourse, or oral-genital contact.

Symptoms Syphilis progresses through several stages. *Primary syphilis* is characterized by an ulcer called a **chancre** that appears within 10–90 days after exposure. Chancres contain large numbers of bacteria and make the disease highly contagious when present; they are often painless and typically heal on their own within a few weeks. If the disease is not treated during the primary stage, about a third of infected individuals progress to chronic stages of infections.

Secondary syphilis is usually marked by mild, flulike symptoms and a skin rash that appears 3–6 weeks after the chancre. The rash may cover the entire body or only a few areas, but the palms of the hands and soles of the feet are usually involved. Areas of skin affected by the rash are

highly contagious but usually heal within several weeks or months. If the disease remains untreated, the symptoms of secondary syphilis may recur over a period of several years; affected individuals may then lapse into an asymptomatic latent stage in which they experience no further consequences of infection. However, in about one-third of cases of untreated secondary syphilis, the individual develops *late,* or *tertiary, syphilis.* Late syphilis can damage many organs of the body, possibly causing severe dementia, cardiovascular damage, blindness, and death.

In infected pregnant women who aren't treated, the probable result is stillbirth, prematurity, or congenital deformity. In many cases, the infant is also born infected (*congenital syphilis*) and requires treatment.

Diagnosis and Treatment Syphilis is diagnosed by examination of infected tissues and with blood tests. All stages can be treated with antibiotics, but damage from late syphilis can be permanent.

Other STDs

Trichomoniasis (often called *trich*) is the most common curable STD among young women. The single-celled organism that causes trich, *Trichomonas vaginalis,* thrives in warm, moist conditions, making women particularly susceptible to these infections in the vagina. Women who become symptomatic with trich develop a greenish, foul-smelling vaginal discharge and severe itching and pain in the vagina. Men usually have no symptoms, but they may have mild irritation after urinating or a slight discharge. Prompt treatment with metronidazole (Flagyl) is important because studies suggest that trich may increase the risk of HIV transmission and, in pregnant women, premature delivery.

syphilis A sexually transmitted bacterial infection caused by the spirochete *Treponema pallidum*.

chancre The sore produced by syphilis in its earliest stage.

trichomoniasis A protozoal infection caused by *Trichomonas vaginalis,* transmitted sexually and externally.

TERMS

Bacterial vaginosis (BV) is the most common cause of abnormal vaginal discharge in women of reproductive age. BV occurs when healthy bacteria that normally inhabit the vagina become displaced by unhealthy species. BV is usually, but not always, associated with sexual activity and often occurs after a change in partners. Symptoms of BV include vaginal discharge with a fishy odor and sometimes vaginal irritation. BV is treated with topical and oral antibiotics.

Pubic lice (commonly known as *crabs*) and **scabies** are highly contagious parasitic infections. Treatment has traditionally been with topical medicines, but in cases where this is ineffective, an oral prescription medicine, called ivermectin, is sometimes used.

Accurate information about HIV/AIDS, including where to go for testing and treatment, is available from health professionals, college clinics, community-based organizations, national hotlines, and many other sources.

WHAT YOU CAN DO

You can take responsibility for your health and contribute to a general reduction in the incidence of STDs in three major areas: education, diagnosis and treatment, and prevention.

Education

Educational campaigns about HIV/AIDS have paid off in changing attitudes and sexual behaviors. Levels of awareness about HIV infection among the general population are quite high, although some segments of the population are harder to reach and continue to engage in very high-risk behaviors. Learning about STDs is still up to every person individually, as is applying that knowledge to personal situations.

Diagnosis and Treatment

Early diagnosis and treatment of STDs can help you and your sex partner(s) avoid unnecessary complications and help prevent the spread of STDs.

Get Vaccinated   Every young, sexually active person should be vaccinated for hepatitis B; vaccines are available for all age groups. Men who have sex with men should be vaccinated for hepatitis A, and girls and women age 9–26 should be vaccinated for HPV.

Be Alert for Symptoms   If you are sexually active, be alert for any sign or symptom of disease, such as a rash, a discharge, sores, or unusual pain, and have a professional examination if you notice such a symptom.

Get Tested   Remember that almost all STDs—including HIV infection—can be completely asymptomatic for long periods of time. The CDC recommends that everyone between the ages of 13 and 64 be tested for HIV at least once during routine medical care. Sexually active young women should have pelvic exams and Pap tests at least once a year, with chlamydia and gonorrhea screening in most cases. Sexually active men, especially if they have had more than one partner, should have periodic STD screenings.

Inform Your Partners   Telling a partner that you have exposed him or her to an STD isn't easy. Despite the awkwardness and difficulty, it is crucial that your sex partner or partners be informed and urged to seek testing and/or treatment as quickly as possible.

Get Treated   With the exception of AIDS treatments, treatments for STDs are safe and generally inexpensive. If you are being treated, follow instructions carefully and complete all the medication as prescribed. Don't stop taking the medication just because you feel better or your symptoms have disappeared.

Prevention

If you choose to be sexually active, think about prevention *before* you have a sexual encounter, and plan accordingly. By thinking and talking about responsible sexual behavior, you are expressing a sense of caring for yourself, your potential partner, and your future children.

Connect to your Choices

Have you ever thought about where you get your behaviors and habits related to infectious diseases and STDs? Many factors can influence our behaviors and habits, some not as obvious as others. Was your family conscientious about making sure you got all the recommended vaccinations when you were growing up? Did you have comprehensive sex education in high school? Do the significant people in your peer group use condoms and practice safer sex? Does your campus health clinic conduct public health campaigns about flu shots and HIV/AIDS awareness?

What are the external factors that influence your choices about infectious diseases and STDs? What are your inner motivations and core values, and how do they affect your choices? Based on what you learned in this chapter, will you make some different choices in the future? If so, what will they be?

Go online to Connect to complete this activity.
www.mcgraw-hillconnect.com

TIPS FOR TODAY AND THE FUTURE

Your immune system is a remarkable germ-fighting network, but it needs your help to work at its best.

RIGHT NOW YOU CAN

- Move your bedtime up 15 minutes, starting tonight, to ensure that you're getting enough sleep.
- Make an appointment with your health care provider if you are worried about possible STD infection.
- Resolve to discuss condom use with your partner if you are sexually active and are not already using condoms.

IN THE FUTURE YOU CAN

- Learn how to communicate effectively with a partner who resists safer sex practices or is reluctant to discuss his or her sexual history. Support groups and educational classes can help.
- Make sure all your vaccinations are up-to-date; ask your doctor if you should be vaccinated against hepatitis A or B, HPV, or any other STDs.

SUMMARY

- The step-by-step process by which infections are transmitted from one person to another involves a pathogen, its reservoir, a portal of exit, a means of transmission, a portal of entry, and a new host.

- The immune response is carried out by white blood cells that are continuously produced in the bone marrow. It has four stages: recognition of the invading pathogen; rapid replication of killer T cells and B cells; attack by killer T cells and macrophages; and suppression of the immune response.

- Immunization is based on the body's ability to remember previously encountered organisms and retain its strength against them.

- Allergic reactions occur when the immune system responds to harmless substances as if they were dangerous antigens.

- Bacteria are single-celled organisms; some cause disease in humans. Bacterial infections include pneumonia, meningitis, strep throat, toxic shock syndrome, tuberculosis, Lyme disease, and ulcers.

- Viruses cannot grow or reproduce themselves; different viruses cause the common cold, influenza, measles, mumps, rubella, chicken pox, cold sores, mononucleosis, encephalitis, hepatitis, polio, and warts.

- Other diseases are caused by certain types of fungi, protozoa, parasitic worms, and prions.

- Autoimmune diseases occur when the body identifies its own cells as foreign.

- HIV affects the immune system, making an otherwise healthy person less able to resist a variety of infections.

- HIV is carried in blood and blood products, semen, vaginal and cervical secretions, and breast milk. HIV is transmitted through the exchange of these fluids.

- There is currently no cure or vaccine for HIV infection. Drugs have been developed to slow the course of the disease and to prevent or treat certain secondary infections.

- Chlamydia causes epididymitis and urethritis in men; in women, it can lead to PID and infertility if untreated.

- Pelvic inflammatory disease (PID), usually a complication of untreated gonorrhea or chlamydia, is an infection of the uterus and oviducts that may extend to the ovaries and pelvic cavity. It can lead to infertility, ectopic pregnancy, and chronic pelvic pain.

- Human papillomavirus (HPV) causes genital warts and cervical cancer. Treatment does not eradicate the virus, which can be passed on by asymptomatic people.

- Genital herpes is a common incurable infection that can be fatal to newborns. After an initial infection, outbreaks may recur at any time.

- Hepatitis B is a viral infection of the liver transmitted through sexual and nonsexual contact.

- Syphilis is a highly contagious bacterial infection that can be treated with antibiotics. If left untreated, it can lead to deterioration of the central nervous system and death.

BOOKS

Engel, J. 2007. *The Epidemic: A Global History of AIDS.* New York: Collins. *A historical, social, and cultural perspective on the AIDS epidemic, from its beginning in 1981 to the present day, from a medical historian.*

Klausner, J. D., and E. W. Hook. 2007. *Current Diagnosis and Treatment of Sexually Transmitted Diseases.* New York: McGraw-Hill. *Written for the clinician; provides an easy-to-use reference of the latest diagnostic and treatment information available on STDs.*

Siegel, M. 2006. *Bird Flu: Everything You Need to Know About the Next Pandemic.* New York: Wiley. *A practicing physician and teacher examines the potential threat of an avian flu outbreak and explains the measures we can take to protect ourselves.*

Sompayrac, L. M. 2008. *How the Immune System Works,* 3rd ed. Malden, Mass.: Blackwell Science. *A highly readable overview of basic concepts of immunity.*

ORGANIZATIONS, HOTLINES, AND WEB SITES

American College Health Association. Offers free brochures on STDs, alcohol use, acquaintance rape, and other health issues.

http://www.acha.org

ASHA/CDC STD and AIDS Hotlines. Callers can obtain information, counseling, and referrals for testing and treatment. The hotlines offer information on more than 20 STDs and include Spanish and TTY service.

800-227-8922

AVERT. An international educational Web site with extensive clinical and epidemiological information on HIV/AIDS in the United States and worldwide. Provides general information for both professionals and the layperson on STDs, sex, and contraception. Also contains games and quizzes geared for teens.

http://www.avert.org/

CDC National Center for Infectious Diseases. Provides extensive information on a wide variety of infectious diseases.

http://www.cdc.gov/ncidod

CDC National Immunization Program. Information and answers to frequently asked questions about immunizations.

http://www.cdc.gov/nip

http://www.cdc.gov/travel

CDC National Prevention Information Network. Provides extensive information and links on HIV/AIDS and other STDs.

http://www.cdcnpin.org

Joint United Nations Programme on HIV/AIDS (UNAIDS). Provides statistics and information on the international HIV/AIDS situation.

http://www.unaids.org

The NAMES Project Foundation AIDS Memorial Quilt. Includes the story behind the quilt, images of quilt panels, and information and links relating to HIV infection.

http://www.aidsquilt.org

National Institute of Allergies and Infectious Disease: Sexually Transmitted Infections. Provides up-to-date fact sheets and brochures.

http://www3.niaid.nih.gov/topics/sti

Planned Parenthood Federation of America. Provides information on STDs, family planning, and contraception.

http://www.plannedparenthood.org

World Health Organization: Infectious Diseases. Provides fact sheets about many emerging and tropical diseases as well as information about current outbreaks.

http://www.who.int/topics/infectious_diseases/en

SELECTED BIBLIOGRAPHY

American Association of Blood Banks. 2007. *Blood Donation Frequently Asked Questions* (http://www.aabb.org/Content/Donate_Blood/Blood_Donation_FAQs/donatefaqs.htm; retrieved October 4, 2010).

American College Health Association. 2009. *American College Health Association—National College Health Assessment II: Reference Group Executive Summary Fall 2009.* Linthicum, Md.: American College Health Association.

American Social Health Association. 2008. *Frequently Asked Questions About Cervical Cancer/HPV Vaccine Access in the U.S.* (http://www.ashastd.org/hpv/hpv_vaccines.cfm; retrieved October 4, 2010).

American Social Health Association. 2010. *Herpes Testing Toolkit* (http://www.ashastd.org/herpes_toolkit/; retrieved October 4, 2010).

Brown, D. R., et al. 2005. A longitudinal study of genital human papillomavirus infection in a cohort of closely followed adolescent women. *Journal of Infectious Diseases* 191(2): 182–192.

Buchbinder, Susan. 2010. HIV epidemiology, testing strategies and prevention interventions. *Topics in HIV Medicine* 18(2): 38–44.

Caskey, Rachel. 2009. Knowledge and early adoption of the HPV vaccine among girls and young women: Results of a national survey. *Journal of Adolescent Health* 45(5): 453–462.

Centers for Disease Control and Prevention. 2008. *BSE (Bovine Spongiform Encephalopathy, or Mad Cow Disease)* (http://www.cdc.gov/ncidod/dvrd/bse; retrieved October 4, 2010).

Centers for Disease Control and Prevention. 2009. Recommended immunization schedules for persons aged 0–18 years—United States, 2009. *Morbidity and Mortality Weekly Report* 57(51): Q1–Q4.

Centers for Disease Control and Prevention. 2009. *Sexually Transmitted Disease Surveillance, 2008.* Atlanta: U.S. Department of Health and Human Services.

Centers for Disease Control and Prevention. 2010. *Asthma: Basic Information* (http://www.cdc.gov/asthma/faqs.htm; retrieved October 3, 2010).

Centers for Disease Control and Prevention. 2010. *Chlamydia Fact Sheet* (http://www.cdc.gov/std/Chlamydia/STDFact-Chlamydia.htm; retrieved October 4, 2010).

Centers for Disease Control and Prevention. 2010. *Expedited Partner Therapy* (http://www.cdc.gov/std/ept/; retrieved October 4, 2010).

Centers for Disease Control and Prevention. 2010. *Genital HPV Infection—CDC Fact Sheet* (http://www.cdc.gov/std/hpv/stdfact-hpv.htm; retrieved October 4, 2010).

Centers for Disease Control and Prevention. 2010. *Hepatitis B Information for Health Professionals* (http://www.cdc.gov/hepatitis/HBV/HBVfaq.htm//overview; retrieved October 4, 2010).

Centers for Disease Control and Prevention. 2010. Recommended adult immunization schedule—United States, January 15, 2010. *Morbidity and Mortality Weekly Report* 59(1).

Centers for Disease Control and Prevention. 2010. Seroprevalence of herpes simplex virus type 2 among persons aged 14 to 49 years, U.S. 2005–2008. *Morbidity and Mortality Weekly Report* 59(15): 456–459.

Fauci, A. S. 2004. Emerging infectious diseases: A clear and present danger to humanity. *Journal of the American Medical Association* 292(15): 1887–1888.

Food and Drug Administration. 2004. *FDA Approves First Oral Fluid Based Rapid HIV Test Kit* (http://www.fda.gov/bbs/topics/news/2004/NEW01042.html; retrieved October 4, 2010).

Garland, S. 2010. Prevention strategies against human papillomavirus in males. *Gynecologic Oncology* 117(2010): S20–25.

Goetz, M. B., et al. 2010. HIV replication capacity is an independent predictor of disease progression in persons with untreated chronic HIV infection. *Journal of Acquired Immune Deficiency Syndrome* 53(4): 472–479.

International AIDS Vaccine Initiative. 2010. *State of the Field* (http://www.iavi.org/research_development/Pages/state-of-field-aspx; retrieved October 4, 2010).

Joint United National Programme on HIV/AIDS (UNAIDS). 2009. *AIDS Epidemic Update 2009*. Geneva: UNAIDS.

Kaiser Family Foundation. 2009. *Survey of Americans on HIV/AIDS* (http://www.kff.org/kaiserpolls/7889.cfm; retrieved October 4, 2010).

Levy, S. B., and B. Marshall. 2004. Antibacterial resistance worldwide: Causes, challenges, and responses. *Nature Medicine* 10(12 Suppl.): S122–S129.

National Immunization Program. 2005. *Epidemiology and Prevention of Vaccine-Preventable Diseases,* 8th ed. Waldorf, Md.: Public Health Foundation.

Voelker, Rebecca. 2010. Experts reconsider wisdom of limiting chlamydia screening only to women. *The Journal of the American Medical Association* 303(9): 823–824.

World Health Organization. 2010. *The World Health Report 2010*. Geneva: World Health Organization.

Xu, F., et al. 2006. Trends in herpes simplex virus type 1 and type 2 seroprevalence in the United States. *Journal of the American Medical Association* 296(8): 964–973.

LOOKING AHEAD...

After reading this chapter, you should be able to:

- Explain how population growth affects the earth's environme and contributes to pollution and climate change

- Discuss the causes and effects of air and water pollution, a describe strategies that people can take to protect these resources

- Discuss the issue of solid waste disposal and the impact it has on the environment and human health

- Identify key sources of chemical and radiation pollution, a discuss methods for preventing such pollution

- Explain how energy use affects the environment, and descri steps everyone can take to use energy more efficiently

Environmental Health

14

We are constantly reminded of our intimate relationship with everything that surrounds us—our environment. Although the planet provides us with food, water, air, and everything else that sustains life, it also provides us with natural occurrences—earthquakes, tsunamis, hurricanes, drought, climate changes—that destroy life and disrupt society. In the past, humans frequently had to struggle against the environment to survive. Today, in addition to dealing with natural disasters, we also have to find ways to protect the environment from the by-products of our way of life. This chapter discusses how the environment affects you and how you affect the environment, and it describes steps you can take to improve your environmental health while reducing your impact on the earth.

ENVIRONMENTAL HEALTH DEFINED

The field of **environmental health** grew out of efforts to control communicable diseases. These efforts led to systematic garbage collection, sewage treatment, filtration and chlorination of drinking water, food inspection, and the establishment of public health enforcement agencies. Cleaning up the environment changed the health profile of the developed world, reducing or eliminating deaths from diseases like typhoid fever and cholera. Unfortunately, infectious diseases continue to take a huge toll worldwide.

In the United States, a complex public health system is constantly at work behind the scenes. Every time the system is disrupted, danger recurs. After any disaster that damages a community's public health system, prompt restoration of basic health services becomes crucial to human survival. And every time we venture beyond the boundaries of our everyday world, we are reminded of the importance of these basics: clean water, sanitary waste disposal, safe food, and insect and rodent control.

Over the last few decades, the focus of environmental health has expanded and become more complex. We now recognize that environmental pollutants contribute not only to infectious diseases but to many chronic diseases as well. Technological advances have increased our ability to affect and damage the environment. Rapid population growth, which has resulted partly from past environmental

Environmental Health Checklist

The following list of statements relates to your effect on the environment. Put a checkmark next to the statements that are true for you.

_____ I ride my bike, walk, carpool, or use public transportation whenever possible.

_____ I keep my car tuned up and well maintained.

_____ My residence is well insulated.

_____ Where possible, I use compact fluorescent bulbs instead of incandescent bulbs.

_____ I turn off lights and appliances when they are not in use.

_____ I avoid turning on heat or air conditioning whenever possible.

_____ I run the washing machine, dryer, and dishwasher only when they have full loads.

_____ I run the clothes dryer only as long as it takes my clothes to dry.

_____ I dry my hair with a towel rather than a hair dryer.

_____ I keep my car's air conditioner in good working order and have it serviced by a service station that recycles CFCs.

_____ When shopping, I choose products with the least amount of packaging.

_____ I choose recycled and recyclable products.

_____ I avoid products packaged in plastic and unrecycled aluminum.

_____ I store food in glass jars and waxed paper rather than plastic wrap.

_____ I take my own bag along when I go shopping.

_____ I recycle newspapers, glass, cans, and other recyclables.

_____ When shopping, I read labels and try to buy the least toxic products available.

_____ I dispose of household hazardous wastes properly.

_____ I take showers instead of baths.

_____ I take short showers and switch off the water when I'm not actively using it.

_____ I do not run the water while brushing my teeth, shaving, or hand-washing clothes.

_____ My faucets have aerators installed in them.

_____ My shower has a low-flow showerhead.

_____ I have a water-saver toilet or a water displacement device in my toilet.

_____ I snip or rip plastic six-pack rings before I throw them out.

_____ When hiking or camping, I never leave anything behind.

Statements you have not checked can help you identify behaviors you can change to improve environmental health.

For an overall estimate of how much land and water your lifestyle requires, take the Ecological Footprint quiz at www.myfootprint.org. You can also determine your "carbon footprint" at the Global Footprint Network Web site (www.footprintnetwork.org/en/index.php/GFN/page/calculators) or at the Nature Conservancy Web site (www.nature.org/initiatives/climatechange/calculator/?src=l12).

---

improvements, means that far more people are consuming and competing for resources than ever before.

Environmental health is therefore seen as encompassing all the interactions of humans with their environment and the health consequences of these interactions. Fundamental to this definition is a recognition that we hold the world in trust for future generations and for other forms of life. Our responsibility is to pass on a world no worse, and preferably better, than the one we live in today (see the box "Environmental Health Checklist").

POPULATION GROWTH AND CONTROL

Throughout most of history, humans have been a minor pressure on the planet. About 300 million people were alive in the year A.D. 1; by the time Europeans were settling in the United States 1600 years later, the world population had increased gradually to a little over 500 million. But then it began rising exponentially—zooming to 1 billion by about 1800, more than doubling by 1930, and then doubling again in just 40 years (Figure 14.1).

The United Nations projects that world population will reach 9.1 billion by 2050 and will continue to increase until it levels off above 10 billion in 2200. Virtually all of this increase is taking place in less-developed regions. This rapid expansion of population, particularly in

environmental health   The collective interactions of humans with the environment and the short-term and long-term health consequences of those interactions.

TERMS

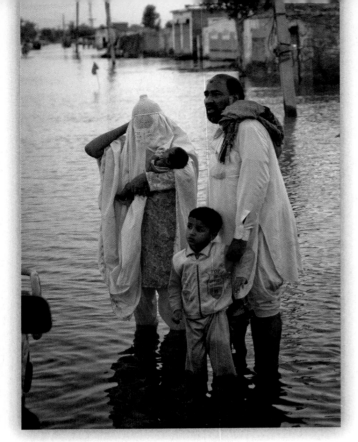

Natural events—such as the flooding in Pakistan in 2010—can directly kill thousands of people while wiping out essential services, polluting water, and facilitating the spread of diseases.

scientists agree that there is a limit. A report from the United Nations Convention on Biological Diversity states that the population's demand for resources already exceed the earth's capacity by 20%. The primary factors that may eventually put a cap on human population are likely to be the limits of the earth's resources—food, land, water, and energy. The mass media have exposed the entire world to the American lifestyle and raised people's expectations of living at a comparable level. But such a lifestyle is supported by levels of energy consumption that the earth cannot support worldwide. The United States has about 5% of the world's population but uses 25% of the world's energy.

Although it is apparent that population growth must be controlled, population trends are difficult to influence and manage. A variety of interconnecting factors fuel the current population explosion, including high fertility rates, lack of family planning resources, and lower death rates.

To be successful, population management policies must change the condition of people's lives, especially poverty, to remove the pressures for having large families. Research indicates that the combination of improved health, better education, and increased literacy and employment opportunities for women works together with family planning to decrease fertility rates. Unfortunately, in the fastest-growing countries, the needs of a rapidly increasing population use up financial resources that might otherwise be used to improve lives and ultimately slow population growth.

AIR QUALITY AND POLLUTION

Air pollution is not a human invention or even a new problem. The air is polluted naturally with every forest fire, pollen bloom, and dust storm, as well as with countless other natural pollutants. To these natural sources,

> *The United States has about 5% of the world's population but uses 25% of the world's energy.*

the past 50 years, is generally believed to be responsible for most of the stress humans put on the environment.

No one knows how many people the world can support, but most

VITAL STATISTICS

FIGURE 14.1 World population growth.
The United Nations estimates that the world's population will continue to increase dramatically until it stabilizes above 10 billion people in 2200.

SOURCE: United Nations Population Division. 2009. *World Population Prospects: The 2009 Revision.* New York: United Nations; U.S. Bureau of the Census.

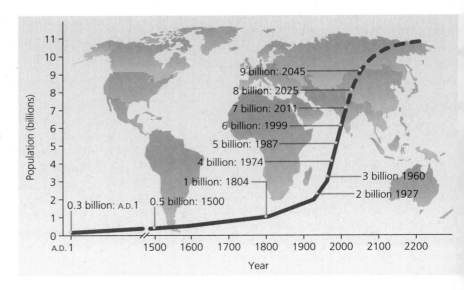

humans have always contributed the by-products of their activities. Air pollution is linked to a wide range of health problems; the very young and the elderly are among those most susceptible to air pollution's effects.

Air Quality and Smog

The U.S. Environmental Protection Agency (EPA) uses a measure called the **Air Quality Index (AQI)** to indicate whether air pollution levels pose a health concern. The AQI is used for five major air pollutants: carbon monoxide (CO), sulfur dioxide (SO_2), nitrogen dioxide (NO_2), particulate matter (PM), and ground-level ozone. A major source of those pollutants is the burning of **fossil fuels** in vehicles and industrial processes. AQI values run from 0 to 500; the higher the AQI, the greater the level of pollution and associated health danger. Local AQI information is often available in newspapers, on television and radio, on the Internet, and from state and local telephone hotlines.

The term **smog** was first used in the early 1900s in London to describe the combination of smoke and fog. What we typically call smog today is a mixture of pollutants, with ground-level ozone being the key ingredient. Major smog occurrences are linked to the combination of several factors: Heavy motor vehicle traffic, high temperatures, and sunny weather can increase the production of ozone. Pollutants are also more likely to build up in areas with little wind and/or where a topographic feature such as a mountain range or valley prevents the wind from pushing out stagnant air.

> ## 175 million
> **Americans live in counties where the air is unhealthy at least some of the time.**
>
> —American Lung Association, 2009

The Greenhouse Effect and Global Warming

The temperature of the earth's atmosphere depends on the balance between the amount of energy the planet absorbs from the sun (mainly as high-energy ultraviolet radiation) and the amount of energy radiated back into space as lower-energy infrared radiation. Key components of temperature regulation are carbon dioxide, water vapor, methane, and other **greenhouse gases**—so named because, like the glass panes in a greenhouse, they let through visible light from the sun but trap some of the resulting infrared radiation and reradiate it back to the earth's surface. This reradiation causes a buildup of heat that raises the temperature of the lower atmosphere, a natural process known as the **greenhouse effect.** Without it, the atmosphere would be far cooler and much more hostile to life (see page T1-5 of the color transparency insert "Touring Lifestyle Behaviors" in Chapter 8).

There is growing consensus that human activity is causing **global warming** or *climate change*. The concentration of greenhouse gases is increasing because of human activity, especially the combustion of fossil fuels. Carbon dioxide levels in the atmosphere have increased rapidly in recent decades. The use of fossil fuels pumps more than 20 billion tons of carbon dioxide into the atmosphere every year. Deforestation, often by burning, also sends carbon dioxide into the atmosphere and reduces the number of trees available to convert carbon dioxide into oxygen.

The overall global temperature rose more than 1 degree Fahrenheit (0.6 degree Celsius) during the twentieth century. There is growing agreement among scientists that temperatures will continue to rise, although estimates vary as to how much they will change. Possible consequences of global warming include increased rainfall and flooding in some regions, increased drought in others; increased mortality from heat stress, urban air pollution, tropical diseases, and extreme weather events; a poleward shift of 50–350 miles in the location of vegetation zones, affecting crop yields, irrigation demands, and forest productivity; and increasingly rapid and drastic melting of

Ask Yourself

QUESTIONS FOR CRITICAL THINKING AND REFLECTION

What is the population of your town or city? Does the sheer number of people in your town make living there difficult, or more enjoyable? In what ways? Do you believe your town has adequate infrastructure and resources to support its residents?

TERMS

Air Quality Index (AQI) A measure of local air quality and what it means for health.

fossil fuels Buried deposits of decayed animals and plants that are converted into carbon-rich fuels by exposure to heat and pressure over millions of years; oil, coal, and natural gas are fossil fuels.

smog Hazy atmospheric conditions resulting from increased concentrations of ground-level ozone and other pollutants.

greenhouse gas A gas (such as carbon dioxide) or vapor that traps infrared radiation instead of allowing it to escape through the atmosphere, resulting in a warming of the earth (the greenhouse effect).

greenhouse effect A warming of the earth due to a buildup of carbon dioxide and certain other gases.

global warming An increase in the earth's atmospheric temperature when averaged across seasons and geographical regions; also called *climate change*.

the earth's polar ice caps. Parties at the 2009 United Nations Climate Change Conference in Copenhagen endorsed the scientific view that keeping the increase in global temperature below 2 degrees Celsius is necessary to stave off the worst effects of climate change.

Thinning of the Ozone Layer

Another air pollution problem is the thinning of the **ozone layer** of the atmosphere, a fragile, invisible layer about 10–30 miles above the earth's surface that shields the planet from the sun's hazardous ultraviolet (UV) rays. Since the mid-1980s, scientists have observed the seasonal appearance and growth of a hole in the ozone layer over Antarctica. More recently, thinning over other areas has been noted.

The ozone layer is being destroyed primarily by **chlorofluorocarbons (CFCs)**, industrial chemicals that rise into the atmosphere and release chlorine atoms, which destroy ozone. In the Northern Hemisphere, ozone levels have declined by about 10% since 1980, and certain areas may be temporarily depleted in late winter and early spring by as much as 40%. Without the ozone layer to absorb the sun's UV radiation, life on earth would be impossible. The potential effects of increased long-term exposure to UV light for humans include skin cancer, wrinkling and aging of the skin, cataracts and blindness, and reduced immune response. UV light may interfere with photosynthesis and cause lower crop yields; it may also kill phytoplankton and krill, the basis of the ocean food chain.

Without the ozone layer to absorb the sun's UV radiation, life on earth would be impossible.

Worldwide production and use of CFCs have declined rapidly since the danger to the ozone layer was recognized. Industrialized nations agreed to end CFC production in 2000. Ozone-depleting substances have very long lifetimes in the atmosphere, however, so despite these efforts, the ozone hole is not expected to recover until 2070. The gradual recovery is masked by annual variations caused by weather fluctuations over Antarctica.

Energy Use and Air Pollution

Americans are the biggest energy consumers in the world, leading China, Russia, Japan, India, and European countries.

ozone layer   A layer of ozone molecules (O_3) in the upper atmosphere that screens out UV rays from the sun.

chlorofluorocarbons (CFCs)   Chemicals used as spray-can propellants, refrigerants, and industrial solvents, implicated in the destruction of the ozone layer.

About 85% of the energy we use comes from fossil fuels—oil, coal, and natural gas. The remainder comes from nuclear power and renewable energy sources (such as hydroelectric, wind, and solar power). Fossil fuel use is at the root of many environmental problems, especially those relating to air pollution and climate change. Every gallon of gas burned puts about 20 pounds of carbon dioxide into the atmosphere. The worst environmental disaster in U.S. history occurred when an oil drilling rig exploded and sank in the Gulf of Mexico in 2010 (see the box "The Gulf Oil Spill of 2010"). Two key strategies for controlling energy use are conservation and the development of nonpolluting, renewable sources of energy (see the box "Renewable Energy").

Alternative Fuels   The U.S. Department of Energy (DOE) is encouraging researchers and automobile manufacturers to produce vehicles that can handle alternative fuels such as ethanol. Ethanol, a form of alcohol, is a renewable and largely domestic transportation fuel produced from fermenting plant sugars such as corn, sugar cane, and other starchy agricultural products. Ethanol use reduces the amount of imported oil required to produce gasoline, reduces overall greenhouse gas emissions from automobiles, and supports the U.S. agricultural industry. Drawbacks of ethanol include the amount of energy required to produce it, which may exceed the amount of energy it yields, and the diversion of corn crops from the food supply to the fuel industry, which is thought to contribute to high food prices and food shortages around the world.

Hybrid and Electric Vehicles   Interest has surged in hybrid electric vehicles (HEVs), such as the Toyota Prius, the Honda Insight, and the Ford Fusion. Hybrid vehicles use two or more distinct power sources to propel the vehicle, such as an on-board energy storage system (batteries, for example) and an internal combustion engine and electric motor. The hybrid vehicle typically realizes greater fuel economy than a conventional car does and produces fewer polluting emissions.

Interest is also growing in all-electric vehicles, including the Nissan Leaf, the GM Volt, and the Tesla. In electric vehicles, electricity is stored in battery packs and then converted into mechanical power that runs the vehicle. These vehicles do not produce tailpipe emissions, but generators that produce the electricity for the batteries do emit pollutants.

Indoor Air Pollution

Although most people associate air pollution with the outdoors, your home may also harbor potentially dangerous pollutants. Some of these compounds trigger allergic responses, and others have been linked to cancer. Common indoor pollutants include environmental tobacco smoke (ETS); carbon monoxide and other combustion

TERMS

In April 2010, the oil rig Deepwater Horizon exploded in the Gulf of Mexico, about 50 miles off the coast of Louisiana. A huge fireball erupted when volatile gases trapped in the well shot up through drilling lines and ignited as they reached the rig. The sudden blast killed 11 of the rig's workers and injured 17 others. The incident disabled and eventually destroyed the drilling platform, and oil began spewing into the waters of the Gulf.

When the smoke cleared, an oil slick covered an area of 5 square miles. Within 4 days, it had grown to 12 square miles. By May 1, it was more than 100 miles long. At first, BP estimated the leak at 1000 barrels a day (more than 40,000 gallons), but estimates rose to 5000, then 10,000, and eventually 60,000 barrels a day. Despite efforts, BP was unable to plug the well or stop the flow of oil from the damaged well head on the ocean floor, 1 mile below the surface.

As oil continued to flow, brigades of volunteers joined professional and military personnel in efforts to capture the oil before it reached shore, to clean up fouled beaches and marshes, and to rescue and clean as many animals as possible. Hundreds of miles of floating booms were put in place to contain patches of oil, specially equipped ships siphoned millions of gallons of sea water and separated the oil from it, and surface oil was corralled and burned.

On shore, workers cleaned beaches and wetlands and attempted to rescue and clean hundreds of sea birds, turtles, and other kinds of wildlife. Relief agencies raised millions of dollars to funnel aid to the clean-up effort. The federal government announced that BP would bear the costs of the clean-up and compensation to individuals and businesses affected by the spill. Government agencies began billing BP millions of dollars to cover various costs, while families and businesses started filing compensation claims.

After several attempts to cap the leak and siphon off the escaping oil, BP was able to plug the leak in mid-July by pumping millions of gallons of mud and cement into the well head. Two relief wells that were drilled to reduce pressure intersected the blown-out well in September, and more cement was pumped in to permanently plug it. On September 19, the well was officially "killed," 5 months after the explosion.

Even after the flow of oil stopped and the well was sealed, the environmental disaster was still just beginning. An estimated 5 million barrels of oil leaked into the Gulf of Mexico, though some scientists say we'll never know for sure just how much oil escaped or what percentage of it will be captured.

Chemical dispersants used to break up the oil had toxic effects and may have caused much of the oil to remain beneath the surface in large plumes or to settle on the ocean floor, where it cannot be reached for clean-up. The disaster killed thousands of birds, hundreds of endangered sea turtles, and many dolphins and other marine mammals. The Gulf's ecosystems may need generations to recover fully, and some parts of it may never recover. Researchers have discovered trace amounts of oil in some fish and shellfish, leading to concerns that oil could reach the human food chain.

The Gulf oil spill raises many questions about oil exploration and the environment. Should oil drilling be permitted in deep water, where leaks are nearly impossible to contain in a short time? Should offshore drilling be halted altogether? Do we have the knowledge and technology to conduct oil exploration and drilling safely? Although the government and industry promise to take steps to make drilling safer, they acknowledge there will always be risks—to the environment, to the economy, and to people's livelihoods.

SOURCES: CNN.com. 2010. *Gulf Coast Oil Disaster* (http://www.cnn.com/SPECIALS/2010/gulf.coast.oil.spill; retrieved October 9, 2010); The New York Times Online. 2010. *Gulf of Mexico Deep Water Horizon Oil Spill* (http://topics.nytimes.com/top/reference/timestopics/subjects/o/oil_spills/gulf_of_mexico_2010/index.html; retrieved October 9, 2010); U.S. Coast Guard. 2010. *Restore The Gulf: Official Web Site* (http://www.restorethegulf.gov/index.shtm; retrieved October 9, 2010); U.S. Environmental Protection Agency. 2010. *EPA Response to BP Spill in the Gulf of Mexico* (http://www.epa.gov/bpspill; retrieved October 9, 2010).

by-products from woodstoves, fireplaces, kerosene heaters and lamps, and gas ranges; formaldehyde gas from certain construction materials, paints, floor finishes, permanent-press clothing, and nail polish; biological pollutants, including bacteria, dust mites, mold, and animal dander; and indoor mold, which can cause health problems when inhaled, especially for people with asthma and other respiratory conditions.

Preventing Air Pollution and Conserving Energy

You can do a great deal to reduce air pollution and conserve energy. Here are a few ideas:

- Cut back on driving. Ride your bike, walk, use public transportation, or carpool in a fuel-efficient vehicle.

Renewable Energy

With fossil fuels becoming increasingly problematic politically, economically, and environmentally, interest and investment in renewable energy sources have grown in recent years. Renewable energy sources are those sources that are naturally replenished and essentially inexhaustible, such as wind and water. Together with technologies that improve energy efficiency, renewable energy sources contribute to *sustainability*, the capacity of natural or human systems to endure and maintain well-being over time. A common definition of sustainable development is development that meets society's present needs without compromising the ability of future generations to meet their needs.

Renewable energy sources include wind power, solar power, water and wave power, geothermal power, and biomass and biofuels from renewable sources, among others.

- Wind power uses the energy of the wind to turn blades that run a turbine, which spins a generator, which produces electricity.

- Solar power uses the heat and light of the sun to produce energy via a variety of technologies. One solar technology is the concentrating solar power (CSP) system, which use mirrors, dishes, or towers to reflect and collect solar heat to generate steam, which runs a turbine to produce electricity. Another solar technology is the photovoltaic (solar cell) system, which converts sunlight directly into electricity by means of semiconducting materials.

- Geothermal power taps the heat in the earth's core. It may be in the form of hot water or steam, which can be used to run a turbine to produce electricity. In some geologically unstable parts of the planet, including Yellowstone Park and parts of northern California, geothermal energy is close to the surface.

- Biomass is plant material, including trees. When biomass is burned, it produces energy. If the plants are produced and harvested sustainably, they are a renewable source of energy.

- Biofuels are fuels based on natural materials, either alcohol or oil. Bioethanol is made primarily from sugar and starch crops like corn, although trees and grasses may be used in the future. Ethanol can be used as a fuel for vehicles or added to gasoline. Biodiesel is made from vegetable oils or animal fats and can be either used in a pure form to power vehicles or added to diesel to reduce carbon emissions.

In 2010, President Obama called for a new energy future, embracing alternative and renewable energy, ending our addiction to foreign oil, and addressing the global climate crisis. The administration's "New Energy for America" plan set a goal of generating 10% of the nation's electricity from renewable sources by 2012 and 25% by 2025, as well as putting 1 million plug-in hybrid cars—cars that can get up to 150 miles per gallon—on the road by 2015.

Worldwide, renewable energy sources were providing one-quarter of the power capacity from all sources and 18% of the global electricity supply in 2009. Between 2005 and 2009, wind power capacity grew an average of 27% annually and ethanol production grew 20% annually. In 2009, both the United States and Europe added more renewable power capacity than conventional (fossil fuel) capacity. By 2010, more than 100 countries had enacted some type of policy target or promotion policy related to renewable energy. Many of these targets call for 15–25% of energy or electricity to be provided by renewable sources by 2020. The pursuit of renewable energy sources is seen as having the potential to create new industries and generate jobs—in addition to benefitting the environment.

SOURCES: REN21. 2010. *Renewables 2010 Global Status Report* (Paris: REN21 Secretariat) (http://www.ren21.net/globalstatusreport/REN21_GSR_2010_full.pdf; retrieved September 27, 2010); RenewableEnergyWorld.com. 2010. *Renewable Energy News* (http://www.renewableenergyworld.com/rea/home; retrieved October 8, 2010); The White House. 2010. *Energy & Environment* (http://www.whitehouse.gov/issues/energy-and-environment; retrieved October 9, 2010).

- Keep your car tuned up and well maintained, and keep your tires inflated at recommended pressures. To save energy when driving, avoid quick starts, stay within the speed limit, limit the use of air conditioning, and don't let your car idle unless absolutely necessary.

- Buy energy-efficient appliances, and run the washing machine, dryer, and dishwasher only when you have full loads. Do laundry in warm or cold water instead of hot. Clean refrigerator coils and clothes dryer lint screens frequently.

- Replace incandescent bulbs with compact fluorescent bulbs (CFLs). Although they cost more initially, they save you money over the long term because they use less electricity to produce light and last up to ten times longer than incandescent bulbs. Burned-out CFLs should be recycled rather than disposed of in the trash because they contain small amounts of mercury.

- Make sure your home is well-insulated, and use insulating shades and curtains. In cold weather, put on a sweater and turn down the thermostat. In hot weather, use a fan instead of an air conditioner to cool yourself.

- Plant and care for trees in your yard and neighborhood. Because they recycle carbon dioxide, trees work against global warming. They also provide shade and cool the air, so less air conditioning is needed.

- Before discarding a refrigerator, air conditioner, or humidifier, check with the waste hauler or your local government to ensure that ozone-depleting refrigerants will be removed prior to disposal. If you use a metered-dose inhaler, ask your physician if an ozone-safe inhaler is available for your medication.

- Keep paints, cleaning agents, and other chemical products tightly sealed in their original containers.

- Clean and inspect chimneys, furnaces, and other appliances regularly. Install carbon monoxide detectors.

WATER QUALITY AND POLLUTION

Few parts of the world have enough safe, clean drinking water, but few things are as important to human health.

Water Contamination and Treatment

Many cities rely at least in part on wells that tap local groundwater, but often it is necessary to tap lakes and rivers to supplement wells. Because such surface water is more likely to be contaminated with both organic matter and pathogenic microorganisms, it is purified in water-treatment plants before being piped into the community.

In most areas of the United States, water systems have adequate, dependable supplies, are able to control waterborne disease, and provide water without unacceptable color, odor, or taste. However, problems do occur. The CDC estimates that 1 million Americans become ill and 900–1000 die each year from microbial illnesses from drinking water.

Water Shortages

Water shortages are a growing concern in many regions of the world. Some parts of the United States are experiencing rapid population growth that outstrips the ability of local systems to provide adequate water to all. Groundwater pumping and the diversion of water from lakes and rivers for irrigation are further reducing the amount of water available to local communities.

Sewage

Most cities have sewage-treatment systems that separate fecal matter from water in huge tanks and ponds and stabilize it so that it cannot transmit infectious diseases. Once treated and biologically safe, the water is released back into the environment. The sludge that remains behind is often contaminated with **heavy metals** and is handled as hazardous waste. If not contaminated, sludge may be used as fertilizer, although this practice is being discouraged by scientists and is not permitted in organic agriculture.

Many cities have now begun expanded sewage-treatment measures to remove heavy metals and other hazardous chemicals. This action has resulted from many studies linking exposure to chemicals such as mercury, lead, and **polychlorinated biphenyls (PCBs)** with long-term health consequences, including cancer and damage to the central nervous system.

Protecting the Water Supply

By taking steps to keep the water supply clean, you reduce pollution overall and help protect the land, wildlife, and other people from illness.

- Take showers, not baths, to minimize your water consumption. Don't let water run when you're not actively using it while brushing your teeth, shaving, or hand-washing clothes.

- Install sink faucet aerators and water-efficient showerheads, which use two to five times less water with no noticeable decrease in performance. Purchase a water-saver toilet, or put a displacement device in your toilet tank to reduce the amount of water used with each flush.

- Fix any leaky faucets in your home. Leaks can waste thousands of gallons of water per year.

- Don't pour toxic materials such as cleaning solvents, bleach, or motor oil down the drain. Store them until you can take them to a hazardous waste collection center.

- Don't pour old medicines down the drain or flush them down the toilet. Some pharmacies will take back unused or expired medications for disposal, and many communities arrange drop-off days for these drugs.

---

heavy metal A metal with a high specific gravity, such as lead, copper, or tin.

polychlorinated biphenyl (PCB) An industrial chemical used as an insulator in electrical transformers and linked to certain human cancers; banned worldwide since 1977 but persistent in the environment.

TERMS

SOLID WASTE POLLUTION

Humans generate huge amounts of waste, which require proper handling to ensure environmental safety.

Solid Waste

QUICK STATS

The average American generates **4.5 pounds** of trash per day; about 1.5 pounds of this is recycled.

—Environmental Protection Agency, 2009

The bulk of the organic food garbage produced in American kitchens is now dumped into the sewage system by way of the garbage disposal. The garbage that remains is not very hazardous from the standpoint of infectious disease because there is very little food waste in it, but it does represent an enormous disposal and contamination problem.

What's In Our Garbage? The biggest single component of household trash by weight is paper products, including junk mail, glossy mail-order catalogs, and computer printouts (Figure 14.2). About 1% of the solid waste is toxic; a new source of toxic waste is the disposal of computer components in both household and commercial waste. Burning, as opposed to burial, reduces the bulk of solid waste, but it may release hazardous material into the air. Manufacturing, mining, and other industries all produce large amounts of potentially dangerous materials that cannot simply be dumped.

Disposing of Solid Waste Since the 1960s, billions of tons of solid waste have been buried in **sanitary landfill** disposal sites. Sometimes protective liners are used around the site, and nearby monitoring wells are now required in most states. Layers of solid waste are regularly covered with thin layers of dirt until the site is filled. Some com-

TERMS

sanitary landfill   A disposal site where solid wastes are buried.

biodegradable   Refers to the ability of some materials to break down naturally and disappear back into the environment.

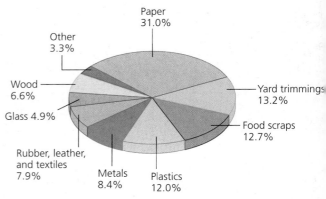

Due to rounding, these numbers do not add up to 100%.

Figure 14.2   Components of municipal solid waste, by weight, before recycling.

SOURCE: Environmental Protection Agency, 2009. *Municipal Solid Waste Generation, Recycling and Disposal in the United States: Facts and Figures* for 2008. Washington, D.C.: Environmental Protection Agency. Pub. No. EPA-530-F-009-021.

munities then plant grass and trees and convert the site into a park. Landfill is relatively stable; almost no decomposition occurs in the solidly packed waste. Much of this waste contains chemicals, ranging from leftover pesticides to paints and oils, which should not be released indiscriminately into the environment. Despite precautions, buried contaminants sometimes leak into the surrounding soil and groundwater. Burial is also expensive and requires huge amounts of space.

The term **biodegradable** means that certain products can break down naturally, safely, and quickly into the raw materials of nature, then disappear back into the environment. Table 14.1 shows the amount of time required for different types of material to biodegrade.

Recycling   In **recycling**, many kinds of waste materials are collected and used as raw materials in the production of new products. Recycling is a good idea because it puts unwanted objects back to good use and it reduces the

Table 14.1	Biodegrading Times of Different Objects
ITEM	TIME REQUIRED TO BIODEGRADE
Banana peel	2–10 days
Paper	2–5 months
Rope	3–14 months
Orange peel	6 months
Wool sock	1–5 years
Cigarette butt	1–12 years
Plastic-coated milk carton	5 years
Aluminum can	80–100 years
Plastic six-pack holder ring	450 years
Glass bottle	1 million years
Plastic bottle	Forever

How to Be a Green Consumer

You can quickly and easily develop habits that direct your consumer dollar toward environmentally friendly products and companies.

● Remember the four Rs of green consumerism:

Reduce the amount of trash and pollution you generate by consuming and throwing away less.

Reuse as many products as possible—either yourself or by selling them or donating them to charity.

Recycle all appropriate materials and buy recycled products whenever possible.

Respond by educating others about reducing waste and recycling, by finding creative ways to reduce waste and toxicity, and by making your preferences known.

● Choose products packaged in refillable, recycled, reusable containers, such as paper, cardboard, aluminum, or glass. Don't buy products that are excessively packaged or wrapped.

● Look for products made with the highest possible content of recycled paper, metal, glass, plastic, and other materials.

● Choose simple products containing the lowest amounts of bleaches, dyes, and fragrances. Look for organic foods from local sources and clothes made from organically grown cotton or Fox Fibre or another naturally colored type of cotton.

● Buy high-quality appliances that have an Energy Star seal from the EPA or some other type of certification indicating that they are energy- and water-efficient.

● Get a reusable cloth shopping bag. If you forget your bag, it doesn't matter much whether you choose paper or plastic—what is important is that you reuse whatever bag you get.

● Look beyond the products to the companies that make them. Support those with good environmental records. If some of your favorite products are overpackaged or contain harmful ingredients, write to the manufacturer.

● Keep in mind that doing something is better than doing nothing. Even if you can't be a perfectly green consumer, doing your best on any purchase *will* make a difference.

SOURCES: U.S. Environmental Protection Agency. 2009. *Consumer Handbook for Reducing Solid Waste* (http://www.epa.gov/osw/wycd/catbook; retrieved October 9, 2010); Natural Resources Defense Council. 2009. *NRDC's Guide to Greener Living* (http://www.nrdc.org/cities/living/gover.asp; retrieved October 9, 2010).

amount of solid waste sitting in landfills, some of which takes decades to decay naturally.

E-Waste Americans scrap about 400 million consumer electronic devices each year. This "e-waste" is the fastest-growing portion of our waste stream. Junked electronic devices are toxic, hazardous waste because they contain varying amounts of lead, mercury, and other heavy metals. Many components of electronic devices are valuable, however, and can be recycled and reused. Local and state e-waste recycling programs are becoming more common, and private companies are betting on the e-waste recycling business. When recycling your electronics, look for a "green" program or one that is certified by e-stewards, an organization that advocates for responsible e-waste recycling (www.e-stewards.org).

Reducing Solid Waste

By recycling more and throwing away less, you can conserve landfill space and put reusable items back into service.

• Buy products with the least amount of packaging you can, or buy products in bulk (see the box "How to Be a Green Consumer") or packaged in recyclable containers.

• Buy recycled or recyclable products. Avoid disposables; instead, use long-lasting or reusable products such as rechargeable batteries.

• Avoid using foam or paper cups and plastic stirrers by bringing your own coffee mug to work or wherever you drink coffee or tea. Pack your lunch in a reusable sack or box.

• To store food, use glass jars and reusable plastic containers rather than foil and plastic wrap.

• Recycle your newspapers, glass, cans, paper, and other recyclables. If you receive something packaged

recycling The use of waste materials as raw materials in the production of new products.

TERMS

Poverty and Environmental Health

Residents of poor and minority communities are often exposed to more environmental toxins than residents of wealthier communities, and they are more likely to suffer from health problems caused or aggravated by pollutants.

Poor neighborhoods are often located near highways and industrial areas that have high levels of air and noise pollution; they are also common sites for hazardous waste production and disposal. Residents of substandard housing are more likely to come into contact with lead, asbestos, carbon monoxide, pesticides, and other hazardous pollutants associated with peeling paint, old plumbing, poorly maintained insulation and heating equipment, and attempts to control high levels of pests such as cockroaches and rodents.

Poor people are more likely to have jobs that expose them to asbestos, silica dust, and pesticides, and they are more likely to catch and consume fish contaminated with PCBs, mercury, and other toxins.

The most thoroughly researched and documented link among poverty, the environment, and health is lead poisoning in children. Many studies have shown that children of low-income black families are much more likely to have elevated levels of lead in their blood than white children. The CDC and the American Academy of Pediatrics recommend annual testing of blood lead levels for all children under age 6, with more frequent testing for children at special risk.

Asthma is another health threat that appears to be linked with both environmental and socioeconomic factors. The number of Americans with asthma has grown dramatically in the past 20 years; most of the increase has occurred in children, with African Americans and the poor hardest hit. Researchers are not sure what accounts for this increase, but suspects include household pollutants, pesticides, air pollution, cigarette smoke, and allergens like cockroaches. These risk factors are likely to cluster in poor urban areas where inadequate health care may worsen asthma's effects.

---

with foam pellets, take them to a commercial mailing center that accepts them for recycling.

- Do not throw electronic items, batteries, or fluorescent lights into the trash. Take all these to state-approved recycling centers.

- If you have a yard, start a compost pile for your organic garbage (non-animal food and yard waste). Some cities, including San Francisco, Dubuque, Iowa, and Portland, Oregon, now collect kitchen scraps for recycling into compost, which is sold to farms and wineries.

CHEMICAL POLLUTION AND HAZARDOUS WASTE

New chemical substances are constantly being introduced into the environment—as pesticides, herbicides, solvents, and hundreds of other products. More people and wildlife are exposed and potentially exposed to them than ever before.

Asbestos

A mineral-based compound, asbestos was widely used for fire protection and insulation in buildings until the late 1960s. Microscopic asbestos fibers can be released into the air when this material is applied or when it later deteriorates or is damaged. These fibers can lodge in the lungs, causing **asbestosis**, lung cancer, and other serious lung diseases. Similar conditions expose workers to risk in the coal mining industry, from coal and silica dust (black lung disease), and in the textile industry, from cotton fibers (brown lung disease).

Lead

Thanks to better preventive efforts, lead poisoning is not as serious a problem today as it was a few years ago. Still, the CDC estimates that about 435,000 children under age 6 may have unsafe lead levels in their blood. Many of these children live in poor, inner-city areas (see the box "Poverty and Environmental Health"). When lead is ingested or inhaled, it can damage the central nervous system, cause permanent mental impairment, hinder oxygen transport in the blood, create digestive problems, and cause coma or even death.

TERMS

asbestosis A lung condition caused by inhalation of microscopic asbestos fibers, which inflame the lung and can lead to lung cancer.

Ask Yourself

QUESTIONS FOR CRITICAL THINKING AND REFLECTION

What are your waste-disposal habits like? Do you recycle everything you possibly can? Do you get rid of items that are still usable? Even if you are conscientious about the way you deal with waste, how could you improve your habits?

Gender and Environmental Health

Although many environmental health risks are shared by all, some risks disproportionately affect women or men. Women and men often have different roles and responsibilities with respect to family, community, and the workforce.

In many societies, women are more often involved in day-to-day activities associated with the environment, including food preparation, agricultural work, and tasks around the home. These activities can expose women to higher levels of indoor air pollution, water pollution, foodborne pathogens, agricultural chemicals, and waste contamination. Indoor pollutants, especially soot from burning wood, charcoal, and other solid fuels used for home heating and cooking, are a particular risk for women. Exposure to this particulate pollution increases the risk of respiratory diseases, lung cancer, and reproductive problems. In 2010, U.S. Secretary of State Hillary Clinton launched a global campaign to introduce clean cookstoves to help hundreds of millions of people, mostly women, avoid the toxic smoke produced by traditional stoves and open fires used in poorly ventilated indoor areas.

All humans are exposed to chemicals in air, food, and drinking water, and we all carry a body load of chemicals. Some of these chemicals bioaccumulate in our bones, blood, or fatty tissues. Women are smaller than men, on average, and have a higher percentage of body fat; so chemicals that accumulate in fatty tissue may pose a relatively greater risk for women. On the other hand, men may be more likely to work in industries that involve significant occupational exposures to disease-related toxins; for example, coal miners have an increased risk of lung cancer (black lung disease).

Although any chemical exposure can be a concern for health, women face the added risk of passing pollutants to a developing fetus during pregnancy or to an infant through breastfeeding. Even relatively low exposure to pollutants can result in a significant chemical body load in an infant or young child because of the small body size. And because infants and children are still developing, the effects of chemical exposure can be significant and devastating. It is not unusual for dangerous environmental toxin exposures to be first recognized through noticeable effects on infants or children. Many chemicals, including PCBs and pesticides, have been found in breast milk.

Studies are ongoing to identify and reduce environmental hazards in the United States and throughout the world. However, many of the people most directly affected by environmental health problems—women, children, and people living in poor communities—have limited economic, social, and political power. It is important that everyone affected by environmental problems be given a voice in determining environmental policies.

SOURCES: McCally, M., ed. 2002. *Life Support: The Environment and Human Health.* Cambridge, Mass.: MIT Press; Population Reference Bureau. 2002. *Women, Men, and Environmental Change: The Gender Dimensions of Environmental Policies and Programs.* Washington, D.C.: Population Reference Bureau.

Young children can easily ingest lead from their environment by picking up dust and dirt on their hands and then putting their fingers in their mouth. Lead-based paints are the chief culprit in lead poisoning of children and were banned from residential use in 1978, but as many as 57 million American homes still contain lead paint. In 2006, the EPA proposed new guidelines requiring contractors to take special lead-containment measures when doing renovations, repairs, or painting in certain buildings. These provisions became law in 2008, with full implementation in 2010. The use of lead in plumbing is now also banned, but some old pipes and faucets contain lead.

Pesticides

Pesticides are used to prevent the spread of insectborne diseases and to maximize food production by killing insects that eat crops. Both uses have risks as well as benefits. Most pesticide hazards to date have been a result of overuse, but there are concerns about the health effects of long-term exposure to small amounts of pesticide residues in foods, especially for children.

Mercury

A naturally occurring metal, mercury is a toxin that affects the nervous system and may damage the brain, kidneys, and gastrointestinal tract; increase blood pressure, heart rate, and heart attack risk; and cause cancer. Mercury slows fetal and child development and causes irreversible deficits in brain function. Coal-fired power plants are the largest producers of mercury; other sources include mining and smelting operations and the disposal of consumer products containing mercury. Mercury persists in the environment and, like pesticides, is bioaccumulative. In particular, large, long-lived fish may carry high levels of mercury. See the box "Gender and Environmental Health" for more on issues affecting pregnant women.

Other Chemical Pollutants

Hazardous wastes are also found in the home and should be handled and disposed of properly. They include automotive supplies (motor oil, antifreeze, transmission fluid), paint supplies (turpentine, paint thinner, mineral spirits), art and hobby supplies (oil-based paint, solvents, acids and alkalis, aerosol sprays), insecticides, batteries, computer and electronic components, and household cleaners containing

> **pesticides** Chemicals used to prevent the spread of diseases transmitted by insects and to maximize food production by killing insects that eat crops.

TERMS

Hazardous chemicals accumulate in many homes, as well as in businesses and industrial sites.

sodium hydroxide (lye) or ammonia. These chemicals are dangerous when inhaled or ingested, when they contact the skin or the eyes, or when they are burned or dumped. Many cities provide guidelines about approved disposal methods and have hazardous waste collection days.

Preventing Chemical Pollution

You can take steps to reduce the chemical pollution in your community.

- When buying products, read the labels, and try to buy the least toxic ones available. Choose nontoxic

nonpetrochemical cleansers, disinfectants, polishes, and other personal and household products.

- Dispose of your household hazardous wastes properly. If you are not sure whether something is hazardous or don't know how to dispose of it, contact your local environmental health office or health department. Don't burn trash.
- Buy organic produce or produce that has been grown locally. Wash, scrub, and, if appropriate, peel fruits and vegetables. Consider eating less meat; animal products require more pesticides, fertilizer, water, and energy to produce.
- If you must use pesticides or toxic household products, store them in a locked place. Don't measure chemicals with food-preparation utensils, and wear gloves whenever handling them.
- If you have your house fumigated for pest control, be sure to hire a licensed exterminator. Keep everyone, including pets, out of the house while the crew works and, if possible, for a few days after.

RADIATION

Radiation can come in different forms and from different sources, such as the sun, uranium, and nuclear weapons. Of most concern to health are gamma rays produced by radioactive sources such as nuclear weapons, nuclear energy plants, and radon gas; these high-energy waves are powerful enough to penetrate objects and break molecular bonds. Although gamma radiation cannot be seen or felt, its effects at high doses can include **radiation sickness** and death; at lower doses, chromosome damage, sterility, tissue damage, cataracts, and cancer can occur. Other types of radiation can also affect health; for example, exposure to UV radiation from the sun or from tanning salons can increase the risk of skin cancer. The effects of some sources of radiation, such as cell phones, remain controversial.

Nuclear weapons pose a health risk of the most serious kind to all species. Reducing the stockpiles of nuclear weapons is a challenge and a goal for the twenty-first century. Power-generating plants that use nuclear fuel also pose health problems. When **nuclear power** was first developed as an alternative to oil and coal, it was promoted

TERMS

radiation   Energy transmitted in the form of rays, waves, or particles.

radiation sickness   An illness caused by excess radiation exposure, marked by low white blood cell counts and nausea; possibly fatal.

nuclear power   The use of controlled nuclear reactions to produce steam, which in turn drives turbines to produce electricity.

Ask Yourself

QUESTIONS FOR CRITICAL THINKING AND REFLECTION

Are there any hazardous chemicals in your home, such as cleaning products, solvents, paint, or batteries? Would you know what to do if one of these chemicals spilled? How would you clean it up?

as clean, efficient, inexpensive, and safe. In general, this has proven to be the case. However, despite all the built-in safeguards and regulating agencies, accidents in nuclear power plants do happen, and the consequences of such accidents are far more serious than those of similar accidents in other types of power-generating plants. An additional, enormous problem is disposing of the radioactive wastes these plants generate. To date, no storage method has been devised that can provide infallible, infinitely durable shielding for nuclear waste. Despite these problems, nuclear power is gaining favor again as an alternative to fossil fuels.

Medical Uses of Radiation

Another area of concern is the use of radiation in medicine, primarily the X ray. Studies have revealed that X ray exposure is cumulative and that no exposure is absolutely safe. From a personal health point of view, no one should ever have a "routine" X ray examination. Each such exam should have a definite purpose, and its benefits and risks should be carefully weighed.

Cell Phones and Radon

A controversy exists today about the effect of radiation from cell phones, which use electromagnetic waves (radio frequency radiation) to send and receive signals. The radiation is not directional, meaning that it travels in all direction equally, including toward the user. Factors such as the type of digital signal coding in the network, the antenna and handset design, and the position of the phone relative to the head all determine how much radiation is absorbed by the user. Because studies to date have not been conclusive, the CDC is beginning a long-term study to determine whether cell phone use exposes users to harmful levels of radiation.

Another area of concern is **radon,** a naturally occurring radioactive gas found in certain soils, rocks, and building materials. When the breakdown products of radon are inhaled, they cling to lungs and bombard sensitive tissue with radioactivity. Radon can enter a home by rising through the soil into the basement through dirt floors, cracks, and other openings. Problem levels can be dealt with through such measures as sealing cracks or installing basement ventilation systems.

Avoiding Radiation

- Use sunscreen to protect yourself from the sun's UV radiation.

- Get X rays only when absolutely necessary, and keep a record of the date and location of every X ray you get.
- Used a hands-free device or wired headset when using your cell phone whenever possible, and carry your phone at least 1 inch from your body.

NOISE POLLUTION

Loud noise in the environment can cause both hearing loss and stress. Prolonged exposure to sounds above 80–85 **decibels** (a measure of the intensity of a sound wave) can cause permanent hearing loss. Hearing damage can occur after 8 hours of exposure to sounds louder than 80 decibels. Regular exposure for longer than 1 minute to more than 100 decibels can cause permanent hearing loss. Children may suffer damage to their hearing at lower noise levels than adults.

Two common sources of excessive noise are the workplace and large gatherings of people at sporting events and concerts. The Occupational Safety and Health Administration (OSHA) sets legal standards for noise in the workplace, but no laws exist regulating noise levels at rock concerts, which can be much louder than most workplaces. Here are some ways to avoid exposing yourself to excessive noise:

- Wear ear protectors when working around noisy machinery.
- When listening to music on a headset with a volume range of 1–10, keep the volume no louder than 6; your headset is too loud if you are unable to hear people around you speaking in a normal tone of voice. Earbuds should not be used more than 30 minutes a day unless the volume is set below 60% of maximum; headphones can be used up to 1 hour.
- Avoid loud music. Don't sit or stand near speakers or amplifiers at a concert, and don't play a car radio or stereo so high that you can't hear the traffic.

YOU AND THE ENVIRONMENT

Faced with a vast array of confusing and complex environmental issues, you may feel overwhelmed and conclude that there isn't anything you can do about global problems. But this is not true. If everyone made individual changes in his or her life, the impact would be tremendous.

radon   A naturally occurring radioactive gas emitted from rocks and natural building materials that can become concentrated in insulated homes, causing lung cancer.

decibel   A unit for expressing the relative intensity of sounds on a scale from 0 for the average least perceptible sound to about 120 for the average pain threshold.

TERMS

TIPS FOR TODAY AND THE FUTURE

Environmental health involves protecting ourselves from environmental dangers and protecting the environment from the dangers created by humans.

RIGHT NOW YOU CAN

- Turn off the lights, televisions, and stereos in any unoccupied rooms.
- Turn off power strips when not in operation.
- Turn down the heat a few degrees and put on a sweater, or turn off the air conditioner and change into cooler clothes.
- Check your trash for recyclable items and take them out for recycling. If your town does not provide curbside pickup for recyclable items, find out where the nearest community recycling center is.

IN THE FUTURE YOU CAN

- As your existing light bulbs burn out, replace them with compact fluorescent light bulbs.
- Have your car checked to make sure it runs as well as it can and puts out the lowest amount of polluting emissions possible.
- Go online and find one of the many calculators available that can help you estimate your environmental footprint. After calculating your footprint, figure out ways to reduce it.

Connect to your Choices

Have you ever thought about where you get your behaviors and habits related to the environment? Many factors can influence our behaviors and habits, some not as obvious as others. When you were growing up, was your family aware of environmental issues and respectful of the environment? Do people in your peer group dispose of their trash when they're outdoors, or do they leave trash behind? Does your school promote environmental awareness and action, such as by participating in the green campus movement, providing for the proper recycling of old computers, cell phones, and other e-waste, and celebrating Earth Day in meaningful ways?

What are the external factors that influence your choices about the environment? What are your inner motivations and core values, and how do they affect your choices? Based on what you learned in this chapter, will you make some different choices in the future? If so, what will they be?

Go online to Connect to complete this activity. www.mcgraw-hillconnect.com

Following the suggestions throughout this chapter will help you make a difference in the environment. In addition, you can become a part of larger community action by sharing what you learn about environmental issues with your friends and family, joining, supporting, or volunteering your time to organizations working on environmental causes that are important to you.

SUMMARY

- Environmental health encompasses all the interactions of humans with their environment and the health consequences of those interactions.

- Factors that may eventually limit human population are food, availability of land and water, energy, and minimum acceptable standard of living.

- Increased amounts of air pollutants are especially dangerous for children, older adults, and people with chronic health problems.

- Heavy motor vehicle traffic, hot weather, and stagnant air contribute to the development of smog.

- Carbon dioxide and other natural gases act as a greenhouse around the earth, increasing the temperature of the atmosphere. Levels of these gases are rising through human activity; as a result, the world's climate could change.

- Environmental damage from energy use can be limited through energy conservation and the development of nonpolluting, renewable sources of energy.

- Indoor pollutants can trigger allergies and illness in the short term and cancer in the long term.

- Concerns with water quality focus on pathogenic organisms and hazardous chemicals from industry and households, as well as on water shortages.

- Sewage treatment prevents pathogens from contaminating drinking water; it often must also deal with heavy metals and hazardous chemicals.

- The amount of garbage is growing all the time; paper is the biggest component. Recycling can help reduce solid waste disposal problems.

- Potentially hazardous chemical pollutants include asbestos, lead, pesticides, mercury, and many household products. Proper handling and disposal are critical.

- Radiation can cause radiation sickness, chromosome damage, and cancer, among other health problems.

- Loud or persistent noise can lead to hearing loss and/or stress.

FOR MORE INFORMATION

BOOKS

Ausenda, F. 2009. *Green Volunteers: The World Guide to Voluntary Work in Nature Conservation*, 7th ed. New York: Universe. *Describes a variety of opportunities to volunteer for environmental causes, in many different parts of the world.*

Cunningham, W. P., et al. 2009. *Environmental Science: A Global Concern*, 11th ed. New York: McGraw-Hill. *A nontechnical survey of basic environmental science and key concerns.*

Maslin, M. 2009. *Global Warming: A Very Short Introduction*, 2nd ed. New York: Oxford University Press. *A survey of the science and politics of global warming.*

Nadakavukaren, A. 2005. *Our Global Environment: A Health Perspective*, 6th ed. Prospect Heights, Ill.: Waveland Press. *A broad survey of major environmental issues and their effects on personal and community health.*

Wright, R. T. 2010. *Environmental Science: Toward a Sustainable Future*. New York: Pearson. *An easy-to-read introduction to the realm of environmental science and its importance to our future.*

ORGANIZATIONS, HOTLINES, AND WEB SITES

CDC National Center for Environmental Health. Provides brochures and fact sheets on a variety of environmental issues.

http://www.cdc.gov/nceh/default.htm

Earth Times. An international online newspaper devoted to global environmental issues.

http://www.earthtimes.org

Ecological Footprint. Calculates your personal ecological footprint based on your diet, transportation patterns, and living arrangements.

http://www.myfootprint.org

Fuel Economy. Provides information on the fuel economy of cars made since 1985 and tips on improving gas mileage.

http://www.fueleconomy.gov

Indoor Air Quality Information Hotline. Answers questions, provides publications, and makes referrals.

800-438-4318

National Lead Information Center. Provides information packets and specialist advice.

http://www.epa.gov/lead/index.html

National Oceanic and Atmospheric Administration (NOAA): Climate. Provides information on a variety of issues related to climate, including global warming, drought, and El Niño and La Niña.

http://www.noaa.gov/climate.html

National Safety Council Environmental Health Center. Provides information on lead, radon, indoor air quality, hazardous chemicals, and other environmental issues.

http://www.nsc.org/international/env_hth_sty/Pages/
EnvironmentalHealthSafety.aspx

Student Environmental Action Coalition (SEAC). A coalition of student and youth environmental groups; the Web site has contact information for local groups.

http://www.seac.org

United Nations. Several U.N. programs are devoted to environmental problems on a global scale; the Web sites provide information on current and projected trends and on international treaties developed to deal with environmental issues.

http://www.un.org/popin (Population Information Network)
http://www.unep.org (Environment Programme)

U.S. Department of Energy: Energy Efficiency and Renewable Energy (EERE). Provides information about alternative fuels and tips for saving energy at home and in your car.

http://www.eere.energy.gov/

U.S. Environmental Protection Agency (EPA). Provides information about EPA activities and many consumer-oriented materials. The Web site includes special sites devoted to global warming, ozone loss, pesticides, and other areas of concern.

http://www.epa.gov

Worldwatch Institute. A public policy research organization focusing on emerging global environmental problems and the links between the world economy and the environment.

http://www.worldwatch.org

There are many national and international organizations working on environmental health problems. A few of the largest and best known are listed below:

Greenpeace: 800-326-0959; http://www.greenpeace.org
National Audubon Society: 212-979-3000; http://www .audubon.org
National Wildlife Federation: 800-822-9919; http://www.nwf.org
Nature Conservancy: 800-628-6860; http://www.nature.org
Sierra Club: 415-977-5500; http://www.sierraclub.org
World Wildlife Fund—U.S.: 800-960-0993; http://www .worldwildlife.org

SELECTED BIBLIOGRAPHY

CDC National Center for Environmental Health. 2010. *Lead* (http://www.cdc.gov/nceh/lead/; retrieved October 8, 2010).

Centers for Disease Control and Prevention. 2006. Adult blood lead epidemiology and surveillance—United States, 2003–2004. *Morbidity and Mortality Weekly Report* 55(32): 876–879.

Centers for Disease Control and Prevention. 2008. Surveillance for waterborne disease and outbreaks associated with drinking water and water not intended for drinking—United States, 2005–2006. *Morbidity and Mortality Weekly Report* 55(SS12): 31–58.

Delworth-Bart, J. E., and C. F. Moore. 2006. Mercy mercy me: Social injustice and the prevention of environmental pollutant exposures among ethnic minority and poor children. *Child Development* 77(2): 247–265.

Dominici, F., et al. 2006. Fine particulate air pollution and hospital admission for cardiovascular and respiratory diseases. *Journal of the American Medical Association* 295(10): 1127–1134.

Energy Information Administration. 2005. *Impacts of Modeled Recommendations of the National Commission on Energy Policy.* Washington, D.C.: U.S. Department of Energy.

Energy Information Agency. 2010. *Gasoline and Diesel Fuel Update* (http://tonto.eia.doe.gov/oog/info/gdu/gasdiesel.asp; retrieved October 8, 2009).

Environmental Protection Agency. 2010. *Municipal Solid Waste* (http://www.epa.gov/waste/nonhaz/municipal/index.htm; retrieved October 8, 2009).

Kunzli, N., et al. 2005. Ambient air pollution and atherosclerosis in Los Angeles. *Environmental Health Perspectives* 113(2): 201–206.

Laden, F., et al. 2006. Reduction in fine particulate air pollution and mortality: Extended follow-up of the Harvard Six Cities study. *American Journal of Respiratory and Critical Care Medicine* 173(6): 667–672.

The National Academies. 2006. *Surface Temperature Reconstructions for the Last 2,000 Years.* Washington, D.C.: National Academies Press.

National Oceanic and Atmospheric Administration. 2008. *Billion Dollar U.S. Weather Disasters, 1980–2007* (http://www.ncdc.noaa.gov/oa/reports/billionz.html; retrieved October 8, 2010).

Parker, J. D., et al. 2005. Air pollution and birth weight among term infants in California. *Pediatrics* 115(1): 121–128.

Trasande, L., P. J. Landrigan, and C. Schechter. 2005. Public health and economic consequences of methylmercury toxicity to the developing brain. *Environmental Health Perspectives* online, 28 February.

United Nations Population Division. 2009. *World Population Prospects: The 2009 Revision.* New York: United Nations.

Virtanen, J. K., et al. 2005. Mercury, fish oils, and risk of acute coronary events and cardiovascular disease, coronary heart disease, and all-cause mortality in men in eastern Finland. *Arteriosclerosis, Thrombosis, and Vascular Biology* 25(1): 228–233.

World Health Organization. 2010. Cholera, 2010. *Weekly Epidemiological Record* 85(13): 1177–1128.

World Health Organization. 2006. *Fuel for Life: Household Energy and Health.* Geneva: WHO Press.

Worldwatch Institute. 2010. *Vital Signs 2010.* New York: Norton.

LOOKING AHEAD...

After reading this chapter, you should be able to:

- Explain the self-care decision-making process and discuss options for self-treatment
- Describe the basic premises, practices, and providers of conventional medicine
- Describe the basic premises, practices, and providers of complementary and alternative medicine
- Explain how to communicate effectively with health care providers and to use their input when evaluating different types of treatment
- Discuss different types of health insurance plans

Conventional and Complementary Medicine

15

Today, people are becoming more empowered and confident in their ability to solve personal health problems on their own. People who manage their own health care gather information and learn skills from a variety of resources; they solicit opinions and advice, make decisions, and take action. They know how to practice safe, effective self-care, and they know how to make decisions about professional medical care, whether conventional Western medicine or complementary and alternative medicine.

This chapter will help you develop the skills both to identify and manage medical problems and to make the health care system work effectively for you.

SELF-CARE

Effectively managing medical problems involves developing several skills. First, you need to learn to be a good observer of your own body and assess your symptoms.

You also must be able to decide when to seek professional advice and when you can safely deal with the problem on your own. You need to know how to safely and effectively self-treat common medical problems. Finally, you need to know how to develop a partnership with physicians and other health care providers and how to carry out treatment plans.

Self-Assessment

Symptoms are often an expression of the body's attempt to heal itself. A fever may be an attempt to make the body less hospitable to infectious agents. A cough can help clear the airways and protect the lungs. Carefully observing symptoms also lets you identify those signals that suggest you need professional assistance. Begin by noting when the symptom began, how often and when it occurs, what makes it worse, what makes it better, and whether you have any associated symptoms or illnesses. You can also monitor your body's vital signs, such as temperature and heart rate. Medical self-tests for blood pressure, blood sugar, pregnancy detection, and urinary tract infections can also help you make a more informed decision about when to seek medical help and when to self-treat.

Knowing When to See a Physician

In general, you should see a physician for symptoms that you would describe as follows:

1. *Severe.* If the symptom is very severe or intense, medical assistance is advised. Examples include severe pains, major injuries, and other emergencies.

2. *Unusual.* If the symptom is peculiar and unfamiliar, it is wise to check it out with your physician. Examples include unexplained lumps, changes in a mole, problems with vision, difficulty swallowing, numbness, weakness, unexplained weight loss, and blood in sputum, urine, or stool.

3. *Persistent.* If the symptom lasts longer than expected, seek medical advice. Examples in adults include fever for more than 5 days, a cough lasting longer than 2 weeks, a sore that doesn't heal within a month, and hoarseness lasting longer than 3 weeks.

4. *Recurrent.* If a symptom tends to return again and again, medical evaluation is advised. Examples include recurrent headaches, stomach pains, and backache.

Sometimes a single symptom is not a cause for concern, but when the symptom is accompanied by other symptoms, the combination suggests a more serious problem. For example, a fever with a stiff neck suggests meningitis.

If you think that you need professional help, you must decide how urgent the problem is. If it is a true emergency, go (or call someone to take you) to the nearest emergency department (ED). Emergencies include the following:

- Major trauma or injury, such as head injury, suspected broken bone, deep wound, severe burn, eye injury, or animal bite
- Uncontrollable bleeding or internal bleeding, as indicated by blood in the sputum, vomit, or stool
- Intolerable and uncontrollable pain or severe chest pain
- Severe shortness of breath
- Persistent abdominal pain, especially if associated with nausea and vomiting
- Poisoning or drug overdose
- Loss of consciousness or seizure
- Stupor, drowsiness, or disorientation that cannot be explained
- Severe or worsening reaction to an insect bite or sting or to a medication, especially if breathing is difficult

If your problem is not an emergency but still requires medical attention, call your physician's office. Often you can be given medical advice over the phone without the inconvenience of a visit.

Self-Treatment

In most cases, your body itself can relieve your symptoms and heal the disorder. Patience and careful self-observation are often the best choices in self-treatment. Nondrug options can be easy, inexpensive, safe, and highly effective. For example, massage, ice packs, and neck exercises may at times be more helpful than drugs in relieving headaches and other pains. Getting adequate rest, increasing exercise, drinking more water, eating more or less of certain foods, using humidifiers, changes in ergonomics when working at a desk, and so on are just some of the hundreds of nondrug options for preventing or relieving many common health problems. For a variety of disorders caused or aggravated by stress, the treatment of choice may be relaxation or other stress-management strategies (see the box "The Health Benefits of Expressive Writing").

Self-Medication Self-treatment with nonprescription medications is an important part of health care. Nonprescription or **over-the-counter (OTC) medications** are medicines that the Food and Drug Administration (FDA) has determined are safe for use without a physician's prescription. There are more than 100,000 OTC drugs on the market; about 60% of all medications are sold over the counter. Hundreds of products sold over the counter today use ingredients or dosage strengths available only by prescription 20 years ago. With this increased consumer choice, however, comes increased consumer responsibility for using OTC drugs safely.

Although many OTC products are effective, others are unnecessary or divert attention from better ways of coping.

Many ingredients in OTC drugs have not been proven effective, a fact the FDA does not dispute.

over-the-counter (OTC) medication A medication or product that can be purchased by the consumer without a prescription.

The Health Benefits of Expressive Writing

The act of writing down feelings and thoughts about stressful life events has been shown to help people improve their health. Investigators remain unsure why writing about one's feelings has beneficial effects. It may be that expressing feelings about a traumatic event helps people work through the event and put it behind them. The resulting sense of release and control may reduce stress levels and have positive physical effects such as reduced heart rate and blood pressure and improved immune function. Alternatively, expressive writing may change the way people think about previous stressful events in their lives and help them cope with new stressors. Whatever the cause, it's clear that expressive writing can be a safe, inexpensive, and effective supplement to standard treatment of certain chronic illnesses.

What about the effects of expressive writing on otherwise healthy individuals? Other studies have found a similar benefit: People who wrote about traumatic experiences reported fewer symptoms, fewer days off work, fewer visits to the doctor, improved mood, and a more positive outlook.

If you'd like to try expressive writing to help you deal with a traumatic event, set aside a special time—15 minutes a day for 4 consecutive days, for example, or 1 day a week for 4 weeks. Write in a place where you won't be interrupted or distracted. Explore your very deepest thoughts and feelings and why you feel the way you do. Don't worry about grammar or coherence or about what someone else might think about what you're writing; you are writing just for yourself. You may find the writing exercise to be distressing in the short term—sadness and depression are common when dealing with feelings about a stressful event—but most people report relief and contentment soon after writing for several days.

Many ingredients in OTC drugs—perhaps 70%—have not been proven to be effective. And any drug may have risks and side effects. Follow these simple guidelines to self-medicate safely:

1. Always read labels and follow directions carefully. The information on most OTC drug labels now appears in a standard format developed by the FDA (Figure 15.1).

2. Do not exceed the recommended dosage or length of treatment unless you discuss this change with your physician.

3. Use caution if you are taking other medications or supplements, because OTC drugs and herbal supplements can interact with some prescription drugs. If you have questions about drug interactions, ask your physician or pharmacist *before* you mix medicines.

4. Try to select medications with one active ingredient rather than combination products. A product with multiple ingredients is likely to include drugs for symptoms you don't even have.

5. When choosing medications, try to buy **generic drugs,** which contain the same active ingredient as the brand-name product but generally at a much lower cost.

6. Never take or give a drug from an unlabeled container or when you can't read the label.

7. If you are pregnant or nursing or have a chronic condition such as kidney or liver disease, consult your health care provider before self-medicating.

8. The expiration date marked on many medications is an estimate of how long the medication is likely to be safe and effective. However, an extensive study by the FDA found that 90% of all prescription and OTC medications are potent for several years after their stated expiration date. Exceptions include the antibiotic tetracycline, liquid antibiotics, nitroglycerine, and insulin. Expiration dates are very conservative. If you have any question about a medicine's expiration date, ask a pharmacist.

9. Store your medications in a cool, dry place that is out of the reach of children.

10. Use special caution with aspirin. Because of an association with a rare but serious problem known as Reye's syndrome, aspirin should not be used by children or adolescents who may have the flu, chicken pox, or any other viral illness. Outdated aspirin that has an acidic odor should be discarded.

Ask Yourself

QUESTIONS FOR CRITICAL THINKING AND REFLECTION

Do you self-medicate for common medical problems, such as headaches or colds? If so, how careful are you about reading product labels and following directions? For example, would you know if you were taking two OTC medications that contained the same ingredient (such as ibuprofen) at the same time?

TERMS

generic drug A drug that is not registered or protected by a trademark; a drug that does not have an exclusive brand name.

PROFESSIONAL CARE

When self-treatment is not appropriate or sufficient, you need to seek professional medical care. The health care system is a broad network of professionals and

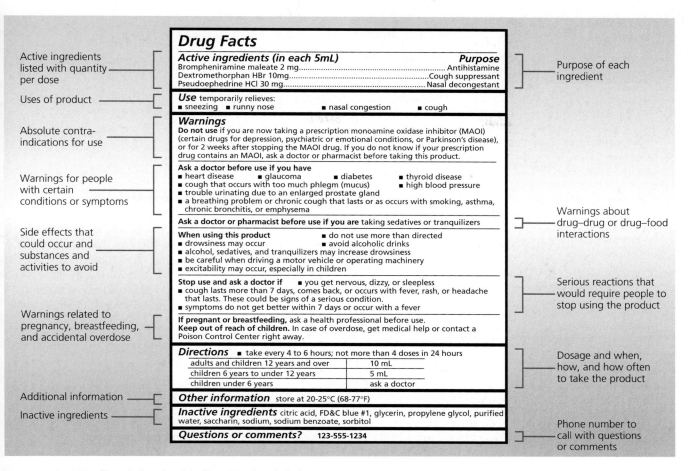

Active ingredients listed with quantity per dose

Uses of product

Absolute contra-indications for use

Warnings for people with certain conditions or symptoms

Side effects that could occur and substances and activities to avoid

Warnings related to pregnancy, breastfeeding, and accidental overdose

Additional information

Inactive ingredients

Drug Facts

Active ingredients (in each 5mL)   ***Purpose***

Brompheniramine maleate 2 mg.. Antihistamine
Dextromethorphan HBr 10mg... Cough suppressant
Pseudoephedrine HCl 30 mg... Nasal decongestant

Use temporarily relieves:
■ sneezing ■ runny nose   ■ nasal congestion   ■ cough

Warnings
Do not use if you are now taking a prescription monoamine oxidase inhibitor (MAOI) (certain drugs for depression, psychiatric or emotional conditions, or Parkinson's disease), or for 2 weeks after stopping the MAOI drug. If you do not know if your prescription drug contains an MAOI, ask a doctor or pharmacist before taking this product.

Ask a doctor before use if you have
■ heart disease   ■ glaucoma   ■ diabetes   ■ thyroid disease
■ cough that occurs with too much phlegm (mucus)   ■ high blood pressure
■ trouble urinating due to an enlarged prostate gland
■ a breathing problem or chronic cough that lasts or as occurs with smoking, asthma, chronic bronchitis, or emphysema

Ask a doctor or pharmacist before use if you are taking sedatives or tranquilizers

When using this product   ■ do not use more than directed
■ drowsiness may occur   ■ avoid alcoholic drinks
■ alcohol, sedatives, and tranquilizers may increase drowsiness
■ be careful when driving a motor vehicle or operating machinery
■ excitability may occur, especially in children

Stop use and ask a doctor if   ■ you get nervous, dizzy, or sleepless
■ cough lasts more than 7 days, comes back, or occurs with fever, rash, or headache that lasts. These could be signs of a serious condition.
■ symptoms do not get better within 7 days or occur with a fever

If pregnant or breastfeeding, ask a health professional before use.
Keep out of reach of children. In case of overdose, get medical help or contact a Poison Control Center right away.

Directions   ■ take every 4 to 6 hours; not more than 4 doses in 24 hours

adults and children 12 years and over	10 mL
children 6 years to under 12 years	5 mL
children under 6 years	ask a doctor

Other information   store at 20-25°C (68-77°F)

Inactive ingredients citric acid, FD&C blue #1, glycerin, propylene glycol, purified water, saccharin, sodium, sodium benzoate, sorbitol

Questions or comments?   **123-555-1234**

Purpose of each ingredient

Warnings about drug–drug or drug–food interactions

Serious reactions that would require people to stop using the product

Dosage and when, how, and how often to take the product

Phone number to call with questions or comments

FIGURE 15.1   Reading and understanding OTC drug labels.

SOURCE: Food and Drug Administration. 1999. Over-the-counter human drugs; Labeling requirements; final rule. *Federal Register* 64(51), 17 March, 13254–13303.

---

organizations, including independent practitioners, health care providers, hospitals, clinics, and public and private insurance programs.

In recent years, many Americans have also sought health care from practitioners of **complementary and alternative medicine (CAM),** defined as those therapies and practices that do not form part of conventional medicine, which is mainstream health care and medical practices as taught in most U.S. medical schools and offered in most U.S. hospitals. The most frequently used CAM therapies are nonvitamin, nonmineral natural products; chiropractic care; deep breathing exercises; meditation; massage, and yoga (Table 15.1). Between 2002 and 2007, there was increased use of many specific CAM treatments as well as increased use of CAM overall (see the box "Evidence Mounting for CAM Therapies"). People often use CAM therapies in addition to their conventional medical treatments, but many do not tell their physicians about it.

Complementary practices are those used *together with* conventional modalities; alternative practices are those used *instead of* conventional modalities. When an alterna-

tive modality is used, there should be a high level of evidence that it is safe and as effective as or more effective than a conventional modality, especially if the condition being treated is serious or life-threatening.

The term **integrative medicine** refers to conventional health care practices (such as physical therapy or dentistry) to which a CAM modality is added (such as hypnosis or music for relaxation). The integrative practitioner is someone who practices conventional medicine and augments it with unconventional modalities.

---

complementary and alternative medicine (CAM) Health care practices and products that are not considered part of conventional, mainstream medical practice as taught in most U.S. medical schools and available at most U.S. health care facilities; examples of CAM practices include acupuncture and herbal remedies.

integrative medicine Conventional health care practice that is sometimes augmented by unconventional (CAM) modalities.

TERMS

Table 15.1	Use of Complementary and Alternative Therapies by Adults	
		PERCENT WHO USED THERAPY IN LAST 12 MONTHS
Natural products (nonvitamin, nonmineral)		17.7
Chiropractic care		8.6
Deep breathing exercises		12.7
Meditation		9.4
Massage		8.3
Yoga		6.1
Diet-based therapies		3.6
Progressive relaxation		2.9
Acupuncture		14.4
Homeopathic treatment		1.8
Guided imagery		2.2
Tai chi		1.0
Hypnosis		0.2
Energy healing therapy/Reiki		0.5
Biofeedback		0.2
Any therapy		38.3

SOURCE: Barnes, P. M., et al. 2008. Complementary and alternative medicine use among adults: United States, 2007. *CDC National Health Statistics Report #12.* Hyattsville, Md.: National Center for Health Statistics.

Ask Yourself

QUESTIONS FOR CRITICAL THINKING AND REFLECTION

What are your views about the use of CAM treatments and therapies? What events or information have shaped those views? Would you consider using complementary or alternative medicine?

Consumers turn to CAM for a large variety of purposes related to health and well-being, such as boosting their immune system, lowering their cholesterol levels, losing weight, quitting smoking, or enhancing their memory. There are indications that people with chronic conditions, including cancer, asthma, autoimmune diseases, and HIV infection, are particularly likely to try CAM therapies. Despite their growing popularity, many CAM practices remain controversial, and consumers need to be critically aware of safety issues.

The following sections examine the principles and providers of both **conventional medicine**—the dominant medical system in the United States and Europe, also referred to as standard Western medicine or biomedicine—and complementary and alternative medicine, with particular attention to consumer issues.

TERMS

conventional medicine A system of medicine based on the application of the scientific method; diseases are thought to be caused by identifiable physical factors and characterized by a representative set of symptoms; also called biomedicine or standard Western medicine.

pharmaceuticals Medical drugs, both prescription and over-the-counter.

CONVENTIONAL MEDICINE

Referring to conventional medicine as standard Western medicine draws attention to the fact that it differs from the various medical systems that have developed in China, Japan, India, and other parts of the world. Calling it "biomedicine" reflects conventional medicine's foundation in the biological and physical sciences.

Premises and Assumptions of Conventional Medicine

One of the important characteristics of Western medicine is the belief that disease is caused by identifiable physical factors. Western medicine identifies the causes of disease as pathogens (such as bacteria and viruses), genetic factors, and unhealthy lifestyles that result in changes at the molecular and cellular levels. In most cases, the focus is primarily on the physical causes of illness rather than mental or spiritual imbalance.

Another feature that distinguishes Western biomedicine from other medical systems is the concept that every disease is defined by a certain set of symptoms and that these symptoms are similar in most patients suffering from this disease. Western medicine tends to treat illnesses as biological disturbances that can occur in human beings, rather than as integral in some way to the individual with the illness.

Related to the idea of illness as the result of invasion by outside factors is the strong orientation toward methods of destroying pathogens or preventing them from causing serious infection. The public health measures of the nineteenth and twentieth centuries—chlorination of drinking water, sewage disposal, food safety regulations, vaccination programs, education about hygiene, and so on—are an outgrowth of this orientation.

The implementation of public health measures is one way to control pathogens; another is the use of drugs and surgery. The discovery and development of sulfa drugs, antibiotics, and steroids in the twentieth century, along with advances in chemistry that made it possible to identify the active ingredients in common plant-derived remedies, paved the way for the current close identification of Western medicine with **pharmaceuticals** (medical drugs, both prescription and over-the-counter). Western medicine also

CAM therapies are slowly but steadily gaining momentum in the United States, as new evidence emerges about the potential value of certain practices and both consumers and health care professionals take notice. According to the National Institutes of Health, nearly 40% of Americans have tried one or more alternative therapies, either in conjunction with or instead of standard Western health care techniques. More than 40 major American universities have added integrative medical centers to their facilities and begun offering courses on integrative therapies to medical students. Although research studies on CAM modalities have been relatively small in size and conservative in their conclusions, some of their results are promising.

Tai Chi and Fibromyalgia

A once mysterious and misunderstood disorder, fibromyalgia causes chronic pain throughout the body and general fatigue. It can be treated with drugs, but exercise is an important component of fibromyalgia therapy because it helps the sufferer maintain muscle strength and build stamina.

Tai chi has long been known to offer many benefits, including gains in strength, flexibility, and stamina, and now it has been shown to be helpful in pain management. A 2010 study published in *The New England Journal of Medicine* tracked the symptoms of two groups of fibromyalgia patients: one that learned a variety of tai chi movements and another that practiced stretching exercises and received wellness counseling. Over the course of the study, the patients who studied tai chi reported significantly less pain than the other group, and the benefits lasted well beyond the study's end.

In another 2010 study, researchers undertook a comprehensive review of existing studies involving tai chi and qigong (a similar practice) to determine whether evidence consistently supported claims that the two practices yield health benefits. In more than 60 studies involving nearly 6500 participants, both tai chi and qigong appeared to enhance cardiorespiratory health, bone health, balance, and overall quality of life. The researchers concluded that tai chi and qigong may be excellent alternatives to conventional forms of exercise for some people.

CAM Therapies and Back Pain

CAM therapies are used more often to treat back pain than for any other condition. A 2010 study showed that about 6% of adult Americans who suffer back pain have tried at least one form of alternative therapy in the hope of finding relief. The therapies most commonly used for back pain are chiropractic, massage, yoga, tai chi, qigong, and acupuncture.

In this study, more than 50% of respondents said they elected to try CAM because conventional medical treatments weren't providing adequate pain relief. Nearly two-thirds said they experienced significantly reduced pain as a result of CAM therapy. Notably, only about one-fourth of the respondents reported getting a doctor's referral to a CAM practitioner.

Chiropractic and Headaches

A new study shows that a specific type of chiropractic technique—called spinal manipulative therapy (SMT)—can be particularly helpful for people who suffer from chronic headaches, especially headaches related to neck problems. The study compared the effects of SMT to those of light massage among two groups of patients who suffered frequent, severe headaches. The group that underwent spinal manipulative therapy from an experienced chiropractor reported less pain and fewer headaches than the group that had light massages. Significantly, the SMT group reported suffering half as many headaches as the massage group during a 24-week period of follow-up.

Despite growing evidence, physicians still advise consumers to use caution when considering any CAM therapy, especially one that has not been studied extensively or that involves the use of herbal remedies. An ever-growing number of studies casts suspicion on the safety and effectiveness of herbal supplements used to treat medical conditions.

SOURCES: Jahnke, R., et al. A comprehensive review of health benefits of qigong and tai chi. *American Journal of Health Promotion* 24(6): e1–e25; Kanodia, A. K., et al. 2010. Perceived benefit of complementary and alternative medicine (CAM) for back pain: A national survey. *Journal of the American Board of Family Medicine* 23(3): 354–362; Voice of America News. 2010. *Almost Half of Americans Use Alternative Medicine* (http://www1.voanews.com/english/news/american-life/Almost-Half-of-Americans-Use-Alternative-Medicine-100980909.html; retrieved August 19, 2010); Wang, C., et al. 2010. A randomized trial of tai chi for fibromyalgia. *New England Journal of Medicine* 363(8): 743–754.

relies heavily on surgery and on advanced medical technology to discover a physical cause of a person's disease and to correct, remove, or destroy it.

Further, Western medicine is based on the scientific method of obtaining knowledge and explaining health-related phenomena. Scientific explanations are:

- *Empirical*—they are based on the evidence of the senses and on objective and systematic observation, often carried out under carefully controlled conditions; they must be capable of verification by others.
- *Rational*—they follow the rules of logic and are consistent with known facts.
- *Testable*—either they are verifiable through direct observation or they lead to predictions about what should occur under conditions not yet observed.
- *Parsimonious*—they explain phenomena with the smallest number of causes.
- *General*—they have broad explanatory power.
- *Rigorously evaluated*—they are constantly evaluated for consistency with the evidence and known principles, for parsimony, and for generality.
- *Tentative*—scientists are willing to entertain the possibility that their explanations are faulty, based on new, better, or connected evidence.

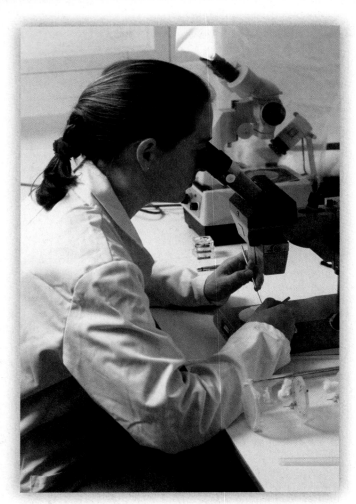

Conventional Western medicine is grounded in scientific explanations resulting from the application of the scientific method or through observable outcomes in randomized controlled studies.

Western medicine translates the scientific method into practice through the research process, a highly refined and well-established approach to exploring the causes of disease and ensuring the safety and efficacy of treatments. Research

ranges from case studies—descriptions of a single patient's illness and treatment—to randomized controlled trials (RTCs) conducted on large populations. The process of drug development is equally rigorous. Drugs are developed and tested through an elaborate course that begins with preliminary research in the lab and continues through trials with human participants, review and approval by the FDA, and monitoring of the drug's effects even after it is on the market. The process may take 12 years or more, and only about 20% of drugs are eventually approved for marketing.

When results of research studies are published in medical journals, a community of scientists, physicians, researchers, and scholars has the opportunity to share the findings and enter a dialogue about the subject. Publication of research often prompts further research designed to replicate and confirm the findings, challenge the conclusions, or pursue a related line of thought or experiment. (See the box "Evaluating Health News.")

The Providers of Conventional Medicine

Conventional medicine is practiced by a wide range of health care professionals in the United States. Several kinds of professionals are permitted to practice specific fields of medicine independently, including medical doctors, osteopaths, podiatrists, optometrists, and dentists.

- **Medical doctors** are practitioners who hold a doctor of medicine (M.D.) degree from an accredited medical school. In the United States, an education in medicine involves 7 to 11 years of study and residency beyond 4 years of undergraduate premedical education.
- **Doctors of osteopathic medicine** (D.O.) receive a medical education similar to that of medical doctors, but their training places special emphasis on musculoskeletal problems and manipulative therapy. M.D.s and D.O.s are the two types of "complete" physicians in the United States, meaning they are trained and licensed to perform surgery and prescribe medication.
- **Podiatrists** are practitioners who specialize in the medical and surgical care of the feet. They hold a doctor of podiatric medicine (D.P.M.) degree.
- **Optometrists** are practitioners trained to examine the eyes, detect eye diseases, and treat vision problems. They hold a doctor of optometry (O.D.) degree.
- **Dentists** specialize in the care of the teeth and mouth. They are graduates of 4-year dental schools and hold the doctor of dental surgery (D.D.S.) or doctor of medical dentistry (D.M.D.) degree.

In addition to these practitioners, there are millions of other trained health care professionals, known as

STATS

Nearly **6.9 million** health care professionals of all types work in the United States.

—U.S. Bureau of Labor Statistics, 2008

Evaluating Health News

Media reports of health-related research studies may oversimplify or exaggerate the results and their meaning to consumers. Researchers do not set out to mislead people, but they must often strike a balance between reporting promising preliminary findings to the public, thereby allowing people to act on them, and waiting 10–20 years until long-term studies confirm (or disprove) a particular finding.

The following questions can help you better assess the health advice that appears in the popular media:

1. *Is the report based on research or on an anecdote?* Information or advice based on one or more carefully designed research studies has more validity than one person's experiences.

2. *What is the source of the information?* A study published in a respected peer-reviewed journal has been examined by editors and other researchers in the field, people who are in a position to evaluate the merits of a study and its results. Many journal articles also include information on the authors and funders of research, alerting readers to any possible conflicts of interest. Research presented at medical meetings should be considered preliminary because the results have not yet undergone a thorough prepublication review; many such studies are never published. It is also wise to ask who funded a study to determine whether there is any potential for bias. Information from universities, government agencies, and national research organizations is usually considered fairly reliable.

3. *How big was the study?* A study involving many subjects is more likely to yield reliable results than a study involving only a few subjects. Another important indication that a finding is meaningful is if several studies conducted by different investigators at different institutions yield the same results.

4. *Who were the participants involved in the study?* Research findings are more likely to apply to you if you share important characteristics with the participants in the study. For example, the results of a study on men over age 50 who smoke may not be particularly meaningful for a 30-year-old nonsmoking woman.

5. *What kind of study was it?* Epidemiological studies involve observation or interviews in order to trace the relationships among lifestyle, physical characteristics, and diseases. While epidemiological studies can suggest links, they do not necessarily establish cause-and-effect relationships. Clinical or interventional studies or trials involve testing the effects of different treatments on groups of people who have similar lifestyles and characteristics. They are more likely to provide conclusive evidence of a cause-and-effect relationship. The best interventional studies share the following characteristics:

- *Controlled.* A group of people who receive the treatment is compared with a comparable group of people (called a *control group*) who do not receive the treatment. The control group receives a placebo and the treatment group receives the treatment being studied.

- *Randomized.* The treatment and control groups are selected randomly.

- *Double-blind.* Researchers and participants are unaware of who is receiving the treatment.

- *Multicenter.* The experiment is performed at more than one institution.

A third type of study, meta-analysis, involves combining the results of individual studies to get an overall view of the effectiveness of a treatment.

6. *What do the statistics really say?* If a study is large and well designed, its results can be deemed statistically significant, meaning there is a 5% or lower chance that the findings resulted from chance.

7. *Is new health advice being offered?* If the media report new guidelines for health behavior or medical treatment, examine the source. Government agencies and national research foundations usually consider a great deal of evidence before offering health advice. Above all, use common sense, and check with your physician before making a major change in your health habits based on news reports.

SOURCES: Stevens, L. M. 2006. Medical journals. *Journal of the American Medical Association* 295(15): 1860; Nemours Foundation. 2006. *Figuring Out Health News* (http://www.kidshealth.org/teen/safety/safebasics/healthnews.html; retrieved September 17, 2006); Tufts University. 2006. Studying research studies: 10 questions you need to ask. *Tufts University Health and Nutrition Letter*, June, 4–5; Patient Inform. 2005. *Understanding Medical Research: What to Look for When Reading Medical Research* (http://www.patientinform.org/understanding-medical-research/; retrieved September 17, 2006).

---

allied health care providers, working in the United States. They include registered nurses (R.N.s), licensed vocational nurses (L.V.N.s), physical therapists, social workers, registered dietitians (R.D.s), physician assistants (P.A.s), nurse practitioners, and certified nurse midwives.

Choosing a Primary Care Physician

Most experts believe it is best to have a primary care physician, someone who gets to know you, who coordinates your medical care, and who refers you to specialists when you need them. Primary care physicians include those certified in family practice, internal medicine, pediatrics, and gynecology. These physicians are able to diagnose and treat the vast majority of common health problems; they also provide many preventive health services. The best time to look for a physician is before you are sick.

> **allied health care providers** Health care professionals who typically provide services under the supervision or control of independent practitioners.

TERMS

To select a physician, begin by making a list of possible choices. If your insurance limits the health care providers you can see, check the plan's list first. Ask for recommendations from family, friends, coworkers, local medical societies, and the physician referral service at a local clinic or hospital. Once you have the names of a few physicians you might want to try, call their offices to find out information such as the following:

- Is the physician covered by your health plan and accepting new patients?
- What are the office hours, and when is the physician or office staff available? What do patients do if they need urgent care or have an emergency?
- Which hospitals does the physician use?
- How many other physicians are available to cover when he or she isn't available, and who are they?
- How long does it usually take to get a routine appointment?
- Does the physician (or a nurse or physician assistant) give advice over the phone for common problems?

Schedule a visit with the physician you think you would most like to use. During that first visit, you'll get a sense of how well matched you are and how well he or she might meet your medical needs.

Getting the Most Out of Your Medical Care

The key to making the health care system work for you lies in good communication with your physician and other members of the health care team.

The Physician-Patient Partnership   The physician-patient relationship is undergoing an important transformation. The image of the all-knowing physician and the passive patient is fading. What is emerging is a physician-patient *partnership,* in which the physician acts more like a consultant and the patient participates more actively. You should expect your physician to be attentive, caring, and able to listen and clearly explain things to you. You also must do your part. You need to be assertive in a firm but nonaggressive manner. You need to express your feelings and concerns, ask questions, and, if necessary, be persistent. If your physician is unable to communicate clearly with you despite your best efforts, you probably need to change physicians.

Your Appointment with Your Physician   Prepare for your visit ahead of time by making a list of your key concerns and questions, along with notes about your symptoms. Present your concerns at the beginning of the visit, to set the agenda. Be specific and concise about your symptoms, and be open and honest about your concerns. Let your physician know if you are taking any drugs, are allergic to any medications, are breast-feeding, or may be pregnant. At the end of the visit, briefly repeat the physician's diagnosis, prognosis, and instructions. Make sure you understand your next steps.

The Diagnostic Process   The first step in the diagnostic process is the medical history, including the primary reason for your visit, your current symptoms, your past medical history, and your social history (job, family life, major stressors, living conditions, and health habits). Keeping up-to-date records of your medical history can help you provide your physician with key facts about your health.

The next step is the physical exam, which usually begins with a review of vital signs: blood pressure, heart rate (pulse), breathing rate, and temperature. Depending on your primary complaint, your physician may give you a complete physical, or the exam may be directed to specific areas, such as your ears, nose, and throat.

Additionally, your physician may order medical tests to complete the diagnosis. Physicians can order X rays, biopsies, blood and urine tests, scans, and **endoscopies** to view, probe, or analyze almost any part of the body. If your physician orders a test for you, be sure you know why you need it, what the risks and benefits of the test are for you, how you should prepare for it, and what the test will involve. Also ask what the test results mean, because no test is 100% accurate—**false positives** and **false negatives** do occur—and interpretation of some tests is subjective.

Medical and Surgical Treatments   Many conditions can be treated in a variety of ways; in some cases, lifestyle changes are enough. In other cases, physicians prescribe a medication. Thousands of lives are saved each year by antibiotics, insulin, and other prescription drugs, but we pay a price for having such powerful tools. A report from the Institute of Medicine (IOM) estimates that 1.5 million prescription drug-related errors—called *adverse drug events,* or ADEs—occur each year in the United States. ADEs happen for several reasons:

> The image of the all-knowing physician and the passive patient is fading. **What is emerging is a physician-patient partnership.**

- *Medication errors:* Physicians may overprescribe drugs, prescribe the wrong drug, or prescribe a dangerous

TERMS

endoscopy   A medical procedure in which a viewing instrument is inserted into a body cavity or opening.

false positive   A test result that incorrectly detects a disease or condition in a healthy person.

false negative   A test result that fails to correctly detect a disease or condition.

combination of drugs; such problems are especially prevalent for older adults, who typically take multiple medications. At the pharmacy, patients may receive the wrong drug or may not be given complete information about drug risks, side effects, and interactions.

• *Off-label drug use:* Once a drug is approved by the FDA for one purpose, it can legally be prescribed (although not marketed) for purposes not listed on the label. Many off-label uses are safe and supported by some research, but both consumers and health care providers need to take special care with off-label use.

• *Online pharmacies:* Some online pharmacies may sell products that are adulterated, expired, ineffective, or counterfeit drugs. The FDA recommends that consumers avoid sites that prescribe drugs without a physical exam, sell prescription drugs without a prescription, or sell medications not approved by the FDA. You should also avoid sites that do not provide access to a registered pharmacist to answer questions or that do not provide a U.S. address and phone number to contact in case of a problem. The National Association of Boards of Pharmacy sponsors a voluntary certification program for Internet pharmacies. To be certified, a pharmacy must have a state license and allow regular inspections.

> **Americans spend more than $200 billion** each year on prescription drugs.
>
> —CDC, 2010

• *Costs:* Spending on prescription drugs is now the fastest-growing portion of U.S. health care spending. Consumers may be able to lower their drug costs by using generic versions of medications; by joining a drug discount program sponsored by a company, organization, or local pharmacy; and by investigating mail-order or Internet pharmacies.

Patients also share some responsibility for problems with prescription drugs. Many people don't take their medications properly, skip doses, take incorrect doses, stop too soon, or do not take the medication at all. An estimated 30–50% of the more than 3 billion prescriptions dispensed annually in the United States are not taken correctly and thus do not produce the desired results. Consumers can increase the safety and effectiveness of their treatment by carefully reading any prescription's label and fact sheets or brochures and by asking the following questions:

• Are there nondrug alternatives?
• What is the name of the medication, and what is it supposed to do, within what period of time?
• How and when do I take the medication, how much do I take, and for how long? What should I do if I miss a dose?
• What other medications, foods, drinks, or activities should I avoid?

• What are the side effects, and what do I do if they occur?
• Can I take a generic drug rather than a brand-name one?
• Is there written information about the medication?

Surgery is another staple of Western medical treatment. Each year, more than 70 million operations and related procedures are performed in the United States. If a health care provider suggests surgery for any reason, ask the following questions:

• Why do I need surgery at this time?
• Are any nonsurgical options available, such as medicine or physical therapy?
• What are the risks and complications of the surgery?
• Can the operation be done on an outpatient basis?
• What can I expect before, during, and after surgery?

COMPLEMENTARY AND ALTERNATIVE MEDICINE

Whereas conventional Western medicine tends to focus on the body, on the physical causes of disease, and on ways to eradicate pathogens in order to restore health, CAM tends to focus on an integration of mind, body, and spirit in seeking ways to restore the whole person to harmony so that he or she can regain health. This approach is referred to as *holistic.* Caution is in order when choosing any mode of treatment—conventional or unconventional—that has not been scientifically evaluated for safety and effectiveness (see the box "Avoiding Health Fraud and Quackery").

The National Center for Complementary and Alternative Medicine (NCCAM), a branch of the National Institutes of Health (NIH), was established in the 1990s to apply rigorous scientific standards for proving or disproving the safety and effectiveness of CAM. NCCAM groups CAM practices into several broad categories: alternative medical systems, mind-body medicine, natural products, manipulative and body-based methods, and other CAM practices. What follows is a general introduction to the types of CAM available and a brief description of some of the more widely used ones.

> ## Ask Yourself
>
> **QUESTIONS FOR CRITICAL THINKING AND REFLECTION**
>
> What sort of relationship do you have with your primary physician? Do you think he or she understands your needs and is familiar enough with your history? Are you satisfied with this relationship?

Alternative Medical Systems

Many cultures elaborated complete systems of medical philosophy, theory, and practice long before the current biomedical approach was developed. The complete systems that are best known in the United States are probably traditional Chinese medicine (TCM), also known as traditional Oriental medicine, and homeopathy. Traditional medical systems have also been developed in many other regions of the world, including North, Central, and South America; the Middle East; India; Tibet; and Australia. In many countries, these medical approaches continue to be used today—frequently alongside Western medicine and quite often by physicians trained in Western medicine.

Alternative medical systems tend to have concepts in common. For example, the concept of life force or energy exists in many cultures. In traditional Chinese medicine, the life force contained in all living things is called *qi* (sometimes spelled chi). Most traditional medical systems think of disease as a disturbance or imbalance not just of physical processes but also of forces and energies within the body, the mind, and the spirit. Treatment aims at re-establishing equilibrium, balance, and harmony. Because the whole patient, rather than an isolated set of symptoms, is treated in most comprehensive alternative medical systems, it is rare that only a single treatment approach is used. Most commonly, multiple techniques and methods are employed and are continually adjusted according to the changes in the patient's health status that occur naturally or are brought about by the treatment.

Traditional Chinese Medicine   In **traditional Chinese medicine (TCM),** the free and harmonious flow of qi produces health—a positive feeling of well-being and vitality in body, mind, and spirit. Illness occurs when the flow of qi is blocked or disturbed. TCM works to restore and balance the flow of blocked qi; the goal is not only to treat illnesses but also to increase energy, prevent disease, and support the immune system.

Two of the primary treatment methods in TCM are **herbal remedies** and **acupuncture.** Chinese herbal remedies number about 5800 and include plant products, animal parts, and minerals. The use of a single medicinal botanical is rare in Chinese herbal medicine; rather, several different plants are combined in very precise proportions, often to make a tea or soup.

Acupuncture works to correct disturbances in the flow of qi through the insertion of thin needles at appropriate points in the skin. Qi is believed to flow through the body along several *meridians*, or pathways, and there are hundreds of acupuncture points located along these meridians. The points chosen for acupuncture are highly individualized for each patient, and they change over the course of treatment as the patient's health status changes.

The World Health Organization has compiled a list of more than 40 conditions in which acupuncture may be

TERMS

traditional Chinese medicine (TCM)   The traditional medical system of China, which views illness as the result of a disturbance in the flow of qi, the life force; therapies include acupuncture, herbal medicine, and massage.

herbal remedy   A medicine prepared from plants.

acupuncture   Insertion of thin needles into the skin at points along meridians, pathways through which qi is believed to flow.

The World Health Organization lists more than 40 conditions that may benefit from acupuncture treatment.

beneficial. At a conference called by the National Institutes of Health (NIH), a panel of experts found evidence that acupuncture was effective in relieving nausea and vomiting after chemotherapy and pain after surgery, including dental surgery. Newer studies show that acupuncture may help relieve the painful symptoms of fibromyalgia and reduce the joint pain and stiffness of osteoarthritis. There is not yet enough evidence to show conclusively that acupuncture is effective for menstrual cramps, tennis elbow, carpal tunnel syndrome, asthma, or certain other conditions. Western researchers typically use a different framework for understanding the effects of acupuncture. For example, they might explain pain relief not in terms of qi but in terms of altering nervous system pathways and the release of hormones and neurotransmitters.

Very few negative side effects have been reported in conjunction with acupuncture. Nonetheless, problems can occur from the improper insertion and manipulation of needles and from the use of unsterile needles. The FDA regulates acupuncture needles like other standard medical devices and requires that they be sterile. Most states require licensing for acupuncture practitioners, but requirements vary widely.

Homeopathy An alternative medical system of Western origin, **homeopathy** is based on two main principles: "Like cures like," and remedies become more effective with greater dilution. "Like cures like" summarizes the concept that a substance that produces the symptoms of an illness in a healthy person can cure the illness when given in very minute quantities. Remedies containing very small quantities of a particular substance are obtained by repeatedly diluting the original solution. The extent of dilution varies, but the final extract is often so dilute that few, if any, of the original molecules are left in it.

More than 1000 different substances (plant and animal parts, minerals, and chemicals) are used to prepare homeopathic remedies, and each of these substances is thought to have different effects at different dilutions. That means a homeopath must not only choose the correct remedy for a particular patient but also decide on the specific dilution of that remedy in order to achieve the desired effect.

In order to assess a patient's condition, homeopaths generally spend quite a bit of time talking with a patient and assessing his or her physical, psychological, and emotional health before deciding on the correct remedy at the proper dilution. This intensive interaction between the practitioner and the patient might play an important role in the success of the therapy. Indeed, critics of homeopathy often attribute its reported effectiveness to this non-specific placebo effect (see the box "The Power of Belief: The Placebo Effect"). However, when the results of 185 homeopathic trials were analyzed recently, it was concluded that the clinical effects of homeopathy could not be completely explained by the placebo effect. Homeopathy remains one of the most controversial forms of CAM.

To date, the FDA has not found any serious adverse events associated with the use of homeopathy, with the possible exception of situations in which a patient might have been successfully treated with standard medical approaches but chose to rely solely on homeopathy. The FDA regulates some homeopathic remedies, but they are subject to many fewer restrictions than prescription or over-the-counter drugs. A few states require practitioners to have special licenses, but most providers practice homeopathy as a specialty under another medical license, such as medical doctor or nurse practitioner.

Naturopathy The health care discipline of **naturopathy** is based on the premise that the body has the ability to restore and maintain optimal health. Naturopathic practitioners help their patients by using holistic approaches, including nutrition, acupuncture, homeopathic medicine, herbology, psychology, and counseling. The most frequently treated conditions are allergies, chronic pain, obesity, heart disease, fertility problems, and cancer. Naturopaths work in hospitals, clinics, and community health centers. They are licensed in several states.

Mind-Body Medicine

Mind-body medicine makes use of the integral connection between mind and body and the effect each can have on the other. They include many of the stress-management techniques discussed in Chapter 2, including meditation, yoga, visualization, taijiquan, and biofeedback. Psychotherapy, support groups, prayer, and music, art, and dance therapy can also be thought of as mind-body interventions. The placebo effect is one of the most widely known examples of mind-body interdependence.

Hypnotherapy is considered to be a CAM therapy, although the use of hypnotherapy for certain conditions was accepted more than 40 years ago by the American Medical Association. Hypnotherapy involves the induction of a state of deep relaxation during which the patient is more likely to accept suggestions to influence health and overcome conditions such as chronic pain, pain during surgery

homeopathy A holistic alternative medical system that treats illnesses by giving very small doses of drugs that in larger doses would produce symptoms like those of the illness.

naturopathy An alternative medical system based on supporting the body's ability to heal itself and maintain optimal health by removing barriers and creating a healing internal and external environment.

The Power of Belief: The Placebo Effect

A placebo is a chemically inactive substance or ineffective procedure that a patient believes is an effective therapy for his or her condition. Researchers frequently give placebos to the control group in an experiment testing the efficacy of a particular drug or other treatment. By comparing the effects of the actual treatment with the effects of the placebo, researchers can judge whether the treatment is effective.

The *placebo effect* occurs when a patient improves after receiving a placebo. In such cases, the effect of the placebo on the patient cannot be attributed to the specific actions or properties of the drug or procedure.

Researchers have consistently found that 30–40% of all patients given a placebo show improvement. This result has been observed for a wide variety of conditions or symptoms, including coughing, seasickness, depression, migraines, and angina. For some conditions, placebos have been effective in up to 70% of patients. In some cases, people given a placebo even report having the side effects associated with an actual drug. Placebos are particularly effective when they are administered by a practitioner whom the patient trusts.

Studies on patients with depression and people with Parkinson's disease have found that treatment with an inactive placebo results in changes in brain function. Such changes in the electrical or chemical activity of the brain may help explain the placebo effect. Other possible explanations for the placebo effect involve relaxation and stress reduction.

The placebo effect can be exploited by unscrupulous people who sell worthless medical treatments to the scientifically unsophisticated public. But placebo power can also be harnessed for its beneficial effects. When a skilled and compassionate medical practitioner provides a patient with a sense of confidence and hope, the positive aspects of placebo power can boost the benefits of standard medical treatment. Getting well, like getting sick, is a complex process. Anatomy, physiology, mind, emotions, and the environment are all inextricably intertwined. But the placebo effect does show that belief can have both psychological and physical effects.

or childbirth, and anxiety and phobias. The hypnotherapist tries to help the patient change unwanted behavior or deal with pain and other symptoms. Hypnosis is sometimes used in smoking cessation programs and as a nondrug approach to anxiety disorders such as phobias and chronic conditions such as irritable bowel syndrome.

Hypnosis can be used by medical professionals (M.D.s, D.O.s, D.D.S.s) but is also offered by hypnotherapists. Physicians are certified by their own associations; many states require hypnotherapists to be licensed, but the requirements for licensing vary.

Natural Products

Natural products, also known as biological-based therapies, consist primarily of herbal therapies or remedies, botanicals, extracts from animal tissues (such as shark cartilage), and dietary supplements. Herbal remedies are a major component of all indigenous forms of medicine; prior to the development of pharmaceuticals at the end of the nineteenth century, people everywhere in the world relied on materials from nature for pain relief, wound healing, and treatment of a variety of ailments. Herbal remedies are also a common element in most systems of traditional medicine. Much of the **pharmacopoeia** of modern scientific medicine originated in the folk medicine of native peoples, and many drugs used today are derived from plants (see the box "Medicine and Drugs from Nature").

A majority of natural products are sold as dietary supplements—that is, in the form of tablets, pills, capsules, liquid extracts, or teas. Like foods, dietary supplements must carry ingredient labels. As with food products, it is the responsibility of the manufacturers to ensure that their dietary supplements are safe and properly labeled prior to marketing. The FDA is responsible for monitoring the labeling and accompanying literature of dietary supplements and for overseeing their safety once they are on the market.

Well-designed clinical studies have been conducted on only a small number of natural products. A few commonly

Medicine and Drugs from Nature

The natural environment is the source of many of the drugs and medicines we use today. Even those synthesized in laboratories are often based on the chemical structure of compounds first found in plants, animals, marine organisms, and microbes.

Many of these compounds have been known to cultures around the world for thousands of years. Medicines made from licorice, myrrh, and poppy are mentioned on clay tablets from Mesopotamia dating to 2600 B.C.—and are still in use today as treatments for various diseases, either as drugs or as herbal preparations. Other natural products include the stimulant and anesthetic cocaine from the coca plant, used in the cultures of Mexico and Central and South America; the anti-malaria drug quinine from the bark of the cinchona tree, also used in Central and South America; products from plants in the nightshade family, ranging from deadly poisons like belladonna to heart stimulants like atropine, used in ancient Greece; the Chinese herb ma huang from the plant genus *Ephedra*, source of ephedra, a stimulant, appetite suppressant, and decongestant; the anti-inflammatory salicin from the bark of the willow tree, source of aspirin, known in medieval England; and digitalis from the foxglove plant, used to treat heart conditions, also known in medieval England.

More recently, penicillin, derived from the fungi *Penicillium*, was famously discovered by accident in 1928 by Scottish scientist Alexander Fleming. Following this discovery, scientists searched water and soil samples from around the world for other antibacterial microbes, eventually discovering the tetracyclins, cephalosporins, and several other agents. Currently, the natural world is yielding compounds used in treating cancer, viral infections, Alzheimer's disease, diabetes, cardiovascular diseases, asthma and other respiratory diseases, high cholesterol, severe chronic pain, and genetic disorders, among others. An analysis of drugs developed between 1981 and 2002 showed that 28% of all new chemical entities launched in the pharmaceutical market were natural products or derived from natural products and that natural products and related drugs are used to treat 87% of all human diseases.

Today, this rich reservoir of biological resources is under threat. The destruction of tropical rainforests is of particular concern. Rainforests cover only about 7% of the planet but are thought to harbor more than half the world's plant and animal species. The International Union for the Conservation of Nature estimates that 70% of the world's plants are now threatened with extinction, along with 21% of the world's mammals, 12% of bird species, and 30% of all amphibians. The main threats are habitat destruction, climate change, and other human activity, with associated loss of biodiversity (the variety of living things on earth). A contributing factor is overharvesting by practitioners of alternative medical systems that use plant and animal parts in their remedies. Environmentalists have called for these practitioners either to stop using endangered plants and animals or to support farming of these species as an alternative to harvesting them from nature.

The loss of natural habitats and species means the potential loss of innumerable yet-to-be discovered drugs. Many organizations worldwide are working to preserve biodiversity, protect endangered species, and maintain healthy ecosystems. The Convention on Biological Diversity, for example, deals specifically with biodiversity and works to commit countries to preserving and managing their biological resources. There are also things you can do as an individual to help preserve natural areas around the world:

- Buy products made only from sustainable resources.

- Don't buy, eat, or use anything from an endangered species.

- Support restrictions on urban sprawl and land clearing for development.

- Buy locally grown food.

- Recycle, reuse, conserve.

In taking steps like these, remember that you are not only supporting the health of the planet but also supporting the possibility of future breakthroughs in human health.

For a detailed description of environmental health—how the environment affects you and how you affect the environment—see Chapter 14.

SOURCES: International Union for the Conservation of Nature. 2009. *Extinction Crisis Continues Apace* (http://www.iucn.org/about/work/programmes/species/red_list/?4143/Extinction-crisis-continues-apace; retrieved October 12, 2010); Chin, Y-W., et al. 2006. Drug discovery from natural sources. *American Association of Pharmaceutical Scientists Journal* 8(2): E239–E253; Convention on Biological Diversity. 2010. *What's New* (http://www.cbd.int; retrieved October 13, 2010).

used herbals, their uses, and the evidence supporting their efficacy are presented in Table 15.2. Participants in clinical trials with St. John's wort, ginkgo, and echinacea experienced only minor adverse events, but the researchers didn't examine the effects of different dosages or how these therapies interact with conventional drugs.

Although most drug-herb interactions are relatively minor compared to conventional drug-drug interactions, some can be potentially serious. An example is the use of herbs that have anticoagulant (anticlotting) properties, such as ginkgo biloba, when used concurrently with the commonly prescribed anticoagulant Coumadin.

Studies have shown that most people do not reveal their use of CAM therapies to their conventional health care providers, a problem that can have severe health consequences. Any herbs or drugs used in combination should be evaluated for safety by a knowledgeable health care provider such as a pharmacist (see the box "Herbal Remedies: Are They Safe?").

Manipulative and Body-Based Practices

Touch and body manipulation are long-standing forms of health care. Manual healing techniques are based on the idea that misalignment or dysfunction in one part of the body can cause pain or dysfunction in that or another part; correcting these misalignments can bring the body back to optimal health.

Table 15.2 — Commonly Used Herbals, Their Uses, Evidence for Their Effectiveness, and Contraindications

BOTANICAL	USE	EVIDENCE	EXAMPLES OF ADVERSE EFFECTS AND INTERACTIONS
Cranberry (*Vaccinium macrocarpon*)	Prevention or treatment of urinary tract disorders	May eliminate and prevent bacteria from infecting the urinary tract	None known
Dandelion (*Taraxacum officinale*)	As a "tonic" against liver or kidney ailments	None yet	May cause diarrhea in some users; people with gallbladder or bile duct problems should not take dandelion
Echinacea (*Echinacea purpurea*, *E. angustifolia*, *E. pallida*)	Stimulation of immune functions; to prevent colds and flulike diseases; to lessen symptoms of colds and flus	Some trials showed that it prevents colds and flus and helps patients recover from colds faster	Might cause liver damage if taken over long periods of time (more than 8 weeks); since it is an immune stimulant, it is not advisable to take it with immune suppressants (e.g., corticosteroids) or during chemotherapy
Evening primrose oil (*Oenothera biennis L.*)	Reduction of inflammation	Long-term supplementation effective in reducing symptoms of rheumatoid arthritis	None known
Feverfew (*Tanacetum parthenium*)	Prevention of headaches and migraines	The majority of trials indicate that it is more effective than placebo	Should not be used by people allergic to other members of the aster family; has the potential to increase the effects of warfarin and other anticoagulants
Garlic (*Allium sativum*)	Reduction of cholesterol	Short-term studies have found a modest effect	May interact with some medications, including anticoagulants, cyclosporine, and oral contraceptives
Ginkgo (*Ginkgo biloba*)	Improvement of circulation and memory	Improves cerebral insufficiency and slows progression of Alzheimer's disease and other types of senile dementia in some patients; improves blood flow in legs	Could increase bleeding time; should not be taken with nonsteroidal anti-inflammatory drugs or anticoagulants; gastrointestinal disturbance
Ginseng (*Panax ginseng*)	Improvement of physical performance, memory, immune function, and glycemic control in diabetes; treatment of herpes simplex 2	No conclusive evidence exists for any of these uses	Interacts with warfarin and alcohol in mice and rats, hence should probably not be used with these drugs; may cause liver damage
St. John's wort (*Hypericum perforatum*)	Treatment of depression	There is strong evidence that it is significantly more effective than placebo, is as effective as some standard antidepressants for mild to moderate depression, and causes fewer adverse effects	Known to interact with a variety of pharmaceuticals and should not be taken together with digoxin, theophylline, cyclosporine, indinavir, and serotonin-reuptake inhibitors
Saw palmetto (*Serenoa repens*)	Improvement of prostate health	Early studies showed that saw palmetto may reduce mild prostate enlargement	Has no known interactions with drugs, but should probably not be taken with hormonal therapies
Valerian (*Valeriana officinalis*)	Treatment of insomnia	Appears to help with sleep disorders	Interacts with thiopental and pentobarbital and should not be used with these drugs

Manual practices are an integral part of physical therapy and osteopathic medicine, although certain practices are not part of conventional health care, such as massage and acupressure. The most commonly used CAM manual healing method is **chiropractic,** a method that focuses on the relationship between structure, primarily of joints and muscles, and function, primarily of the nervous system, to maintain or restore health. An important therapeutic procedure is the manipulation of joints, particularly those of the spinal column. However, chiropractors also use a variety of other techniques, including exercise, patient education and lifestyle modification, nutritional supplements, and orthotics (mechanical supports and braces) to treat patients.

TERMS

chiropractic A system of manual healing most frequently used to treat musculoskeletal problems; the primary treatment is manipulation of the spine and other joints.

Chiropractors, or doctors of chiropractic, are trained for a minimum of four full-time academic years at accredited chiropractic colleges and can go on to postgraduate training in many countries. Chiropractic is accepted by many health care and health insurance providers to a far greater extent than the other types of CAM therapies. Chiropractic is effective in managing acute low-back pain, and promising results have been reported with the use of chiropractic techniques in neck pain and headaches.

Spinal manipulation performed by a person without proper chiropractic training can be extremely dangerous. The American Chiropractic Association can help you find a licensed chiropractor near you.

Exercise for health maintenance, health promotion, and disease prevention currently fits the definition of a CAM modality. However, an initiative called *Exercise Is Medicine* is under way, launched by the American College of Sports Medicine (ACSM) and the American Medical Association (AMA), to make physical activity and exercise a standard part of the health care paradigm in the United States. The program encourages physicians to record level of physical activity as a standard vital sign in every patient visit and to become proficient at counseling patients regarding their physical activity needs. A study has found that 65% of Americans would be more interested in using exercise for health purposes if advised to do so by their physicians. Exercise Is Medicine suggests that physicians advise patients to participate in 150 minutes per week of moderate-intensity physical activity, to stretch, and to do light muscle training. Through efforts such as this, exercise is likely to transition from a CAM modality to a conventional modality and to become part of the mainstream health care system.

Other CAM Practices

Energy therapies are forms of treatment that use energy originating either within the body (biofields) or from other sources (electromagnetic fields). Biofield therapies are based on the idea that energy fields surround and penetrate the body and can be influenced by movement, touch, pressure, or the placement of hands in or through the fields. **Qigong**, a component of traditional Chinese medicine, combines movement, meditation, and regulation of breathing to enhance the flow of qi, improve blood circulation, and enhance immune function. **Therapeutic touch** is derived from the ancient technique of laying-on of hands; it is based on the premise that healers can identify and correct energy imbalances by passing their hands over the patient's body. **Reiki** is one form of therapeutic touch; it is intended to correct disturbances in the flow of life energy (*ki* in the Japanese tradition) and enhance the

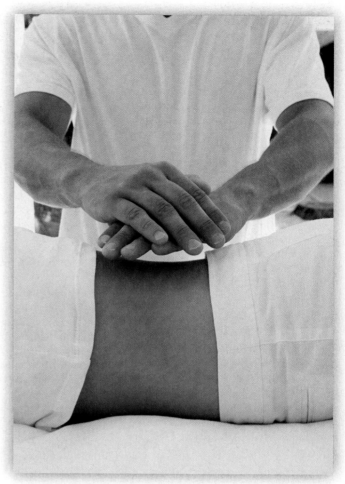

One of several touch therapies, Reiki massage has a spiritual, as well as physical, component.

body's healing powers through the use of specific hand positions on or near the patient.

Bioelectromagnetics is the study of the interaction between living organisms and electromagnetic fields, both those produced by the organism itself and those produced by outside sources. The recognition that the body produces electromagnetic fields has led to the development of many diagnostic procedures in Western medicine,

---

energy therapies Forms of CAM treatment that use energy fields originating either within the body or from outside sources to promote health and healing.

qigong A component of traditional Chinese medicine that combines movement, meditation, and regulation of breathing to enhance the flow of qi, improve blood circulation, and enhance immune function.

therapeutic touch A CAM practice based on the premise that healers can identify and correct energy imbalances by passing their hands over the patient's body.

Reiki A CAM practice intended to correct disturbances in the flow of life energy and enhance the body's healing powers through the use of 13 hand positions on the patient.

TERMS

Herbal Remedies: Are They Safe?

Consider the following research findings and FDA advisories:

- St. John's wort interacts with drugs used to treat HIV infection and heart disease; the herb may also reduce the effectiveness of oral contraceptives, antirejection drugs used with organ transplants, and some medications used to treat infections, depression, asthma, and seizure disorders.

- Supplements containing kava kava have been linked to liver damage, and anyone who has liver problems, drinks large amounts of alcohol, or takes medications that can affect the liver are advised to consult a physician before using kava kava–containing supplements.

- In a sample of ayurvedic herbal medicine products, 20% were found to contain potentially harmful levels of lead, mercury, and/or arsenic.

These findings highlight safety concerns about dietary supplements, which now represent annual sales of more than $15 billion in the United States.

Drug Interactions

Botanicals may decrease the effects of drugs, making them ineffective, or increase their effects, in some cases making them toxic. Most patients do not tell their physicians about their use of CAM

modalities. Botanicals can also interact with alcohol, usually heightening alcohol's effects. Many manufacturers are offering new combinations of botanical preparations without empirical or scientific information about the interactions of the individual products.

Lack of Standardization

The Dietary Supplement Health and Education Act of 1994 requires that dietary supplement labels list the name and quantity of each ingredient. However, confusion can result because different plant species—with distinct chemical compositions and effects— may have the same common name. The

content of herbal preparations is also variable. Botanicals are naturally grown products. Herb producers do not have complete control over natural processes any more than farmers have control over the vitamin content of fruit.

As an attempt toward standardization, herb producers have identified one or two substances that indicate quality; these substances should be listed on a product's label with their corresponding concentrations, lot numbers, and purity analysis data. Avoid any herbal product whose label is missing this information. Reputable retailers sell only products with this identifying information, and some send qualified inspectors to the site of production to verify the label information.

The Role of Government in Safety Issues

In the United States, because herbs are considered supplements rather than food or drug products, they do not have to meet FDA food and drug standards for safety or effectiveness, nor do they currently have to meet any manufacturing standards. The manufacturer is responsible for ensuring that a supplement is safe before it is marketed; the FDA has the power to restrict a substance if it is found to pose a health risk after it is on the market.

---

including electroencephalography (EEG), electrocardiography (ECG), and nuclear magnetic resonance (NMR) scans. **Bioelectromagnetic-based therapies** involve the use of electromagnetic fields to manage pain and to treat conditions such as asthma. Although promising, the available research is still very limited and does not allow firm conclusions about the efficacy of these therapies.

Evaluating Complementary and Alternative Therapies

Because there is less information available about complementary and alternative therapies, as well as less regulation of associated products and providers, consumers need to take an active role when they are thinking about using them.

Working with Your Physician The NCCAM advises consumers not to seek complementary therapies without first visiting a conventional health care provider for an evaluation and diagnosis of their symptoms. It's usually best to become informed about and discuss conventional treatments that have been shown to be beneficial for your condition. If you are thinking of trying any alternative therapies, it is important to tell your physician, pharmacist, or other conventional provider who is knowledgeable about your health status and also informed about CAM. Areas to discuss with your physician or pharmacist include the *safety* of the complementary treatment; evidence for its effectiveness, if any; issues of timing; and likely cost.

> The NCCAM advises consumers not to seek CAM treatment *without talking to their usual health care provider first.*

If appropriate, schedule a follow-up visit with your physician to assess your condition and your progress after a certain amount of time using a complementary therapy. Keep a symptom diary to more accurately track your symptoms and gauge your progress. (Symptoms such as pain and fatigue are very difficult to recall with accuracy, so an ongoing symptom diary is an important tool.) If you plan to pursue a therapy against your physician's advice, you need to tell him or her.

Questioning the CAM Practitioner   You can also get information from individual practitioners and from schools, professional organizations, and state licensing boards. Ask about education, training, licensing, and certification. If appropriate, check with local or state regulatory agencies or the consumer affairs department to determine if any complaints have been lodged against the practitioner. Some guidelines for talking with a CAM practitioner include the following:

- Ask the practitioner why he or she thinks the therapy will be beneficial for your condition. Ask for a full description of the therapy and any potential side effects. In all cases, demand an evidence-based approach.

- Describe in detail any conventional treatments you are receiving or plan to receive.

- Ask how long the therapy should continue before it can be determined if it is beneficial.

- Ask about the expected cost of the treatment. Does it seem reasonable? Will your health insurance pay some or all of the costs?

If anything an alternative practitioner says or recommends directly conflicts with advice from your physician, discuss it with your physician before making any major changes in any current treatment regimen or in your lifestyle.

Doing Your Own Research   You can investigate CAM therapies on your own by going to the library or doing research online, although caution is in order when using Web sites for the various forms of CAM. A good place to start is the Web sites of government agencies like the FDA or NCCAM and of universities and similar organizations that conduct government-sponsored research on CAM approaches. Perhaps more so than for any other consumer

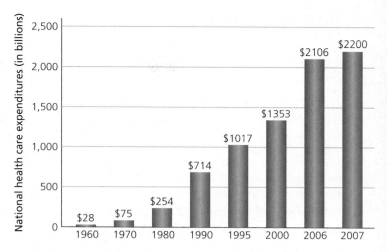

FIGURE 15.2   National health care expenditures (public and private) 1960–2007.

SOURCE: National Center for Health Statistics. 2010. *Health, United States: 2009.* Hyattsville, Md.: National Center for Health Statistics.

products and services, the use of CAM calls for consumer skills, critical thinking, and caution.

PAYING FOR HEALTH CARE

The American health care system is one of the most advanced and comprehensive in the world, but it is also the most expensive (Figure 15.2). In 2007, the United States spent $2.2 trillion on health care, or more than $7400 per person. Many factors contribute to the high cost of health care in the United States, including the cost of advanced equipment and new technology, expensive treatments for some illnesses, the aging of the population, and the demand for profits by insurance companies and many commercial health care providers.

The Current System

Health care is financed by a combination of private and public insurance plans, patient out-of-pocket payments, and government assistance. Currently, private insurance and individual patients pay about 55% of the total; the government pays the rest, mainly through Medicare and Medicaid. Most nonelderly Americans receive health insurance through their employers.

By some estimates, as many as 50 million Americans—the vast majority of them employed—have no health insurance at all. Many more are underinsured, meaning they may be uninsured for periods of time, have health insurance that does not cover all needed services, and/or have high out-of-pocket costs. New and extended government health insurance programs for children have reduced the number of Americans under age 18 who lack health insurance; still, 8.9 million American children were uninsured as of June 2009.

Health Insurance

Health insurance enables people to receive health care they might not otherwise be able to afford. Health insurance plans are either fee-for-service or managed care.

Traditional Fee-for-Service (Indemnity) Plans In a fee-for-service, or indemnity, plan, you can use any medical provider (such as a physician or a hospital) you choose. You or the provider sends the bill to your insurance company, which pays part of it. Usually you have to pay a deductible amount each year, and then the plan will pay a percentage—often 80%—of what is considered the "usual and customary" charge for covered services.

Managed-Care Plans Managed-care plans have agreements with a network of specified physicians, hospitals, and health care providers to offer a range of services to plan members at reduced cost. In general, you have lower out-of-pocket costs and less paperwork with a managed-care plan than with an indemnity plan, but you also have less freedom in choosing health care providers. Managed-care plans may follow different models:

• **Health maintenance organizations (HMOs)** offer members a range of services for a set monthly fee. You choose a primary care physician who manages your care and refers you to specialists if you need them.

• **Preferred provider organizations (PPOs)** have arrangements with physicians and other providers who have agreed to accept lower fees.

• **Point-of-service (POS) plans** are options offered by many HMOs in which you can see a physician outside the plan and still be partially covered.

Many managed-care plans try to reduce costs over the long term by paying for routine preventive care, such as regular checkups, screening tests, and prenatal care; they may also encourage prevention by offering health education and lifestyle modification programs for members.

Government Programs Americans who are 65 or older and younger people with certain disabilities can be covered by **Medicare,** a federal health insurance program that helps pay for hospitalization, physician services, and prescription drugs. **Medicaid** is a joint federal-state health insurance program that covers some low-income people, especially children, pregnant women, and people with certain disabilities.

Health Care Reform

In March 2010, Congress passed the Affordable Care Act, a sweeping reform of the health care industry that could ultimately extend health insurance coverage to some 32 million Americans who are currently uninsured. The law aims to make medical coverage more affordable and widely available through two broad types of action:

• *Subsidizing insurance coverage for Americans who cannot afford it.* Millions of Americans live without health care insurance simply because they cannot pay the premiums. This is particularly true for low-income Americans, large families, the unemployed, and people with serious health conditions. The act provides federal and state funding to subsidize insurance coverage for qualified Americans who cannot access health care coverage through employer-sponsored or private plans. (However, not everyone will qualify for free or low-cost coverage under the federal law. For more information, see the box "Health Care Reform: Who's Left Out?.") The law also opens Medicaid to more Americans by loosening income requirements and other restrictions.

• *Placing tighter restrictions on the insurance industry.* As described in Chapter 1, the Affordable Care Act restricts or bans certain insurance-industry practices that have prevented millions of Americans from getting health care insurance. Some restrictions (such as banning lifetime coverage limits and prohibiting discrimination against children with preexisting health conditions) began in 2010; other regulations will gradually take effect through 2014.

The act also creates health care insurance "exchanges," where qualified Americans can purchase affordable coverage. Each state will ultimately have its own exchange; states can choose to manage their own exchanges or allow the federal government to manage them. Exchanges will offer a variety of coverage options from private insurance companies, with the goal of creating competitive rates to make plans more affordable. In 2010, the federal government began working with individual states to create exchanges, and every state should have its own exchange in place by no later than 2014.

For more information on the Affordable Care Act, visit the U.S. government's health care Web site at www.healthcare.gov.

TERMS

managed-care plan A health care program that integrates the financing and delivery of services by using designated providers, utilization review, and incentives for following the plan's policies; HMOs, PPOs, and POS plans are managed-care plans.

health maintenance organization (HMO) A prepaid health insurance plan that offers health care from designated providers.

preferred provider organization (PPO) A prepaid health insurance plan in which providers agree to deliver services for discounted fees; patients can go to any provider, but using nonparticipating providers results in higher costs to the patient.

point-of-service (POS) plan A managed-care plan that covers treatment by an HMO physician but permits patients to seek treatment elsewhere with a higher copayment.

Medicare A federal health insurance program for people 65 or older and for younger people with certain disabilities.

Medicaid A federally subsidized state-run plan of health care for people with low income.

The Affordable Care Act of 2010 is expected to expand health care coverage to some 32 million of the 50 million Americans who were uninsured at the time of the law's passage. Under the law, federal and state governments will use a variety of methods to help qualified Americans find and pay for affordable medical insurance, while placing tough new regulations on insurance companies and banning certain practices that have effectively blocked many American families from getting health insurance.

Still, the plan may leave as many as 20 million individuals uninsured, for a variety of reasons. Who won't be covered under the Affordable Care Act? Here are some examples:

● Illegal immigrants: The law states that illegal immigrants may not participate in government-run health insurance exchanges or qualify for tax credits to purchase private insurance. However, the act does not bar individual states or localities from providing assistance to undocumented immigrants or their families in need of medical care.

● Americans who don't want medical insurance coverage: Many Americans—particularly young adults and recent college graduates—feel they don't want or need health insurance. Depending on their income level, individuals who don't participate in employer-provided insurance plans or who refuse to purchase private insurance may have to pay a penalty at tax time.

● People who fall "outside the system": People who have no permanent address or are itinerant may not stay in one place long enough to learn about services or benefits available where they currently live or may not meet residency requirements for some services. In rural areas with few or no health care services available, residents may be eligible for coverage but unable to access adequate medical care.

As well-intentioned as the Affordable Care Act is, the law's passage may actually make it difficult for some Americans to continue their current health care coverage. Examples include the following:

● Some early retirees: Many Americans retire from work before reaching age 65, when they are eligible for Medicare coverage. Some of these people are able to continue their medical coverage through their former employer, but with the passage of health care reform legislation, some companies have announced that they will no longer provide such coverage. This change leaves thousands of retirees without medical insurance until they reach 65.

● Workers covered by an employer's "mini med" plans: Some large companies pay their workers low hourly wages but offer minimal health care coverage. Workers may opt into these "mini med" plans for a few dollars a week, but their benefits may be capped at only a few thousand dollars per year. Because of some requirements in the Affordable Care Act, such employers may be forced to eliminate this minimal coverage

and workers may be required to purchase private insurance at much higher costs.

As the Affordable Care Act's provisions become real (taking full effect in 2014), Americans will need to make sure they understand what their insurance options are. One good way to find out is to visit the federal government's new health care Web site at www.healthcare.gov.

SOURCES: HealthCare.gov. 2010. *Your Health Care, Explained* (http://www. healthcare.gov; retrieved October 2, 2010); The Henry J. Kaiser Family Foundation. 2010. *Insurance* (http://www.kaiseredu.org/topics/insurance. aspx; retrieved October 2, 2010); The New York Times Online. 2010. *Health Care Reform News* (http://topics.nytimes.com/top/news/health/ diseasesconditionsandhealthtopics/health_insurance_and_managed_ care/health_care_reform/index.html; retrieved October 2, 2010); The White House. 2010. *The Affordable Care Act* (http://www.whitehouse.gov/ healthreform/healthcare-overview; retrieved October 2, 2010).

TIPS FOR TODAY AND THE FUTURE

Most of the time, you can take care of yourself without consulting a health care provider. When you need professional care, you can still take responsibility for yourself by making informed decisions.

RIGHT NOW YOU CAN

- Make sure that you have enough of your prescription medications on hand, and that your prescriptions are up-to-date.
- If you take any supplements (dietary or herbal), ask your pharmacist if they can interact with any prescription drugs you are taking.

IN THE FUTURE YOU CAN

- Thoroughly research any form of complementary or alternative medical treatments you are using or considering; make sure it is considered safe and effective.
- Review your medical insurance policy and make sure you are familiar with your coverage and the policy's terms. If you have any questions about your policy, contact your insurance agent. If you don't have any medical insurance, start investigating your options.

Connect to your Choices

Have you ever thought about where you get your attitudes toward conventional medicine and complementary and alternative medicine? Many factors can influence our attitudes, some not as obvious as others. When you were growing up, was your family respectful of the medical establishment, or were they skeptical of it? Did your parents or grandparents use herbal remedies? Do any of your peers express strong opinions about doctors or about CAM practices? Are there CAM practitioners in your community? Do you know people who see chiropractors or get acupuncture or massages?

What are the external factors that influence your choices about medicine? What are your inner motivations and core values, and how do they affect your choices? Based on what you learned in this chapter, will you make some different choices in the future? If so, what will they be?

Go online to Connect to complete this activity.
www.mcgraw-hillconnect.com

SUMMARY

- Informed self-care requires knowing how to evaluate symptoms. It's necessary to see a physician if symptoms are severe, unusual, persistent, or recurrent.

- Self-treatment doesn't necessarily require medication, but OTC drugs can be a helpful part of self-care.

- Conventional medicine is characterized by a focus on the external, physical causes of disease; the identification of a set of symptoms for different diseases; the development of public health measures to prevent disease and of drugs and surgery to treat them; the use of rational, scientific thinking to understand phenomena; and a well-established research methodology.

- Conventional practitioners include medical doctors, doctors of osteopathic medicine, podiatrists, optometrists, and dentists, as well as allied health care providers.

- The diagnostic process involves a medical history, a physical exam, and medical tests. Patients should ask questions about medical tests and treatments recommended by their physicians.

- Safe use of prescription drugs requires knowledge of what the medication is supposed to do, how and when to take it, and what the side effects are.

- Complementary and alternative medicine (CAM) is defined as those therapies and practices that do not form part of conventional health care and medical practice as taught in most U.S. medical schools and offered in most U.S. hospitals.

- CAM is characterized by a view of health as a balance and integration of body, mind, and spirit; and a body of knowledge based on accumulated experience and observations of patient reactions.

- Alternative medical systems such as traditional Chinese medicine and homeopathy are complete systems of medical philosophy, theory, and practice.

- Mind-body medicine includes meditation, biofeedback, group support, hypnosis, and prayer.

- Natural products include herbal remedies, botanicals, animal-tissue products, and dietary supplements.

- Manipulative and body-based practices include massage and other physical healing techniques; the most frequently used is chiropractic.

- Other CAM practices include movement therapies, traditional healing practices, and energy therapies.

- Because there is less information available about CAM and less regulation of its practices and providers, consumers must be proactive in researching and choosing treatments, using critical thinking skills and exercising caution.

- Health insurance plans are usually described as either fee-for-service (indemnity) or managed-care plans. Indemnity plans allow consumers more choice in medical providers, but managed-care plans are less expensive.

BOOKS

Committee on the Use of Complementary and Alternative Medicine by the American Public. 2005. *Complementary and Alternative Medicine in the United States.* Washington, D.C.: National Academy Press. *Outlines ways of integrating conventional and complementary therapies, and proposes changes to dietary supplement laws.*

Mayo Clinic. 2007. *The Mayo Clinic Book of Alternative Medicine.* New York: Time-Life. *A concise review of currently popular CAM therapies and treatments.*

PDR. 2007. *PDR for Nonprescription Drugs, Dietary Supplements, and Herbs, 2008,* 29th ed. Montvale, N.J.: Thomson Healthcare. *A reference covering the safety and efficacy of over-the-counter medications.*

Thompson, W. G. 2005. *The Placebo Effect and Health: Combining Science and Compassionate Care.* New York: Prometheus Books. *Describes the placebo effect and how it may be used to benefit health.*

ORGANIZATIONS AND WEB SITES

American Board of Medical Specialties. Provides information on board certification, including information on specific physicians.
   http://www.abms.org
American Chiropractic Association. Provides information on chiropractic care, consumer tips, and a searchable directory of certified chiropractors.
   http://www.amerchiro.org
American Medical Association (AMA). Provides information about physicians, including their training, licensure, and board certification.
   http://www.ama-assn.org
American Osteopathic Association. Provides information on osteopathic physicians, including board certification.
   http://www.osteopathic.org
Food and Drug Administration: Information for Consumers. Provides materials on dietary supplements, foods, prescription and OTC drugs, and other FDA-regulated products.
   http://www.fda.gov/consumer/default.htm
National Center for Complementary and Alternative Medicine (NCCAM). Provides general information packets, answers to frequently asked questions about CAM, consumer advice for safer use of CAM, research abstracts, and bibliographies.
   http://nccam.nih.gov
National Council Against Health Fraud. Provides news and information about health fraud and quackery and links to related sites.
   http://www.ncahf.org
Quackwatch. Provides information on health fraud, quackery, and health decision making.
   http://www.quackwatch.org

U.S. Treasury Department: Health Savings Accounts. Provides information about HSAs and links to relevant IRS forms.
   http://www.treas.gov/offices/public-affairs/hsa/

SELECTED BIBLIOGRAPHY

American Medical Association. 2004. *Health Savings Accounts at a Glance.* Chicago: American Medical Association.

Babones, S. J. 2008. Income inequality and population health: Correlation and causality. *Social Science and Medicine* 66(7): 1614–1626.

Burke, A., et al. 2006. Acupuncture use in the United States: Findings from the national health interview survey. *Journal of Alternative and Complementary Medicine* 12(7): 639–648.

Cyna, A. M., et al. 2006. Antenatal self-hypnosis for labour and childbirth: A pilot study. *Anaesthesia and Intensive Care* 34(4): 464–469.

Ernst, E. 2004. Prescribing herbal medications appropriately. *Journal of Family Practice* 53(12): 985–988.

Frazier, S. C. 2005. Health outcomes and polypharmacy in elderly individuals: An integrated literature review. *Journal of Gerontological Nursing* 31(9): 4–11.

Grzywaca, J. G., et al. 2008. Age-related differences in the conventional health care–complementary and alternative medicine link. *American Journal of Health Behavior* 32(6): 650–663.

Kaiser Family Foundation. 2005. *Trends and Indicators in the Changing Health Care Marketplace.* Menlo Park, Calif.: Kaiser Family Foundation.

National Academy of Sciences, Institute of Medicine. 2006. *Preventing Medication Errors.* Washington, D.C.: National Academies Press.

National Center for Health Statistics. 2005. Trends in health insurance and access to medical care for children under age 19 years. *Advance Data from Vital Health Statistics* No. 355.

National Center for Health Statistics. 2008. *Early Release of Selected Estimates Based on Data from the 2007 National Health Interview Survey.* Hyattsville, Md.: National Center for Health Statistics.

National Center for Health Statistics. 2009. *Health, United States, 2008.* Hyattsville, Md.: National Center for Health Statistics.

Radley, D. C., et al. 2006. Off-label prescribing among office-based physicians. *Archives of Internal Medicine* 166(9): 1021–1026.

Remler, D. K., and S. A. Glied. 2006. How much more cost sharing will health savings accounts bring? *Health Affairs* 25(4): 1070–1078.

Saha, S., et al. 2008. Racial and ethnic disparities in the VA health care system: A systematic review. *Journal of General Internal Medicine* 23(5): 654–671.

Schoen, C., et al. 2008. How many are underinsured? Trends among U.S. adults, 2003 and 2007. *Health Affairs,* 10 June [epub].

U.S. Department of the Treasury. 2008. *Health Savings Accounts (HSAs)* (http://www.ustreas.gov/offices/public-affairs/hsa; retrieved February 20, 2009).

Wahbeh, H., S. M. Elsas, and B. S. Oken. 2008. Mind-body interventions: Applications in neurology. *Neurology* 70(24): 2321–2328.

LOOKING AHEAD...

After reading this chapter, you should be able to:

- Identify factors that contribute to unintentional injuries
- List the most common types of unintentional injuries and strategies for preventing them
- Describe factors that contribute to violence and intentional injuries
- Discuss different forms of violence and how to protect yourself from intentional injuries
- List strategies for helping others in an emergency situation

16

Personal Safety

Each year, more than 182,000 Americans die from injuries, and many more are temporarily or permanently disabled. The economic cost of injuries is high, with more than $700 billion spent each year for medical care and rehabilitation of injured people. Injuries also cause emotional suffering for injured people and their families, friends, and colleagues.

Engineering strategies such as safety belts can help lower injury rates, as can the passage and enforcement of safety-related laws, such as those requiring tamper-proof containers for OTC medications. Public education campaigns about risky behaviors such as texting while driving or driving under the influence of alcohol can also help prevent injuries. Ultimately, though, it is up to each person to take responsibility for his or her actions and make wise choices about safety behaviors.

DIFFERENTIATING INJURIES

An **intentional injury** is one that is purposely inflicted, by oneself or by another person. If an injury occurs when no harm is intended, it is considered an **unintentional injury.**

Motor vehicle crashes, falls, and fires often result in unintentional injuries. (Public health officials prefer not to use the word *accidents* to describe unintentional injuries because it suggests events beyond human control. *Injuries* are predictable outcomes of factors that can be controlled or prevented.) Although Americans tend to express more concern about intentional injuries, unintentional injuries are actually far more common. For example, the National Safety Council (NSC) estimates that in 2008, 333 Americans died each day from unintentional injuries, whereas 91 died of suicide and 35 died from homicide. Unintentional injuries are the fifth leading cause of death among all Americans and the leading cause of death for Americans under age 45.

UNINTENTIONAL INJURIES

Injury situations are generally categorized into four general classes, based on where they occur: motor vehicle injuries, home injuries, public injuries, and work injuries. The greatest number of deaths occur in motor vehicle crashes, but the greatest number of disabling injuries occur in the home (Table 16.1).

Table 16.1   Unintentional Injuries in the United States

	DEATHS	DISABLING INJURIES
Motor vehicle	39,000	2,100,000
Home	54,500	13,100,000
Public	22,200	7,400,000
Work	4,303	3,200,000
All classes*	118,000	25,700,000

*Deaths and injuries for the four separate classes total more than the "All classes" figures because of rounding and because some deaths and injuries are included in more than one class.

SOURCE: National Safety Council. 2010. *Injury Facts, 2010 Edition*. Itasca, Ill.: National Safety Council.

What Causes an Injury?

Most injuries are caused by a combination of human and environmental factors. Human factors are inner conditions or attitudes that lead to an unsafe state, whether physical, emotional, or psychological. Environmental factors are external conditions and circumstances, such as poor road conditions, a slippery surface, or the undertow of the ocean at the beach. A common human factor that leads to injuries is risk-taking behavior. Young men are especially prone to taking risks (see the box "Injuries Among Young Men"). Alcohol and drug use is another common risk factor that leads to many injuries and deaths.

Psychological and emotional factors can also play a role in injuries. People sometimes act on the basis of inadequate or inaccurate beliefs about what is safe or unsafe. However, many people who have accurate information still decide to engage in risky behavior. Young people often have unsafe attitudes, such as "I won't get hurt" or "It won't happen to me." Attitudes like this can lead to risk taking and ultimately to injuries.

Environmental factors leading to injury may be natural (weather conditions), social (a drunk driver), work-related (defective equipment), or home-related (faulty wiring) (see the box "Extreme Weather and Personal Safety"). Making the environment safer is an important aspect of safety. Laws are often passed to try to make our environment safer; examples include speed limits on highways and workplace safety requirements.

Motor Vehicle Injuries

According to the Centers for Disease Control and Prevention (CDC), more than 43,000 Americans were killed and nearly 2.5 million injured in motor vehicle crashes in 2008. Worldwide, motor vehicle crashes kill 1.2 million and injure up to 50 million people each year, making motor vehicle injuries the eleventh leading cause of death overall. **Motor vehicle injuries** also result in the majority of cases of paralysis due to spinal injuries, and they are the leading cause of severe brain injury in the United States.

Factors Contributing to Motor Vehicle Injuries

Common causes of motor vehicle injuries are speeding, aggressive driving, fatigue, inexperience, cell phones and other distractions, the use of alcohol and other drugs, and the incorrect use of safety belts and other safety devices.

SPEEDING   Nearly 63% of all motor vehicle crashes are caused by bad driving, especially speeding. As speed increases, momentum and the force of impact increase, and the time allowed for the driver to react (reaction time) decreases. Speed limits are posted to establish the safest maximum speed limit for a given area under ideal conditions; if visibility is limited or the road is wet, the safe maximum speed may be considerably lower.

AGGRESSIVE DRIVING   Aggressive driving includes frequent, erratic, and abrupt lane changes; tailgating; running red lights or stop signs; passing on the shoulder; and blocking other cars trying to change lanes or pass. Aggressive drivers increase the risk of crashes for themselves and others. Injuries may also occur if aggressive drivers stop their vehicles and confront each other following an incident.

FATIGUE AND SLEEPINESS   Driving requires mental alertness and attentiveness. Studies have shown that sleepiness causes slower reaction time, reduced coordination and vigilance, and delayed information processing. Research shows that even mild sleep deprivation causes a deterioration in driving ability comparable to that caused by a 0.05% blood alcohol concentration—a level considered hazardous when driving.

CELL PHONES AND OTHER DISTRACTIONS   Anything that distracts a driver can increase the risk of a motor vehicle

TERMS

intentional injury   An injury that is purposely inflicted, by either oneself or another person.

unintentional injury   An injury that occurs without harm being intended.

motor vehicle injuries   Unintentional injuries and deaths involving motor vehicles in motion, both on and off the highway or street; incidents causing motor vehicle injuries include collisions between vehicles and collisions with objects or pedestrians.

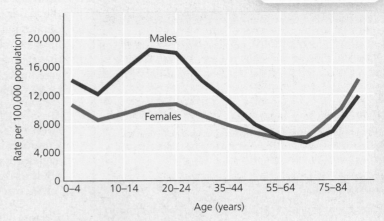

Injures Among Young Men

GENDER MATTERS

Overall, rates of injury are highest among young adults and seniors over age 85. Except among the oldest group of adults, the nonfatal injury rate is substantially higher in males than in females—and it peaks among young adult males (see figure). Males also significantly outnumber females in injury deaths—whether unintentional or intentional.

Why do men, especially young men, have such high rates of injury? Gender roles may be a key factor: Traditional gender roles for males may associate masculinity with risk-taking behavior and a disregard for pain and injury, and risk-taking behavior may be particularly common among young men. Men are more likely to drive dangerously, drink and drive, binge-drink, and use aggressive behavior to control situations—all of which can lead to higher rates of fatal and nonfatal injury. Men may also have a lower perception of risk of dangerous behaviors compared with women.

Traditional gender roles may also make it more difficult for men to admit to injury or emotional vulnerability. Physical injuries may worsen or become chronic if care is not sought promptly. Untreated depression can lead to suicide.

In addition, men may have greater exposure to some injury situations. Compared with women, men may drive more miles, have greater access to fire-

arms, and be more likely to ride motorcycles, operate machinery, and have jobs associated with high rates of workplace injuries. They may be more likely to engage in sports and other recreational activities associated with high rates of injuries. Greater access and use of firearms play a role in higher rates of deaths among men from assault and suicide; as described in Chapter 3, women are more likely than men to attempt suicide, but men are much more likely to succeed, primarily because they are more likely to use firearms.

Some researchers suggest that the male hormone testosterone may play a role in risky and aggressive behavior. Differences in brain structure and activity may also influence how men and

women respond to stressors and how quickly and to what degree they become verbally or physically aggressive in response to anger.

Further studies are needed to identify all the factors underlying excessive risk-taking among men and how these risk behaviors can be changed to lower the rates of fatal and nonfatal injury among men.

SOURCES: Centers for Disease Control and Prevention. 2004. Surveillance for fatal and nonfatal injuries—United States, 2001. *MMWR Surveillance Summaries* 53(SS7): 1–57; World Health Organization. 2002. *Gender and Road Traffic Injuries.* Geneva: World Health Organization; Courtenay, W. 1998. College men's health: An overview and a call to action. *Journal of American College Health* 46(6): 279–290.

Nonfatal injury rate by age and sex.

injury. Common distractions include talking to someone on a cell phone or in the vehicle, texting, eating, smoking, and reaching for controls in the car. Objects and activities outside the vehicle are a source of distraction as well: more than a dozen U.S. cities have banned digital billboards because of their potential to distract drivers.

Several common causes of crashes, such as disregarding stop signs, have been linked to driver distraction. Distraction is a contributing factor in 25–50% of all crashes. About 70% of distracted driver crashes involve noncollision (single-vehicle) or rear-end crashes. One study showed that drivers who use cell phones are nearly six times as likely to be involved in a crash as drivers who don't. The same study showed that sober drivers using cell phones can perform worse than drivers who are inebriated. Eight states (New York, New Jersey, California, Washington, Oregon, Delaware, Maryland, and Connecticut), the District of Columbia, and the U.S. Virgin Islands have

banned the use of handheld phones while driving (see the box "Cell Phones, Texting, and Distracted Driving").

ALCOHOL AND OTHER DRUGS Alcohol is involved in about 31% of all fatal crashes. Alcohol-impaired driving is illegal in all states; the legal limit for blood alcohol concentration (BAC) is 0.08%, but people can be impaired at much lower BACs. The combination of fatigue and alcohol use increases the risk even further. Because alcohol affects reason and judgment as well as the ability to make fast, accurate, and coordinated movements, a person who has been drinking will be less likely to recognize that he or she is impaired. Use of many over-the-counter and all psychoactive drugs is potentially dangerous if you drive.

SAFETY BELTS, AIR BAGS, AND CHILD SAFETY SEATS Although some type of mandatory safety belt law is in effect in 49 states (excluding New Hampshire) and the District of Columbia, only about 83% of motor vehicle occupants

Extreme Weather and Personal Safety

According to the U.S. Environmental Protection Agency, climate change has the potential to affect the frequency and intensity of extreme weather events, such as heat waves, cold waves, storms, floods, and droughts. In the second half of the twentieth century there were increases in the number of heat waves, the number of droughts, the intensity and duration of tropical storms and hurricanes, and the incidence of heavy precipitation and flooding.

Although it isn't possible to directly link a specific weather event to human-caused climate change, scientists project that certain changes are likely in the next 100 years. These changes include warmer days and nights, more heat waves, more heavy precipitation events, more droughts, more and more intense tropical storms, and more occasions of extreme high sea levels. All of these changes have the potential to adversely affect human health and mortality by increasing the risk of injury, infectious disease, foodborne illness, and stress-related disorders, among others.

Since you can't control the weather, the best approach is to be prepared for whatever event may occur in your area.

Heat: Extreme heat is the leading weather-related killer in the United States, according to the National Weather Service. Heat-related illness such as heat stroke and heat exhaustion can be fatal, especially for children, older adults, and people with certain health conditions. The best way to deal with excessive heat is to stay indoors as much as possible, with a fan or air conditioner on. Wear lightweight, light-colored clothing, drink plenty of water to stay hydrated, and avoid heavy meals. If you must go out, move slowly and rest frequently in the shade. See Chapter 10 for advice on exercising in hot weather.

Cold: Each year, dozens of Americans die from exposure to cold temperatures. Conditions such as hypothermia (low body temperature) and frostbite (frozen skin or flesh) can be deadly. Most injuries and deaths in cold weather are due to a lack of preparedness or understanding of the dangers of low temperatures and wind chill. If you must go outdoors in very cold weather, dress in layers and cover your face, fingers, and ears to protect them from frostbite. Make sure your home and car are prepared with plenty of fuel, drinking water, warm clothes and blankets, batteries, and other emergency supplies. See Chapter 10 for advice on exercising in cold weather.

Wind: Sustained winds as slow as 30 miles an hour can make it difficult or impossible to walk or stand. In severe hurricanes and tornadoes, sustained winds near the storm's center can blow at speeds in excess of 200 mph—strong enough to sweep a house off its foundations. In extremely windy conditions, take cover in a sturdy shelter, preferably a permanent structure with a foundation. In a severe storm such as a tornado, move to the lowest portion of the building or to a small interior room away from windows. If you're outdoors when a severe storm or tornado strikes, lie flat in a low spot or ditch. Don't stay inside a car or hide under an open-sided structure such as a bridge; such structures can act as a funnel and make wind more intense.

Lightning: About 400 Americans are struck by lightning every year, and about 60 of them die. Lightning can strike even when it's not raining, and it often strikes with no warning. If you hear thunder, you are close enough to the lightning's source to be struck. When conditions are right for lightning, go indoors. Stay out of water, even indoors, because water pipes can conduct electricity. Don't use corded telephones or appliances because their wiring can also conduct the power from a lightning strike.

Flooding: Stay away from rapidly rising or moving water—it can carry you away in an instant. Even fairly shallow water can sweep a car away if the current is fast enough. If you're near rapidly rising water, move to higher ground and call for help. Don't attempt to drive or walk through flooded streets, and don't traverse a bridge if it is being pounded by high, fast-moving water. During heavy rain, stay alert for flash flood warnings and be ready to evacuate if necessary.

For a detailed discussion of environmental health—how the environment affects you and how you affect the environment—see Chapter 14.

SOURCES: National Severe Storms Laboratory. 2009. *Education: Severe Weather* (http://www.nssl.noaa.gov/edu/safety/; retrieved October 8, 2010); National Weather Service. 2010. *Weather Safety* (http://www.weather.gov/safety.php; retrieved October 8, 2010); U.S. Environmental Protection Agency. 2010. *Extreme Events* (http://www.epa.gov/climatechange/effects/extreme.htm; retrieved October 10, 2010).

use safety belts even though they are the single most effective way to reduce the risk of crash-related death. If you wear a combination lap and shoulder belt, your chance of surviving a crash is three to four times better than that of a person who doesn't wear one.

Some people think that if they are involved in a crash they are better off being thrown free of their vehicle. In fact, the chances of being killed are 25 times greater if you are thrown from a vehicle. Safety belts also provide protection from the second collision: If a car is traveling at 65 mph and hits another vehicle, the car stops first; then the occupants stop because they, too, are traveling at 65 mph.

The second collision occurs when occupants hit something inside the car, such as the dashboard or windshield. The safety belt stops the second collision from occurring and spreads the collision's force over the body.

Since 1998, all new cars and light trucks have been equipped with dual air bags—one for the driver and one for the front passenger. Many vehicles also offer optional side air bags, which further reduce the risk of injury. Although air bags provide supplementary protection in the event of a collision, most are useful only in head-on collisions. They also deflate immediately after inflating and therefore do not provide protection in collisions involving

Cell Phones, Texting, and Distracted Driving

At any given moment, about 5% of drivers are talking or texting on a cell phone. In 2001, New York became the first state to ban the use of hand-held cellular phones while driving; drivers there must use hand-free equipment or face fines of up to $100. Since then, five other states, the District of Columbia, and the U.S. Virgin Islands have passed similar bans, and many other states have bans under consideration. Around the world, many countries have laws against the use of handheld cell phones while driving.

Available evidence indicates that use of a cell phone while driving can increase the risk of motor vehicle crashes. In a study using a driver-training simulator, cell phone users were about 20% slower to respond to sudden hazards than were other drivers, and they were about twice as likely to rear-end a braking car in front of them. Among young adult drivers who used a cell phone, reaction time was reduced to the level of a 70-year-old driver who was not using a phone. It is unclear, however, if bans such as those in New York will help reduce the risk: Studies have not found much, if any, benefit in the use of headsets. It appears that the mental distraction of

talking is a factor in crashes rather than holding the phone.

The safest strategy is not to use your phone while driving. For people who live in areas where cell phone use is legal

while driving and who choose to use a phone, the following strategies may help increase safety:

- Be familiar with your phone and its functions, especially speed dial and redial.

- Store frequently called numbers on speed dial so you can place calls without looking at the phone.

- If your phone has voice-activated dialing, use it.

- Use a hands-free device so you can keep both hands on the steering wheel.

- Let the person you are speaking to know you are driving and be prepared to end the call at any time.

- Don't place or answer calls in heavy traffic or hazardous weather conditions.

- Don't take notes or look up phone numbers while driving.

- Time calls so that you can place them when you are at a stop.

Text messaging is potentially even more distracting than talking on a cell phone. Washington, Minnesota, Alaska, California, Connecticut, Louisiana, New Jersey, and the District of Columbia prohibit texting while driving.

multiple impacts. Air bags are not a replacement for safety belts; everyone in a vehicle should buckle up.

Air bags deploy forcefully and can injure a child or short adult who is improperly restrained or sitting too close to the dashboard, although second-generation air bags are somewhat safer for children than the older devices. To ensure that air bags work safely, always follow these basic guidelines: Place infants in rear-facing infant seats in the back seat, transport children age 12 and under in the back seat, always use safety belts or appropriate safety seats, and keep 10 inches between the air bag cover and the breastbone of the driver or passenger. If necessary, adjust the steering wheel or use seat cushions to ensure that an inflating air bag will hit a person in the chest and not in the face. Children who have outgrown child safety seats but are still too small for adult safety belts alone (usually age 4–8)

should be secured using booster seats that ensure that the safety belt is positioned low across the waist.

Preventing Motor Vehicle Injuries   About 75% of all motor vehicle collisions occur within 25 miles of home and at speeds lower than 40 mph. Strategies for preventing motor vehicle injuries include the following:

- Obey the speed limit.
- Always wear a safety belt.
- Never drive under the influence of alcohol or other drugs, or ride with a driver who is.
- Keep your car in good working order.
- Always allow enough following distance. Use the 3-second rule: When the vehicle ahead passes a

reference point, count out 3 seconds. If you pass the reference point before you finish counting, drop back and allow more following distance.

- Always increase your following distance and slow down if weather or road conditions are poor.
- Choose interstate highways rather than rural roads. Highways are much safer because of better visibility, wider lanes, fewer surprises, and other factors.
- Always signal when turning or changing lanes.
- Stop completely at stop signs. Follow all traffic laws.
- Take special care at intersections. Look left, right, and then left again. Make sure you have time to complete your maneuver in the intersection.
- Don't pass on two-lane roads unless you're in a designated passing area and have a clear view ahead.

Motorcycles and Motorized Scooters   About one out of every ten traffic fatalities among people age 15–34 involves someone riding a motorcycle. Injuries from motorcycle collisions are generally more severe than those involving automobiles because motorcycles provide little, if any, protection. People riding motorized scooters face additional challenges. Such vehicles usually have a maximum speed of 30–35 mph and have less power for maneuverability, especially in an emergency. Strategies for preventing motorcycle and motor scooter injuries include the following:

> *Airbags are not a replacement for safety belts; everyone in a vehicle should buckle up.*

- Wear light-colored clothing, drive with your headlights on, and correctly position yourself in traffic.
- Develop the necessary skills. Lack of skill is a major factor in motorcycle and motor scooter injuries. Skidding from improper braking is the most common cause of loss of control.
- Wear a helmet. Helmets should be marked with the DOT symbol, certifying that they conform to federal safety standards established by the Department of Transportation. Helmet use is required by law in nearly half of the states.
- Protect your eyes with goggles, a face shield, or a windshield.
- Drive defensively, particularly when changing lanes and at intersections, and never assume that other drivers can see you.

Bicycles   Bicycle injuries result primarily from riders not knowing or understanding the rules of the road, failing to follow traffic laws, not having sufficient skill or experience to handle traffic conditions, or being intoxicated. Bicycles are considered vehicles; bicyclists must obey all traffic laws that apply to automobile drivers, including stopping at traffic lights and stop signs.

Head injuries are involved in about two-thirds of all bicycle-related deaths. Wearing a helmet reduces the risk of head injury by 85% (see the box "Choosing a Bicycle Helmet"). Safe cycling strategies include the following:

- Wear safety equipment, including a helmet, eye protection, gloves, and proper footwear. Secure the bottom of your pant legs with clips, so they don't get tangled in the chain.
- Wear light-colored, reflective clothing. Equip your bike with reflectors, and use lights, especially at night or when riding in wooded or other dark areas.
- Ride with the flow of traffic, not against it, and follow all traffic laws. Use bike paths when they are available.
- Ride defensively; never assume that drivers have seen you. Be especially careful when turning or crossing at corners and intersections. Watch for cars turning right.
- Stop at all traffic lights and stop signs. Know and use hand signals.
- Continue pedaling at all times when moving (no coasting) to help keep the bike stable and to maintain your balance.

Home Injuries

The most common fatal **home injuries** are the result of falls, fires, poisoning, suffocation, and unintentional shootings.

Falls   Most deaths occurring from falls involve falling on stairs or steps or from one level to another. Falls also occur on the same level, from tripping, slipping, or stumbling. Alcohol is a contributing factor in many falls. Strategies for preventing falls include the following:

- Install handrails and nonslip surfaces in the shower and bathtub.

home injuries   Unintentional injuries and deaths that occur in the home and on home premises to occupants, guests, domestic servants, and trespassers; falls, burns, poisonings, suffocations, unintentional shootings, drownings, and electrical shocks are examples.

TERMS

Choosing a Bicycle Helmet

Wearing a bicycle helmet can help you avoid serious head injury, brain damage, or even death in the event of a collision or fall. Helmets have a layer of stiff foam, which absorbs shock and cushions a blow to your head, covered by a thin plastic shell that will skid along the ground. For maximum protection, it's important to select a correctly fitting helmet. When you go shopping, remember the four S's: size, strap, straight, and sticker.

- *Size:* Try on several different sizes before making your selection; it may take several tries before you find the most comfortable fit. The helmet should be very snug but not overly tight on your head. Pads are usually provided to help adjust the fit. A good salesperson can also help you get the right fit. When the helmet is strapped onto your head, it should not move more than an inch in any direction, and you should not be able to pull or twist it off no matter how hard you try.

- *Strap:* Be sure that the chin strap fits snugly under your chin and that the V in the strap meets under your ear. Avoid thin straps, which can be uncomfortable. Check to be sure that the buckle is strong and won't pop open and that the straps are sturdy.

- *Straight:* The helmet should sit straight on your head, not tilted back or forward. A rule of thumb is that the rim should be about two finger widths above your eyebrows (depending on the height of your forehead).

- *Sticker:* Since March 1999, helmets sold in the United States must meet uniform safety standards established by the U.S. Consumer Product Safety Commission (CPSC). Look for a sticker or label that says the helmet meets the CPSC standard. If a helmet does not have one, it does not meet federal safety standards and should not be used.

You are more likely to wear your helmet if it is comfortable, so be sure that vents on the helmet provide airflow to promote cooling and sweat control. You will be safer with a brightly colored helmet that makes you more visible to drivers, especially in rainy, foggy, or dark conditions. Reflective tape will also increase your visibility. Finally, a helmet is a good place to put emergency information (your name, address, and phone number, plus any emergency medical conditions and an emergency contact).

If you are involved in a crash, replace your helmet. Even if the helmet doesn't have any visible signs of damage, its ability to protect your head may be compromised.

SOURCES: Bicycle Helmet Safety Institute. 2009. *A Consumer's Guide to Bicycle Helmets* (http://www.helmets.org/guide.htm; retrieved February 21, 2009); Bicycle Helmet Safety Institute. 2007. *How to Fit a Bicycle Helmet* (http://www.helmets.org/fit.htm; retrieved February 21, 2009).

- Keep floors, stairs, and outside areas clear of objects or conditions that could cause slipping or tripping, such as ice, snow, electrical cords, and toys.

- Put a light switch by the door of every room so no one has to walk across a room to turn on a light. Use night lights in bedrooms, halls, stairs, and bathrooms.

- When climbing a ladder, use both hands. Never stand higher than the third step from the top. When using a stepladder, make sure the spreader brace is in the locked position. With straight ladders, set the base out 1 foot for every 4 feet of height. Don't use chairs to reach things.

- If there are small children in the home, place gates at the top and bottom of stairs. Never leave a baby unattended on a bed or table. Install window guards to prevent children from falling out of windows.

Fires A death caused by a residential fire occurs every 143 minutes. Cooking is the leading cause of home fire injuries; careless smoking is the leading cause of fire deaths, followed by problems with heating equipment and arson. To prevent fires, it's important to dispose of all cigarettes in ashtrays and to never smoke in bed. Other strategies include proper maintenance of fireplaces, furnaces, heaters, chimneys, and electrical outlets, cords, and appliances. If you use a portable heater, keep it at least 3 feet away from curtains, bedding, or anything else that might catch fire. Never leave heaters on unattended.

It's important to be adequately prepared to handle fire-related situations. Plan at least two escape routes out of each room, and designate a location outside the home as a meeting place. For practice, stage a home fire drill; do it at night, as that's when most deadly fires occur.

Install smoke detectors on every level of your home. Your risk of dying in a fire is almost twice as high if you do not use them. Clean the detectors and check the batteries once a month, and replace the batteries at least once a year. These strategies can help prevent injuries in a fire:

- Get out as quickly as possible, and go to the designated meeting place. Don't stop for a keepsake or a pet. Never hide in a closet or under a bed. Once outside, count heads to see if everyone is out. If you think someone is still inside the burning building, tell the firefighters. Never go back inside a burning building.

- If you're trapped in a room, feel the door. If it is hot or if smoke is coming in through the cracks, don't open it; use the alternative escape route. If you can't get out, go to the window and shout for help.
- Smoke inhalation is the primary cause of death and injury in fires. To avoid inhaling smoke, crawl along the floor away from the heat and smoke. Cover your mouth and nose, ideally with a wet cloth, and take short, shallow breaths.
- If your clothes catch fire, don't run. Drop to the ground, cover your face, and roll back and forth to smother the flames. Remember: stop-drop-roll.

Poisoning More than 2.4 million poisonings and more than 30,000 poison-related deaths occur every year in the United States. Poisons come in many forms, some of which are not typically considered poisons. Medications are safe when used as prescribed, but overdosing or incorrectly combining medications with another substance may result in poisoning. Other poisonous substances include cleaning agents, petroleum-based products, insecticides and herbicides, cosmetics, nail polish and remover, and many houseplants. All potentially poisonous substances should be used only as directed and stored out of the reach of children.

The most common type of poisoning by gases is carbon monoxide poisoning. Carbon monoxide gas is emitted by motor vehicle exhaust and some types of heating equipment. The effects of exposure to this colorless, odorless gas include headache, blurred vision, and shortness of breath, followed by dizziness, vomiting, and unconsciousness. Carbon monoxide detectors (similar to smoke detectors) are available for home use. To prevent poisoning by gases, never operate a vehicle in an enclosed space, have your furnace inspected yearly, and use caution with any substance or device that produces potentially toxic fumes.

Keep the national poison control hotline number (800-222-1222) in a convenient location. A call to the national hotline will be routed to a local Poison Control Center, which provides expert emergency advice 24 hours a day. If a poisoning does occur, it's important that you act quickly. Remove the poison from contact with the victim's eyes, skin, or mouth, or move the victim away from contact with poisonous gases. Call the Poison Control Center immediately for instructions; do not follow the emergency instructions on product labels because they may be incorrect. Do not induce vomiting. If you are advised to go to an emergency room, take the poisonous substance or container with you.

Suffocation and Choking Suffocation and choking account for about 5000 deaths annually. Children can suffocate if they put small items in their mouth, get tangled in their crib bedding, or get trapped in airtight appliances like old refrigerators. Keep small objects out of reach of children under age 3, and don't give them raw carrots, hot dogs, popcorn, gum, or hard candy. Examine toys carefully for small parts that could come loose; don't give plastic bags or balloons to small children.

Many choking victims can be saved with the **Heimlich maneuver.** The American Red Cross recommends abdominal thrusts as the easiest and safest thing to do when an adult is choking. Back blows in conjunction with abdominal thrusts are an acceptable procedure for dislodging an object from the throat of an infant.

Firearms About 40% of all unintended firearm deaths occur among people age 5–29. People who use firearms should remember the following:

- Always treat a gun as though it were loaded, even if you know it isn't.
- Never point a gun—loaded or unloaded—at anything you do not intend to shoot.
- Always unload a gun before storing it. Store unloaded firearms under lock and key, in a place separate from the ammunition.
- Always inspect firearms carefully before handling.
- If you ever plan to handle a gun take a firearms safety course first.
- If you own a gun, buy and use a gun lock designed specifically for that weapon.

Proper storage is critical. Do not assume that young children cannot fire a gun. Every year, about 120 Americans are unintentionally shot to death by children under age 6. If you plan to handle a gun, avoid alcohol and drugs, which affect judgment and coordination.

Leisure Injuries

Leisure activities encompass a large part of our free time, so it is not surprising that **leisure injuries** are a significant health-related problem in the United States. Specific safety strategies for activities associated with leisure injuries include the following:

- Don't swim alone, in unsupervised places, under the influence of alcohol, or for an unusual length of time. Use caution when swimming in unfamiliar surroundings or in water colder than 70°F. Check the depth of water before diving. Make sure that residential pools are fenced and that children are never allowed to swim unsupervised.

Heimlich maneuver A maneuver developed by Henry J. Heimlich, M.D., to help force an obstruction from the airway.

leisure injuries Unintentional injuries and deaths that occur in public places or places used in a public way, not involving motor vehicles; includes most sports and recreation deaths and injuries; falls, drownings, burns, and heat and cold stress are examples.

- Always use a **personal flotation device** (also known as a life jacket) when on a boat.

- For all sports and recreational activities, make sure facilities are safe, follow the rules, and practice good sportsmanship. Develop adequate skill in the activity, and use proper safety equipment, including, where appropriate, a helmet, eye protection, correct footwear, and knee, elbow, and wrist pads.

- If using equipment such as skateboards, snowboards, mountain bikes, or all-terrain vehicles, wear a helmet and other safety equipment, and avoid excessive speeds and unsafe stunts. Playground equipment should be used only for those activities for which it is designed.

- If you are active in excessively hot and humid weather, drink plenty of fluids, rest frequently in the shade, and slow down or stop if you feel uncomfortable. Danger signals of heat stress include excessive perspiration, dizziness, headache, muscle cramps, nausea, weakness, rapid pulse, and disorientation.

- Do not use alcohol or other drugs during recreational activities—such activities require coordination and sound judgment.

Work Injuries

According to the Bureau of Labor Statistics, 4.1 million Americans suffered injuries on the job in 2006. Certain types of **work injuries**, including skin disorders and repetitive strain injuries, are increasing. Although laborers make up less than half of the workforce, they account for more than 75% of all work-related injuries and illnesses. Most fatal occupational injuries

> *Laborers make up less than half the American workforce but **suffer 75% of all work-related injuries.***

FIGURE 16.1 Correct lifting technique. Stay upright, bending at the knees and hips.

involve crushing injuries, severe lacerations, burns, and electrocutions; among women, the leading cause of work-place injury deaths is homicide.

Back problems accounted for more than 450,000 work injuries in 2007; many of these could be prevented through proper lifting technique (Figure 16.1).

- Avoid bending at the waist. Remain in an upright position and crouch down if you need to lower yourself to grasp the object. Bend at the knees and hips.

- Place feet securely about shoulder-width apart; grip the object firmly.

- Lift gradually, with straight arms. Avoid quick, jerky motions. Lift by standing up or pushing with your leg muscles. Keep the object close to your body.

- If you have to turn, change the position of your feet. Twisting is a common and dangerous cause of injury. Plan ahead so that your pathway is clear and turning can be minimized.

- Put the object down gently, reversing the steps for lifting.

Musculoskeletal injuries and disorders in the workplace include **repetitive strain injuries (RSIs)**. RSIs are caused by repeated strain on a particular part of the body. Twisting, vibrations, awkward postures, and other

Repetitive Strain Injury

Repetitive strain injuries (RSI) impact the musculoskeletal and nervous systems. Other terms to describe this condition include *repetitive motion disorder (RMD)*, *cumulative trauma disorder (CTD)*, and *occupational overuse syndrome (OOS)*.

An RSI can be caused by a combination of physical and psychosocial stressors, but the injury typically involves some kind of repetitive action or forceful exertion on the body over time. Pain in the extremities as well as the back and shoulders is commonly cited and tends to worsen with extended activity.

The task associated with an RSI may be something relatively simple and nonexertive like typing, writing, or clicking a computer mouse. One of the most common work-related injuries is *carpal tunnel syndrome (CTS)*, which is characterized by pressure on the median nerve in the wrist that also affects tendons and ligaments in the forearm. Symptoms of CTS include numbness, tingling, burning, and/or aching in the hand, particularly in the thumb and the first three fingers. The pain may worsen at night and may shoot up from the hand as far as the shoulder. If it does not clear up on its own, immobilization of the joint at night can be helpful; other options may involve anti-inflammatory drugs or even surgery in extreme cases.

There are complex and more physically destructive examples of an RSI. If a person is operating a jackhammer, the vibration of the equipment and the position in which it must be operated are contributory factors often recognized for that RSI. In terms of physical activity by an athlete, examples include conditions commonly referred to as "golfer's elbow" or "tennis elbow," in which the joints are continually exposed to extreme stress in order to complete an action accurately with speed and force. With new technologies being introduced every day, another type of RSI is now being recognized. Many people who use their thumbs to text are suffering form a condition referred to as "Blackberry thumb." Similarly, people who spend countless hours using handheld controls to play video games are experiencing "gamer's thumb."

In all cases, research indicates the primary risk factors are usually associated with poor posture, improper techniques for completing the activity, and overuse of a certain part of the body. The good news is that a person can make adjustments to reduce the risk of an RSI, either by modifying the action or by modifying the environment. Warm up your wrists before you begin any repetitive motion activity, and take frequent breaks to stretch and flex your wrists and hands:

- Extend your arms out in front of you and stretch your wrists by pointing your fingers to the ceiling; hold for a count of five. Then straighten your wrists and relax your fingers for a count of five.

- With arms extended, make a tight fist with both hands and then bend your

wrists so your knuckles are pointed toward the floor; hold for a count of five. Then straighten your wrists and relax your fingers for count of five.

Repeat these stretches several times, and finish by letting your arms hang loosely at your sides and shaking them gently for several seconds. It's also important to maintain a physically active lifestyle, take plenty of breaks to avoid hours of sedentary activity, continue stretching during an activity, apply proper ergonomic principles, and try to minimize other stress factors.

---

stressors may contribute to RSIs. **Carpal tunnel syndrome** is one type of RSI that has increased in recent years due to increased use of computers (see the box "Repetitive Strain Injury").

Ask Yourself

QUESTIONS FOR CRITICAL THINKING AND REFLECTION

Think of one injury you have suffered. What were you doing when you were injured? Thinking back on the injury, was there anything you could have done to avoid or minimize it? How did the experience change your attitudes or behaviors?

VIOLENCE AND INTENTIONAL INJURIES

Violence—the use of physical force with the intent to inflict harm, injury, or death upon oneself or another—is a major public health concern in the United States. According to the Federal Bureau of Investigation (FBI), over 1.3 million violent crimes occurred in the United States in 2009. In comparison to other industrialized countries, U.S. rates of violence are unusually high in only two areas—homicide and firearm-related deaths. The U.S. homicide death rate is four to ten times that of similar countries, and the firearm death rate is eight times that of other developed countries.

Factors Contributing to Violence

Most intentional injuries and deaths are associated with an argument or the committing of another crime. However, there are many forms of violence, and no single factor can explain all of them.

Social Factors Rates of violence vary by geographic region, neighborhood, socioeconomic level, and many other factors. According to the FBI, violence was highest in the South in 2009, followed by the West. Neighborhoods that are disadvantaged in status, power, and economic resources are typically the ones with the most violence. Rates of violence are highest among young people and minorities, groups that have relatively little power. In 2009, people under age 25 accounted for 45% of the arrests for violent crime in the United States and 50% of the arrests for property crime.

People who feel a part of society (have strong family and social ties), who are economically integrated (have a reasonable chance at getting a decent job), and who grow up in areas where there is a feeling of community (good schools, parks, and neighborhoods) are significantly less likely to engage in violence.

Studies have shown that the environment on college campuses can contribute to violence. The nature of college campuses—transitory communities rather than permanent places where people work and live together over the long term—means that there is less incentive for people to cooperate and coexist amicably.

Violence in the Media The mass media play a major role in exposing audiences of all ages to violence as an acceptable and effective means of solving problems. Children may view as many as 10,000 violent acts on television and in movies each year. Computer and video games also include many violent acts, leading to concern that children's exposure to violence will make them more accepting or tolerant of it. The consequences of violence are depicted much less frequently.

Researchers have found that exposure to media violence at least temporarily increases aggressive feelings in children, making them more likely to engage in violent or fearful behavior; the direct, short-term effects on teens and adults are less clear. Parents should monitor the TV shows, movies, video games, music, and other forms of media to which children are exposed. Watching programs with children gives parents the opportunity to talk to children about violence and its consequences, to explain that violence is not the best way to resolve conflicts or solve problems, and to point out examples of positive behaviors such as kindness and cooperation.

Gender In most cases, violence is committed by men (Figure 16.2). Males are nine times more likely than females to commit murder and three times more likely than females to be murdered. Male college students are twice as likely to be the victim of violence as female students.

Women do commit acts of violence, including a small but substantial proportion of murders of spouses. This fact has been used to argue that women have the same capacity to commit violence as men, but most researchers note substantial differences. Men often kill their wives as the culmination of years of violence or after stalking them; they may kill their entire family and themselves at the same time. Women virtually never kill in such circumstances; rather, they kill their husbands after repeated victimization or while being beaten.

Interpersonal Factors Although most people fear attack from strangers, the majority of victims are acquainted with their attacker. More than half of murders of women and three-fourths of sexual assaults are committed by someone the woman knows. Crime victims and violent criminals tend to share many characteristics—that is, they are likely to be young, male, in a minority, and poor.

Studies of the effects of violent video games and movies—such as *The Expendables* from 2010— have had mixed results. Some experts believe violent entertainment desensitizes young viewers and leads to increased violence in society.

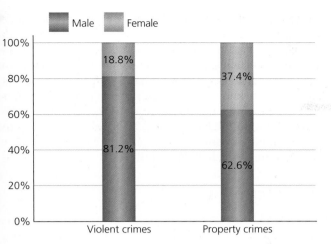

FIGURE 16.2 **Arrests in the United States, 2009.** Males were arrested significantly more often than females for both violent and property crimes.

SOURCE: Federal Bureau of Investigation. 2010. *Crime in the United States 2009.* Washington, D.C.: U.S. Department of Justice.

Alcohol and Other Drugs Substance abuse and dependence are consistently associated with interpersonal violence and suicide. Intoxication affects judgment and may increase aggression in some people, causing a small argument to escalate into a serious physical confrontation. On college campuses, alcohol is involved in about 95% of all violent crimes.

Firearms Many criminologists feel that the high rate of homicide in the United States is directly related to the fact that we are the only industrialized country in which handguns are widespread and easily available. The use of a handgun can change a suicide attempt into a completed suicide and a violent assault into a murder.

> **21%** of aggravated assaults involve the use of a firearm.
>
> —FBI, 2008

Over 100,000 deaths and injuries occur in the United States each year as a result of the use of firearms. Firearms are used in more than two-thirds of homicides, and studies reveal a strong correlation between the incidence of gun ownership and homicide rates for a given area of the country. Over half of all suicides involve a firearm, and people living in households in which guns are kept have a risk of suicide that is five or more times greater than that of people living in households without guns.

Assault

Assault is the use of physical force by a person or persons to inflict injury or death on another; homicide, aggra-

vated assault, and robbery are examples of assault. The victims of assaultive injuries and their perpetrators tend to resemble one another in terms of ethnicity, educational background, psychological profile, and reliance on weapons. In many cases, the victim actually magnifies the confrontation through the use of a weapon.

Homicide

The FBI estimates that more than 15,000 Americans were murdered in 2009. Men, teenagers, young adults, and members of minority groups, particularly African Americans and Latinos, are most likely to be murder victims. The murder rate for black males is several times higher than the rate for the U.S. population as a whole. Poverty and unemployment have been identified as key factors in homicide, and this may account for the high rates of homicide among blacks and other minority groups. Most homicides are committed with a firearm, occur during an argument, and occur among people who know one another. Intrafamilial homicide, where the perpetrator and victim are related, accounts for about one out of every eight homicides. About 40% of family homicides are committed by spouses, usually following a history of physical and emotional abuse directed at the woman.

Gang-Related Violence

Gangs are most frequently associated with large cities, but gang activity also extends to the suburbs and even to rural areas. It is estimated that more than 1 million Americans belong to gangs; the average age for joining a gang is 14. Gang members are more likely than non–gang members to possess weapons, and violence may result from conflicts over territory or illegal activities. Gangs are more common in areas that are poor and suffer from high unemployment, population density, and crime. In these areas, an individual may feel that his or her hope of legitimate success in life is out of reach and know that involvement in the drug market makes some gang members rich. Often, gangs serve as a mechanism for companionship, self-esteem, support, and security; indeed, in some areas gang membership may be viewed as the only possible means of survival.

Hate Crimes

When bias against another person's race or ethnicity, national origin, religion, sexual orientation, or disability motivates a criminal act, the offense is classified as a hate crime. Hate crimes may be committed against people or property. Those against people may include intimidation, assault, and even rape or murder. Crimes against property most frequently involve graffiti, the desecration of churches or synagogues, cross burnings, and other acts of vandalism or property damage.

Nearly 7900 hate crimes were reported in 2008; many more go unreported. Crimes against people made up about 60% of all incidents; intimidation and assault are the most common offenses. Racial or ethnic bias was cited as a motivation in 51% of the hate crimes reported in 2008. National origin or ethnicity was cited in 13% of cases, religion in 18%, and sexual orientation in 18%. But research indicates that a substantial number of hate crimes are committed by males under age 20. Hate crimes are frequently, but not always, associated with fringe groups that have extremist ideologies, such as the Ku Klux Klan and neo-Nazi groups. The rapid growth of hate sites on the Internet is another area of concern.

School Violence

According to the National School Safety Center, about 468 school-associated violent deaths of students, faculty, and administrators have occurred since 1992. Most of these deaths occurred in urban areas, at high schools, and involved use of a firearm. As with other types of violence, both victims and offenders were predominantly young men. Homicide and suicide are the most serious but least common types of violence in schools; an estimated 400,000 less serious incidents of violence and crime occur each year, including theft, vandalism, and fights not involving weapons.

Being a victim of teasing, bullying, or rejection may lead to aggressive behavior or violence.

Children are actually much safer at school than away from it. Less than 1% of all homicides among youths age 5–19 occur at school, and 90% of schools report no incidents of serious violence. Children and adolescents are more likely to be killed by an adult in their own home or away from school than they are to die as a result of school-associated violence. According to the CDC, the overall number of violent incidents has decreased steadily since 1992, but the number of multiple-victim events may have increased.

Schools are basically safe places overall, but there are ways to identify at-risk youths and improve safety for all students. Characteristics associated with youths who have caused school-associated violent deaths include uncontrollable angry outbursts, violent and abusive language and behavior, isolation from peers, depression and irritability, access to and preoccupation with weapons, and lack of support and supervision from adults. Being a victim of teasing, bullying, or social exclusion (rejection) may lead to aggressive behavior and violence.

Recommendations for reducing school violence include offering classroom training in anger management, social skills, and improved self-control; providing mental health and social services for students in need; developing after-school programs that help students build self-esteem and

make friends; and keeping guns out of the hands of children and out of schools.

Being bullied and harassed also leads some teens to suicide, especially gay teens who see no other solution. In 2010, the "It Gets Better" campaign was launched to let LGBT youth know that they are not alone and to give them hope about the possibility of a better future. The campaign was criticized, however, for failing to take steps to stop the harassment and homophobia that in many cases continue unchallenged and unabated in schools.

Workplace Violence

Each year U.S. workers experience an average of 1.5 million minor assaults, 400,000 serious assaults, 85,000 robberies, 50,000 sexual assaults, and 700 homicides. Most of the perpetrators of workplace violence are white males over age 21. Firearms are used in more than 80% of workplace homicides, and the majority of these homicides occur during the commission of a robbery or other crime. Police and corrections officers have the most dangerous jobs, followed by taxi drivers, security guards, bartenders, mental health professionals, and workers at gas stations and convenience and liquor stores. General crime prevention strategies, including use of surveillance cameras and silent alarms and limiting the amount of cash on hand, can help reduce workplace violence related to robberies. Clear guidelines about acceptable behavior and prompt action after any threats or incidents of violence can help control workplace violence.

Terrorism

In 2001, more Americans died as a result of terrorism than in any year before or since; the attacks on September 11 killed more than 3000 people, including citizens of 78 countries. The FBI defines terrorism as the unlawful use of force or violence against persons or property to intimidate or coerce a government, the civilian population, or any segment thereof in furtherance of political or social objectives (see the box "Violence and Health: A Global View"). Terrorism can be either domestic, carried out by groups based in the United States, or international. It comes in many forms, including biological, chemical, nuclear, and cyber. Its intent is to promote helplessness by instilling fear of harm or destruction.

Terrorism-prevention activities occur at all levels of government. U.S. government efforts include close work with the diplomatic, law-enforcement, intelligence, economic, and military communities. The mission of the Department of Homeland Security is to help prevent, protect against, and respond to acts of terrorism on U.S. soil. It is coordinating efforts to protect electric and water supply systems, transportation, gas and oil, emergency services, the computer infrastructure, and other systems.

One step you can take is to put together an emergency plan and kit for your family or household that can serve

The World Health Organization (WHO) estimates that more than 1.6 million people die from violent acts each year. Suicide claims a life every 40 seconds, homicide every minute, and armed conflict every 2 minutes. Violence is among the leading causes of death for people age 15–44, accounting for 14% of deaths among males and 7% of deaths among females. Millions more victims of violence survive but are left with physical, psychological, and reproductive problems. Beyond individual misery, violence has devastating social and economic consequences.

Interpersonal Violence

WHO defines *interpersonal violence* as the intentional use of physical force or power, threatened or actual, against another person that is likely to result in injury, death, psychological harm, or deprivation. Each year, more than 500,000 people die from interpersonal violence, and more than 60 million children and elderly adults are maltreated. It's estimated that 10–70% of women experience physical violence at the hands of an intimate partner during their lifetime; in addition, forced prostitution, child marriage, sexual trafficking, and female genital mutilation are prevalent in some areas of the world.

Worldwide, adolescents and young adults are the primary victims and perpetrators of interpersonal violence. Individual risk factors for violence highlighted in the WHO report include being young, male, and poor; being intoxicated; and having easy access to firearms. At the community and social levels, risk factors include low social capital (norms and networks that promote coordination and cooperation), high crime rates, rapid social change, poverty, poor rule of law and corruption, gender inequality, firearm availability, and armed conflict.

Collective Violence

WHO applies the term *collective violence* to violence inflicted by one group against another group to achieve political, economic, or social objectives. Collective violence includes armed conflict within or between states; genocide, repression, and other human rights abuses; terrorism; and organized violent crime. Characteristics of countries with increased risk of violent conflict include long-standing tensions between groups, a lack of democratic processes, unequal access to power, unequal distribution and control of resources, and rapid demographic changes.

In the twentieth century, an estimated 191 million people—well over half of them civilians—lost their lives directly or indirectly as a result of armed conflict, and many more were injured. In addition to directly causing deaths and injuries, collective violence destroys infrastructure and disrupts trade, food production, and vital services, thus setting the stage for famine, increased rates of infectious diseases, and mass movements of refugees. The resulting social turmoil also increases rates of interpersonal violence.

What Can Be Done?

The WHO report emphasizes that violence is neither an inevitable part of the human condition nor an intractable social problem. Rather, the wide variation in violence within and among nations over time suggests that violence is the product of a complex but modifiable set of social and environmental factors. Potential strategies to reduce violence include the following:

- Individual and relationship approaches to encourage healthy attitudes and behaviors, such as training in social, parenting, and relationship skills and conflict resolution.

- Community-based efforts to raise public awareness and address local social and material causes of violence, such as creating safe places for children to play and adopting community policing

- Societal approaches to change underlying cultural, social, and economic factors, such as new laws and international treaties, policy changes to reduce poverty and inequality, efforts to change harmful social and cultural norms (for example, ethnic discrimination or gender inequality), and disarmament and demobilization programs in countries emerging from conflict.

SOURCES: World Health Organization. 2002. *The World Health Report 2002: Reducing Risks, Promoting Healthy Life.* Geneva: World Health Organization; World Health Organization. 2002. *World Report on Violence and Health.* Geneva: World Health Organization.

---

for any type of emergency or disaster (see the box "The Human Dimension in Antiterrorism Efforts").

Family and Intimate Violence

Family violence generally refers to any rough and illegitimate use of physical force, aggression, or verbal abuse by one family member toward another. Such abuse may be physical and/or psychological in nature. Based on reported cases, an estimated 5–7 million women and children are abused each year in the United States.

Battering   Studies reveal that 95% of domestic violence victims are women. Violence against wives or intimate partners, or battering, occurs at every level of society but is more common at lower socioeconomic levels. It occurs more frequently in relationships with a high degree of conflict—an apparent inability to resolve arguments through negotiation and compromise. About 25% of women report having been physically assaulted or raped by an intimate partner. In more than 10% of cases, the domestic violence continues for 20 years or longer. The problem of intimate violence is even apparent among young people; each year, 1.5 million high school students are victims of physical violence while on a date.

At the root of much of this abusive behavior is the need to control another person. Abusive partners are controlling partners. They not only want to have power over another person, but also believe they are entitled to it, no matter what the cost to the other person. Abuse includes

The Human Dimension in Antiterrorism Efforts

People in the United States were shocked when terrorist attacks resulted in deaths and destruction on American soil in 2001. But since then, Americans have taken more responsibility in the hope of preventing similar incidents in the future.

One immediate result of the attacks on September 11, 2001, was increased restriction on travel. In particular, airline security was elevated to include daily alerts, invasive security checks of luggage and devices, increased random personal searches of passengers, and restrictions on family members in waiting and boarding areas. The initial response to these measures was frustration and anger, especially about delays and the extra time needed for security check-in. Gradually, however, people adjusted to the changes and accepted that the measures were for their own protection.

Terrorist attacks on the Internet—as well as attacks by hackers—have resulted in heightened cybersecurity as well. The importance of having firewalls established and protocols in place to identify or filter viruses and other destructive programs is no longer questioned. Instead of opening every document they receive, most people are now a little more skeptical when their e-mail has unusual or inappropriate identifiers in the sender or domain names. Increased security provisions are offset by more peace of mind.

Individual Americans have also demonstrated courage and resourcefulness in response to terrorist acts. Even on September 11, one of the planes hijacked by terrorists was brought down in a field in Pennsylvania by passengers who organized themselves to prevent another disaster like the ones unfolding at the World Trade Center and the Pentagon. As a result of their actions, onboard security measures have increased dramatically through increased training of flight personnel and pre-boarding procedures.

An incident in New York City's Times Square on May 1, 2010, is another example of individual Americans demonstrating their willingness to be proactive against terrorist acts. Street vendors, many of whom were war veterans, detected a homemade bomb smoldering in a parked SUV. Acting on their slogan "If you see something, say something," they alerted police, and as a result many lives were saved and injuries avoided.

The world is changing, and the unfortunate truth is that terrorism has become part of our existence. International groups like the Organization for Security and Co-operation in Europe have been established to fight terrorism and meet its challenge through preventive efforts worldwide, including North America.

Part of its strategy is to identify any potential gaps that could weaken a country if attacked by terrorists so that countermeasures can be put in place. Its proactive efforts focus on providing technical assistance and help in developing the human dimension of antiterrorism projects. The belief is that by working together with common goals in mind, people worldwide can effectively address terrorism.

What can you do to help combat terrorism? Be aware that danger can exist, and be willing to take personal responsibility to act. At the same time, don't let yourself be immobilized by fear or hypervigilance. Inform yourself, and work locally within your community so you know what to do in case of emergency. Make sure you have an emergency supply kit and a household or family emergency plan in place. Take a first aid class and see whether your community has an emergency response group you can join. More information about what you can do in case of a terrorist attack or any kind of disaster is available from the following sources:

American Red Cross (www.redcross.org)

Federal Emergency Management Agency (www.fema.gov)

U.S. Department of Homeland Security (www.ready.gov)

---

behavior that physically harms, arouses fear, prevents a person from doing what she wants, or compels her to behave in ways she does not freely choose.

In abusive relationships, the abuser (in most cases a man) usually has a history of violent behavior, traditional beliefs about gender roles, and problems with alcohol abuse. He has low self-esteem and seeks to raise it by dominating and imposing his will on another person. Research has revealed a three-phase cycle of battering, consisting of a period of increasing tension, a violent explosion and loss of control, and a period of contriteness in which the man begs forgiveness and promises it will never happen again. The batterer is drawn back to this cycle over and over again, but he never succeeds in changing his feelings about himself.

Battered women often stay in violent relationships for years. They may be economically dependent on their partners, feel trapped or fear retaliation if they leave, believe their children need a father, or have low self-esteem themselves. They may love or pity their husband, or they may believe they'll eventually be able to stop the violence. They usually leave the relationship only when they become determined that the violence must end. Battered women's shelters offer physical protection, counseling, support, and other assistance.

Stalking and Cyberstalking Battering is closely associated with **stalking**, characterized by harassing behaviors such as following or spying on a person and making verbal, written, or implied threats. In the United States, it is estimated that 1 million women and 400,000 men are stalked each year; about 87% of stalkers are men. About half of female victims are stalked by current or former

stalking Repeatedly harassing or threatening a person through behaviors such as following a person, appearing at a person's residence or workplace, leaving written messages or objects, making harassing phone calls, or vandalizing property; frequently directed at a former intimate partner.

intimate partners; of these, 80% had been physically or sexually assaulted by that partner during the relationship. Stalking among female college students may be greater than that experienced by the general population. A stalker's goal may be to control or scare the victim or to keep her or him in a relationship. Most stalking episodes last a year or less.

The use of the Internet, e-mail, chat rooms, Facebook, and other electronic means to stalk another person is known as **cyberstalking.** As with offline stalking, the majority of cyberstalkers are men, and the majority of victims are women, although there have been same-sex cyberstalking incidents. Cyberstalkers may send harassing or threatening e-mails or chat room messages to the victim, or they may encourage others to harass the victim—for example, by impersonating the victim and posting inflammatory messages and personal information on bulletin boards or in chat rooms. Guidelines for staying safe online include the following:

- Avoid using your real name on the Internet. Select an age- and gender-neutral identity.
- Avoid filling out profiles for accounts with information that could be used to identify you.
- Do not share personal information in public spaces anywhere online or give it to strangers.
- Learn how to filter unwanted e-mail messages.
- If you experience harassment online, do not respond to the harasser. Log off or go to a different site.

Educational campaigns can help raise awareness about child abuse. Support and therapy, including family therapy, can help the victims.

If harassment continues, contact the harasser's Internet service provider (ISP) by identifying the domain of the stalker's account (after the "@" sign); most ISPs have an e-mail address for complaints. Often, an ISP can try to stop the conduct by direct contact with the harasser or by closing his or her account. Save all communications for evidence, and contact your ISP and your local police department.

Violence Against Children Every year, at least 1 million American children are physically abused by their parents, and another 1 to 2 million are victims of neglect. Parents who abuse children tend to have low self-esteem, to believe in physical punishment, to have a poor marital relationship, and to have been abused themselves (although many people who were abused as children do not grow up to abuse their own children). Poverty, unemployment, and social isolation are characteristics of families in which children are abused. External stressors related to socioeconomic and environmental factors are most closely associated with neglect, whereas stressors related to interpersonal issues are more closely associated with physical abuse. Single parents, both men and women, are at especially high risk for abusing their children.

Elder Abuse Each year, 1–2 million older adults are abused, exploited, or mistreated by someone who is supposed to be giving them care and protection; only one in six incidents is reported. Most abusers are family members who are serving as caregivers. Elder abuse can take different forms: physical, sexual, or emotional abuse; financial exploitation; neglect; or abandonment. Neglect accounts for about 55% of reported cases. Physical abuse accounts for about 15% of reported cases, and financial exploitation for about 13%. Abuse often occurs when caring for a dependent adult becomes too stressful for the caregiver, especially if the elder is incontinent, has suffered mental deterioration, or is violent. Abuse may become an outlet for frustration. Many believe that the solution to elder abuse is support in the form of greater social and financial assistance, such as adult day-care centers and education and public care programs.

Sexual Violence

The use of force and coercion in sexual relationships is one of the most serious problems in human interactions. The most extreme manifestation of sexual coercion is rape, but sexual coercion occurs in many subtler forms, including sexual harassment.

cyberstalking The use of e-mail, chat rooms, bulletin boards, or other electronic communications devices to stalk another person.

Sexual Assault: Rape   Sexual coercion that relies on the threat and use of physical force or takes advantage of circumstances that render a person incapable of giving consent (such as when drunk) constitutes **sexual assault** or **rape**. When the victim is younger than the legally defined age of consent, the act constitutes **statutory rape**, whether or not coercion is involved. Coerced sexual activity in which the victim knows or is dating the rapist is often referred to as **date rape**, or *acquaintance rape*. Most victims know their assailant, but less than one-third of all sexual crimes are reported.

Any woman—or man—can be a rape victim. Between 100,000 and 130,000 cases of rape are reported each year. It is estimated that nearly 700,000 women are raped each year and that 1 in 6 women and 1 in 33 men have experienced an attempted or completed rape at some point in their lives. A study of college students found that between 1 in 4 and 1 in 5 college women experienced a completed or attempted rape during their college years. Most male-on-male rapes do not occur in prison.

WHO COMMITS RAPE?   Men who commit rape may be any age and come from any socioeconomic group. Some rapists are exploiters in the sense that they rape on the spur of the moment and mainly want immediate gratification. Some attempt to compensate for feelings of sexual inadequacy and an inability to obtain satisfaction otherwise. Others are more hostile and sadistic and are primarily interested in hurting and humiliating a particular woman or women in general. Often, the rapist is more interested in dominance, control, and power than in sexual satisfaction.

Most women are in much less danger of being raped by a stranger than of being sexually assaulted by a man they know or date. Surveys suggest that as many as 25% of women have had experiences in which the men they were dating persisted in trying to force sex despite pleading, crying, screaming, or resisting. Surveys have also found that more than 60% of all rape victims were raped by a current or former spouse, boyfriend, or date.

Most cases of date rape are never reported to the police, partly because of the subtlety of the crime. Usually no weapons are involved, and direct verbal threats may not have been made. Victims of date rape tend to shoulder much of the responsibility for the incident, questioning their own judgment and behavior rather than blaming the aggressor.

FACTORS CONTRIBUTING TO DATE RAPE   Although the general status of women in society has improved, it is still a commonly held cultural belief that nice women don't say yes to sex (even when they want to) and that real men don't take no for an answer.

Men and women also differ in their perception of romantic encounters and signals. In one study, researchers found that men interpreted women's actions on dates, such as smiling or talking in a low voice, as indicating an interest in having sex, whereas the women interpreted the same actions as just being friendly. Men's thinking about forceful sex also tends to be unclear. One psychologist reports that men find "forcing a woman to have sex against her will" more acceptable than "raping a woman," even though the former description is the definition of rape.

DATE-RAPE DRUGS   The drugs used in date rapes include flunitrazepam (Rohypnol), gamma hydroxybutyrate (GHB), and ketamine hydrochloride ("Special K"). These drugs have a variety of effects, including sedation; if slipped surreptitiously into a drink, they can incapacitate a person within about 20 minutes and make her or him more vulnerable to assault. Rohypnol, GHB, and other drugs also often cause anterograde amnesia, meaning victims have little memory of what happened while they were under the influence of the drug. The Drug-Induced Rape Prevention and Punishment Act of 1996 adds up to 20 years to the prison sentence of any rapist who uses a drug to incapacitate a victim. Strategies such as the following can help ensure that your drink is not tampered with at a bar or party:

- Check with campus or local police to find out if drug-facilitated sexual assault has occurred in your area and, if so, where.
- Drink moderately and responsibly. Avoid group drinking and drinking games.
- Be wary of opened beverages—alcoholic or non-alcoholic—offered by strangers. When at an unfamiliar bar, watch the bartender pour your drink.
- If an opened beverage tastes, looks, or smells strange, do not drink it. If you leave your drink unattended, obtain a fresh drink when you return to your table.
- If you go to a party, club, or bar, go with friends. Have a prearranged plan for checking on each other visually and verbally. If you feel giddy or lightheaded, get assistance.

Both males and females can take actions that will reduce the incidence of acquaintance rape; see the box "Preventing Date Rape" for specific suggestions.

DEALING WITH A SEXUAL ASSAULT   Each situation is unique, and a woman should respond to the threat of rape in

TERMS

sexual assault, or rape   The use of force to have sex with someone against that person's will.

statutory rape   Sexual interaction with someone under the legal age of consent.

date rape   Sexual assault by someone the victim knows or is dating; also called *acquaintance rape*.

Preventing Date Rape

Guidelines for Women

- Believe in your right to control what you do. Set limits, and communicate these limits clearly, firmly, and early. Say no when you mean no.

- Be assertive with someone who is sexually pressuring you. Men often interpret passivity as permission.

- If you are unsure of a new acquaintance, go on a group date or double date. If possible, provide your own transportation.

- Remember that some men assume sexy dress and a flirtatious manner mean a desire for sex.

- Remember that alcohol and drugs interfere with clear communication about sex.

- Use the statement that has proven most effective in stopping date rape: "This is rape, and I'm calling the police."

Guidelines for Men

- Be aware of social pressure. It's OK to not score.

- Understand that no means no. Don't continue making advances when your date resists or tells you she wants to stop. Remember that she has the right to refuse sex.

- Don't assume sexy dress and a flirtatious manner are invitations to sex, that previous permission for sex applies to the current situation, or that your date's relationships with other men constitute sexual permission for you.

- Remember that alcohol and drugs interfere with clear communication about sex.

whatever way she thinks best. If a woman chooses not to resist, it does not mean that she has not been raped. If you are threatened by a rapist and decide to fight back, here is what Women Organized Against Rape (WOAR) recommends:

- Trust your gut feeling. If you feel you are in danger, don't hesitate to run and scream. It is better to feel foolish than to be raped.

- Yell—and keep yelling. It will clear your head and start your adrenaline going; it may scare your attacker and also bring help. Don't forget that a rapist is also afraid of pain and afraid of getting caught.

- If an attacker grabs you from behind, use your elbows for striking his neck, his sides, or his stomach.

- Try kicking. Your legs are the strongest part of your body, and your kick is longer than his reach. Kick with your rear foot and with the toe of your shoe. Aim low to avoid losing your balance.

- His most vulnerable spot is his knee; it's low, difficult to protect, and easily knocked out of place. Don't try to kick a rapist in the crotch; he has been protecting this area all his life and will have better protective reflexes there than at his knees.

- Once you start fighting, keep it up. Your objective is to get away as soon as you can.

- Remember that ordinary rules of behavior don't apply. It's OK to vomit, act crazy, or claim to have a sexually transmitted disease.

If you are raped, tell what happened to the first friendly person you meet. Call the police, tell them you were raped, and give your location. Try to remember as many facts as you can about your attacker; write down a description as soon as possible. Don't wash or change your clothes, or you may destroy important evidence. The police will take you to a hospital for a complete exam; show the physician any injuries. Tell the police simply, but exactly, what happened. Be honest, and stick to your story.

If you decide that you don't want to report the rape to the police, be sure to see a physician as soon as possible. You need to be checked for pregnancy and STDs.

THE EFFECTS OF RAPE Rape victims suffer both physical and psychological injury. For most, physical wounds heal within a few weeks. Psychological pain may endure and be substantial. Even the most physically and mentally strong are likely to experience shock, anxiety, depression, shame, and a host of psychosomatic symptoms after being victimized. Some victims experience rape trauma syndrome, a form of PTSD, characterized by fear, nightmares, fatigue, crying spells, and digestive upset. Self-blame is very likely; society has contributed to this tendency by perpetuating the myths that women can actually defend themselves and that no one can be raped if she doesn't want to be. Fortunately, these false beliefs are dissolving in the face of evidence to the contrary.

Many organizations offer counseling and support to rape victims. Look online or in the telephone directory under Rape or Rape Crisis Center for a hotline number to call. Your campus may have counseling services or a support group.

Child Sexual Abuse Child sexual abuse is any sexual contact between an adult and a child who is below the legal age of consent. Adults and older adolescents are able to coerce children into sexual activity because of their authority and power over them. Threats, force, or the promise of friendship or material rewards may be used to manipulate a child. Sexual contacts are typically brief and consist of genital manipulation; genital intercourse is much less common. Sexual abusers are usually

Most rape victims are assaulted by someone they know, not by a stranger.

male, heterosexual, and known to the victim. The abuser may be a relative, a friend, a neighbor, or another trusted adult acquaintance. Child abusers are often pedophiles, people who are sexually attracted to children. They may have poor interpersonal and sexual relationships with other adults and feel socially inadequate and inferior. One highly traumatic form of sexual abuse is **incest,** sexual activity between people too closely related to legally marry.

Child sexual abuse is often unreported. Surveys suggest that as many as 27% of women and 16% of men were sexually abused as children. An estimated 150,000–200,000 new cases of child sexual abuse occur each year. It can leave lasting scars; as adults, victims are more likely to suffer from low self-esteem, depression, anxiety, eating disorders, self-destructive tendencies, sexual problems, and difficulties in intimate relationships.

If you were a victim of sexual abuse as a child and feel it may be interfering with your functioning today, you may want to address the problem. A variety of approaches can help, such as joining a support group of people who have had similar experiences, confiding in a partner or friend, or seeking professional help.

Sexual Harassment Unwelcome sexual advances, requests for sexual favors, and other verbal, visual, or physical conduct of a sexual nature constitute **sexual harassment** if such conduct explicitly or implicitly affects academic or employment decisions or evaluations; interferes with an individual's academic or work performance; or creates an intimidating, hostile, or offensive academic, work, or student living environment.

Extreme cases of sexual harassment occur when a manager, professor, or other person in authority uses his or her ability to control or influence jobs or grades to coerce people into having sex or to punish them if they refuse. A hostile environment can be created by conduct such as sexual gestures, displaying of sexually suggestive objects or pictures, derogatory comments and jokes, sexual remarks about clothing or appearance, obscene letters, and unnecessary touching or pinching.

If you have been the victim of sexual harassment, you can take action to stop it. Be assertive with anyone who uses language or actions you find inappropriate. If possible, confront your harasser in writing, over the telephone, or in person, informing him or her that the situation is unacceptable to you and you want the harassment to stop. If assertive communication doesn't work, assemble a file or log documenting the harassment, noting the details of each incident and information about any witnesses. You may discover others who have been harassed by the same person, which will strengthen your case. Then file a grievance with the harasser's supervisor or employer.

If your attempts to deal with the harassment internally are not successful, you can file an official complaint with your city or state Human Rights Commission or Fair Employment Practices Agency, or with the federal Equal Employment Opportunity Commission. You may also wish to pursue legal action under the Civil Rights Act or under local laws prohibiting employment discrimination. Very often, the threat of a lawsuit or other legal action is enough to stop the harasser.

What You Can Do About Violence

Violence in our society is a serious threat to our collective health and well-being. This is especially true on college campuses (see the box "Staying Safe on Campus"). Schools are now providing training for conflict resolution and are educating people about the diverse nature of our society, thereby encouraging tolerance and understanding.

Reducing gun-related injuries may require changes in the availability, possession, and lethality of the 8–12 million firearms sold in the United States each year. As part of the Brady gun control law, computerized instant background checks are performed for most gun sales to prevent purchases by convicted felons, people with a history of mental instability, and certain other groups. In some states, waiting periods are required in addition to the background checks. Some groups advocate a complete and universal federal ban on the sale of all handguns.

Safety experts also advocate the adoption of consumer safety standards for guns, including features such as child-proofing and indicators to show if a gun is loaded. Technologies are now available to personalize handguns to help prevent unauthorized use. Education about proper storage is also important.

QUICK STATS

About **12,000** sexual harassment charges are filed with the EEOC each year.

—U.S. Equal Employment Opportunity Commission, 2008

Ask Yourself

QUESTIONS FOR CRITICAL THINKING AND REFLECTION

Have you or anyone you know ever been the victim of a violent act? If so, what were the circumstances surrounding the event? What was the outcome? How did the event affect your life? In hindsight, what steps could have been taken to avoid or prevent the incident?

Staying Safe on Campus

College campuses can be the site of criminal activity and violence just as any other environment or living situation can be—and so they require the same level of caution and awareness that you would use in other situations. Two key points to remember: 80% of campus crimes are committed by a student against a fellow student, and alcohol or drug use is involved in 90% of campus felonies. Drinking or drug use can affect judgment and lower inhibitions, so be aware if you or another person is under the influence. Here are some suggestions for keeping yourself safe on campus:

- Don't travel alone after dark. Many campuses have shuttle buses that run from spots on campus such as the library and the dining hall to residence halls and other locations. Escorts are often available to walk with you at night.

- Be familiar with well-lit and frequently traveled routes around campus if you do need to walk alone.

- If you have a car, follow the usual precautions about parking in well-lit areas, keeping the doors locked while you are driving, and never picking up hitchhikers.

- Always have your keys ready as you approach your residence hall, room, and car. Don't lend your keys to others.

- Let friends and family members know your schedule of classes and activities to create a sort of buddy system.

- Be sure the doors and windows of your dorm room have sturdy locks, and use them.

- Don't prop open doors or hold doors open for nonstudents or nonresidents trying to enter your dorm. Be aware of nonresidents around your dorm. If someone says that he or she is meeting a friend inside, that person should be able to call the friend from outside the building.

- Keep valuables and anything containing personal information—credit cards, wallets, jewelry, and so on—

hidden. Secure expensive computer and stereo equipment with cables so that it can't be easily stolen. Use a quality U-shaped lock whenever you leave a bicycle unattended.

- Be alert when using an ATM, and don't display large amounts of cash.

- Stay alert and trust your instincts. Don't hesitate to call the police or campus security if something doesn't seem or feel right.

The Jeanne Clery Disclosure of Campus Security Policy and Campus Crime Statistics Act, named for a Lehigh University student who was murdered in her residence hall in 1986, requires colleges and universities to collect and report campus crime statistics. You can now review this information online at the Crime Statistics Web site of the U.S. Department of Education's Office of Postsecondary Education (http://ope.ed.gov/security/Search.asp).

PROVIDING EMERGENCY CARE

A course in **first aid** can help you respond appropriately when someone is injured. One important benefit of first aid training is learning what *not* to do in certain situations. For example, a person with a suspected neck or back injury should not be moved unless other life-threatening conditions exist. A trained person can assess emergency situations accurately before acting.

Emergency rescue techniques can save the lives of people who are choking, who have stopped breathing, or whose hearts have stopped beating. As described earlier, the Heimlich maneuver is used when a victim is choking. Pulmonary resuscitation (also known as rescue breathing, artificial respiration, or mouth-to-mouth resuscitation) is used when a person is not breathing. Cardiopulmonary resuscitation (CPR) is used when a pulse cannot be found. Training is required before a person can perform CPR; courses are offered by the American Red Cross and the

American Heart Association. In 2008 the American Heart Association issued new guidelines for hands-only CPR, which has been found to be as effective as CPR with rescue breathing (see the inside back cover).

A new feature of some of these courses is training in the use of automated external defibrillators (AEDs), which monitor the heart's rhythm and, if appropriate, deliver an

incest Sexual activity between close relatives, such as siblings or parents and their children.

sexual harassment Unwelcome sexual advances, requests for sexual favors, and other conduct of a sexual nature that affects academic or employment decisions or evaluations; interferes with an individual's academic or work performance; or creates an intimidating, hostile, or offensive academic, work, or student living environment.

first aid Emergency care given to an ill or injured person until medical care can be obtained.

TERMS

electrical shock to restart the heart. Because of the importance of early use of defibrillators in saving heart attack victims, these devices are being installed in public places, including casinos, airports, and many office buildings.

As a person providing assistance, you are the first link in the **emergency medical services (EMS) system.** Your responsibility may be to render first aid, provide emotional support for the victim, or just call for help. The basic pattern for providing emergency care is check-call-care:

- *Check the situation:* Make sure the scene is safe for both you and the injured person.
- *Check the victim:* Conduct a quick head-to-toe examination. Assess the victim's signs and symptoms, such as level of responsiveness, pulse, and breathing rate. Look for bleeding and any indications of broken bones or paralysis.
- *Call for help:* Call 9-1-1 or a local emergency number. Identify yourself and give as much information as you can about the condition of the victim and what happened.
- *Care for the victim:* If the situation requires immediate action (no pulse, shock, etc.), provide first aid if you are trained to do so.

Connect to your Choices

Have you ever thought about where you get your behaviors and habits related to your personal safety? Many factors can influence our behaviors and habits, some not as obvious as others. Does your social circle include people who are risk takers, who think they're invincible, or who drink excessively? Are there unsafe places in your community, such as swimming pools or waterways without lifeguards? Does your residence have smoke alarms or sprinklers? Does your school have an emergency warning system in case of a terrorist attack or a dangerous situation on campus?

What are the external factors that influence your choices about personal safety? What are your inner motivations and core values, and how do they affect your choices? Based on what you learned in this chapter, will you make some different choices in the future? If so, what will they be?

Go online to Connect to complete this activity. www.mcgraw-hillconnect.com

TIPS FOR TODAY AND THE FUTURE

Protecting yourself from injuries means taking sensible safety precautions every day and preparing yourself to deal with an emergency.

RIGHT NOW YOU CAN

- Check your home for any object or situation that could cause an injury, such as a tripping hazard, top-heavy shelves, and so on.
- Test the batteries in your home's smoke detectors, and change them if necessary. Test the detectors to make sure they work properly.
- If you ride a bike, check your helmet to ensure that it still fits properly and will protect you in a crash. If you have any doubts, throw it away and buy a new one.

IN THE FUTURE YOU CAN

- Get trained in CPR, rescue breathing, and the use of an automated external defibrillator. If you have already had such training, take a refresher course.
- Be watchful for hazardous situations at your school and workplace. If you notice anything suspicious, report it to an appropriate person right away.

SUMMARY

- Key factors in motor vehicle injuries include aggressive driving, speeding, a failure to wear safety belts, alcohol and drug intoxication, fatigue, and distraction.

- Motorcycle, motor scooter, and bicycle injuries can be prevented by developing appropriate skills, driving or riding defensively, and wearing proper safety equipment.

- Most fall-related injuries are a result of falls at floor level, but stairs, chairs, and ladders are also involved in a significant number of falls.

- Careless smoking and problems with cooking or heating equipment are common causes of home fires. Being prepared for fire emergencies means planning escape routes and installing smoke detectors.

- The home can contain many poisonous substances, including medications, cleaning agents, plants, and fumes from cars and appliances.

- Performing the Heimlich maneuver can prevent someone from dying from choking.

- The proper storage and handling of firearms can help prevent injuries; assume that any gun is loaded.

- Many injuries during leisure activities result from the misuse of equipment, lack of experience, use of alcohol, and a failure to wear proper safety equipment.

Adopting Safer Habits

For the next 7–10 days, keep track of any mishaps you are involved in or injuries you receive, recording them on a daily behavior record like the one shown in Chapter 1. Count each time you cut, burn, or injure yourself, fall down, run into someone, or have any other potentially injury-causing mishap, no matter how trivial. Also record any risk-taking behaviors, such as failing to wear your safety belt or bicycle helmet, drinking and driving, exceeding the speed limit, putting off home or bicycle repairs, and so on. For each entry (injury or incidence of unsafe behavior), record the date, the time, what you were doing, who else was there and how you were influenced by him or her, what your motivations were, and what you were thinking and feeling at the time.

At the end of the monitoring period, examine your data. For each incident, determine both the human factors and the environmental factors that contributed to the injury or unsafe behavior. Were you tired? Distracted? Did you not realize this situation was dangerous? Did you take a chance? Did you think this incident couldn't happen to you? Was visibility poor? Were you using defective equipment? Then consider each contributing factor carefully, determining why it existed and how it could have been avoided or changed. Finally, consider what preventive actions you could take to avoid such incidents or to change your behaviors in the future.

As an example, let's say that you usually don't use a safety belt when you run local errands in your car and that several factors contribute to this behavior: You don't really think you could be involved in a crash so close to home, you go on only short trips, you just never think to use it, and so on. One of the contributing factors to your unsafe behavior is inadequate knowledge. You can change this factor by obtaining accurate information about auto crashes (and their usual proximity to a victim's home) from this chapter and from library or Internet research. Just acquiring information about auto crashes and safety belt use may lead you to examine your beliefs and attitudes about safety belts and motivate you to change your behavior.

Once you're committed, you can use behavior change techniques described in Chapter 1, such as completing a contract, asking family and friends for support, and so on, to build a new habit. Put a note or picture reminding you to buckle up in your car where you can see it clearly. Recruit a friend to run errands with you and to remind you about using your safety belt. Once your habit is established, you may influence other people—especially people who ride in your car—to use safety belts all the time. By changing this behavior, you have reduced the chances that you or your passengers will suffer a serious injury or even die in a vehicle crash.

- Most work-related injuries involve extensive manual labor; back problems and repetitive strain injuries are most common.

- Factors contributing to violence include poverty, the absence of strong social ties, the influence of the mass media, cultural attitudes about gender roles, problems in interpersonal relationships, alcohol and drug abuse, and the availability of firearms.

- Types of violence include assault, homicide, gang-related violence, hate crimes, school violence, workplace violence, and terrorism.

- Battering and child abuse occur at every socioeconomic level. The core issue is the abuser's need to control other people.

- Most rape victims are women, and most know their attackers. Factors in date rape include different standards of appropriate sexual behavior for men and women and different perceptions of actions.

- Sexual harassment is unwelcome sexual advances or other conduct of a sexual nature that affects academic or employment performance or evaluations or that creates an intimidating, hostile, or offensive academic, work, or student living environment.

- Steps in giving emergency care include making sure the scene is safe for you and the injured person, conducting a quick examination of the victim, calling for help, and providing emergency first aid.

FOR MORE INFORMATION

BOOKS

American Medical Association. 2009. *American Medical Association Handbook of First Aid and Emergency Care.* New York: Random House Reference. *An everyday guide to the most current first aid and emergency resuscitation techniques, with instructions for using automatic defibrillators.*

Dacey, J. S., and L. B. Fiore. 2006. *The Safe Child Handbook.* San Francisco: Jossey-Bass. *A practical handbook for keeping your family safe and coping with the stress and fear associated with many real-world dangers.*

Henry, J., H. Larson, and J. Rubin. 2007. *Home Emergency Pocket Guide.* Tigard, OR.: Informed Publishing. *A small, spiral-bound guide that provides critical information to help in dealing with a variety of emergencies.*

Lipman, I. A. 2010. *How to Be Safe: Survival Tactics to Protect Yourself, Your Home, Your Business and Your Family.* New York: Readers Digest Books. *A wide-ranging guide to safety, covering topics from home security to dealing with a terrorist attack.*

World Health Organization. 2010. *Preventing intimate partner and sexual violence against women: Taking action and generating evidence.* Geneva: World Health Organization. *The latest volume in a series of publications addressing the varying types of violence affecting our global society.*

ORGANIZATIONS, HOTLINES, AND WEB SITES

American Bar Association: Domestic Violence. Provides information on statistics, research, and laws relating to domestic violence.

    http://www.abanet.org/publiced/practical/domviol.html

Consumer Product Safety Commission. Provides information and advice about safety issues relating to consumer products.

    http://www.cpsc.gov

Insurance Institute for Highway Safety. Provides information about crashes on the nation's highways, as well as reports on topics such as speeding and crashworthiness of vehicles.

    http://www.iihs.org

National Center for Injury Prevention and Control. Provides consumer-oriented information about unintentional injuries and violence.

    http://www.cdc.gov/injury

National Center for Victims of Crime. An advocacy group for crime victims; provides statistics, news, safety strategies, tips on finding local assistance, and links to related sites.

    http://www.ncvc.org

National Highway Traffic Safety Administration. Supplies materials about reducing deaths, injuries, and economic losses from motor vehicle crashes.

    http://www.nhtsa.gov

National Safety Council. Provides information and statistics about preventing unintentional injuries.

    http://www.nsc.org

National Violence Hotlines. Provide information, referral services, and crisis intervention.

    800-799-SAFE (domestic violence)
    800-422-4453 (child abuse)
    800-656-HOPE (sexual assault)

Occupational Safety and Health Administration. Provides information about topics related to health and safety issues in theworkplace.

    http://www.osha.gov

Prevent Child Abuse America. Provides statistics, information, and publications relating to child abuse, including parenting tips.

    http://www.preventchildabuse.org

Rape, Abuse, and Incest National Network (RAINN). Provides guidelines for preventing and dealing with sexual assault and abuse.

    http://www.rainn.org

Tolerance.Org. Offers suggestions for fighting hate and promoting tolerance; sponsored by the Southern Poverty Law Center.

    http://www.tolerance.org

World Health Organization: Violence and Injury Prevention. Provides statistics and information about the consequences of intentional and unintentional injuries worldwide.

    http://www.who.int/violence_injury_prevention

The following sites provide statistics and background information on violence and crime in the United States:

Bureau of Justice Statistics: http://bjs.ojp.usdoj.gov
Federal Bureau of Investigation: http://www.fbi.gov
Justice Information Center: http://www.ncjrs.org

SELECTED BIBLIOGRAPHY

Anderson, C. A., et al. 2010. Violent video game effects on aggression, empathy, and prosocial behavior in eastern and western countries: A meta-analytic review. *Psychological Bulletin* 136(2): 151–173.

Carr, J. L. 2005. *American College Health Association Campus Violence White Paper.* Baltimore, Md.: American College Health Association.

Centers for Disease Control and Prevention. 2010. *Unintentional Drug Poisoning in the United States.* Atlanta, Ga.: Centers for Disease Control and Prevention.

Centers for Disease Control and Prevention. 2008. Nonfatal, unintentional, non-fire-related carbon monoxide exposures—United States, 2004–2006. *Morbidity and Mortality Weekly Report* 57(33): 896–899.

Centers for Disease Control and Prevention. 2006. Nonfatal injuries and restraint use among child passengers—United States, 2004. *Morbidity and Mortality Weekly Report* 55(22): 624–627.

Centers for Disease Control and Prevention. 2010. Youth Risk Behavior Surveillance—United States, 2009. *Morbidity and Mortality Weekly Report Surveillance Summaries* 59(SS05): 1–142.

FIA Foundation for the Automobile and Society. 2010. *U.N. Decade of Action for Road Safety, 2001–2020* (http://www.fiafoundation.org/publications/Documents/decade_is_action_booklet.pdf; retrieved October 8, 2010).

Cummings, P., et al. 2006. Changes in traffic crash mortality rates attributed to use of alcohol, or lack of a seat belt, air bag, motorcycle helmet, or bicycle helmet, United States, 1982–2001. *Injury Prevention* 12(3): 148–154.

Federal Bureau of Investigation. 2009. *Hate Crime Statistics, 2008.* Washington, D.C.: U.S. Department of Justice.

Federal Bureau of Investigation. 2010. *Crime in the United States, 2009.* Washington, D.C.: U.S. Department of Justice.

Governors' Highway Safety Association. 2010. *Cell Phone and Texting Laws: October, 2010* (http://www.ghsa.org/html/stateinfo/laws/cellphone_laws.html; retrieved October 8, 2010).

Iudice, A., et al. 2005. Effects of prolonged wakefulness combined with alcohol and hands-free cell phone divided attention tasks on simulated driving. *Human Psychopharmacology* 20(2): 125–132.

Narang, P., et al. 2010. Do guns provide safety? At what cost? *Southern Medical Journal* 103(2): 151–153.

National Center for Health Statistics. 2009. Deaths: Final data for 2007. *National Vital Statistics Reports* 58(19).

National Safety Council. 2010. *In0jury Facts 2010.* Itasca, Ill.: National Safety Council.

National School Safety Center. 2010. *School Associated Violent Deaths.* Oak Park, Ca.: National School Safety Center.

National Traffic Safety Administration. 2007. *Traffic Safety Facts Research Note: Driver Cell Phone Use in 2006—Overall Results.* Washington, D.C.: National Traffic Safety Administration.

Olson, C. M., et al. 2006. Association of first- and second-generation air bags with front occupant death in car crashes: A matched cohort study. *American Journal of Epidemiology* 164(2): 161–169.

Roudsari, B., et al. 2009. Ethnicity, age, and trends in alcohol-related driver fatalities in the United States. *Traffic Injury Prevention* 10(5): 410–414.

Strayer, D. L., et al. 2006. A comparison of the cell phone driver and the drunk driver. *Human Factors* 48(2): 381–391.

Thompson, R. S., et al. 2006. Intimate partner violence: Prevalence, types and chronicity in adult women. *American Journal of Preventive Medicine* 30(6): 447–457.

UC Berkeley School of Public Health. 2006. Cycling: Use your head. *University of California, Berkeley, Wellness Letter* 22(9): 6.

Zimmerman, F. J., et al. 2005. Early cognitive stimulation, emotional support, and television watching as predictors of subsequent bullying among grade-school children. *Archives of Pediatrics and Adolescent Medicine* 59(4): 384–388.

LOOKING AHEAD...

After reading this chapter, you should be able to:

- List strategies for healthful aging
- Explain the physical, social, and mental changes that may accompany aging and discuss how people can best confront these changes
- Describe practical considerations of older adults and caregivers, including housing, finances, health care, communication, and transportation
- Understand personal considerations in preparing for death, including making a will, assessing choices for end-of-life care, and making arrangements for a funeral or memorial service
- Describe the experience of living with a life-threatening illness and list ways to support a person who is dying
- Explain the grieving process and how support can be offered to adults and children who have experienced a loss

The Challenge of Aging

17

A ging does not begin at some specific point in life, and there is no precise age at which a person becomes "old." Rather, aging is a normal process of development that occurs throughout life. If you optimize wellness during young adulthood, you can exert great control over the physical and mental aspects of aging, and you can better handle your response to events that might be out of your control. This chapter discusses the aging process, and it also addresses the process of dying and issues that arise around death.

GENERATING VITALITY AS YOU AGE

Biological aging includes all the normal, progressive, irreversible changes to one's body that begin at birth and continue until death. Psychological aging and social aging usually involve more abrupt changes in circumstance and emotion: relocating, changing homes, losing a spouse and friends, retiring, having a lower income, and changing roles and social status. These changes represent opportunities for growth throughout life.

Successful aging requires preparation. People need to establish good health habits in their teens and twenties. During their twenties and thirties, they usually develop important relationships and settle into a particular lifestyle. By their mid-forties, they generally know how much money they need to support the lifestyle they've chosen. At this point, they must assess their financial status and perhaps adjust their savings in order to continue enjoying that lifestyle after retirement. In their mid-fifties, they need to reevaluate their health insurance plans and may want to think about retirement housing. In their seventies and beyond, they need to consider ways of sharing their legacy with the next generation.

What Happens as You Age?

A significant number of older Americans describe themselves as being in poor health. Many of the characteristics associated with aging are due not to aging but to neglect and abuse of our bodies and minds. These assaults lay the foundation for later psychological problems and chronic conditions like arthritis, heart disease, diabetes, hearing loss, and hypertension. But even with the healthiest behavior and environment, aging inevitably occurs as a result of biochemical processes we don't yet fully understand. Studies of healthy people indicate that functioning remains essentially constant until after age 70. Further research may help pinpoint the causes of aging and aid in the development of therapies to repair damage to aging organs.

Life-Enhancing Measures: Age-Proofing

You can prevent, delay, lessen, or even reverse some of the changes associated with aging through good habits. Simple things you can do daily will make a vast difference to your level of energy and vitality—your overall wellness.

Challenge Your Mind Numerous studies show that older adults who stay mentally active have a lower risk of developing dementia. Reading, doing puzzles, learning a language, and studying music are good ways to stimulate the brain. The more complex the activity, the more protective it may be.

Develop Physical Fitness Exercise significantly enhances both psychological and physical health. A review of more than 70 scientific studies cited in the 2008 *Physical Activity Guidelines Advisory Committee Report* found that physically active people have about a 30% lower risk of dying prematurely compared with inactive people. Poor fitness and low physical activity levels were found to be better predictors of premature death than smoking, diabetes, or obesity. The committee found that about 150 minutes (2.5 hours) of physical activity per week is sufficient to decrease all causes of mortality and that it is the overall volume of energy expended, regardless of what kinds of activities produce the energy expenditure, that makes a difference in risk of premature death. The positive effects of exercise include lower blood pressure and healthier cholesterol levels; better protection against heart attacks and an increased chance of survival should one occur; sustained or increased lung capacity; weight control through less accumulation of fat; maintenance of strength, flexibility, and balance; protection against osteoporosis and type 2 diabetes; increased effectiveness of the immune system; and maintenance of mental agility and flexibility, response time, memory, and hand-eye coordination.

The stimulation that exercise provides also seems to protect against the loss of **fluid intelligence,** the ability to find solutions to new problems. Fluid intelligence depends on rapidity of responsiveness, memory, and alertness. Individuals who exercise regularly are also less susceptible to depression and dementia.

TERMS

fluid intelligence The ability to develop a solution when confronted with a new problem.

Regular exercise is a key to successful, healthy aging.

Regular physical activity is essential for healthy aging, as it is throughout life. The 2008 *Physical Activity Guidelines for Americans* includes recommendations for older adults that are the same as for all adults:

- All older adults should avoid inactivity. Some physical activity is better than none.
- For substantial health benefits, older adults should do at least 150 minutes a week of moderate-intensity activity, or 75 minutes a week of vigorous-intensity activity, or a combination of both. For additional and more extensive health benefits, older adults should increase their aerobic physical activity to 300 minutes a week of moderate-intensity, or 150 minutes a week of vigorous-intensity, aerobic physical activity.
- Older adults should also do muscle-strengthening activities that are moderate or high intensity and involve all major muscle groups on 2 or more days a week, as these activities provide additional health benefits.

There are also guidelines just for older adults:

- When older adults cannot do 150 minutes of moderate-intensity aerobic activity a week because of chronic conditions, they should be as physically active as their abilities and conditions allow.

Can Exercise Delay the Effects of Aging?

As people age, they often experience declines in functional health—the ability to perform the tasks of everyday life—and related declines in the quality of life. According to the CDC, more than 25% of Americans over age 65 report their health as only "fair" or "poor." Similarly, according to a Medicare survey, 31% of men and 42% of women age 65–74 reported some sort of mobility limitation in 2003 (meaning they had difficulty walking one-quarter mile).

Can physical activity and exercise combat the degenerative effects of aging in middle-aged and older adults? The evidence indicates that they can. In reviewing the research, the U.S. government's Physical Activity Guidelines Advisory Committee concluded that physical activity can prevent or delay the onset of limitations and declines in functional health in older adults, can maintain or improve functional health in those who already have limitations, and can reduce the incidence of falls and fall-related injuries.

One mechanism by which physical activity prevents declines in functional health is through maintenance or improvement of the physiological capacities of the body, such as aerobic power, muscular strength, and balance—in other words, through improvements in physical fitness. Declines in these physiological capacities occur with biological aging and are often compounded by disease-related disability. But evidence shows that older adults who participate in regular aerobic exercise are 30% less likely than inactive individuals to develop functional limitations (such as a limited ability to walk or climb stairs) or role limitations (such as a limited ability to be the family grocery shopper). Although studies found that both physical activity and aerobic fitness were associated with reduced risk of functional limitations, aerobic fitness was associated with a greater reduction of risk. Evidence also suggests that regular physical activity is safe and beneficial for older adults who already have functional limitations.

Numerous studies have shown that regular exercise—particularly strength training, balance training, and flexibility exercises—can improve muscular strength, muscular endurance, and stability and provide some protection against falls. Aerobic activity, especially walking, also helps reduce risk of falls, and some evidence indicates that tai chi exercise programs are beneficial as well. Regular exercise not only reduces the incidence of falls but also greatly enhances mobility, allowing older people to live more independently and with greater confidence. Research also shows that regular physical activity can reduce anxiety and depression in older adults. Exercise stimulates blood flow to the brain and can even increase brain mass, helping the brain to function more efficiently and improving memory. There is some evidence that exercise may stave off mental decline and the occurrence of age-related dementia.

Current physical activity recommendations for older adults from the American Heart Association and the American College of Sports Medicine include moderate- to vigorous-intensity aerobic activity, strength training, and flexibility exercises, as well as balance exercises for older adults at risk for falls. Unfortunately, more than 75% of Americans age 65 and older do not get the recommended amounts of physical activity, and many get no exercise at all beyond the activities of daily living. Older adults are the least active group of Americans. Although it is important to exercise throughout life, the evidence indicates that older adults who become more active even late in life can experience improvements in physical fitness and functional health.

SOURCES: Centers for Disease Control and Prevention. 2007. Prevalence of regular physical activity among adults—United States, 2001 and 2005. *Morbidity and Mortality Weekly Re*port 56 (46): 1209–1212; Physical Activity Guidelines Advisory Committee. 2008. *Physical Activity Guidelines Advisory Committee Report, 2008.* Washington, DC: U.S. Department of Health and Human Services.

- Older adults should do exercises that maintain or improve balance if they are at risk of falling.
- Older adults with chronic conditions should understand whether and how their conditions affect their ability to do regular physical activity safely.
- Older adults should maintain the flexibility necessary for regular physical activity and activities of daily life.

For more on the beneficial effects of exercise for older adults, see the box "Can Exercise Delay the Effects of Aging?"

Eat Wisely   Good health at any age is enhanced by eating a varied diet full of nutrient-rich foods. Special guidelines for older adults include the following:

- Get enough vitamin B-12 and extra vitamin D from fortified foods or supplements.
- Limit sodium intake to 1500 mg per day (as is now recommended for the entire population), and get enough potassium (4700 mg per day).

- Eat foods rich in dietary fiber and drink plenty of water to help prevent constipation.
- Pay special attention to food safety; older adults tend to be more susceptible to foodborne illness.

Maintain a Healthy Weight   Weight management is especially difficult if you have been overweight most of your life. A sensible program of expending more calories through exercise, cutting calorie intake, or a combination of both will work for most people who want to lose weight, but there is no magic formula. Obesity is not physically healthy, and it leads to premature aging.

Control Drinking and Overdependence on Medications   Alcohol abuse ranks with depression as a common hidden mental health problem, affecting about 10% of older adults. (The ability to metabolize alcohol decreases with age.) The problem is often not identified because the effects of alcohol or drug dependence can mimic disease, such as Alzheimer's disease. Signs of potential alcohol or drug dependence include unexplained falls or frequent injuries, forgetfulness, depression, and malnutrition. Problems can be avoided by not using alcohol to relieve anxiety or emotional pain and not taking medication when safer forms of treatment are available.

Don't Smoke   The average pack-a-day smoker can expect to live about 13–14 years less than a nonsmoker. Furthermore, smokers suffer more illnesses that last longer, and they are subject to respiratory disabilities that limit their total vigor for many years before their death. Premature balding, skin wrinkling, and osteoporosis have been linked to cigarette smoking.

Schedule Physical Examinations to Detect Treatable Diseases   When detected early, many diseases, including hypertension, diabetes, and many types of cancer, can be successfully controlled by medication and lifestyle changes. Regular testing for **glaucoma** after age 40 can prevent blindness from this eye disease. Recommended immunizations, including those for influenza and pneumococcus, can protect you from preventable infectious diseases. An immunization against shingles, a painful condition caused by the herpes zoster virus, is recommended for adults 60 and older.

Recognize and Reduce Stress   Stress-induced physiological changes increase wear and tear on your body. Cut down on the stresses in your life. Don't wear yourself out through lack of sleep, substance abuse or misuse, or overwork. Practice relaxation, using the techniques described in Chapter 2.

QUICK STATS

One older American dies every 35 minutes from a fall.

—National Council on Aging, 2010

DEALING WITH THE CHANGES OF AGING

Just as you can act now to prevent or limit the physical changes of aging, you can also begin preparing yourself psychologically, socially, and financially for changes that may occur later in life.

Planning for Social Changes

Retirement marks a major change in the second half of life. As Americans' longevity has increased, people spend a larger proportion of their lives in retirement.

TERMS

glaucoma   A disease in which fluid inside the eye is under abnormally high pressure; can lead to the loss of peripheral vision and blindness.

Ask Yourself

QUESTIONS FOR CRITICAL THINKING AND REFLECTION
How do you feel about the prospect of growing old? Would you say that you look forward to it, or are you anxious about it? What influences have shaped your feelings about aging?

Changing Roles and Relationships   Changes in social roles are a major feature of life as we age. Children become young adults and leave home, putting an end to daily parenting. Parents experiencing this empty-nest syndrome must adapt to changes in their customary responsibilities and personal identities. And although retirement may be a desirable milestone for most people, it may also be viewed as a threat to prestige, purpose, and self-respect—the loss of a valued or customary role—and often requires some adjustment.

Retirement and the end of child rearing also bring about changes in the relationship between partners. The amount of time a couple spends together will increase and activities will change. Couples may need a period of adjustment, in which they get to know each other as individuals again. Discussing what types of activities each partner enjoys can help couples set up a mutually satisfying routine of shared and independent activities.

Increased Leisure Time   Although retirement confers the advantages of leisure time and freedom from deadlines, competition, and stress, many people do not know how to enjoy their free time. If you have developed diverse interests, retirement can be a joyful and fulfilling period of your life. It can provide opportunities for expanding your horizons by giving you the chance to try new activities, take classes, and meet new people. Volunteering in your community can enhance self-esteem and allow you to be a contributing member of society.

The Economics of Retirement   Financial planning for retirement should begin early in life. People in their twenties and thirties should estimate how much money they need to support their standard of living, calculate their projected income, and begin a savings program. The earlier people begin such a program, the more money they will have at retirement.

Financial planning for retirement should begin early in life—as early as your twenties.

Financial planning for retirement is especially critical for women. American women are much less likely than men to be covered by pension plans, reflecting the fact that many women have lower-paying jobs or work part-time during their childbearing years. They tend to have less money vested in other types of retirement plans as well. Although the gap is narrowing, women currently outlive men by about 5–6 years, and they are more likely to develop chronic conditions that impair their daily activities later in life. The net result of these factors is that older women are almost twice as likely as older men to live in poverty. Women should investigate their retirement plans and take charge of their finances to be sure they will be provided for as they get older.

Adapting to Physical Changes

Some changes in physical functioning are inevitable, and successful aging involves anticipating and accommodating these changes. Decreased energy and changes in health mean that older people have to develop priorities for how to use their energy. Rather than curtailing activities to conserve energy, they need to learn how to generate energy. This usually involves saying yes to enjoyable activities and paying close attention to the need for rest and sleep. Adapting, rather than giving up, favorite activities may be the best strategy for dealing with physical limitations. For example, if **arthritis** interferes with playing an instrument, a person can continue to enjoy music by taking up a different instrument or attending concerts.

Hearing Loss   The loss of hearing is a common physical change that can have a particularly strong effect on the lives of older adults. Hearing loss affects a person's ability to interact with others and can lead to a sense of isolation and depression. Hearing loss should be assessed and treated by a health care professional; in some cases, hearing can be completely restored by dealing with the underlying cause of hearing loss. In other cases, hearing aids may be prescribed.

Vision Changes   Vision usually declines with age. For some individuals this can be traced to conditions such as glaucoma or **age-related macular degeneration (AMD)** that can be treated medically. Glaucoma is caused by increased pressure within the eye due to built-up fluid. The optic nerve can be damaged by this increased pressure, resulting in a loss of side vision and, if untreated, blindness. Medication can relieve the pressure by decreasing the amount of fluid produced or by helping it drain more efficiently. Laser and conventional surgery are other options. People over 60, African Americans over 40, and anyone with a family history of glaucoma are at risk.

120,000 Americans are blind due to glaucoma, accounting for 9–12% of all blindness.

—Glaucoma Research Foundation, 2010

AMD is a slow disintegration of the *macula*, the tissue at the center of the retina where fine, straight-ahead detail is distinguished. AMD affects more than 1.5 million Americans over 40 and is the leading cause of blindness in people over age 75. Losing this vision makes it difficult to read, drive, or perform other close-up activities. Risk factors for AMD are age, gender (women may be at higher risk than men), smoking, elevated cholesterol levels, and family history. Some cases of AMD can be treated with laser surgery. Both glaucoma and AMD can be detected with regular screening.

By the time they reach their forties, many people have developed **presbyopia**, a gradual decline in the ability to focus on objects close to them. **Cataracts,** a clouding of the lens caused by lifelong oxidation damage (a by-product of normal body chemistry), may dim vision by the sixties.

Arthritis   More than 46 million American adults are estimated to have some form of arthritis. This degenerative disease causes joint inflammation leading to chronic pain, swelling, and loss of mobility. There are more than 100 different types of arthritis; osteoarthritis (OA) is by far the most common. In a person with OA, the cartilage that caps the bones in joints wears away, forming sharp spurs. It most often affects the hands and weight-bearing joints of the body—knees, ankles, and hips.

Strategies for reducing the risk of arthritis and, for those who already have OA, for managing it include exercise, weight management, and avoidance of heavy or repetitive muscle use. Exercise lubricates joints and strengthens the muscles around them, protecting them from further damage. Swimming, walking, cross-country skiing, cycling, and tai chi are good low-impact exercises. Maintaining an appropriate weight is important to avoid placing stress on the hips, knees, and ankles.

Many people with OA take medication to relieve inflammation and reduce pain. Nonsteroidal anti-inflammatory drugs like ibuprofen can help but can irritate the digestive tract; prescription drugs that relieve pain without damaging the stomach have been found to have other dangerous side effects. Acetaminophen can also reduce pain without upsetting the stomach, but exceeding the recommended dosage can cause liver damage.

arthritis   Inflammation of a joint or joints, causing pain and swelling.

age-related macular degeneration (AMD)   A deterioration of the macula (the central area of the retina) leading to blurred vision and sensitivity to glare; some cases can lead to blindness.

presbyopia   The inability of the eyes to focus sharply on nearby objects, caused by a loss of elasticity of the lens that occurs with advancing age.

cataracts   Opacity of the lens of the eye that impairs vision and can cause blindness.

TERMS

Menopause   The natural process of menopause usually occurs during a woman's forties or fifties. The ovaries gradually stop functioning, estrogen levels drop, and eventually menstruation ceases. Several years before a woman stops menstruating, her periods usually become irregular, and she may experience hot flashes, vaginal dryness, sleep disturbances, and mood swings. This period, called *perimenopause,* can be troublesome for many women, some more than others. For more on menopause see Chapters 5 and 12.

Lifestyle strategies for reducing menopause-related problems include eating a healthy diet, exercising, losing excess weight, avoiding tobacco, and managing stress.

Osteoporosis   As described in Chapter 9, **osteoporosis** is a condition in which bones become dangerously thin and fragile over time. Fractures are the most serious consequence of osteoporosis. Other problems associated with osteoporosis are loss of height and a stooped posture due to vertebral fractures, severe back and hip pain, and breathing problems.

Osteoporosis affects about 10 million Americans, 80% of whom are women. Women are at greater risk than men for osteoporosis because they have 10–25% less bone in their skeleton, and bone loss accelerates in women during the first 5–10 years after the onset of menopause because of the drop in estrogen production. Black women have higher bone density and fewer fractures than white or Asian women but may be at increased risk of osteoporosis due to lack of vitamin D (a condition caused by high levels of melatonin). Other risk factors include a family history of osteoporosis, early menopause (before age 45), abnormal or irregular menstruation, a history of anorexia, and a thin, small frame. Thyroid medication, corticosteroid drugs for arthritis or asthma, and long-term use of certain contraceptives can also have a negative effect on bone mass.

> *A key to avoiding osteoporosis is to build as much bone mass as you can while you're young.*

Preventing osteoporosis requires building as much bone mass as possible during your young years and then maintaining it as you age. Diet and exercise play key roles. Weight-bearing aerobic activities must be performed regularly throughout life to have lasting effects. Strength training improves bone density, muscle mass, strength, and balance, protecting against both bone loss and falls, a major cause of fractures. Even for people in their seventies, low-intensity strength training has been shown to improve bone density. Two other lifelong strategies for reducing the effects of osteoporosis are avoiding tobacco use and managing depression and stress. Bone mineral density testing can be used to gauge an individual's risk of fracture and help determine if any treatment is needed.

Handling Psychological and Mental Changes

Most older adults in good health remain mentally alert and retain their full capacity to learn and remember new information. Many people become smarter as they become older and more experienced.

Dementia   Severe and significant brain deterioration in elderly individuals, termed **dementia,** affects about 7% of people under age 80 (the incidence rises sharply for people in their eighties and nineties). Early symptoms include slight disturbances in a person's ability to grasp the situation he or she is in. As dementia progresses, memory failure becomes apparent, and the person may forget conversations, the events of the day, or how to perform simple tasks. It is important to have any symptoms evaluated by a health care professional because some of the over 50 known causes of dementia are treatable.

The two most common forms of dementia among older people—multi-infarct dementia and **Alzheimer's disease**—are irreversible. Multi-infarct dementia results from a series of small strokes or changes in the brain's blood supply that destroy brain tissue. Alzheimer's disease is characterized by changes in brain nerve cells. About 5.3 million Americans have Alzheimer's disease, and that number is expected to quadruple in the next 50 years, as more people live into their eighties and nineties. Alzheimer's disease usually occurs in people over 60 but can occur in people as young as 40.

Ask Yourself

QUESTIONS FOR CRITICAL THINKING AND REFLECTION

Have you watched someone you know grow old? How did the aging process affect that person? In what ways did the person's physical and mental health change? In what ways were you affected, as you watched him or her age?

There is evidence that some cases of dementia are hereditary, but experts say genetics are not always a sure sign that a person will develop the disease. You can also take lifestyle steps to help ward off dementia, such as controlling weight and blood pressure, eating a balanced diet (including adequate B vitamins and omega-3 fatty acids), exercising, practicing stress reduction techniques, maintaining social contacts, and cultivating a variety of mental pursuits, such as doing crossword puzzles. Strong evidence links the Mediterranean diet with reduced risk of Alzheimer's disease.

Grief   Another psychological and emotional challenge of aging is dealing with grief and mourning. Aging is associated with loss—the loss of friends, peers, physical appearance, possessions, and health. Grief is the process of getting through the pain of loss, and it can be one of the loneliest and most emotionally intense times in a person's life. It can take years to completely come to terms with the loss of a loved one. Unresolved grief can have serious physical and psychological or emotional health consequences and may require professional help.

Depression   Unresolved grief can lead to depression, a common problem in older adults. If you notice the signs of depression in yourself or someone you know, consult a mental health professional. A marked loss of interest in usually pleasurable activities, decreased appetite, insomnia, fatigue, and feelings of worthlessness are signs of depression. Listen carefully when an older friend or relative complains about being depressed; it may be a request for help. Suicide rates are relatively high among the elderly, and depression should be taken seriously.

AGING AND LIFE EXPECTANCY

Life expectancy is the average length of time we can expect to live. In 2007, life expectancy for the total population was 77.9 years, but those who reach age 65 can expect to live even longer—18.5 more years or longer—because they have already survived hazards to life in the younger years. Women have a longer life expectancy than men (see the box "Why Do Women Live Longer?"). As life expectancy increases, a larger proportion of the population will be in their later years. This change will necessitate new government policies and changes in our general attitudes toward older adults.

> The life expectancy of white Americans is **78.2 years;** the life expectancy of black Americans is **73.2 years.**
>
> —National Center for Health Statistics, 2010

Some individuals defy all preconceived ideas about age and continue to live vigorous and productive lives into their seventies, eighties, and beyond.

America's Aging Minority

People over 65 are a large minority in the American population—over 37.3 million people, about 12% of the total population in 2006. That number is expected to nearly double by the year 2030. The enormous increase in the over-55 population is markedly affecting our stereotypes of what it means to grow old. The misfortunes associated with aging—frailty, forgetfulness, poor health, isolation—occur in fewer people in their sixties and seventies and are shifting instead to burden the very old, those over 85.

More than 80% of older Americans own their homes. Their living expenses are lower after retirement because they no longer support children and have fewer work-related expenses; they consume and buy less food. They are more likely to continue practicing their expertise for years after retirement: Thousands of retired consultants, teachers, technicians, and craftspeople work until their middle and late seventies. They receive greater amounts of assistance, such as Medicare, pay proportionately lower taxes, and have greater net worth from lifetime savings. As the aging population increases proportionately, however, the number of older people who are ill and dependent rises. Health care remains the largest expense for older adults. Most older Americans have at least one chronic condition; many have more than one.

Why Do Women Live Longer?

GENDER MATTERS

Women live longer than men in most countries around the world, even in places where maternal mortality rates are high. In the United States, women on average can expect to live about 5 years longer than men. Worldwide, among people over age 100, women outnumber men about 9 to 1.

The reason for the gender gap in life expectancy is not entirely understood but may be influenced by biological, social, and lifestyle factors. Estrogen production and other factors during a woman's younger years may protect her from early heart disease and from age-related declines in the pumping power of the heart. Women may have lower rates of stress-related illnesses because they cope more positively with stress by seeking social support.

The news for women is not all good, however, because not all their extra years are likely to be healthy years. They are more likely than men to suffer from chronic conditions like arthritis and osteoporosis. Women's longer life spans, combined with the facts that men tend to marry younger women and that widowed men remarry more often than widowed women, means there are many more single older women than

men. Older men are more likely to live in family settings, whereas older women are more likely to live alone. Older women are also less likely to be covered by a pension or to have retirement savings, so they are more likely to be poor.

Increased male mortality can be traced in part to higher rates of behaviors such as smoking and alcohol and drug abuse. Testosterone production may be partly responsible in that it is linked to aggressive and risky behavior and to unhealthy cholesterol levels. Men have much higher rates of death from car crashes and other unintentional injuries, firearm-related deaths, homicide, suicide, AIDS, and early heart attack. Gender roles that promote risky behavior among young men are a factor in many of these causes of death. Indeed, among people who have made it to age 65, the gender longevity gap is smaller.

Social and behavioral factors may be more important than physiological causes in explaining the gender gap; for example, among the Amish, a religious sect that has strict rules against smoking and drinking, men usually live as long as women. This suggests that the longevity gap could be substantially narrowed through lifestyle changes.

SOURCES: National Center for Health Statistics. 2009. *Health, United States, 2009*. Hyattsville, Md.: National Center for Health Statistics; U.S. Census Bureau. 2005. *We the People: Women and Men in the United States*. Washington, D.C.: U.S. Census Bureau; World Health Organization. 2003. *Gender, Health, and Aging*. Geneva: World Health Organization.

Retirement finds many older people with their incomes reduced to subsistence levels. The majority of older Americans live with fixed sources of income, such as pensions, that are eroded by inflation. **Social Security** benefits constitute 90% of the total income for one-third of Americans over age 65. Social Security was intended to serve as a supplement to personal savings and private pensions, not as a sole source of income. It is vital to plan for an adequate retirement income.

Family and Community Resources for Older Adults

With help from friends, family members, and community services, people in their later years can remain active and independent. About 66% of noninstitutionalized older Americans live with a spouse or other family member; the other 30% live alone. Only 4% live in institutional settings, but among those over age 85, about 15% live in a nursing home. In about three out of four cases, a spouse, a grown daughter, or a daughter-in-law assumes a caregiving role for elderly relatives. Recent surveys indicate that the average woman will spend about 17 years raising children and 18 years caring for an aging relative.

Caregiving can be rewarding, but it is also hard work. If the experience is stressful and long-term, family members may become emotionally exhausted. Corporations are increasingly responsive to the needs of their employees who are family caregivers by providing services such as referrals, flexible schedules and leaves, and on-site adult care. Professional health care advice is another critical part of successful home care.

The best thing a family can do is talk honestly about the obligations, time, and commitment required by caregiving. Families should also explore the community resources and professional assistance that may be available to reduce the stress in this difficult job.

TERMS

Social Security   A government program that provides financial assistance to people who are unemployed, disabled, or retired (and over a certain age); financed through taxes on business and workers.

Government Aid and Policies

The federal government helps older Americans through several programs, such as food stamps, housing subsidies, Social Security, Medicare, and Medicaid. Medicare is a major health insurance program for older adults and disabled persons, paying about 30% of the medical costs of older Americans. It provides basic health care coverage for acute episodes of illness that require skilled professional care, and it pays for some preventive services. Medicare pays less than 2% of nursing home costs, and private insurers pay less than 1%, creating a tremendous financial burden for nursing home residents and their families. When their financial resources are exhausted, people may apply for Medicaid, which provides medical insurance to low-income people of any age.

> In 2005, Social Security benefits accounted for **37%** of the aggregate income of the older population.
>
> —AOA, 2008

Health care policy planners hope that rising medical costs for older adults will shrink dramatically through education and prevention. Health care professionals, including **gerontologists** and **geriatricians,** are beginning to practice preventive medicine, just as pediatricians do. They advise older people about how to avoid and, if necessary, how to manage disabilities.

There can be benefits to aging, but they don't come automatically. They require planning and wise choices earlier in life. One octogenarian, Russell Lee, founder of a medical clinic in California, perceived the advantages of aging as growth: "The limitations imposed by time are compensated by the improved taste, sharper discretion, sounder mental and esthetic judgment, increased sensitivity and compassion, clearer focus—which all contribute to a more certain direction in living. . . . The later years can be the best of life for which the earlier ones were preparation."

Ask Yourself

QUESTIONS FOR CRITICAL THINKING AND REFLECTION

What do you want your life to be like when you are old? Do you hope to retire, or keep working indefinitely? Where would you like to live? How much time do you spend thinking about these questions? Have you done any planning yet for old age?

Death awaits all of us at the end of our lives, and accepting and dealing with death are difficult but important tasks.

WHAT IS DEATH?

Whether it is an earthquake devastating Haiti, a man having a heart attack in a crowded restaurant, or an elderly woman dying peacefully with her family close by, images of death are easy to envision. Nevertheless, rarely do we think about the inevitability of death in our own lives. Accepting and dealing with death are important tasks that present unique challenges to our sense of self, our relationships with others, and our understanding of the meaning of life itself. Although times of pain and distress may accompany the dying process, facing death also presents an opportunity for growth as well as affirmation of the preciousness of simple aspects of our daily lives.

gerontologist   One who studies the biological, psychological, and social phenomena associated with aging and old age.

geriatrician   A physician specializing in the diseases, disabilities, and care of older adults.

TERMS

Questions about the meaning of death and what happens when we die are central concerns of the great religions and philosophies. Some promise a better life after death. Others teach that everyone is evolving toward perfection or divinity, a goal reached after successive rounds of death and rebirth. There are also those who suggest that it is not possible to know what happens—if anything—after death and that any judgment about life's worth must be made on the basis of satisfactions or rewards that we create for ourselves in our lifetime.

Defining Death

Traditionally, death has been defined as cessation of the flow of vital body fluids. This occurs when the heart stops beating and breathing ceases. These traditional signs are adequate for determining death in most cases. However, the use of respirators and other **life-support systems** in modern medicine allows some body functions to be artificially sustained. The concept of **brain death** was developed to determine whether a person is alive or dead when the traditional signs are inadequate because of supportive medical technology.

According to the standards published by a Harvard Medical School committee, brain death involves four characteristics: (1) lack of receptivity and response to external stimuli, (2) absence of spontaneous muscular movement and spontaneous breathing, (3) absence of observable reflexes, and (4) absence of brain activity, as signified by a flat **electroencephalogram (EEG).** The Harvard criteria require a second set of tests to be performed after 24 hours have elapsed, and they exclude cases of hypothermia (body temperature below 90°F) and situations involving central nervous system depressants, such as barbiturates.

In contrast to **clinical death**, which is determined by either the cessation of heartbeat and breathing or the criteria for establishing brain death, **cellular death** refers to a gradual process that occurs when heartbeat, respiration, and brain activity have stopped. It encompasses the breakdown of metabolic processes and results in complete nonfunctionality at the cellular level.

The way in which death is defined has potential legal and social consequences in a variety of areas, including criminal prosecution, inheritance, taxation, treatment of the corpse, and even mourning. It also affects the practice of organ transplantation, because some organs—hearts, most obviously—must be harvested from a human being who is legally determined to be dead.

Learning About Death

Our understanding of death changes as we grow and mature, as do our attitudes toward it. A child's understanding of death evolves greatly from about age 5 to age 9. During this period, most children come to understand that death is final, universal, and inevitable. A child who consciously recognizes these facts is said to possess a **mature understanding of death.** This understanding of death is further refined during the years of adolescence and young adulthood by considering the impact of death on close relationships and contemplating the value of religious or philosophical answers to the enigma of death.

It is important to add, however, that individuals who possess a mature understanding of death commonly hold nonempirical ideas about it as well. Such nonempirical ideas—that is, ideas not subject to scientific proof—deal mainly with the notion that human beings survive in some form beyond the death of the physical body. What happens to an individual's personality after he or she dies? Does the self or soul continue to exist after the death of the physical body? If so, what is the nature of this afterlife? Developing personally satisfying answers to such questions is also part of the process of acquiring a mature understanding of death.

> **70% of Americans believe the soul survives after the body's death.**
> —Harris Interactive, 2005

Denying Versus Welcoming Death

Our ability to find meaning and comfort in the face of mortality depends not only on our having an understanding of the facts of death, but also on our attitudes toward it. Many people seek to avoid any thought or mention of death. The sick and old are often isolated in hospitals and nursing homes. Relatively few Americans have been present at the death of a loved one. Instead of facing death directly, we tend to amuse ourselves with unrealistic portrayals on television and movie screens.

TERMS

life-support systems Medical technologies, such as the respirator, that allow vital body functions to be artificially sustained.

brain death A medical determination of death as the cessation of brain activity indicated by various diagnostic criteria, including a flat EEG reading.

electroencephalogram (EEG) A record of the electrical activity of the brain (brain waves).

clinical death A determination of death made according to accepted medical criteria.

cellular death The breakdown of metabolic processes at the level of the cell.

mature understanding of death The recognition that death is universal and irreversible, that it involves the cessation of all physiological functioning, and that there are biological reasons for its occurrence.

El Día de los Muertos: The Day of the Dead

In contrast to the solemn attitude toward death so prevalent in the United States, a familiar and even ironic attitude is more common among Mexicans and Mexican Americans. In the Mexican worldview, death is another phase of life, and those who have passed into it remain accessible. Ancestors are not forever lost, nor is the past dead. This sense of continuity has its roots in the culture of the Aztecs, for whom regeneration was a central theme. When the Spanish came to Mexico in the sixteenth century, their beliefs about death, along with symbols such as skulls and skeletons, were absorbed into the native culture.

Mexican artists and writers confront death with humor and even sarcasm, depicting it as the inevitable fate that all— even the wealthiest—must face. At no time is this attitude toward death livelier than at the beginning of each November on the holiday known as Día de los Muertos, "the Day of the Dead." This holiday coincides with All Souls' Day, the Catholic commemoration of the dead, and represents a unique blending of indigenous ritual and religious dogma.

The celebration in honor of the dead typically spans two days—one day devoted to dead children, one to adults. It reflects the belief that the dead return to earth in spirit once a year to rejoin their families and partake of holiday foods prepared especially for them. The fiesta usually begins at midday on October 31, with flowers and food—candies, cookies, honey, milk—set out on altars in each house for the family's dead. The next day, family groups stream to the graveyards, where they have cleaned and decorated the graves of their loved ones, to celebrate and commune with the dead. They bring games, music, and special food; they sit on the graves, eat, sing, and talk with the departed ones. Tears may be shed as the dead are remembered, but mourning is tempered by the festive mood of the occasion.

During the season of the dead, graveyards and family altars are decorated with yellow candles and yellow marigolds—the "flower of death." In some Mexican villages, yellow flower petals are strewn along the ground, connecting the graveyard with all the houses visited by death during the year. Wherever Mexican Americans have settled in the United States, Día de los Muertos celebrations keep the traditions alive.

Keeping death in the forefront of consciousness may provide solace to the living, reminding them of their loved ones and assuring them that they themselves will not be forgotten when they die. Yearly celebrations and remembrances may help people keep in touch with their past, their ancestry, and their roots. The festive atmosphere may help dispel the fear of death, allowing people to look at it more directly. Although it is possible to deny the reality of death even when surrounded by images of it, such practices as Día de los Muertos may help people face death with more equanimity.

SOURCE: Adapted from DeSpelder, L., and A. Strickland. 2007. *The Last Dance*, 8th ed. New York: McGraw-Hill.

Although some commentators characterize the predominant attitude toward death in the United States as "death denying," others are reluctant to paint society as a whole with such a broad brush. Individuals often maintain conflicting or ambivalent attitudes toward death. Those who come to view death as a relief or release from insufferable pain may have at least a partial sense of welcoming death, but few people wholly avoid or wholly welcome death. Problems can arise, however, when avoidance or denial fosters the notion that death happens to others but not to you or me. (For another perspective, see the box "El Día de los Muertos: The Day of the Dead.")

PLANNING FOR DEATH

Acknowledging the inevitability of death allows us to plan for it. Adequate planning can help ensure that a sudden, unexpected death is not made even more difficult for survivors. Even when death is not sudden, many decisions can be anticipated, considered, and discussed with close relatives and friends.

Making a Will

Surveys indicate that about seven out of ten Americans die without leaving a will. A **will** is a legal instrument expressing a person's intentions and wishes for the disposition of his or her property after death. It is a declaration of how one's **estate**—that is, money, property, and other possessions—will be distributed after death. During the life of the **testator** (the person

will A legal instrument expressing a person's intentions and wishes for the disposition of his or her property after death.

estate The money, property, and other possessions belonging to a person.

testator The person who makes a will.

TERMS

making the will), a will can be changed, replaced, or revoked. Upon the testator's death, it becomes a legal instrument governing the distribution of the testator's estate.

When a person dies **intestate**—that is, without having left a valid will—property is distributed according to rules set up by the state. If you haven't yet made a will, start thinking about how you'd like your property distributed in the case of your death. If you have a will, consider whether it needs to be updated in response to a key life event such as marriage, the birth of a child, or the purchase of a home.

You can also help your family members by completing a *testamentary letter;* this document includes information about your personal affairs, such as bank accounts, credit cards, the location of documents and keys, the names of your professional advisers, the names of people who should be notified of your death, and so on.

Considering Options for End-of-Life Care

An appropriate balance in end-of-life care may involve a combination of home care, hospital stays, and hospice or palliative care.

Home Care Many people express a preference to be cared for at home during the end stage of a terminal illness. An obvious advantage of home care is the fact that the dying person is in a familiar setting, ideally in the company of family and friends. For home care to be an option, however, support generally must be provided not only by family and friends, but also by skilled, professional caregivers.

Hospital-Based Palliative Care Although hospitals are primarily organized to provide short-term intensive treatment for acute injury and illness, they are also adopting the principles of **palliative care** for patients who require comprehensive care at the end of life. Unlike acute care, which involves taking active measures to sustain life, palliative care focuses on controlling pain and relieving suffering by caring for the physical, psychological, spiritual, and existential needs of the patient. Although the

Ask Yourself

QUESTIONS FOR CRITICAL THINKING AND REFLECTION

What situations or events make you think seriously about your own mortality? Is this something you consider often, or do you avoid thinking about death? What has influenced your willingness or reluctance to think about death?

emphasis is generally placed on comfort care, palliative therapies can be combined with cure-oriented treatment approaches in some cases. In all cases, the goal of palliative care is to achieve the best possible quality of life for patients and their families.

Hospice Programs As a comprehensive program of care offering a set of services designed to support terminally ill patients and their families, **hospice** is a well-known form of palliative care. Although the term *hospice* sometimes refers to a freestanding medical facility to which terminally ill patients are admitted, most hospice care takes place in patients' homes with family members as primary caregivers.

Hospice care allows many people to choose where they die, a comforting fact for patients and families. Nursing home residents who chose hospice care are 50% less likely to spend their final 30 days of life in a hospital. Hospitalization can negatively influence a dying person's quality of life.

*Hospitalization can **negatively impact** a dying person's quality of life.*

Deciding to Prolong Life or Hasten Death

Modern medicine can keep the human organism alive despite the cessation of normal heart, brain, respiratory, or kidney function. But should a patient without any hope of recovery be kept alive by means of artificial life support? What if a patient has fallen into a **persistent vegetative state,** a state of profound unconsciousness, lacking any sign of normal reflexes and unresponsive to external stimuli, with no reasonable hope of improvement?

Ethical questions about a person's right to die have become prominent since the landmark case of Karen Ann Quinlan in 1975. At age 22, she was admitted to an intensive care unit in a comatose state. There, her breathing was sustained by a respirator. When she remained unresponsive, her parents asked that the respirator be disconnected. The request to withdraw treatment eventually reached the New Jersey Supreme Court, which ruled that artificial respiration could be discontinued.

Since then, courts have ruled on removing other types of life-sustaining treatment, including artificial feeding mechanisms that provide nutrition and hydration to permanently comatose patients who are able to breathe on their own. Notable was the case of Terri Schiavo in 2003.

Terri had been diagnosed as being in a persistent vegetative state. Contending that she would not want to continue living on life support, Terri's husband requested that her feeding tube be removed. Terri's parents contested the request, and a series of legal actions ensued. Finally, in 2005, after intervention by the U.S. Supreme Court, doctors were allowed to remove the tube. Cases like this highlight the importance of expressing one's wishes about life-sustaining treatment, in writing, before the need arises.

Withholding or Withdrawing Treatment   The right of a competent patient to refuse unwanted treatment is now generally established in both law and medical practice. The consensus is that there is no medical or ethical distinction between withholding (not starting) a treatment and withdrawing (stopping) a treatment once it has been started. The choice to forgo life-sustaining treatment involves refusing treatments that would be expected to extend life. The right to refuse treatment remains constitutionally protected even when a patient is unable to communicate. Although specific requirements vary, all states authorize some type of written advance directive to honor the decisions of individuals unable to speak for themselves but who have previously recorded their wishes in an appropriate legal document.

> **95** prescriptions were written for lethal drugs under Oregon's Death with Dignity Act in 2009; **53** patients took the drugs.
>
> —Oregon Department of Human Services, 2009

The practice of withholding or withdrawing a treatment that could potentially sustain life is sometimes termed **passive euthanasia,** although many people consider this term a misnomer because it tends to confuse the widely accepted practice of withholding or withdrawing treatment with the generally unacceptable and unlawful practice of taking active steps to cause death.

Assisted Suicide and Active Euthanasia   In contrast to withdrawing or withholding treatment, assisted suicide and active euthanasia refer to practices that intentionally hasten a person's death. In **physician-assisted suicide (PAS),** a physician provides lethal drugs or other interventions—at the patient's request—with the understanding that the patient plans to use them to end his or her life. The patient administers the fatal dose.

In 1997, the Supreme Court reviewed two cases relating to physician-assisted suicide. The decisions in these cases (*Washington v. Glucksberg* and *Vacco v. Quill*) are important for several reasons. First, the Court upheld the distinction between, on the one hand, withholding or withdrawing treatment and, on the other hand, physician-assisted suicide. Second, the Court affirmed the rights of states to craft policy concerning physician-assisted suicide, either prohibiting it, as most states now do, or permitting it under a regulatory system.

Oregon is currently the only state where PAS is permitted. The Death with Dignity Act, a ballot initiative, was passed by Oregon voters in 1994 and, after surviving judicial challenges, was reaffirmed in 1997. During its first 9 years of implementation, 292 people were reported to have legally committed suicide with the assistance of their physicians. These patients exhibited strong beliefs in personal autonomy and a determination to control the end of their lives. The Death with Dignity Act withstood Supreme Court scrutiny in 2006, when the Court ruled that the federal government could not block Oregon physicians from prescribing lethal drugs to patients who qualified for PAS under the act's provisions.

A third finding of importance in the Supreme Court's 1997 rulings about PAS relates to the concept of **double effect** in the medical management of pain. The doctrine of double effect states that a harmful effect of treatment, even if it results in death, is permissible if the harm is not intended and occurs as a side effect of a beneficial action. Sometimes the dosages of medication needed to relieve a patient's pain must be increased to levels that can cause respiratory depression, resulting in the patient's death. Such medication for pain, even if it hastens death, is not physician-assisted suicide if the intent is to relieve pain.

Unlike physician-assisted suicide, **active euthanasia** is the intentional act of killing someone who would otherwise suffer from an incurable and painful disease. *Voluntary euthanasia* (also known as voluntary active euthanasia, or VAE) is the intentional termination of life at the patient's request. In practice, this generally means that a

---

passive euthanasia   The practice of withholding (not starting) or withdrawing (stopping) treatment that could potentially sustain a person's life, with the recognition that, without such treatment, death is likely to occur.

physician-assisted suicide (PAS)   The practice of a physician intentionally providing, at the patient's request, lethal drugs or other means for a patient to hasten death with the understanding that the patient plans to use them to end his or her life.

double effect   A situation in which a harmful effect occurs as an unintended side effect of a beneficial action, such as when medication intended to control a patient's pain has the unintended result of causing the patient's death.

active euthanasia   A deliberate act intended to end another person's life; voluntary active euthanasia involves the practice of a physician administering—at the request of a patient—medication or some other intervention that causes death.

TERMS

competent patient requests direct assistance to die, and he or she receives assistance from a qualified medical practitioner. Voluntary active euthanasia is legal in Belgium and the Netherlands but is currently unlawful in the United States. Taking active steps to end someone's life is a crime—even if the motive is mercy.

Completing an Advance Directive

To make your preferences known about medical treatment, you need to document them through a written **advance directive.** Two forms of advance directives are legally important. First is the **living will,** which enables individuals to provide instructions about the kind of medical care they wish to receive if they become incapacitated or otherwise unable to participate in treatment decisions. The second important form of advance directive is the **health care proxy,** which is also known as a *durable power of attorney for health care.* This document makes it possible to appoint another person to make decisions about medical treatment if you become unable to do so. This decision maker, also known as a **surrogate,** may be a family member, close friend, or attorney with whom you have discussed your treatment preferences. The proxy is expected to act in accordance with your wishes as stated in an advance directive or as otherwise made known.

For advance directives to be of value, you must do more than merely complete the paperwork. Discuss your wishes ahead of time with caregivers and family members as well as with your physician.

 Organ/Tissue Donor Card

I wish to donate my organs and tissues. I wish to give:

☐ any needed organs and tissues   ☐ only the following organs and tissues:

_____

Donor Signature _____ Date _____
Witness _____
Witness _____

FIGURE 17.1 A sample organ/tissue donor card.

SOURCE: U.S. Department of Health and Human Services (http://www.organdonor.gov/donor/index.htm; retrieved November 29, 2010).

Becoming an Organ Donor

Each day about 77 people receive an organ transplant while another 19 people on the waiting list die because not enough organs are available. As of July 2010, nearly 110,000 Americans were waiting for organ transplants.

If you decide to become a donor, the first step is to indicate your wish by completing a **Uniform Donor Card** (Figure 17.1); alternatively, you can indicate your wish on your driver's license. Be sure to discuss your decision with your family.

Planning a Funeral or Memorial Service

Funerals and memorial services are rites of passage that commemorate a person's life and acknowledge his or her passing from the community. Funerals and memorials allow survivors to support one another as they cope with their loss and express their grief. The presence of death rites in every human culture suggests that they serve innate human needs.

Disposition of the Body People generally have a preference about the final disposition of their body. For most Americans, the choice is either burial or cremation. *Burial* usually involves a grave dug into the soil or entombment in a mausoleum. For personal and environmental reasons, some people choose a natural, or green, burial (see the box "Green Burials"). *Cremation* involves subjecting a body to intense heat. Cremated remains can be buried, placed in a columbarium niche, put into an

450,000
Americans have benefited from organ transplants.

—United Network for Organ Sharing, 2009

urn kept by the family or interred in an urn garden, or scattered at sea or on land. If the body is to be viewed during a wake or will be present at the funeral, **embalming** is generally done.

Green Burials

By some estimates, there are more than 22,000 cemeteries in the United States, covering hundreds of thousands of acres of land. These burial grounds hold millions of graves, some of which are hundreds of years old. In the face of long-standing burial traditions, however, many Americans are rethinking the notion of burying the dead in sealed caskets, placed in permanent stone or concrete vaults. This practice, say environmentalists, needlessly consumes vast tracts of land, and chemicals from embalmed bodies and caskets slowly leach into the soil and water.

Despite the notion that cremation avoids these problems, cremation actually uses a great deal of energy and contributes to air pollution. For example, a typical cremation releases dioxin, hydrochloric acid, hydrofluoric acid, sulfur dioxide, and carbon dioxide into the atmosphere. Foreign materials in the body—such as metal fillings and artificial joints—may release other compounds into the air during cremation.

One solution to the environmental impact of burials and cremations is the natural, or "green," burial now being offered in a growing number of communities. In a green burial, the body is wrapped in cloth or a biodegradable coffin and buried directly in the ground. There is no embalming or use of chemicals, and there is no vault to prevent decomposition.

Until recently, many states did not allow green burials, especially in areas outside a government-regulated cemetery. These rules are intended to control hazardous wastes that might leach from burial sites and to make sure that human remains are disposed of in a manner that is legal, meets safety standards, and ensures dignity for the deceased and his or her family.

Today, however, more states and local governments are easing restrictions on green burials, for a few key reasons. First, a growing number of organizations support green burials, and more mortuaries offer preparation services that are appropriate for natural interment. More public and private cemeteries are making space available exclusively for green burials, and they are taking steps to ensure that the grounds can never be sold for development or used for any other purposes.

Another advantage to natural burials is their relatively low cost. The family does not have to pay for embalming or cremation, an expensive casket, or a concrete vault. Instead, advocates of green burials encourage families to invest in caring for the funeral plot by planting grass, trees, and shrubs on and around it. Planting preserves the natural essence of the site while preventing erosion and encouraging the natural decomposition of the body. Green cemeteries are also maintained differently than traditional ones. Natural overgrowth is encouraged, the land's topography is not disturbed, and chemical applications are prohibited.

If you are interested in a green burial, experts suggest plenty of advance planning to make sure that the family is fully aware of your wishes and so that appropriate arrangements can be made. Arrangements should include finding a funeral home or mortuary that offers green burial preparations and biodegradable coffins or wraps. Even more important is finding a burial site that is properly zoned and licensed for natural burials. The family should talk to everyone involved in the planning, preparation, and performance of the burial service to ensure that only licensed, qualified individuals and service providers are used.

SOURCES: Funeral Consumers Alliance. 2007. *Green Burial* (http://www.funerals.org/ frequently-asked-questions/56-green-burial; retrieved October 10. 2010); Green Burial Council. 2010. *FAQs and Fictions* (http://www. greenburialcouncil.org/faqs-fiction/; retrieved October 10, 2010); GreenBurials.org. 2008. *What Is a Green Burial?* (http://www. greenburials.org/; retrieved October 10, 2010).

Arranging a Service   Although it is becoming more common for individuals and families to express a preference for no services, bereaved relatives and friends can derive important benefits from having an opportunity to honor the deceased and express their grief through ceremony. Decisions about your last rites are ideally made with a view to the needs and wishes of your survivors. Religious and cultural or ethnic traditions play a major role in shaping the way people honor their dead. The diversity of life and death in the United States calls for a diversity of rites. A meaningful funeral or memorial service can be designed in many ways. Making at least some plans ahead of time and discussing the options with family members can help reduce the burden on survivors who find themselves facing a number of tasks and decisions once death occurs.

COPING WITH DYING

There is no one right way to live with or die of a life-threatening illness. Every disease has its own set of problems and challenges, and each person copes with these

Ask Yourself

QUESTIONS FOR CRITICAL THINKING AND REFLECTION

Have you ever been involved in a funeral? What role did you play? Did you feel that the service reflected the values and beliefs of the deceased person? Did the experience cause you to think about your own funeral and what it should be like?

In Search of a Good Death

Participants in a recent study were asked to discuss the deaths of family members, friends, or patients and reflect on what made their deaths good or bad. From these discussions, six major themes emerged as components of a good death.

● Pain and symptom management. Many people fear dying in pain, and portrayals of bad deaths usually included inadequate pain management. When reassured that pain could be managed, patients were less anxious.

● Clear decision making. Both providers and families feared entering a medical crisis without knowing the patient's preferences. Patients and families who had good communication with health care providers and had discussed treatment decisions ahead of time felt empowered, and providers felt they were giving good care. Tolerance for uncertainty may increase if values and preferences are clarified.

● Preparation for death. Patients expressed satisfaction when they had time to prepare their wills and help plan their funeral arrangements. Patients and families also wanted to know what to expect during the course of the illness and what physical and psychosocial changes would take place as death approached.

● Completion, the opportunity to review one's life, resolve conflicts, spend time with loved ones, and say good-bye. Participants confirmed the deep importance of spirituality or meaningfulness at the end of life. Many times, patients were able to view their experience of dying as part of a broader life trajectory and thus continue to grow emotionally and spiritually in their last days. Issues of faith were often mentioned as important to healing.

● Contributing to others. Patients wanted to know that they still had something to offer to others, whether it was making someone laugh or lightening the load of someone closer to death. Many patients found that as they reflected on their lives, what they valued most was their personal relationships with family and friends, and they were anxious to impart this wisdom to others.

● Affirmation of the whole person. Patients appreciated empathic health care providers, and family members were comforted by those who treated their loved ones as unique and whole people, rather than as a disease. The quality of dying is related to the acknowledgment that people die in character, that is, as an extension of who they have been in their lives.

The study affirmed that most people think of death as a natural part of life, not as a failure of technology. Although the biomedical aspects of end-of-life care are crucial, they merely provide a point of departure toward a good death. When pain is properly managed and the practical aspects of dying are taken care of, patients and their families have the opportunity to address the important emotional, psychological, and spiritual issues that all human beings face at the end of life.

---

problems and challenges in his or her own way. Living with an illness that is life-threatening and incurable can be described as a living-dying experience. Hope and honesty are often delicately balanced—honesty to face reality as it is, hope for a positive outcome. The object of hope changes. The early hope that the symptoms are not really serious gives way to hope that a cure is possible. When the illness is deemed incurable, there is hope for more time. As time begins to run out, one hopes for a pain-free death, a "good death" (see the box "In Search of a Good Death").

The Tasks of Coping

In her 1969 book *On Death and Dying,* Elisabeth Kübler-Ross suggested that the response to an awareness of imminent death involves five psychological stages: denial, anger, bargaining, depression, and acceptance. Individuals go back and forth among the stages during the course of an illness, and different stages can occur simultaneously. More recently, the notion of stages has been deemphasized in favor of highlighting the tasks that deserve attention in coping with a life-threatening illness. Psychologist Charles Corr, for example, distinguishes four primary dimensions in coping with dying:

1. *Physical:* Satisfying bodily needs and minimizing physical distress

2. *Psychological:* Maximizing a sense of security, self-worth, autonomy, and richness in living

3. *Social:* Sustaining significant relationships and addressing the social implications of dying

4. *Spiritual:* Identifying, developing, or reaffirming sources of meaning and fostering hope

People who apparently cope best with life-threatening illness often exhibit a fighting spirit that views the illness not only as a threat but also as a challenge. These people strive to inform themselves about their illness and take an active part in treatment decisions. They are optimistic and have a capacity to discover positive meaning in ordinary events. Holding to a positive outlook despite distressing circumstances involves creating a sense of meaning that is bigger than the threat. In the context of life-threatening illness, this encompasses a person's ability to comprehend the implications an illness has for the future as well as for his or her ability to accomplish goals, maintain relationships, and sustain a sense of personal vitality, competence, and power.

Supporting a Dying Person

People often feel uncomfortable in the presence of a person who is close to dying. What can we say? How should we act? It may seem that any attempt to be comforting could result only in words that are little more than stale platitudes. Yet we want to express concern and establish meaningful contact with the person who is facing death. In such circumstances, the most important gift we can bring is that of listening. Offering the dying person opportunities to speak openly and honestly about his or her experience can be crucial, even when such conversation is initially painful.

We tend to place dying people in a special category, but the reality is that their needs are not fundamentally different from anyone else's, although their situation is perhaps more urgent. Dying people need to know that they are valued, that they are not alone, that they are not being unfairly judged, and that those closest to them are also striving to come to terms with a difficult situation. As with any relationship, there are opportunities for growth on both sides.

COPING WITH LOSS

Even if we have not experienced the death of someone close, we are all survivors of losses that occur in our lives because of changes and endings. The loss of a job, the ending of a relationship, transitions from one school or neighborhood to another—these are examples of the kinds of losses that occur in all our lives. Such losses are sometimes called little deaths and, in varying degrees, they all involve grief.

Experiencing Grief

Grief is the reaction to loss. It encompasses thoughts and feelings, as well as physical and behavioral responses. Mental distress may involve disbelief, confusion, anxiety, disorganization, and depression. The emotions that can be present in normal grief include not only sorrow and sadness, but also relief, anger, and self-pity, among others. Common behaviors associated with grief include crying, searching for the deceased, and talking incessantly about the deceased and the circumstances of the death. Bereaved people may be restless, as if not knowing what to do with themselves. Physically, grief may involve frequent sighing, insom-

The loss of a loved one—particularly a spouse—generates a broad range of emotional, physical, and behavioral reactions.

nia, and loss of appetite. Grief may also evoke a reexamination of religious or spiritual beliefs as a person struggles to make meaning of the loss. All such manifestations of grief can be present as part of one's total response to **bereavement**—that is, the event of loss.

Mourning is closely related to grief and is often used as a synonym for it. However, mourning refers not so much to the *reaction* to loss but to the *process* by which a bereaved person adjusts to loss and incorporates it into his or her life. How this process is managed is determined, at least partly, by cultural and gender norms for the expression of grief.

Tasks of Mourning Experiencing grief is part of the process by which a bereaved person integrates a significant loss into his or her life. Psychologist William Worden has identified four tasks that must be attended to:

1. *Accepting the reality* of the loss
2. *Working through the pain* of grief
3. *Adjusting to a changed environment* in which the deceased is absent
4. *Emotionally relocating the deceased and moving on with life*

Accomplishing the fourth task does not mean dishonoring the deceased's memory or denying normal feelings

grief   A person's reaction to loss as manifested physically, emotionally, mentally, and behaviorally.

bereavement   The objective event of loss.

mourning   The process whereby a person actively copes with grief in adjusting to a loss and integrating it into his or her life.

TERMS

of connection that persist beyond death. Making the journey of grief and attending to the various tasks along the way, we come to a place where we learn how to keep a special place for the deceased in our hearts and memories while moving forward with our lives.

The Course of Grief   Grieving, like dying, is highly individual. In the first hours or days following a death, a bereaved person is likely to experience overwhelming shock and numbness, as well as a sense of disbelief. The cause or mode of death—natural, accidental, homicide, or suicide—has an influence on how grief is experienced (see the box "Profound Trauma and Loss"). Even when a death is anticipated, grief is not necessarily diminished when the loss becomes real.

The sense of disorganization experienced by survivors during the early period of grief is set against the need to attend to decisions and actions surrounding the disposition of the deceased's body. As family and friends gather to offer mutual support, funeral ceremonies are held. Engaging in such activities promotes accepting the reality of the death and moving beyond the initial shock and numbness.

In its middle phase, the course of grief is characterized by anxiety, apathy, and pining for the deceased. The pangs of grief are felt as the bereaved person deeply experiences the pain of separation. There is often a sense of despair as a person repeatedly goes over the events surrounding the loss, perhaps fantasizing that somehow everything could be undone and be as it was before.

In moving toward the restoration of one's well-being, the last phase of active grief involves resolution. The acute pain and emotional turmoil of grief subside. Physical and mental balance is reestablished. The bereaved becomes increasingly reintegrated into his or her social world. Sadness doesn't go away completely, but it recedes into the background.

Some people, however, have more trouble resolving their grief than others. Such people may get stuck in the grieving process for months or even years, sometimes becoming so burdened with loss that they lose the ability to cope with daily living. Experts call this long-term, unresolved grief *complicated grief* and describe it as truly debilitating. Complicated grief is most likely to occur when a person has lost a loved one in a sudden, violent manner (such as homicide) or experienced an untimely death (such as the loss of a child). Grief counseling or therapy can help people work through complicated grief.

Supporting a Grieving Person

In experiencing a significant loss, a person initially may feel and behave much like a frightened, helpless child. He or she may respond best to the kind of loving support that is given by a parent. A hug may be more comforting than any words. Also, because talking about a loss is an important way that survivors cope with the changed reality, simply listening can be very helpful. The key to being

Ask Yourself

QUESTIONS FOR CRITICAL THINKING AND REFLECTION

Have you ever been in the position of being supportive to a bereaved person? What kind of support did he or she seem to appreciate most? Why do you think that was the case? How did the experience affect you?

a good listener is to refrain from making judgments about whether the feelings expressed by a survivor are right or wrong, good or bad.

Funerals and other ceremonies generally help survivors gain a sense of closure and begin to integrate a loss into their lives. Social support for the bereaved is as critical during the later course of grief as it is during the first days after a loss. In offering support, we can reassure them that grief is normal, permissible, and appropriate. They may also need permission to occasionally give themselves a break from grieving. An extended need for support often continues through the first year or two of mourning. Bereaved people also may want to share their stories and concerns through organized support groups, such as those for widows and widowers. Many support groups are organized around some specific type of bereavement.

Children tend to cope with loss in a healthier fashion when they are included as part of their family's experience of grief and mourning. In talking about death with children, the most important guideline is to be honest. Set the explanation you are offering at the child's level of understanding. In general, it's advisable to keep the explanation simple, stick to basics, and verify what the child has understood from your explanation. A child's readiness for more details can usually be assessed by paying attention to his or her questions.

COMING TO TERMS WITH DEATH

We may wish we could keep death out of view and not make a place for it in our lives. But this wish cannot be fulfilled. With the death of a beloved friend or relative, we are confronted with emotions and thoughts that relate not only to the immediate loss but also to our own mortality. Our encounters with dying and death teach us that relationships are more important than things and that life offers no guarantees. In discovering the meaning of death in our own lives, we find that life is both precious and precarious. Allowing ourselves to make room for death, we discover that it touches not only the dying or bereaved person and his or her family and friends but also the wider community of which we are all part. We recognize that dying and death offer opportunities for extraordinary growth in the midst of loss.

Profoundly traumatic events—the terrorist attacks of September 11, 2001, Hurricane Katrina, the Haiti earthquake, the 2010 floods in Pakistan—all represent a category of loss far beyond normal comprehension. Experiencing traumatic loss in such extraordinary circumstances can cause severe and disruptive reactions in emotion and behavior.

Many World War I veterans developed psychological symptoms that collectively were described as shell shock. However, it was not until after the Vietnam War that the medical community became fully aware of how disruptive and enduring the psychological effects could be for those experiencing profound traumatic loss.

It is now widely recognized that significant psychological symptoms can follow the experiencing of loss in traumatic circumstances. Elements commonly seen in a customary reaction to grief, such as sadness, disbelief, crying, insomnia, and loss of appetite, are frequently exaggerated in the aftermath of profoundly traumatic events and will often include more pronounced symptoms, such as overwhelming distress, numbness, doubt, despair, guilt, and disabling depression and anxiety.

Depending on the severity of exposure and a person's underlying vulnerability, the symptoms can persist long after the original trauma. Memories and images of the event may suddenly pop into the victim's mind, causing anxiety, depression, and anger. Insomnia and nightmares can disrupt the sleep-wake cycle. The person may start avoiding everything that serves as a reminder of the event and, as a kind of self-protection, may begin to become numb, to lose all feelings. Such people may startle easily and have difficulty concentrating. Their work life, social life, and intimate relationships may become markedly impaired. People experiencing these severe symptoms most likely have PTSD, which can persist for months or years.

The events of September 11, 2001, are an example of a profound trauma that caused PTSD in affected people. As described in Chapter 3, PTSD symptoms occurred among survivors, rescue workers, passersby, residents of Manhattan, and some people exposed to the events through repeated television images. Researchers who interviewed residents of Manhattan found that about 7.5% reported symptoms consistent with a diagnosis of PTSD and 9.7% reported symptoms consistent with new onset of depression; these numbers are about twice as high as the expected rates in surveys of this type. Among people who lived closest to the World Trade Center, the prevalence of PTSD was as high as 20%.

Many people experience disabling depression or anxiety but do not meet the full criteria for PTSD. More persistent and severe grief reactions, unexplained physical symptoms, and the increased use of alcohol and drugs are frequent occurrences for people who have undergone such trauma. In addition, family and interpersonal conflict and financial strain are commonly seen. All too frequently, in war or natural disasters, the primary wage earner of the family dies or the family's house and belongings are destroyed.

How long will an individual's symptoms last after experiencing an event like September 11 or witnessing a friend killed by a roadside bomb in Iraq? Factors such as the severity of the trauma, the individual's proximity to the event, and his or her emotional closeness to those who have died can all play important roles in the magnitude and duration of the reaction to traumatic loss. In general, though, symptoms will diminish with time, especially in the absence of new threats and traumatic losses. Studies of those who have developed full-blown PTSD suggest that approximately half of the cases resolve within 2 years but that nearly a third never fully recover.

Psychological support and treatment can greatly help many of those who suffer from disabling emotional symptoms in reaction to traumatic loss. Building on research and work done with Vietnam veterans in the 1970s and 1980s, clinicians have developed multiple therapeutic strategies involving group therapy, individual psychological support, and pharmacologic intervention to treat persistent symptoms.

SOURCES: Coker, A. L., et al. 2006. Social and mental health needs assessment of Katrina evacuees. *Disaster Management and Response* 4(3): 88–94; Watanabe, T., et al. 2006. Acute stress syndrome in a victim of the Indian Ocean Tsunami. *Psychiatry and Clinical Neurosciences* 60(5): 644; Galea, S., and H. Resnick. 2005. Posttraumatic stress disorder in the general population after mass terrorist incidents: Considerations about the nature of exposure. *CNS Spectrums* 10(2): 107–115; Galea, S., et al. 2002. Psychological sequelae of the September 11 terrorist attacks in New York City. *New England Journal of Medicine* 346(13): 982–987.

Connect to Your Choices

Have you ever thought about where you get your attitudes toward aging, older adults, and dying? Many factors can influence our attitudes, some not as obvious as others. Were your grandparents part of your life when you were growing up? Have they or your parents talked to you about their end-of-life wishes? Are older adults present and visible in your community, or are you surrounded primarily by young adults? How susceptible are you to ageism, and how strongly are you influenced by the youth orientation of the media? Have you gotten the idea from the mainstream culture that it's best not to think about death?

What are the external factors that influence your attitudes toward aging and death? What are your inner motivations and core values, and how do they affect your choices? Based on what you learned in this chapter, will you make some different choices in future? If so, what will they be?

Go online to Connect to complete this activity.
www.mcgraw-hillconnect.com

TIPS FOR TODAY AND THE FUTURE

The best way to ensure a high-quality life in later years is by cultivating healthy habits in your younger years.

RIGHT NOW YOU CAN

- Think about any unhealthy habits you have and resolve to change them. Set a timetable and start developing a plan.
- Think about how you want your body to be disposed of when you die.
- Think about how you would want your worldly goods to be distributed if you were to die soon.
- Think about organ donation. If you want to be an organ donor, start making the appropriate arrangements now, as described in this chapter.

IN THE FUTURE YOU CAN

- Learn a new skill, such as a language or a game of strategy.
- Talk to your parents or grandparents about their wishes for end-of-life care and funeral arrangements, and discuss ways you can be involved.

SUMMARY

- People who take charge of their health during their youth have greater control over the physical and mental aspects of aging.

- A lifetime of interests and hobbies helps maintain creativity and intelligence. Exercise and a healthy diet throughout life enhance physical and psychological health.

- Retirement can be a fulfilling and enjoyable time of life for those who adjust to their new roles, enjoy participating in a variety of activities, and have planned ahead for financial stability.

- Slight confusion and forgetfulness are not signs of a serious illness; however, severe symptoms may indicate Alzheimer's disease or another form of dementia.

- Resolving grief and mourning and dealing with depression are important tasks for older adults.

- People over 65 form a large minority in the United States, and their status is improving.

- Family and community resources can help older adults stay active and independent.

- Government aid to the elderly includes food stamps, housing subsidies, Social Security, Medicare, and Medicaid.

- Dying and death are more than biological events; they have social and spiritual dimensions.

- The traditional criteria for determining death focus on vital signs such as breathing and heartbeat. Brain death is characterized by a lack of physical responses other than breathing and heartbeat.

- A will is a legal instrument that governs the distribution of a person's estate after death.

- End-of-life care may involve a combination of home care, hospital stays, and hospice or palliative care.

- The practice of withholding or withdrawing potentially life-sustaining treatment is sometimes termed passive euthanasia.

- Physician-assisted suicide occurs when a physician provides lethal drugs or other interventions, at a patient's request, with the understanding that the patient plans to use them to end his or her life.

- Advance directives, such as living wills and health care proxies, are used to express one's wishes about the use of life-sustaining treatment.

- People can donate their bodies or specific organs for transplantation and other medical uses after death.

- Bereaved people usually benefit from participating in a funeral or memorial service to commemorate a loved one's death.

- Coping with dying involves physical, psychological, social, and spiritual dimensions.

- In offering support to a dying person, the gift of listening can be especially important.

- Grief encompasses thoughts and feelings as well as physical and behavioral responses.

- Mourning, the process by which a person integrates a loss into his or her life, is determined partly by social and cultural norms for expressing grief.

FOR MORE INFORMATION

BOOKS

Batuello, J. T. 2003. *End of Life Decisions: A Practical Guide.* College Station, Tex.: Virtualbookworm. *A guide to end-of-life decisions, including those related to pain relief and palliative and hospice care.*

DeSpelder, L. A., and A. L. Strickland. 2009. *The Last Dance: Encountering Death and Dying,* 8th ed. New York: McGraw-Hill. *A comprehensive and readable text highlighting a broad range of topics related to dying and death.*

Johns Hopkins Medical Center. 2007. *The Johns Hopkins Medical Guide to Health After 50.* New York: Black Dog & Leventhal. *A practical guide to healthy aging for all wellness dimensions.*

National Institute on Aging. 2006. *Fitness Over Fifty: An Exercise Guide from the National Institute on Aging,* book and DVD ed. New York: Hatherleigh Press. *A practical guide to physical activity and exercise, with specific guidelines for safe exercise for older adults.*

Weil, A. 2007. *Healthy Aging: A Lifelong Guide to Your Physical and Spiritual Well-Being.* New York: Anchor. *One of America's best-known complementary care physicians discusses the aging process and explains methods for maintaining health during the latter years of life.*

ORGANIZATIONS AND WEB SITES

AARP. Provides information on all aspects of aging, including health promotion, health care, and retirement planning.
http://www.aarp.org

Alzheimer's Association. Offers tips for caregivers and patients and information on the causes and treatment of Alzheimer's disease.
http://www.alz.org

Association for Death Education and Counseling (ADEC). Provides resources for education, bereavement counseling, and care of the dying.
http://www.adec.org

Dying Well. A Web site focused on wellness through the end of life.
http://www.dyingwell.org

Hospice Foundation of America. Promotes the hospice concept of care through education and leadership.
http://www.hospicefoundation.org

Medicare. Provides information about Medicare.
http://www.medicare.gov

National Council on Aging. Provides helpful information on retirement planning, health promotion, and lifelong learning.
http://www.ncoa.org

National Funeral Directors Association (NFDA). Provides resources related to funerals and funeral costs, body disposition, and bereavement support.
http://www.nfda.org

National Institute on Aging. Provides fact sheets and brochures on aging-related topics.
http://www.nia.nih.gov
http://nihseniorhealth.gov

Nolo Press: Wills and Estate Planning. Provides answers to questions about planning for death, from writing a basic will to organ donation.
http://www.nolo.com

On Our Own Terms: Public Broadcasting System. A companion Web site to the Bill Moyers PBS series on improving end-of-life care.
http://www.pbs.org/wnet/onourownterms

Oregon Department of Health and Human Services. Provides information about Oregon's Death with Dignity Act.
http://egov.oregon.gov/DHS/ph/pas

SELECTED BIBLIOGRAPHY

Anderson, K., et al. 2005. Depression and the risk of Alzheimer's disease. *Epidemiology* 16(2): 233–238.

Annas, G. J. 2005. "Culture of life" politics at the bedside—the case of Terri Schiavo. *New England Journal of Medicine,* 23 March [epub].

Beyond menopause: Life after estrogen. 2005. *Mayo Clinic Health Letter Supplement,* February.

Centers for Disease Control and Prevention. 2006. Prevalence of doctor-diagnosed arthritis and arthritis-attributable activity limitation—United States, 2003–2005. *Morbidity and Mortality Weekly Report* 55(40): 1089–1092.

Chochinov, H. M. 2006. Dying, dignity, and new horizons in palliative end-of-life care. *CA: A Cancer Journal for Clinicians* 56(2): 84–103.

Christ, G. H., and A. E. Christ. 2006. Current approaches to helping children cope with a parent's terminal illness. *CA: A Cancer Journal for Clinicians* 56(4): 197–212.

Donatelli, L. A., et al. 2006. Ethical issues in critical care and cardiac arrest: Clinical research, brain death, and organ donation. *Seminars in Neurology* 26(4): 452–459.

DuBois, J. M., and E. E. Anderson. 2006. Attitudes toward death criteria and organ donation among healthcare personnel and the general public. *Progress in Transplantation* 16(1): 65–73.

Field, N. P. 2006. Unresolved grief and continuing bonds: An attachment perspective. *Death Studies* 30(8): 739–756.

Harvard Medical School. 2006. Minding your mind: 12 ways to keep your brain young with proper care and feeding. *Harvard Men's Health Watch* 10(10): 1–4.

Heyn, P. C., et al. 2008. Endurance and strength training outcomes on cognitively impaired and cognitively intact older adults: A meta-analysis. *Journal of Nutrition, Health & Aging* 12(6): 401–409.

Jager, R. D., et al. 2008. Age-related macular degeneration. *New England Journal of Medicine* 258(24): 2606–2617.

Lipkin, K. M. 2006. Identifying a proxy for health care as part of routine medical inquiry. *Journal of General Internal Medicine,* 17 July [online early ed.].

Mudge, A. M., et al. 2008. Exercising body and mind: An integrated approach to functional independence in hospitalized older people. *Journal of the American Geriatrics Society* 56(4): 630–635.

Oregon Department of Health and Human Services, Public Health Division. 2008. *"Death With Dignity Act" Annual Report: Year 9—2006 Summary* (http://www.oregon.gov/dhs/ph/pas/index.shtml; retrieved November 29, 2010).

Rietjens, J. A., et al. 2006. Terminal sedation and euthanasia: A comparison of clinical practices. *Archives of Internal Medicine* 166(7): 749–753.

Rosengren, A., et al. 2005. Body mass index, other cardiovascular risk factors, and hospitalization for dementia. *Archives of Internal Medicine* 165(3): 321–326.

Satel, S. 2006. Death's waiting list. *New York Times,* 15 May.

Scarmeas, N., et al. 2006. Mediterranean diet, Alzheimer disease, and vascular mediation. *Archives of Neurology* 63: December [early online release].

Schulz, R., et al. 2006. Predictors of complicated grief among dementia caregivers: A prospective study of bereavement. *American Journal of Geriatric Psychiatry* 14(8): 650–658.

Siminoff, L. A., et al. 2006. Racial disparities in preferences and perceptions regarding organ donation. *Journal of General Internal Medicine* 21(9): 995–1000.

Sorrell, J. M. 2008. As good as it gets? Rethinking old age. *Journal of Psychosocial Nursing and Mental Health Services* 46(5): 21–24.

Tufts University. 2006. Pendulum swings on estrogen and women's heart health risk. *Tufts University Health & Nutrition Letter* 24(3): 1–2.

U.S. Department of Health and Human Services. 2008. *Organ Donor Card* (http://www.organdonor.gov/donor/index.htm; retrieved November 21, 2010).

Ward, E. M. 2006. A weekly to-do list to help delay or prevent dementia. *Environmental Nutrition* 29(5): 2.

Wolfe, M. S. 2006. Shutting down Alzheimer's. *Scientific American* 294(5): 72–79.

APPENDIX

NUTRITION RESOURCES

Nutritional Content of Common Foods

If you are developing a behavior change plan to improve your diet, or if you simply want to choose healthier foods, you may want to know more about the nutritional content of common food items. You can look up the nutrient content of the foods you eat in the USDA Agricultural Research Service National Nutrient Database, which lists foods both by description and by nutrient content. For example, under "protein," you can find out how much protein there is in a chicken pot pie or what foods have the most protein per serving. Although cumbersome, the database is comprehensive. **www.ars.usda.gov/Services/docs.htm?docid=17477**

You can also track your daily food intake, calculate your nutrient intake from foods, and compare your intake with MyPyramid recommendations for your age, sex, height, and weight at the MyPyramid Web site (**www.mypyramidtracker.gov**).

Nutritional Content of Popular Items from Fast-Food Restaurants

Although most foods served at fast-food restaurants are high in calories, fat, saturated fat, cholesterol, sodium, and sugar, some items are healthier than others. If you eat at fast-food restaurants, knowing the nutritional content of various items can help you make better choices. Fast-food restaurants provide nutritional information both online and in print brochures available at most restaurant locations. To learn more about the items you order, visit the restaurant Web sites:

Arby's:	**www.arbysrestaurant.com**	McDonald's:	**www.mcdonalds.com**
Burger King:	**www.burgerking.com**	Subway:	**www.subway.com**
Domino's Pizza:	**www.dominos.com**	Taco Bell:	**www.tacobell.com**
Hardees:	**www.hardees.com**	Wendy's:	**www.wendys.com**
KFC:	**www.kfc.com**	White Castle:	**www.whitecastle.com**

PHOTO CREDITS

Chapter One
p. 1, © Marcy Maloy/PhotoDisc/Getty Images; p. 4, Comstock Images; p. 7, Getty Images/Digital Vision; p. 9, © Tim Platt/Iconica/Getty Images; p. 12, © AP Photo/J. Scott Applewhite; p. 15, © Getty Images; p. 20, © Cindy Charles/PhotoEdit

Chapter Two
p. 24, © Jonathan Daniel/Getty Images; p. 29, Jonnie Miles/Getty Images; p. 31, © Tom Grill/Corbis; p. 33, © Tim Boyle/Getty Images; p. 34, © Scott Olson/Getty Images; p. 36, © Nick Daly/PhotoDisc/Getty Images; p. 42, BananaStock/Jupiterimages

Chapter Three
p. 47, © Image Source/PunchStock; p. 48, © Fancy Photography/Veer; p. 51, © Purestock/PunchStock; p. 54, © PhotoAlto/Laurence Mouton/Getty Images; p. 57, © Peter Cade/Iconica/Getty Images; p. 60, © SW Productions/PhotoDisc/Getty Images; p. 63, © Ken Bank/Corbis

Chapter Four
p. 70, Jack Hollingsworth/Getty Images; p. 71, © Chris Robbins/Digital Vision/Getty Images; p. 73, © JLP/Jose L. Pelaez/Corbis; p. 75, © Mike Iannace/Corbis; p. 77, © Elie Bernager/ONOKY/Getty Images; p. 78, © Brooke Slezak/Stone/Getty Images; p. 79, © Michael J. Doolittle/The Image Works; p. 83, © AP Photo/Eric Risberg; p. 87, © Royalty-Free/Corbis

Chapter Five
p. 91, © Stockbyte/Punchstock; p. 94, Photodisc Collection/Getty Images; p. 96, Ingram Publishing/SuperStock; p. 99, © Royalty-Free/Corbis; p. 104, © Image Source/SuperStock; p. 106, © Joe Raedle/Getty Images; p. 112, © Bananastock/PictureQuest; p. 113, © rubberball/Getty Images

Chapter Six
p. 125, © CKerrigan/McGraw-Hill Companies; p. 129, © Joel Gordon; p. 134, © The McGraw-Hill Companies, Inc./Christopher Kerrigan, photographer; p. 143, © Diane McDonald/Photographer's Choice RF/Getty Images; p. 145, © Alex Wong/Getty Images

Chapter Seven
p. 152, © Peter Dazeley/Photographer's Choice/Getty Images; p. 154, © Dex Images/Corbis; p. 163, Tracy Montana/PhotoLink/PhotoDisc/Getty Images; p. 166, © AP Photo/Daily Post-Athenian, Ben Benton; p. 168, Doug Menuez/Getty Images; p. 171, © SW Productions/PhotoDisc/Getty Images

Chapter Eight
p. 177, © John Rensten/Riser/Getty Images; p. 181, © AP Photo/Reed Saxon; p. 184, © Rachel Weill/UpperCut Images/Getty Images; p. 190, © Brother Luck/Alamy; p. 193, Twentieth Century-Fox Film Corporation/The Kobal Collection; p. 197, © Donn Thompson/DK Stock/Getty Images; p. 198, © Jeff Greenberg/The Image Works

Chapter Nine
p. 206, © Ron Levine/The Image Bank/Getty Images; p. 217, Getty Images/Lifesize; p. 225, © Stockbyte/Masterfile; p. 233, © Nancy R. Cohen/Getty Images

Chapter Ten
p. 241, © Hans Neleman/Taxi/Getty Images; p. 242, © artparadigm/Digital Vision/Getty Images; p. 246T, Chair: © Stockbyte/PunchStock; p. 246TML, Weight lifter: Ryan McVay/Getty Images; p. 246TMR, Stretching: The McGraw-Hill Companies, Inc/Ken Karp photographer; p. 246M, Biking: Joaquin Palting/Getty Images; p. 246BL, Walking to work: Doug Menuez/Getty Images; p. 246BR, Raking: UpperCut Images/Alamy; p. 247, © Brendan Smialowski/Getty Images; p. 249L, Dancing: RubberBall Productions; p. 249M, Biking: © Royalty-Free/Corbis; p. 249R, Weights: Thinkstock Images/Jupiterimages; p. 252, © Glow Wellness RM 26/Alamy; p. 257, © Justin Sullivan/Getty Images

Chapter Eleven
p. 263, Blend Images/Getty Images; p. 264, Scale: Ryan McVay/Getty Images; p. 264, Bike: © Royalty-Free/Corbis; p. 264, Orange: © Stockdisc/PunchStock; p. 264, Cheese: © Photodisc/PunchStock; p. 264, Beans: C Squared Studios/Getty Images; p. 264, Cookie: © Brand X Pictures/PunchStock; p. 264, Broccoli: © Stockdisc/PunchStock; p. 264, Tomato: © Comstock/Jupiter Images; p. 266, © 3660 Group, Inc./Getty Images; p. 268, TRBfoto/Getty Images; p. 270, © Ramin Talaie/Corbis; p. 276, © PNC/Digital Vision/Getty Images; p. 277, © Comstock/PunchStock

Chapter Twelve
p. 282, Photodisc/Getty Images; p. 284, © 2007 Getty Images, Inc.; p. 286, © Jeff J. Mitchell/Getty Images; p. 293, © Paul Seheult/Eye Ubiquitous/Corbis; p. 305, © AP Photo/John Amis; p. 306, © Stockbyte/Getty Images; p. 311, © Mitchell Funk/Photographer's Choice/Getty Images

Chapter Thirteen
p. 317, © BSIP/Phototake; p. 322, © AP Photo/Matt Rourke; p. 327, Doug Menuez/Getty Images; pp. 334, 342, © Joel Gordon

Chapter Fourteen
p. 346, Courtesy NASA; p. 348, © Daniel Berehulak/Getty Images; p. 351, © Saul Loeb/AFP/Getty Images; p. 352, Digital Vision/PunchStock; p. 355, Photodisc/Getty Images; p. 358, © Tony Hobbs/Alamy

Chapter Fifteen
p. 362, © Botanica/Jupiterimages/Getty Images; p. 368, Andrew Wakeford/Getty Images; p. 374, © Comstock/Alamy; p. 377, © Image Source/Getty Images; p. 378, © Marc Schlossman/The Image Bank/Getty Images; p. 381, © Mark Richards/PhotoEdit

Chapter Sixteen
p. 384, © Dorling Kindersley/Getty Images; p. 388, Glowimages/Getty Images; p. 390, © Michael Blann/PhotoDisc/Getty Images; p. 392, Ken Karp for MMH; p. 394, Karen Ballard/© Lionsgate/Courtesy Everett Collection; p. 399, © Rachel Epstein/PhotoEdit; p. 403, © Owaki/Kulla/Corbis

Chapter Seventeen
p. 407, PhotoLink/PhotoDisc/Getty Images; p. 408, © Markku Heikkilä/Flickr/Getty Images; p. 413, © AP Photo/The Salt Lake Tribune/Scott Sommerdorf; p. 414, © Mary Kate Denny/Photographer's Choice/Getty Images; p. 415, © Tom Mareschal/Photographer's Choice/Getty Images; p. 417, FogStock LLC/age footstock; p. 421, © AP Photo/Orlin Wagner; p. 423, © Johner Royalty Free/Getty Images; p. 425, © Eitan Abramovich/AFP/Getty Images

Transparency Insert One
Students talking: Photodisc Red/Getty Images; Drinking on couch: George Doyle/Getty Images; Beer: ©iStockphoto.com/Bjorn Heller; Tequila: © iStockphoto.com/Chris Hutchison; Wine: © iStockphoto.com/plainview; Girl smoking: Image Source; Girl running: Rubberball/Getty Images; View of Earth from Space: © Planetary Vision Limited; Globe in space: © Planetary Vision Limited; Carrying bike: Creatas/PictureQuest; CFL bulb: Mike Kemp/Getty Images; Electric car: © iStockphoto.com/Christian Waadt; Produce stand: Blend Images/Getty Images; Girl on computer: Comstock/Corbis; Bike rack: Masterfile/Royalty Free

Transparency Inset Two
Mountain Biking: Joaquin Palting/Getty Images; Girl eating: ©iStockphoto.com/webphotographeer; Jumping jacks: Mike Powell/Getty Images

INDEX

Boldface numbers indicate pages on which key terms are defined.

A

ABCD test for melanoma, 307
abortifacient, **137**
abortion, **142**–149
    complications of, 148–149
    information resources on, 150
    legal status of, 142, 144
    methods of, 146–148
    personal considerations on, 145
    public opinion on, 144–145
    risks of, 128, 148–149
    spontaneous, 118, 142, 143
    statistics on, 145–146
    summary points about, 149–150
abstinence, 104, **135**–136
abuse
    alcohol, **185**
    child, 399, 401–402
    elder, 399
    physical, 397–398
    sexual, 400–402
    substance, **155**
abusive relationships, 397–398
academic stress, 32
acamprosate, 188
acceptance, 48
accidents, 384
acquaintance rape. *See* date rape
acquired immune deficiency syndrome.
    See AIDS
acquired immunity, **319**
action plan, 19, 20
active euthanasia, **419**–420
active immunity, 321
acupuncture, **372**–373
acute stress, **30**
addiction, 152, **153**
addictive behaviors, **152**–155
    characteristics of, 153
    description of, 152–153
    development of, 153
    examples of, 154
    sex addiction, 106, 154–155
    summary points about, 175
addicts, 154
Adequate Intake (AI), 218
adipose tissue, **264**
adolescents
    antidepressant use by, 60
    dietary challenges for, 225–226
    leading causes of death among, 5
    See also children; young people
adoption, 146
adrenal androgens, 253
adrenal glands, **95**
adult identity, 50
advance directives, **420**
adverse drug events (ADEs), 370–371

advertising, false, 372
AEDs. *See* automated external defibrillators
affirmations, 39
Affordable Care Act (2010), 380–382
African Americans
    alcohol use by, 189
    cardiovascular disease in, 290
    genetic diseases in, 114
    health concerns of, 9
age-related macular degeneration (AMD), **411**
aggressive driving, 385
aging, 407–415
    characteristics of, 407–408
    delaying the effects of, 408–410
    exercise and, 408–409
    family/community and, 414
    government programs and, 414, 415
    information resources on, 427
    life expectancy and, **412**, 413, 414
    mental changes with, 412
    physical changes with, 411–412
    population shift due to, 413–414
    psychological changes with, 413
    sexuality and, 99–100
    social changes with, 410–411
    summary points about, 426
    See also older adults
aging male syndrome, 99–100
agoraphobia, **56**
AIDS (acquired immune deficiency
    syndrome), **329**
    diagnosis of, 331
    global epidemic of, 330–331
    See also HIV infection
air bags, 387–388
air pollution, 348–353
    energy use and, 350
    global warming and, **349**–350
    indoor, 350–351
    ozone layer and, **350**
    prevention of, 351–353
    smog as, **349**
Air Quality Index (AQI), **349**
Al-Anon, 188
alarm reaction, 28
Alaska Natives
    alcohol use by, 190
    health concerns of, 9
alcohol, 177, **178**
    absorption of, 178
    abuse vs. dependence, 185
    blood concentration of, 178–180
    dose-response function of, 182
    drug interactions with, 180–181
    metabolism of, **178**, 179
alcohol abuse, **185**
alcohol dependence, **185**, 186–188
alcoholic beverages
    caffeinated, 181
    common types of, 177–178
Alcoholics Anonymous (AA), 172, 188

alcoholism, **185**, 186–188
    causes and effects of, 187
    ethnicity and, 189–190
    gender and, 188–189
    helping others with, 190
    older adults and, 409–410
    treatments for, 187–188
alcohol-related neurodevelopmental disorder
    (ARND), **185**
alcohol use, 177–190
    aggression and, 182
    benefits related to, 185
    binge drinking and, **186**, 187
    cancer and, 184, 309
    cardiovascular disease and, 287, 297
    chemistry of, 177–180
    connecting to choices about, 202
    deaths associated with, 177, 182, 184, 186
    demographics of, 188
    dependence and, 185, 186–188
    driving and, 182–183
    drug use with, 180–181
    emergencies related to, 180
    gender differences in, 178, 188–189
    health effects of, 180–185, 187
    hooking up fueled by, 81
    immediate effects of, 180–182, 183
    information resources on, 203, 205
    injuries related to, 181–183, 386
    long-term effects of, 183–184
    older adults and, 409–410
    pregnancy and, 116, 184–185
    recommended guidelines for, 220
    responsibility and, 189
    sexual behavior and, 182
    stress and, 42–43
    summary points about, 202
    violence and, 182
    See also drug use
allergens, **321**
allergies, **321**–323
    dealing with, 322–323
    food, 234
allied health care providers, **369**
allostatic load, 29–**30**
altered states of consciousness, **169**
alternative medical systems, 372–373
    See also complementary and alternative medicine
altruism, 35
Alzheimer's disease, **412**
amenorrhea, **269**
American Academy of Pediatrics (AAP), 121, 122
American Cancer Society (ACS), 299–300, 311
American College of Obstetricians and Gynecologists
    (ACOG), 117
American College of Sports Medicine (ACSM), 248,
    255, 377
American Heart Association (AHA), 283, 314, 403
American Indians
    alcohol use by, 190
    health concerns of, 9

American Medical Association (AMA), 377
amino acids, **207**, 253
amnesia, 164
amniocentesis, **115**
amniotic sac, **113**
amphetamines, 165–166
anabolic steroids, **253**
anal intercourse, 104
anaphylaxis response, 234, **322**
androgens, **95**
andropause, 99
anemia, **216**
aneurysm, **294**
anger, 54–55, 78, 287, 288, 298
angina pectoris, **292**
angiogram, **294**
anorexia nervosa, **276**
anterograde amnesia, 164
antibiotics, **325**, 328
antibodies, **319**
anticarcinogens, **310**
antidepressants, 59, 60, 63
antigenic drift, 321
antigenic shift, 321
antigens, **319**
antioxidants, **213**, 216–217
antisocial personality disorder, 182
antiterrorism efforts, 398
antiviral drugs, 333–335
anxiety, **56**
    heart disease and, 287
    social, 67
    test, 44
anxiety disorders
    gender and, 63
    therapies for, 58
    types of, 56, 58
aorta, **283**
aortic aneurysm, 195
Apgar score, **121**
appreciation, expression of, 88
arrhythmia, **292**
arteries, **283**
arthritis, 247, **411**
artificial (intrauterine) insemination, **109**
asbestos, 311, 356
asbestosis, **356**
Asian Americans
    alcohol use by, 189
    cardiovascular disease in, 290
    health concerns of, 9
aspirin, 292, 294
assault, 395
assertiveness, **54**
assisted reproductive technology (ART), **109**
asthma, 247, **322**
asymptomatic diseases, **331**
atherosclerosis, **194**, **284**, 291
athletes, 226, 253
athletic injuries, 258–259
athletic shoes, 256
atrial fibrillation, 294
atrium, 282, **283**
attachment, **71**, 122
attention deficit hyperactivity disorder (ADHD), 64, 167
auditory hallucinations, 61
authenticity, 48
authoritarian parents, 86
authoritative parents, 86
autoeroticism, **104**
autoimmune diseases, **319**, 329
automated external defibrillators (AEDs), 292, 403–404
autonomic nervous system, **25**

autonomy, **48**
ayurvedic products, 378

B
back pain, 246, 367
bacteria, **323–325**
    diseases caused by, 324–325
    foodborne, 229
bacterial vaginosis (BV), **342**
balloon angioplasty, **294**
bariatric surgery, 275
barrier methods, 125, **126**
basal cell carcinoma, **307**
battering, 397–398
B cells, 319
beans, 224
beer, 177
behavioral therapy, 65
behavior change, **14–20**
    beverage choices and, 235
    building motivation for, 15–17
    choosing target behaviors for, 14–15
    drug habits and, 174
    enhancing readiness for, 17
    examining pros and cons of, 15–16
    personal contract for, 19–20
    plan of action for, 17–20
    relapses related to, 17
    self-efficacy and, 16–17
    stages of, 17
benign tumors, **298**
bereavement, **423**
beverage consumption, 235
bicycle helmets, 390
bicycle injuries, 389
bidis, 197
binge drinking, **186**, 187
binge-eating disorder, 278
biodegradability, **354**
bioelectromagnetic-based therapies, 378
biofield therapies, 377
biofuels, 352
biomass, 352
biopsy, **298**
bipolar disorder, **61**
birth control, 125, **126**
    See also contraception
blastocyst, **112**
blood alcohol concentration (BAC), **178–180**
blood pressure, 284, 297–298
blood tests
    HIV infection, 333
    prenatal care and, 115
    prostate-specific antigen, **304**
BMI (body mass index), **265–266**
Bod Pod, 266
body-based practices, 375–377
body composition, **243**, 244, 263–264, 266
body dysmorphic disorder (BDD), 275
body fat
    body composition and, 263–264
    distribution of, 267
    excess, 266–267, 269–270
    low levels of, 267, 269
    wellness and, 266–269
body image, **267**, 275, 277
body mass index (BMI), **265–266**
bone health, 216
bone marrow, **299**
borderline disordered eating, 278
bottled water, 257
brain
    alcohol abuse and, 184
    drug effects on, 159
    nicotine and, 194

brain death, **416**
Braxton Hicks contractions, 111
breakthrough bleeding, 127
breast cancer, 301–302
breastfeeding, 122
breast self-exam (BSE), 302, 303
breathing exercises, 41
budgets, 4
bulimia nervosa, **276–278**
bupropion, 201
burials, 420, 421
burnout, **32**

C
caffeinated alcoholic beverages (CABs), 181
caffeine, 42, 167
    alcoholic beverages with, 181
    content in popular beverages, 167
    decreasing your consumption of, 174
    pregnancy and, 116
calcium, 297
calendar methods of contraception, 136
calories
    discretionary allowance for, 224
    recommended intake of, 223, 297
    weight management and, 271, 272
CAM. See complementary and alternative medicine
campus violence, 34, 403
cancer, **298–313**
    alcohol use and, 184, 309
    breast, 301–302
    causes of, 309–310
    cervical, 304
    colorectal, 301
    diagnosis of, 311
    diet and, 309–310, 314
    early detection of, 310, 312
    endometrial, 306
    environment and, 310, 311
    exercise and, 245
    female reproductive tract, 304–306
    head and neck, 307
    HPV and, 304, 305
    immune system and, 329
    incidence of, 299–300
    information resources on, 315
    lifestyle choices and, 313
    lung, 300–301
    metastasis of, **298**
    obesity and, 310
    ovarian, 306
    prostate, 302–304
    remission from, **298**
    skin, 306–307
    summary points about, 313, 315
    testicular, 308, 309
    tips for preventing, 313
    tobacco use and, 195, 197, 300–301, 307, 309
    treatments for, 311, 313
    tumors and, **298**
    types of, 299
    uterine, 306
candida albicans, 327
cannabis products, 162, 167–168
capillaries, **283**
carbohydrates, **209–212**, 219
    diets low in, 273
    recommended intake of, 212, 297
    setting intake goals for, 211
    sources of, 210–211, 219
carbon monoxide, 391
carcinogens, **193**, 310, 311
carcinomas, **299**
cardiac arrest, 292, 293
cardiac defibrillation, 292

cardiac myopathy, **184**
cardiopulmonary resuscitation (CPR), **292**, 403
cardiorespiratory endurance, 241–**242**
cardiorespiratory endurance training, 241, **242**, 250–251
cardiovascular disease (CVD), 282, **283**–298
  alcohol use and, 287, 297
  cholesterol and, 285–286, 298
  death rates for, 291
  diabetes and, 286–287
  diet and, 285, 290, 296–297, 314
  drug use and, 287
  ethnicity and, 290
  exercise and, 244, 245, 247, 286, 297, 299
  gender differences in, 288, 289
  heredity and, 287–288
  homocysteine levels and, 290–291
  hypertension and, **284**–285
  inflammation and, 288–289
  information resources on, 315
  insulin resistance and, 289–290
  lifestyle choices and, 313
  major forms of, 291–296
  metabolic syndrome and, 289–290
  nutrition and, 219
  obesity and, 286
  prevalence of, 282
  protecting yourself against, 296–298
  psychological factors in, 287, 288, 298
  risk factors for, 283–291
  stress and, 30, 287, 289, 298
  summary points about, 313
  tips for preventing, 313
  tobacco use and, 194–195, 283, 297
  triglycerides and, **287**
cardiovascular system, 282–**283**
  alcohol use and, 184, 185
  exercise and, 244
caregiving, 414
carotenoids, **310**
carpal tunnel syndrome, **392**, 393
cataracts, **411**
Caucasians
  genetic diseases in, 114
  skin cancer in, 306
CD4 T cells, **330**–331, 333
celibacy, **103**–104
cell health, 244
cell phones
  motor vehicle injuries and, 385–386, 388
  radiation from, 359
cellular death, **416**
Centers for Disease Control and Prevention (CDC), 5
central nervous system (CNS), **161**
cerebral cortex, **194**
cerebrovascular accident (CVA), 294
cervical cancer, 304, 305
cervical cap, 134
cervical dysplasia, 304
cervix, **92**
cesarean section, **121**–122
chancre, **341**
changing behavior. *See* behavior change
Chantix, 201
CHD. *See* coronary heart disease
chemical pollution, 356–358
chemotherapy, **301**, 311
chicken pox, 326
childbirth
  choices related to, 119–120
  information resources on, 123–124
  labor and delivery in, 120–122
  postpartum period after, **122**
  preparing for, 117
  summary points about, 123

children
  adoption of, 146
  antidepressant use by, 60
  choices about having, 122
  death understood by, 416
  dietary challenges for, 225–226
  divorce and, 85–86
  safety seats for, 388
  sexual abuse of, 401–402
  tobacco smoke and, 198–199
  violence against, 399
chiropractic, 367, **376**–377
chlamydia, **336**–337
chlorofluorocarbons (CFCs), **350**
choking, 391
cholesterol, **208**–209, 285–286, 297, 298
chorionic villus sampling (CVS), **115**
chromium picolinate, 253
chronic bronchitis, **195**
chronic diseases, **3**
chronic obstructive pulmonary disease (COPD), 195
chronic stress, **30**
cigarettes
  clove/bidis, 197
  e-cigarettes, 197–198
  menthol, 194
  "reduced harm," 194
  toxic chemicals in, 193–194
  See also tobacco use
cigarette tar, **193**
cigars, 197
cilia, 318
circumcision, **93**, 94
cirrhosis, **183**
civil unions, 83
climate change, 13, 349–350, 387
clinical death, **416**
clitoris, **92**
clove cigarettes, 197
club drugs, 164
cluster headaches, 31
cocaine, 164–165
cocarcinogens, **193**
codependency, 172–173
cognitive distortions, **52**
cognitive techniques, 38–39
cognitive therapy, 65
cohabitation, **81**–82
coitus interruptus, 136
cold sores, 326
cold viruses, 325–326
cold weather safety, 387
collective violence, 397
college students
  binge drinking by, 186, 187
  campus violence and, 34, 403
  contraceptive use by, 140
  dietary challenges for, 226
  drug use among, 156
  eating strategies for, 226
  stressors for, 32
colorectal cancer, 301
colostrum, **122**
combination pill, 127
commercial sex, 105–106
commitment
  family life and, 88
  marriage and, 85
  unequal/premature, 73
communication
  contraception and, 141
  family life and, 88
  gender differences in, 76–77
  guidelines for effective, 76

nonverbal, 75–76
  psychological health and, 54
  relationships and, 75–78
  sexual behavior and, 106, 107
  skills related to, 76
  stress management and, 36
community resources, 414
competitiveness, 74
complementary and alternative medicine (CAM), **365**–366, 371–379
  alternative medical systems and, 372–373
  energy therapies and, **377**–378
  evaluation of, 378–379
  information resources on, 383
  manual healing techniques and, 375–377
  mind-body medicine and, 373–374
  natural products and, **374**–375
  research supporting, 367
  statistics on use of, 366
  summary points about, 382
complete proteins, 207
complex carbohydrates, 210
complicated grief, 424
compulsions, **58**, 153, 154, 155
computed tomography (CT) scan, **295**
conception, 107–108, 125, **126**
condoms
  female, 132–133
  male, **131**–132
conflict in relationships, 77–78
congenital heart defects, **296**
congenital malformations, 116
congestive heart failure, **296**
Consumer Product Safety Commission (CPSC), 390
contagion, 319–320
contemplation, 17
continuation rate, **126**
contraception, **125**–142
  abstinence as, **135**–136
  American women and, 140
  choosing methods of, 140–141, 149
  combining methods of, 137
  definition of, **126**
  effectiveness of, 126, 138
  emergency, **137**
  failure rate for, 126
  fertility awareness-based, **136**
  information resources on, 150
  men's involvement in, 142
  permanent methods of, 138–139
  principles of, 125–126
  responsible sex and, 107
  reversible methods of, 126–138
  risks of, 128, 140–141
  STDs and, 125, 132, 138, 141
  summary points about, 149
  talking with partners about, 141
  withdrawal method of, **136**
contraceptive failure rate, **126**
contraceptives, 125, **126**
  diaphragms, **133**–134
  female condoms, 132–133
  FemCap, **134**
  implanted, 129–130
  injectable, 130
  intrauterine devices, **130**–131
  male condoms, **131**–132
  oral, **126**–128
  skin patch, 128–129
  sponge, **134**–135
  vaginal ring, 129
  vaginal spermicides, 135
contractions, **120**
control groups, 369

conventional medicine, **366**–371
  choosing physicians for, 369–370
  getting the most out of, 370–371
  information resources on, 383
  premises and assumptions of, 366–368
  providers of, 368–369
  summary points about, 382
coping mechanisms, 53, 272, 422
core training, 254
coronary arteries, **283**
coronary bypass surgery, **294**
coronary heart disease (CHD), **194**, **291**
  alcohol use and, 185
  tobacco use and, 194–195
corpus luteum, **97**
Corr, Charles, 422
cortisol, **25**
Cowper's glands, **93**
CPR (cardiopulmonary resuscitation), **292**, 403
crabs (pubic lice), 342
C-reactive protein (CRP), 288–289
creatine monohydrate, 253
creativity, 48
credit cards, 4
cremation, 420, 421
crimes, hate, 395
cross-training, **259**
cruciferous vegetables, **217**
culture
  lifestyle and, 10
  psychological disorders and, 57
  stress and, 28
cunnilingus, **104**
CVD. *See* cardiovascular disease
cybersex, **105**
cyberstalking, **399**
cystic fibrosis, 114
cytokines, **320**

D
Daily Values, **218**
dairy products, 224
DASH diet, 221, 285, 297
date rape, **400**
  drugs used in, 400
  prevention of, 401
dating, 80–81
death, 415–425
  advance directives for, **420**
  characteristics of a good, 422
  coming to terms with, 424
  coping with dying and, 421–423
  definitions of, 416
  denying vs. welcoming, 416–417
  disposition of the body at, 420–421
  end-of-life care and, 418
  euthanasia and, 419–420
  funeral/memorial after, 420–421
  grief as reaction to, **423**–424
  information resources on, 427
  leading causes of, 3, 5, 282, 397
  life-sustaining treatment vs., 418–419
  mature understanding of, **416**
  Mexican view of, 417
  organ donation at, 420
  planning for, 417–421
  summary points about, 426–427
  trauma and, 425
  wills and, **417**–418
debt, 4
decibels, **359**
deep breathing, 41
defense mechanisms, **53**
Defense of Marriage Act (DOMA), 83
delirium tremens (DTs), **187**

delusions, 61
demandingness, 86
dementia, **412**
demoralization, 51–52
dendritic cells, 319
dentists, **368**
Department of Energy (DOE), 350
Department of Health and Human Services
  (DHHS), 218, 243
dependence
  alcohol, **185**, 186–188
  drug, **155**–156
  See also substance dependence
depersonalization, **168**
Depo-Provera, 130
depressants, **161**, 162, 163–164
depression, **58**–61
  aging process and, 413
  cardiovascular disease and, 287
  postpartum, **122**
  suicide and, 62, 63
  symptoms of, 58–59
  treatments for, 59–61
designated drivers, 182
diabetes mellitus, **267**, 268
  cardiovascular disease and, 286–287
  excess body fat and, 267
  exercise and, 245, 247
  gestational, **119**, 268
  types of, 268
*Diagnostic and Statistical Manual of Mental
  Disorders* (APA), 155
diagnostic process, 370
diaphragms, **133**–134
diastole, **283**
diet
  beverages in, 235
  cancer and, 309–310, 314
  cardiovascular disease and, 285, 290,
    296–297, 314
  choices about, 234
  DASH-style, 221, 285, 297
  exercise and, 255
  information resources on, 236–237
  Mediterranean, 221
  MyPyramid, **218**, 221–224
  nutritional guidelines for, 217–227
  personal plan for, 227–235
  special populations and, 225–227
  stress management and, 36
  summary points about, 235–236
  vegetarian, 224–225
  weight management and, 271, 273, 279
  See also food; nutrition
dietary fats, 208–209, 210
  cancer and, 309
  diets low in, 273
  hydrogenated, 208, 220
  recommended intake of, 209, 296–297, 314
  setting intake goals for, 211
dietary fiber, **212**–213, 273, 297
Dietary Guidelines for Americans, **218**
Dietary Reference Intakes (DRIs), **217**–218, 227,
    238–240
Dietary Supplement Health and Education Act
    (1994), 378
dietary supplements, 227, 229
  athletic performance and, 253
  club drugs sold as, 164
  information resources on, 230
  labels on, 227, 229, 230
  weight loss and, 272–273
  See also herbal remedies
diet soda consumption, 270
digestion, 206, **207**

digestive system
  alcohol use and, 183
  illustration of, 207
dilation and curettage (D & C), 147
dilation and evacuation (D & E), **147**–148
disability, 9
discretionary calories, 224
discrimination, 10, 33, 290
disease
  autoimmune, **319**, 329
  chronic, **3**
  genetic, 114
  physical activity and, 244–245
  prevention of, 5–6
  testing for, 410
  See also infectious diseases
distress, **28**
disulfiram, 188
diversity
  stress and, 33
  wellness and, 7–10, 12
divorce, 85–86
doctor of osteopathic medicine, **368**
domestic violence, 397–399
dominant genes, 114
dose-response function, **160**, 182
double effect, **419**
douche, **135**
drinking
  binge, **186**, 187
  driving after, 182–183
  water during exercise, 255–256
  See also alcohol use
DRIs. *See* Dietary Reference Intakes
driving
  aggressive, 385
  distracted, 385–386, 388
  drinking and, 182–183, 386
drug abuse. *See* substance abuse
drug dependence. *See* substance dependence
drugs, **153**
  addiction to, 152–155
  alcohol used with, 180–181
  date-rape, 400
  dependence on, 155–156, 157, 158
  generic, 364, **365**
  herbal interactions with, 378
  off-label use of, 371
  over-the-counter, 163, **363**–364, 365
  pharmacological properties of, **159**–160
  widespread use of, 152
  See also medications; psychoactive drugs
drug use
  alcohol use with, 180–181
  changing a habit of, 174
  club drugs and, 164
  college students and, 156
  connecting to choices about, 174
  cost to society of, 170
  demographics of, 156–158
  dependence and, 155–156, 157, 158
  effects of, 159–161, 162
  ethnicity and, 171
  gender differences in, 157
  information resources on, 175–176
  injuries related to, 386
  legalization debate, 170
  methods of, 160
  personal history of, 160
  pregnancy and, 116–117
  prevalence of, 152, 153
  reasons for, 158
  risks of, 158–159
  signs of, 173
  social factors and, 160–161

spirituality and, 158
stress and, 42–43
summary points about, 175
treating dependence on, 172–173
workplace testing for, 170, 172
See also alcohol use
ysmenorrhea, **98**
yspareunia, 102
ysthymic disorder, 58

ating
borderline disordered, 278
coping with stress through, 43
strategies for college students, 226
weight management and, 270, 271, 279
See also diet; nutrition
ating disorders, **275–278**
anorexia nervosa, **276**
binge-eating disorder, **278**
bulimia nervosa, **276–278**
treatment of, 278
bola hemorrhagic fever (EHF), 328
-cigarettes, 197–198
.coli bacteria, 328
cstasy (MDMA), 164, 169
ctopic pregnancy, **118**
cumenical partnerships, 79
ducational attainment
contraceptive use and, 140
drug use and, 171
wellness and, 9, 10
jaculation, **131**
jaculatory ducts, **93**
lder abuse, 399
lderly. *See* older adults
lectrical impedance analysis, 266
lectric vehicles, 350
lectrocardiogram (ECG/EKG), 248, **292**
lectroconvulsive therapy (ECT), **59**
lectroencephalogram (EEG), **416**
ELISA test, **333**
mbalming, **420**
mbolus, **294**
mbryo, **113**
differentiation of, 95
early development of, 113
mergency care, 403–404
mergency contraception (EC), **137**
mergency department (ED), 363
mergency medical services (EMS) system, **404**
merging infections, 328–329
motional intelligence, **49**
motional wellness, 2
exercise and, 245–246
weight management and, 272
motions, **49**
mphysema, **195**
mployment status
drug use and, 171
sexual harassment and, 402
ending relationships, 75
endocrine disrupting chemicals (EDCs), 96–97
endocrine system, 25
end-of-life care, 418
endometrial cancer, 306
endometriosis, 101
endometrium, **96**
endorphins, **25**
endoscopies, **370**
endurance training, 241, **242**, 251–253
energy
carbohydrates for, 209–212, 219
weight management and, 219, 264–265, 273, 279

energy consumption
air pollution and, 350
renewable energy and, 352
energy therapies, **377–378**
entry inhibitors, **334**
environment
bottled water and, 257
carcinogens in, 310, 311
climate change and, 13, 239–250
drug development and, 375
methamphetamine and, 166
oil exploration and, 351
stressors in, 33
tobacco use and, 199
wellness and, 3, 12
Environmental Defense Fund (EDF), 257
environmental hazards
cancer and, 310, 311
pregnancy and, 143, 357
reproductive system and, 96–97
environmental health, 346–361
air pollution and, 348–353
chemical pollution and, 356–358
connecting to choices about, 360
definition of, 346–**347**
gender and, 357
information resources on, 361
noise pollution and, 359
oil exploration and, 351
population growth and, 347–348
poverty and, 356
radiation and, **358**–359
self-assessment checklist, 347
solid waste pollution and, 354–356
summary points about, 360
tips related to, 360
water quality and, 353
Environmental Protection Agency (EPA),
199, 387
environmental tobacco smoke (ETS), 177, 194,
198–199, 301
Environmental Working Group
(EWG), 257
epidemics, **321**
epididymis, **93**
epididymitis, 101
epinephrine, **25**
epithelia, **299**
erectile dysfunction, **102**
erogenous zones, **100**
erotic fantasy, **104**
erythropoietin (EPO), 253
essential fat, 263, **264**
essential nutrients, 206, **207**
estate, **417**
estrogen, **95**, 289
estrogenic phase, 96
ethanol, 350
ethnicity
alcohol abuse and, 189–190
body image and, 277
cardiovascular disease and, 288, 290
contraceptive use and, 140
diabetes and, 268
drug use and, 171
genetic diseases and, 114
HIV infection and, 332
psychological disorders and, 57
suicide rate by, 62
wellness and, 9, 10
ETS. *See* environmental tobacco smoke
euphoria, **161**
eustress, **28**
euthanasia, 419–420
e-waste, 355

exercise, **243**, 244–260
ACSM guidelines for, 248
aging process and, 408–409
benefits of, 244–246, 249
CAM modalities and, 377
cardiorespiratory endurance, 250–251
cardiovascular disease and, 244, 245, 247, 286,
297, 299
compulsive use of, 154
connecting to choices about, 259
core training, 254
designing a program of, 246, 248–255
dietary supplements and, 253
eating and drinking for, 255–256
flexibility, 253–254
footware for, 256
immune system and, 246
information resources on, 261
injuries and, 246, 258–259
isometric, **251**
isotonic, **251**
levels of, 246, 248
physical health and, 244–245, 249
pregnancy and, 117
psychological health and, 59, 245–246
resistance, **251**
special health concerns and, 247
strength/endurance, 251–253
stress management and, 36
summary points about, 260–261
tips related to, 259
weight management and, 271–272
See also physical fitness
Exercise Is Medicine initiative, 377
exercise program, 246, 248–259
activity selection for, 250, 260
consistency with, 256, 258
cross-training in, 259
designing, 246, 248–255
equipment for, 251, 255
FITT principle, 249, 254–255
frequency of, 250, 251–252, 254
injury management/prevention, 258–259
instructors/facilities for, 255
intensity of, 250, 252–253, 254
management/maintenance of, 256, 258–259, 260
medical clearance for, 248
planning a personal, 260
specific skills training in, 254
three phases of, 256
time allotted to, 250, 252–253, 254
training principles for, 248–249
warm-up and cool-down, 251
exhaustion, 29
expectations in relationships, 73–74
expedited partner therapy, 337
expressive writing, 364
external locus of control, 16

F
fallopian tubes, **92**
falls, injury from, 389–390
false negatives, **370**
false positives, **370**
families, 86–88
older adults in, 414
parenting in, 86–87
qualities of successful, 88
sexual abuse in, 402
stepfamilies as, 87
violence in, 397–399
fast-food restaurants, 226
fat. *See* body fat; dietary fats
fat-free mass, **243**
fatigue, 385

fat-soluble vitamins, 214
FDA. *See* Food and Drug Administration
Federal Bureau of Investigation (FBI), 393
Federal Trade Commission (FTC), 372
feedback, 76
fee-for-service plans, 380
fellatio, **104**
female athlete triad, **269**
female condoms, 132–133
female genital cutting (FGC), 94
female reproductive tract cancers, 304–306
females
　infertility in, 108
　sex organs in, 91–92
　sexual maturation in, 95–98
　sterilization of, 139
　See also women
FemCap, **134**
fertility, 107–109, **127**
fertility awareness-based methods, **136**
fertilization, **107**, 108
fertilized egg, **107**
fetal alcohol spectrum disorder (FASD), 185
fetal alcohol syndrome (FAS), **116**, 184–185
fetal development, 111–115
　diagnosing abnormalities in, 114–115
　stages or trimesters of, 111–114
fetal programming theory, 115
fiber, 212–213, 273, 297
fibromyalgia, 367
fight-or-flight reaction, **25–27**
financial issues
　concerns about, 32
　wellness related to, 3, 4
firearms, 62, 391, 393, 395, 402
fires, 390–391
first aid, **403**
fish consumption, 231
fitness. *See* physical fitness
FITT principle, 249, 254–255
flashbacks, **169**
Fleming, Alexander, 375
flexibility, 242–**243**
flexibility exercises, 253–254
flood safety, 387
fluid intelligence, **408**
flushing syndrome, 179
flu viruses, 326
folic acid, 297
follicle, **96**
food
　additives in, 231–232
　allergies to, **234**
　antioxidants in, 216–217
　beverages and, 235
　carcinogens in, 310
　considering choices of, 234
　genetically modified, **233**–234
　illnesses from, 229
　intolerances to, **234**, 235
　irradiation of, **232**–233
　labels on, 227, 228
　nutrient-dense, 219, 224
　organic, **229**, 231, 232–233
　personal plan for, 227–235
　phytochemicals in, **217**
　safe handling of, 220, 231
　vegetarian, 225
　See also diet; nutrition
food allergies, **234**
Food and Drug Administration (FDA), 60, 218,
　229, 363
food intolerances, **234**, 235
food irradiation, **232**–233
footware, exercise, 256

foreplay, **104**
fortified wines, 178
fossil fuels, **349**, 352
fraternal twins, **108**
fraud, health, 372
free radicals, **216**–217
fried foods, 309
friendships, 71–72
fruits, 223–224, 309–310, 314
functional fiber, **212**
fungus, **326**–327

G
gambling, compulsive, 154
gamete intrafallopian transfer (GIFT), **109**
gamma globulin, 321
gang-related violence, 395
gender
　alcohol use and, 178, 188–189
　body image and, 277
　cardiovascular disease and, 288, 289
　communication and, 76–77
　definition of, **7**
　drug use and, 157
　environmental health and, 357
　HIV infection and, 332
　injury rates and, 386
　life expectancy and, 414
　muscular strength and, 252
　nutritional needs and, 225
　psychological disorders and, 63
　sex distinguished from, 7
　STD infection and, 337
　stress and, 28, 29
　suicide rate by, 62
　tobacco use and, 196
　violence and, 394
　wellness and, 7–9
gender roles, **28**, 71
general adaptation syndrome (GAS), **28–29**
generalized anxiety disorder (GAD), **56**
generic drugs, 364, **365**
genes, **12**, **108**, 114
genetically modified (GM) organisms, **233**–234
genetic diseases, 114
genetics
　body weight and, 269
　cancer and, 309
　cardiovascular disease and, 287–288
　psychological disorders and, 55–56
　wellness and, 12
genital alteration, 94
genital herpes, **339**–340
genital warts, 305, **338**
genome, **12**
geographic location, 9, 171
geothermal power, 352
geriatricians, **415**
germ cells, 91, **92**
gerontologists, **415**
gestational diabetes (GDM), **119**, 268
GHB (gamma hydroxybutyrate), 164, 400
giardiasis, **327**
gingivitis, 197
glans, **93**
glaucoma, **410**
global warming, 13, **349**–350
glucose, **210**
glycemic index, **211**
glycogen, **210**
goal setting
　exercise, 260
　SMART criteria for, 18
　weight management, 279
gonads, 91, **92**

gonococcal conjunctivitis, **337**
gonorrhea, **337**–338
government aid, 415
grains
　recommended intake of, 222–223
　whole, **210**–211, 212
green burials, 421
green consumerism, 355
greenhouse effect, **349**
greenhouse gases, **349**
grief, 413, **423**–424
groups, self-help, 172
Gulf oil spill, 351

H
H1N1 flu pandemic, 322
HAART therapy, 334
hallucinations, 61, **187**
hallucinogens, 162, **168**–169
hangover, 180
hantavirus pulmonary syndrome (HPS), 328
happiness, 48–49
hardiness, 27
hard liquor, 178
harm reduction strategies, 172
hassles, 32
hate crimes, 395–396
hatha yoga, 41–42
hazardous waste, 356–358
HDL (high-density lipoprotein), **209**, **285**
headaches, 31, 367
health
　alcohol use and, 180–185
　altruism and, 35
　beverage consumption and, 235
　definition of, 1, **2**
　dietary fats and, 208–209
　evaluating news about, 369
　excess body fat and, 266–267
　expressive writing and, 364
　habits related to, 12, 14
　intimate relationships and, 84
　promotion of, **5**
　stress and, 28–31
　tobacco use and, 193–198
　See also wellness
health care, 362–383
　access to, 10, 12
　allied providers of, 369
　avoiding fraud and quackery in, 372
　complementary and alternative, 365–366, 367,
　　371–379
　connecting to choices about, 382
　conventional, 366–371
　costs of, 379
　drug use and, 170
　getting the most out of, 370–371
　information resources on, 383
　insurance plans/programs, 379–380
　primary care physician for, 369–370
　professional options for, 364–366
　reform bill on, 11, 380–382
　self-care and, 362–364
　summary points about, 382
Health Care and Education Reconciliation Act
　(2010), 11
health care proxy, **420**
health information
　evaluating sources of, 15
　See also information resources
health insurance, 379–380
health journal, 17–18
health maintenance organizations (HMOs), **380**
health-related fitness, 241, **242**
Healthy Campus 2010 program, 7

Healthy People 2020 initiative, 6–7
hearing loss, 411
heart
    cardiovascular system and, 282–283
    congenital defects in, 296
heart attack, 292–294
    helping a victim of, 292
    warning signs of, 293
heart disease, 292–294
    anger/hostility and, 288
    angina pectoris and, 292
    arrhythmias and, 292
    congestive heart failure and, 296
    detecting and treating, 292, 294
    exercise and, 247
    less common forms of, 296
    See also cardiovascular disease
heavy metals, 353
Hegar's sign, 110
Heimlich maneuver, 391
hemochromatosis, 114
hemorrhagic stroke, 294, 295
hepatitis, 326, 340
hepatitis A virus (HBA), 326, 340
hepatitis B virus (HBV), 326, 340–341
hepatitis C virus (HCV), 159, 326, 340
herbal remedies, 372, 374–375
    overview of commonly used, 376
    safety issues related to, 378
    traditional Chinese, 372
    weight loss and, 273
    See also dietary supplements
heredity. *See* genetics
herpesvirus, 326
heterosexual relationships, 82
hierarchy of needs, 47–48
high, drug-induced, 160
high blood pressure, 284–285
high-density lipoprotein (HDL), 209, 285
histamine, 319, 321
HIV antibody test, 333
HIV infection, 330–335
    AIDS and, 329–330
    diagnosis of, 333
    education about, 342
    getting tested for, 334, 342
    global epidemic of, 330–331
    injection drug use and, 159, 332
    populations of special concern for, 332
    progression/stages of, 330–331
    protecting yourself from, 335, 336
    symptoms of, 332–333
    transmission of, 331–332
    treatments for, 333–335
HIV-positive diagnosis, 333
HIV RNA assay, 333
holistic approach, 371
home care, 418
home injuries, 389–391
homeopathy, 373
homeostasis, 26
homeostatic resilience, 28
homicide, 393, 395
homocysteine, 290–291
homophobia, 82
homosexual relationships, 82
honesty, 73
hooking up, 81
hormonal methods of contraception, 125, 126
hormones, 25
    sex, 95
    stress-related, 25, 37
hormone therapy (HT), 99
hospice, 418
hostility, 287, 288

hot weather safety, 387
HPV. *See* human papillomavirus
human chorionic gonadotropin (HCG), 109
human immunodeficiency virus (HIV), 329
    stages of infection by, 330–331
    transmission of, 331–332
    See also HIV infection
human papillomavirus (HPV), 132, 304, 305, 326, 338–339
humor, sense of, 39
hybrid electric vehicles (HEVs), 350
hydrogenation, 208
hydrostatic weighing, 266
hymen, 92
hypertension, 247, 284–285, 299
hypertrophic cardiomyopathy (HCM), 296
hypertrophy, 286
hypnotherapy, 373–374
hypothalamus, 95
hysterectomy, 139

I
identical twins, 108
identity crisis, 50
illness
    foodborne, 229
    risk factors for, 1
    See also disease
imagery, 40
immune response, 319, 320
immune system, 318–320
    allergies and, 321–323
    autoimmune diseases and, 319, 329
    cancer and, 329
    exercise and, 246
    guidelines for supporting, 329
    immune response of, 318–320
    stress and, 30, 31, 340
immunity, 319, 321
immunization, 321
implants, contraceptive, 129–130
impotence, 102
incest, 402, 403
income inequality, 9, 10
incomplete proteins, 207
incontinence, 304
incubation, 319–320
indemnity plans, 380
indoor air pollution, 350–351
infant mortality, 119
infants
    HIV infection in, 332
    mortality rate for, 119
    safety seats for, 388
    syphilis in, 341
    tobacco smoke and, 198–199
    See also children
infatuation, 72
infection, 317, 318
infectious diseases, 3, 317–345
    bacterial, 323–325
    emerging, 328–329
    epidemics of, 321
    fungal, 326–327
    immune response to, 318–320
    immunization against, 321
    inflammatory response to, 319
    information resources on, 344
    pandemics of, 321, 322
    parasitic worms and, 327
    pathogens associated with, 323–329
    prevention guidelines, 329
    prions and, 327–328
    protozoal, 327
    sexually transmitted, 329–342

    summary points about, 343
    transmission of, 317–318
    viral, 325–326
infertility, 108–109
inflammation, 288–289
inflammatory response, 319
influenza, 321, 322, 326
information resources
    on abortion, 150
    on aging, 427
    on alcohol use, 203, 205
    on cancer, 315
    on cardiovascular disease, 315
    on contraception, 150
    on death and dying, 427
    on diet and nutrition, 236–237
    on drug use/abuse, 175–176
    on environmental health, 361
    on exercise and fitness, 261
    on health care, 383
    on infectious diseases, 344
    on intimate relationships, 89–90
    on personal safety, 405–406
    on pregnancy and childbirth, 123–124
    on psychological health, 68
    on sexuality, 123–124
    on STDs, 344
    on stress, 45–46
    on tobacco use, 203, 205
    on weight management, 280–281
    on wellness, 21–22
inhalants, 162, 169–170
injectable contraceptives, 130
injection drug users (IDUs), 159
injuries, 384–393
    athletic, 258–259
    bicycle, 389, 390
    care of common, 258
    causes of, 385
    home, 389–391
    inflammatory response to, 319
    intentional, 384, 385, 393–402
    leisure, 391–392
    motor vehicle, 385–389
    preventing, 246, 259
    self-inflicted, 62
    statistics on, 385
    summary points about, 404–405
    unintentional, 384–393
    work, 392–393
insomnia, 37
Institute of Medicine (IOM), 370
insulin resistance, 289–290
intact dilation and extraction, 148
integration, 51
integrative medicine, 365
intellectual wellness, 2
intentional injuries, 384, 385, 393–402
    See also violence
interfaith partnerships, 79
intermittent explosive disorder (IED), 54
internal locus of control, 16
Internet
    addiction to, 155
    health information on, 15
    unlawful sales on, 372
interpersonal stress, 32
interpersonal violence, 397
interpersonal wellness, 2
intersex individuals, 82
intestate, 418
intimate relationships, 70–90
    capacity for, 48
    challenges in, 73–74
    choosing partners for, 78–80

intimate relationships (*Cont.*)
    commitment to, 73, 85
    communication in, 75–78
    conflict in, 77–78
    connecting to choices about, 88
    contraceptive use in, 141
    dating and, 80–81
    development of, 50, 70–75
    ending, 75
    enhancing support in, 74
    family life and, 86–88
    friendships and, 71–72
    health benefits of, 84
    information resources on, 89–90
    living together in, 81–82
    love and sex in, 72–73
    marriage and, 84–86
    same-sex partners in, 82, 83
    sense of self in, 70–71
    singlehood and, 82, 84
    summary points about, 88–89
    tips related to, 88
    unhealthy, 75
    violence in, 397–399
intoxication, 152, **153**, 158–159
intra-abdominal fat, 264
intracerebral hemorrhage, 294
intrafaith partnerships, 79
intrauterine devices (IUDs), **130–131**
intrauterine insemination, 109
in vitro fertilization (IVF), **109**
irradiated foods, 232–233
ischemic stroke, **294**, 295
isometric (static) exercises, **251**
isotonic (dynamic) exercises, **251**

J
jaundice, **326**
jealousy, 74
job-related stressors, 32
journals
    health, 17–18
    self-help using, 64
    stress, 43

K
Kaposi's sarcoma, **333**
kava kava, 378
Kegel exercises, 117
ketamine, 164, 400
kilocalories, **207**
Koop, C. Everett, 148
Kübler-Ross, Elisabeth, 422

L
labels
    dietary supplement, 227, 229, 230
    food, 227, 228
    OTC drug, 365
    reporting false, 372
labor, **120**
    induction of, 119
    pain relief during, 121
    stages of, 120–121
lactation, **122**
lacto-ovo-vegetarians, 225
lactose intolerance, 114
lacto-vegetarians, 225
laparoscopy, **139**
Latinos
    alcohol use by, 189
    cardiovascular disease in, 290
    health concerns of, 9
LDL (low-density lipoprotein), **208**–209, **285**
lead poisoning, 356–357

Lee, Russell, 415
legislation
    abortion, 142, 144
    banning same-sex marriage, 83
    health care reform, 11, 380–382
    tobacco use, 199–200
leisure injuries, **391**–392
leisure time, 410
leukemia, **299**
leukoplakia, 197
life changes, 32
life expectancy, 3, **412**, 413, 414
lifestyle choices, **5**
    culture and, 10
    exercise on connecting to, 21
    weight management and, 269–270
    wellness and, 14–20, 21
life-support systems, **416**
lifting technique, 392
lightening, **110**, 111
lightning strikes, 387
limit setting, 174
lipids, 208
lipoproteins, **285**
listening, 76
living together, 81–82
living will, **420**
locus of control, **16**
loneliness, 54
love
    intimacy and, 72–73
    pleasure and pain of, 72–73
    transformation of, 73
low-back pain, 246
low birth weight (LBW) babies, **119**
low-carbohydrate diets, 273
low-density lipoprotein (LDL), **208**–209, **285**
low-fat diets, 273
LSD (lysergic acid diethylamide), 164, 168–169
lung cancer, 195, 300–301
Lyme disease, 325
lymphatic system, **298**
lymphocytes, 319
lymphomas, **299**

M
macronutrients, 206
macrophages, 319
mad cow disease, 229
magnetic resonance imaging (MRI), **294**
mainstream smoke, **198**
malaria, **327**
male condoms, **131**–132
male menopause, 99
males
    infertility in, 108
    injury rate for, 386
    sex organs in, 92–93
    sexual maturation of, 98–99
    sterilization of, 138–139
    See also men
malignant tumors, **298**
mammogram, **302**
managed-care plans, **380**
management
    anger, 54–55
    lifestyle, 14–20
    stress, 34–44
mania, **61**
manual healing techniques, 375–377
manual vacuum aspiration (MVA), **147**
marijuana, 42–43, 162, 167–168
marriage, 84–86
    benefits of, 84
    cohabitation vs., 81–82

    commitment in, 85
    contraception in, 140
    divorce and, 85–86
    family life and, 86–88
    interfaith/intrafaith, 79
    issues in, 84–85
    same-sex, 83
    statistics on, 82
    wellness and, 84
    See also intimate relationships
Maslow, Abraham, 47
mast cells, 321
masturbation, **103**
mature understanding of death, **416**
maximal oxygen consumption (VO$_{2max}$), **250**
MDMA (ecstasy), 164, 169
mealasma, 127
meaning, 49
meat consumption, 224
media
    health information in, 369
    smoking portrayed in, 192–193
    violence in, 394
Medicaid, **380**, 415
medical abortion, 148
medical doctors, **368**
Medicare, **380**, 415
medications
    alcoholism, 188
    antiviral, 333–335
    drug dependence, 172, 409–410
    errors prescribing, 370–371
    generic, 364, **365**
    herbal interactions with, 378
    over-the-counter, 163, **363**–364, 365
    teenage abuse of, 163
    weight loss, 274
medicine
    alternative systems of, 372–373
    complementary and alternative, **365**–366, 367, 371–379
    conventional, 366–371
    integrative, **365**
    mind-body, 373–374
    See also health care
meditation, 40–**41**
Mediterranean diet, 221
melanoma, **306**, 307
men
    alcohol abuse by, 188
    communication advice for, 77
    contraception involvement by, 142
    health issues for, 8
    injuries among young, 386
    life expectancy of, 414
    nutritional needs of, 225
    stress and, 29
    See also males
menarche, **96**
meningitis, 324
menopause, **99**, 412
menses, **96**
menstrual cycle, 95–97
menstrual problems, 98
mental challenges, 408
mental health. *See* psychological health
menthol cigarettes, 194
mercury, 231, 357
meridians, 372
mescaline, 169
metabolic rate, 244
metabolic syndrome, 289–290
metabolism, **178**, 244
metastasis, **298**
methamphetamine, 165, 166

micronutrients, 206
migraines, 31
milk products, 224
mind-body medicine, 373–374
mindfulness meditation, 41
minerals, **215**–216
  bone health and, 216
  facts about, 215
minipill, 127
miscarriage
  definition of, **142**
  environmental hazards and, 143
mitral valve prolapse (MVP), **296**
monoclonal antibodies, **302**
monounsaturated fats, 209, 210
mood disorders, 58–61
morbidity rate, **3**
morning-after pill, 137
morning sickness, 110
mortality rate, **3**
motorcycles/scooters, 389
motor vehicle injuries, **385**–389
  alcohol use and, 182–183, 386
  cell phone use and, 385–386, 388
  factors contributing to, 385–388
  motorcycles/scooters and, 389
  prevention of, 388–389
mourning, **423**–424
MRI (magnetic resonance imaging), **294**
mucus method of contraception, 136
multifaith partnerships, 79
multi-fetal pregnancy reduction (MFPR), **147**
multiple births, 108
murmur, **296**
muscle dysmorphia, 275
muscular endurance, **242**
muscular strength, **242**, 252
music, listening to, 42
myocardial infarction, **195**, 292
MyPyramid, **218**, 221–224
  daily calorie intake, 223
  food intake patterns, 222–224
  key messages of, 221–222

N

naltrexone, 188
narcotics, 161
Narcotics Anonymous (NA), 172
National Cancer Institute (NCI), 314
National Center for Complementary and
    Alternative Medicine (NCCAM), 371
National Cholesterol Education Program (NCEP),
    296–297
National Highway Transportation Safety
    Administration (NHTSA), 182
National Institute for Occupational Safety and
    Health (NIOSH), 311
National Institutes of Health (NIH), 5, 263,
    371, 373
National Safety Council (NSC), 384
National Sleep Foundation (NSF), 37
National Strength and Conditioning Association
    (NSCA), 255
National Survey on Drug Use and Health
    (NSDUH), 163
Native Americans. *See* American Indians
natural killer cells, 319
natural methods of contraception, 125, **126**
natural products, **374**–375
nature
  ADHD and exposure to, 64
  stress and exposure to, 40
nature deficit disorder, 64
naturopathy, **373**
needs, hierarchy of, 47–48

negative self-talk, 52
neoplasm, 298
nervous system
  autonomic, **25**
  central, **161**
  somatic, **27**
neuropeptides, 30
neurotransmitters, **159**
neutrophils, 319
newsletters on health, 21
nicotine, **191**
nicotine replacement products, 201
noise pollution, 359
non-rapid eye movement (non-REM) sleep, 36–37
nonreactive resilience, 28
nonverbal communication, 75–76
norepinephrine, **25**
normality, **49**
nuclear power, **358**–359
nutrient-dense foods, 219, 224
nutrition, 206–240
  antioxidants and, 216–217
  beverages and, 235
  bone health and, 216
  carbohydrates and, **209**–212, 219
  connecting to choices about, 234
  definition of, **207**
  Dietary Reference Intakes, **217**–218, 227,
      238–240
  essential nutrients and, 206–**207**
  fats and, 208–209
  fiber and, 212–213
  gender differences and, 225
  guidelines for, 217–227
  information resources on, 236–237
  minerals and, **215**–216
  personal food plan for, 227–235
  phytochemicals and, **217**
  prenatal, 115–116
  proteins and, **207**–208, 219
  special population groups and, 225–227
  stress management and, 36
  summary points about, 235–236
  vegetarian diets and, 224–225
  vitamins and, **213**–215
  water and, 216
  See also diet; food
NuvaRing, 129

O

obesity
  cancer and, 310
  cardiovascular disease and, 286
  definition of, 264, **265**
  exercise and, 247
  factors contributing to, 269–270
  health risks of, 266–267
  options for overcoming, 272–275
  See also weight management
obsessions, **56**
obsessive-compulsive disorder (OCD), **56**, 58, 63
Occupational Safety and Health Administration
    (OSHA), 359
off-label drug use, 371
oil exploration, 351
oils, dietary, 224
older adults
  dietary issues for, 226, 409
  elder abuse and, 399
  exercise for, 408–409
  family/community resources for, 414
  government programs for, 414, 415
  increasing numbers of, 413
  life-enhancing measures for, 408–410
  mental changes in, 412

physical changes in, 411–412
  psychological changes in, 413
  social changes for, 410–411
  See also aging
omega-3 fatty acids, **209**, 297
On Death and Dying (Kübler-Ross), 422
one drink (standard drink), **178**
online pharmacies, 371
online relationships, 80
open adoption, 146
openness, 73
opioids, 43, **161**, 162
opportunistic infections, **331**, 335
optimism, **53**
optometrists, **368**
oral cancer, 197
oral contraceptives (OCs), **126**–128
  advantages/disadvantages of, 127–128
  effectiveness of, 128
oral sex, 104
organ donation, 420
organic farming, 232–233
organic foods, **229**, 231, 232–233
organizational resources. *See* information resources
orgasm, **101**
orgasmic dysfunction, **102**
oropharyngeal cancer, 305
Ortho Evra patch, 128–129
osteoarthritis (OA), 411
osteopaths, 368
osteoporosis, **216**, 245, 247, 412
ova, 91, **92**, 107
ovarian cancer, 306
ovaries, **92**
over-the-counter (OTC) medications, 163,
    363–364, 365
overweight
  definition of, 264, **265**
  options for overcoming, 272–275
  See also weight management
ovulation, 96–**97**
oxytocin, 29
ozone layer, **350**

P

Pacific Islander Americans, 9
palliative care, **418**
pandemics, **321**, 322
panic disorder, **56**, 63
Pap test, **128**, **304**
parasitic worms, **327**
parasympathetic division, **25**
parenting, 86–87
  family life cycle and, 86–87
  single parents and, 87
  styles of, 86
partial birth abortion, 148
partners
  choosing, 78–80
  interfaith/intrafaith, 79
  same-sex, 82, 83
passive euthanasia, **419**
passive immunity, 321
pathogens, **320**, 323–329
  bacteria, **323**–325
  body's defenses against, 318–320
  chain of infection by, 317–318
  fungi, **326**–327
  immunization against, **321**
  parasitic worms, 327
  prions, **327**–328
  protozoa, **327**
  viruses, **325**–326
  See also infectious diseases
PCP (drug), 169

peer counseling, 44, 64
pelvic inflammatory disease (PID), 101, 131, **338**
penicillin, 375
penis, **92**
percent body fat, **264**
perimenopause, 412
peripheral arterial disease, 291
permissive parents, 86
persistent vegetative state, **418**
personal contract, 19
personal flotation device, **392**
personality, **27–28**
personal safety, 384–406
    adopting habits for, 405
    bicycles and, 389, 390
    college campuses and, 403
    connecting to choices about, 404
    emergency care and, 403–404
    extreme weather and, 387
    home-based, 389–391
    information resources on, 405–406
    leisure activities and, 391–392
    motor vehicle operation and, 385–389
    summary points about, 404–405
    unintentional injuries and, 384–393
    violence and, 393–402
    workplace and, 392–393
pessimism, 53
pesticides, **357**
pharmaceuticals, **366**
pharmacological properties, **159**–160
pharmacological therapy, 65
pharmacopoeia, **374**
phobias, 56
physical activity, **243–244**
    aging and, 408–409
    benefits of, 244–246, 249
    cardiovascular disease and, 286, 297, 299
    connecting to choices about, 259
    guidelines for adults, 243–244
    levels of, 246, 248
    making time for, 245
    pregnancy and, 117
    weight management and, 270, 271–272
    See also exercise
Physical Activity Guidelines for Americans (DHHS), 243–244, 408
physical activity pyramid, 246, 248
physical dependence, **155**
physical fitness, 241–243
    aging and, 408–409
    assessment of, 258
    body composition and, **243**
    cardiorespiratory endurance and, 241–**242**
    definition of, **242**
    flexibility and, 242–**243**
    health-related, 241, **242**
    information resources on, 261
    muscular strength/endurance and, **242**
    skill-related, **243**
physical wellness, 2
physician-assisted suicide (PAS), **419**
physicians
    choosing primary care, 369–370
    discussing CAM therapies with, 378–379
    partnership of patients and, 370
    when to see, 363
phytochemicals, **217**, 310
pipe smoking, 197
pituitary gland, **95**
PKC enzyme, 31
placebo effect, **160**, 373, 374
placenta, **113**
placental abruption, **118**

placenta previa, **118**
plant stanols/sterols, 297
plaque, **194**, 291
platelets, **283**
Pneumocystis pneumonia, **333**
pneumonia, 324, 333
podiatrists, **368**
point-of-service (POS) plans, **380**
poisoning, 391
    alcohol, 180
    lead, 356–357
pollution
    air, 348–353
    chemical, 356–358
    industrial, 310, 311
    noise, 359
    solid waste, 354–356
    water, 353
polychlorinated biphenyls (PCBs), **353**
polypeptide supplements, 253
polyps, **301**
polyunsaturated fats, 209, 210
population growth, 347–348
pornography, **105**
positive growth resilience, 28
positive psychology, 47–49
positron emission tomography (PET), 294
postmenopausal women, 289
postpartum depression, **122**
postpartum period, **122**
post-traumatic stress disorder (PTSD), 31, 34, **58**, 63, 425
potassium, 219–220, 297
poverty
    environmental health and, 356
    health/wellness and, 9, 10, 328
    See also socioeconomic status
precontemplation, 17
pre-diabetes, 268
preeclampsia, **118**
preferred provider organizations (PPOs), **380**
pregnancy, 109–119
    alcohol use during, 116, 184–185
    caffeine use during, 116
    childbirth classes during, 117
    cocaine use during, 165
    complications of, 118–119
    drug use during, 116–117
    ectopic, **118**
    environmental hazards and, 143, 357
    fathers' tasks during, 112
    fetal development and, 111–115
    HIV infection and, 335
    home tests for, 109
    information resources on, 123–124
    miscarriage and, **142**, 143
    nutrition during, 115–116
    physical activity during, 117
    physiological changes during, 110–111
    prenatal care during, 115–117
    preventing unwanted, 125
    risks of, 128
    smoking during, 116, 199
    summary points about, 123
    trimesters of, **109**–110, 111–114
    unintended, 140, 141
prejudice, 10
premature babies, **119**
premature ejaculation, **102**, 103
premenstrual dysphoric disorder (PMDD), 98
premenstrual syndrome (PMS), **98**
premenstrual tension, 98
prenatal care, 115–117
prepuce, **92**
presbyopia, **411**

prescription drugs
    errors related to, 370–371
    teenage abuse of, 163
    weight loss using, 274
    See also medications
preterm labor, 119
prevention
    air pollution, 351–353
    date rape, 401
    diabetes, 268
    disease, 5–6
    drug abuse, 173
    injury, 246, 259, 388–389
    pregnancy, 125
primary care physicians, 369–370
primary tumor, 298
prions, **327**–328
problem solving, 39
pro-choice groups, 145
prodromal period, 320
professional care, 364–366
professional help, 65–66
    choosing a therapist for, 66
    determining the need for, 65
profound trauma, 425
progestagens, **95**
progestational phase, 97
progesterone, **95**
progressive overload, **249**
progressive relaxation, 40
pro-life groups, 145
proof value, **178**
prostaglandins, 98
prostate cancer, 302–304
prostate gland, **93**, 302
prostate-specific antigen (PSA) blood test, **304**
prostatitis, 101
prostitution, **105**–106
protease inhibitors, **334**
proteins, **207**–208
    athletic performance and, 253
    recommended intake of, 208
    setting intake goals for, 211
    sources of, 207–208, 219
protozoa, **327**
psychoactive drugs, **152**
    abuse of, 155
    addiction to, 152–155
    chart of commonly used, 162
    club drugs as, 164
    definition of, **153**
    dependence on, 155–156, 157, 158
    depressants, **161**, 163–164
    effects of, 159–161, 162
    hallucinogens, **168**–169
    information resources on, 175–176
    inhalants, 169–170
    legalization debate, 170
    marijuana, 167–168
    opioids, **161**
    statistics on use of, 153
    stimulants, **164**–165, 167
    summary points about, 175
    treating dependence on, 172
    workplace testing for, 170, 172
    See also drug use
psychodynamic therapy, 65
psychological disorders, 55–63
    anxiety disorders, 56, 58
    ethnicity/culture and, 57
    factors influencing, 55–56
    gender and, 63
    mood disorders, **58**–61
    prevalence of, 55
    professional help for, 65–66

schizophrenia, **61**
suicide and, 61–62
treatments for, 65
psychological health, 47–69
abortion and, 148–149
altruism and, 35
anger and, 54–55
communication and, 54
connecting to choices about, 66
defense mechanisms and, **53**
definition of, 47–**48**
development of, 50
disorders related to, 55–63
exercise and, 59, 245–246
happiness and, 48–49
help related to, 63–65
information resources on, 68
loneliness and, 54
normality vs., **49**
optimism and, **53**
self-actualization and, **48**
self-esteem and, **48**, 51–52
summary points about, 66–68
tips related to, 65
psychological problems
alcohol use and, 187
cardiovascular disease and, 287, 288, 298
peer counseling for, 64
professional help for, 65–66
self-help for, 63–64
stress related to, 30–31
support groups for, 65
therapies for, 65
psychoneuroimmunology (PNI), **30**
psychotherapy
choosing professionals for, 66
types of, 65
PTSD. *See* post-traumatic stress disorder
puberty, **95**
pubic lice, **342**
pulmonary circulation, 282, **283**
pulmonary edema, **296**
pulmonary heart disease, 195
purging, **276**

Q
qigong, **377**
quadruple marker screen (QMS), **115**
quantity vs. quality of life, 6
Quinlan, Karen Ann, 418
quitting tobacco use, 200–202, 204

R
racial differences
contraceptive use and, 140
health care disparities and, 10
See also ethnicity
radiation, **358**
carcinogenic, 310
environmental health and, 358–359
medical uses of, 311, 359
ultraviolet, **306**–307
radiation sickness, **358**
radon, 311, **359**
randomized controlled trials (RTCs), 368
rape, **400**–401
rapid eye movement (REM) sleep, **36**–37
realism, 48
realistic self-talk, 52
recessive genes, 114
Recommended Dietary Allowance (RDA), 218
recycling, **354**, 355
"reduced harm" cigarettes, 194
reframing situations, 54–55
Reiki, **377**

reinforcement, 153
relapse, 17
relationships
abusive, 397–398
aging process and, 410
friendship, 71–72
online, 80
See also intimate relationships
relaxation response, **39**, 41
relaxation techniques, 39–42
religion
contraceptive methods and, 141
drug use and, 158
intimate relationships and, 79
tobacco use and, 192
REM (rapid eye movement) sleep, **36**–37
remission, **298**
renewable energy, 352
repetitive strain injuries (RSIs), **392**–393
reproductive system, 95–100
aging and, 99–100
environmental hazards and, 96–97
female, 95–98
male, 98–99
reservoir, 317, **318**
resilience, 28
resistance, 28
resistance exercise, **251**
resources. *See* information resources
responsiveness, 86
resting metabolic rate (RMR), **269**
retarded ejaculation, **102**
retirement, 410–411
reverse transcriptase inhibitors, **333**–334
reversibility, exercise, **249**
rheumatic fever, **296**
rheumatic heart disease (RHD), 296
Rh factor, **115**
R-I-C-E principle, 258
rickets, 213
risk factors, **2**
abortion, 128, 148–149
cardiovascular disease, 283–291
contraception, 128, 140–141
drug use, 158–159
eating disorder, 276, 277–278
excess body fat, 266–267
HIV transmission, 335
illness/injury, 1
physical inactivity, 244
pregnancy, 128
suicide, 62
ritalin, 167
Roe v. Wade (1973), 142, 145
rohypnol, 164, 400
role models, 16
rotavirus, 328

S
safer sex, 107
safety. *See* personal safety
safety belts, 386–387
same-sex partnerships, 82, 83
sanitary landfill, **354**
sarcomas, **299**
saturated fat, 208–209, 210, 314
saving money, 4
scabies, **342**
Schiavo, Terri, 419
schizophrenia, **61**
school violence, 34, 396, 403
scientific method, 367–368
scrotum, **92**, 93
scurvy, 213
seasonal affective disorder (SAD), **59**, 61

secondary tumors, 298
secondhand smoke, 198–199
sedation, **161**
sedative-hypnotics, **161**
selective estrogen-receptor modulators
(SERMs), 302
self-actualization, **48**
self-assessment
of bodily symptoms, 362–363
of caffeine consumption, 174
self-care, 362–364
self-concept, **48**, 51, 70–71
self-disclosure, 76
self-efficacy, **16**–17
self-esteem, **48**, 51–52, 70–71
self-help, 63–64
self-help groups, 172
self-image, 48
self-injury, 62
self-medication, 363–364
self-monitoring, 174, 279
self-talk, 16, **52**, 272
self-treatment, 363–364
Seligman, Martin, 48
Selye, Hans, 28
semen, **101**
seminal vesicles, **93**
separation and divorce, 85–86
severe acute respiratory syndrome (SARS), 328
sewage treatment, 353
sex
definition of, 7
wellness and, 7–9
See also gender
sex chromosomes, **95**
sex hormones, 95
sexting, 105
sexual anatomy
female, 91–92
male, 92–93
sexual assault, **400**–401
sexual behavior, 103–107
addiction to, 106, 154–155
alcohol use and, 182
atypical/problematic, 105
commercial forms of, 105–106
communicating about, 106, 107
hooking up as, 81
responsible, 106–107
safe and sober, 107
sexual orientation and, 103
varieties of, 103–105
sexual coercion, **105**
sexual dysfunctions, **101**, 102–103
sexual functioning, 100–103
problems with, 101–102
response cycle for, 100–101
stimulation and, 100
sexual harassment, 402, **403**
sexual intercourse, **104**–105
abstaining from, 135–136
HIV transmission via, 332
sexuality, 91, **92**
aging and, 99–100
communicating about, 106, 107
information resources on, 123–124
summary points about, 123
tips related to, 123
sexually transmitted diseases (STDs), **126**,
329–342
bacterial vaginosis, **342**
chlamydia, **336**–337
choices about, 343
condoms and, 132
contraception and, 125, 132, 138

sexually transmitted diseases (STDs) (*Cont.*)
   diagnosis of, 342
   education about, 342
   genital herpes, **339**–340
   gonorrhea, **337**–338
   hepatitis B virus, 326, 340–341
   HIV/AIDS, 329–335
   human papillomavirus, 132, 304, 305, 326, **338**–339
   information resources on, 344
   pelvic inflammatory disease, 101, 131, **338**
   preventing infection by, 336, 342, 343
   prostitution and, 105
   pubic lice and scabies, **342**
   summary points about, 343
   syphilis, **341**
   treatments for, 342
   trichomoniasis, **341**
   vaccinations for, 342
   women and, 337
sexual orientation, **82**
   same-sex partnerships and, 82
   sexual behavior and, 103
   wellness and, 9, 12
sexual privacy, 106
sexual response cycle, 100–101
sexual stimulation, 100
sexual violence, 399–402
   child sexual abuse, 401–402
   rape and date rape, **400**–401
   sexual harassment, **402**
shopping addiction, 155
shyness, 67
sickle-cell disease, 114
sidestream smoke, **194**, 198
simple (specific) phobia, **56**
simple carbohydrates, 210
singlehood, 82, 84
single parents, 87
skill-related fitness, **243**
skin cancer, 300, 306–307
skinfold measurements, 266
skin patch, contraceptive, 128–129
sleep
   phases of, 36–37
   problems related to, 37
   stress and, 37
sleep apnea, **37**
sleep deprivation, **37**, 385
SMART criteria, 18
smog, **349**
smokeless tobacco, 196–197
smoking
   cessation products, 201
   effects on nonsmokers, 198–199
   immediate effects of, 194
   laws and regulations on, 199–200
   long-term effects of, 194–196
   media portrayal of, 192–193
   pregnancy and, 116, 199
   quitting, 200–202, 204
   See also tobacco use
sober sex, 107
social anxiety, 67
social isolation, 287
social networks, 32–33
social phobia, **56**
Social Security, **414**
social stressors, 32–33
social support
   behavior change and, 16
   stress management and, 34
socioeconomic status
   cardiovascular disease and, 287, 290
   contraceptive use and, 140

drug use and, 171
environmental health and, 356
obesity and, 270
soda consumption, 270
sodium, 219–220, 297
solar power, 352
solid waste, 354–356
   disposing of, 354–355
   green consumerism and, 355
   reducing, 355–356
somatic nervous system, **27**
sonograms, **114**–115
soy protein, 297
specificity, exercise, **249**
sperm, 91, **92**, 108
spermicide, **132**, 133–134, 135, 332
sphygmomanometer, 284
spinal manipulative therapy (SMT), 367
spirituality
   drug use and, 158
   See also religion
spiritual wellness, 2, 38, 88
spit tobacco, 196–197
sponge, contraceptive, **134**–135
spontaneous abortion, 118, 142, 143
spotting, 127
squamous cell carcinoma, **307**
stability, 51
stages of change, 17
stalking, **398**–399
staphylococcus, **324**
state dependence, **165**
statutory rape, **400**
STDs. *See* sexually transmitted diseases
stepfamilies, 87
sterilization, 138, **139**
   female, 139
   male, 138–139
steroids, 253
stillbirth, 118
stimulants, 162, 164–**165**, 167, 253
St. John's wort, 378
strength training, 251–253
strep throat, 324
streptococcus, **324**
stress, 24–46
   academic, 32
   acute vs. chronic, 30
   aging process and, 410
   allostatic load and, 29–**30**
   burnout and, **32**
   campus violence and, 34
   cardiovascular disease and, 30, 287, 289, 298
   cultural background and, 28
   definition of, 24–**25**
   diversity and, 33
   endocrine system and, **25**
   fight-or-flight reaction and, **25**–27
   GAS model of, 28–29
   gender and, 28, 29
   genital herpes and, 340
   headaches and, 31
   health and, 28–31
   hormones related to, 25, 37
   immune system and, 30, 31, 340
   information resources on, 45–46
   interpersonal, 32
   management of, 34–44
   nervous system and, 25, 27
   past experiences and, 28
   perceptions of, 29
   personality and, **27**–28
   psychological problems and, 30–31
   sleep patterns and, 37
   sources of, 32–34

summary points about, 45
   test anxiety and, 44
stress journal, 43
stress management, 34–44
   altruism and, 35
   cognitive techniques and, 38–39
   communication and, 36
   connecting to choices about, 45
   counterproductive, 42–43
   exercise and, 36
   nature and, 40
   nutrition and, 36
   personal plan for, 43–44
   relaxation techniques and, 39–42
   sleep and, 36–37
   social support and, 34
   spiritual wellness and, 38
   time management and, 38
   tips related to, 44
   writing and, 38, 364
stressors
   college, 32
   definition of, 24, **25**
   environmental, 33
   identifying, 43
   job-related, 32
   responses to, 25–28
   social, 32–33
stress response, 24, **25**
stretching exercises, 253–254
stroke, 195, 293, **294**–296, 299
subarachnoid hemorrhage, 294
subcutaneous fat, **264**
substance abuse, **155**
   alcohol and, 185
   prevention of, 173
   resources on, 175
   treatments for, 172
Substance Abuse and Mental Health Services Administration (SAMHSA), 156
substance dependence, **155**–156
   alcohol, **185**, 186–188
   amphetamine, 165
   codependency and, **172**–173
   drug potential for, 157
   marijuana, 168
   older adults and, 409–410
   risk factors for, 158
   state dependence, **165**
   treatments for, 172
suction curettage, **146**, 147
sudden cardiac death, **292**
sudden infant death syndrome (SIDS), **119**, 198
suffocation, 391
suicide, 61–62
   depression and, 62, 63
   physician-assisted, **419**
   rates and warning signs, 62
sunburns, 307
suncreens, 307, 308
sun exposure, 307, 308
sun-protective clothing, 307, 308
supplements. *See* dietary supplements
support groups, 65
supportiveness, 74
surgery, 371
   cancer, 311
   coronary bypass, **294**
   weight loss, 274–275
surgical methods of contraception, 125, **126**
surrogate, **420**
sustainability, 352
swimming safety, 391
sympathetic division, **25**
synesthesia, **169**

syphilis, **341**
syringe exchange programs (SEPs), 159
systemic circulation, 282, **283**
systemic infection, **318**
systole, **283**

T
tai chi, 42, 367
tanning salons, 306, 308
target behavior, **14**
target heart rate range, **250**
Tay-Sachs disease, 114
T cells, 319
teenagers. *See* adolescents
temperature methods of contraception, 136
tension headaches, 31
teratogens, **116**
terrorism, 396–397, 398
testamentary letter, 418
test anxiety, 44
testator, **417**–418
testes, **92**, 93
testicle self-examination, 309
testicular cancer, 101, 308, 309
testicular torsion, 101
testosterone, 29, **95**, 99–100
text messaging, 388
therapeutic touch, **377**
therapy. *See* psychotherapy
thrombus, **294**
tickborne infections, 325
time-action function, **160**
time management, 38
time pressures, 32
tobacco, 177, **178**
tobacco use, 190–202
    aging process and, 410
    cancer and, 195, 197, 300–301, 307, 309
    cardiovascular disease and, 194–195, 283, 297
    demographics of, 190–191
    environmental smoke from, 177, 198–199
    gender differences in, 196
    health hazards of, 193–198
    immediate effects of, 194
    information resources on, 203, 205
    laws and regulations on, 199–200
    long-term effects of, 194–196
    mainstream smoke from, **198**
    media portrayal of, 192–193
    nicotine addiction and, 191
    pregnancy and, 116, 199
    psychology of, 191
    quitting, 200–202, 205
    reasons for, 191–193
    religion and, 192
    smokeless, 196–197
    stress and, 42
    summary points about, 203
Tolerable Upper Intake Level (UL), 218, 227
tolerance, 152, **153**
    alcohol, 187
    drug, 152, 155
    tobacco, 191
total fiber, **212**
touching
    sexual, 104
    therapeutic, 377
Toward a Psychology of Being (Maslow), 47
toxic shock syndrome (TSS), **134**, 324
traditional Chinese medicine (TCM), **372**–373
tranquilizers, **161**
trans fatty acids, **208**, 210, 220, 314
transgender individuals, 82
transient ischemic attack (TIA), **295**
transition stage of labor, **120**–121

traumatic events, 425
treatments
    for alcoholism, 187–188
    for cancer, 311, 313
    for depression, 59–61
    for diabetes, 268
    for drug dependence, 172
    for eating disorders, 278
    for HIV infection, 333–335
    for psychological disorders, 65
    for sexually transmitted diseases, 342
trichomoniasis, **341**
triglycerides, 208, **287**
trimesters, pregnancy, **109**–110, 111–114
tropical rainforests, 375
tubal sterilization, **139**
tuberculosis (TB), **324**
tumors, **298**
twins, 108
type 1 diabetes, 268
type 2 diabetes, 245, 268
Type A/B/C personalities, 27

U
ulcers, 325
ultrasonography, **114**–115, **302**
ultraviolet (UV) radiation, **306**–307, 350
umbilical cord, **113**
unhealthy relationships, 75
Uniform Donor Card, **420**
unintended pregnancies, 140
unintentional injuries, 384, **385**–393
    See also injuries
uninvolved parents, 86
unsaturated fats, 209
urethra, **92**, 93
urethritis, **336**
U.S. Department of Agriculture (USDA), 218, 221
U.S. Supreme Court, 142, 144, 148, 419
uterine cancer, 306
uterus, **92**

V
vaccines, **321**
    for HPV, 305
    for STDs, 342
vagina, 92
Vaginal Contraceptive Film (VCF), 135
vaginal ring, 129
vaginal spermicides, 135
vaginitis, 101
values, **50**
vas deferens, **93**
vasectomy, **138**–139
vasocongestion, **100**
vegetables, 223, 309–310, 314
vegetarian diets, 224–225
veins, **283**
venae cavae, 282, **283**
ventricle, 282, **283**
ventricular fibrillation, 292
viable fetus, **142**
Viagra, 102–103
violence, 393–402
    assault, 395
    campus, 34, 403
    collective, 397
    definition of, 393
    drug- and alcohol-related, 170, 182, 395
    factors contributing to, 394–395
    family and intimate, 397–399
    gang-related, 395
    gender differences in, 394
    global view of, 397
    hate crimes, 395–396

homicides, 395
    interpersonal, 397
    resources on, 405–406
    school, 34, 396
    sexual, 399–402
    summary points about, 405
    terrorism, 396–397, 398
    workplace, 396
virtual sex, 105
viruses, **325**–326
visceral fat, **264**
vision changes, 411
visualization, 16, **40**
vitamins, **213**–215
    facts about, 214
    homocysteine levels and, 291, 297
    prenatal care and, 116
volunteering, 35
vulva, 91, **92**

W
water
    bottled, and the environment, 257
    consuming during exercise, 255–256
    nutritional importance of, 216
    quality/pollution of, 353
water-soluble vitamins, 214
weather safety, 387
Web resources. *See* information resources;
        Internet
weight management, 263–281
    accepting limits of, 275
    aging process and, 409
    basic concepts of, 263–269
    body composition and, 263–264, 266
    body image and, **267**, 275, 277
    body mass index and, **265**–266
    connecting to choices about, 280
    coping strategies and, 272
    creating a personal plan for, 279
    diabetes prevention and, 268
    dietary supplements for, 272–273
    diet/eating habits and, 270, 271, 279
    diet soda consumption and, 270
    do-it-yourself approach to, 272
    eating disorders and, **275**–278
    energy balance and, 219, 264–265, 273, 279
    genetic factors and, 269
    information resources on, 280–281
    lifestyle factors and, 269–270
    physical activity and, 270, 271–272
    physiological factors and, 269
    prescription drugs for, 274
    psychosocial factors and, 270
    summary points about, 280
    surgical approaches to, 274–275
    thinking/emotions and, 272
    tips related to, 280
    weight-loss programs for, 273–274
    wellness and, 266–269
wellness, 1–23
    body fat and, 266–269
    continuum of, 2
    definition of, 1, **2**
    dimensions of, 1–3
    diversity and, 7–10, 12
    ethnicity and, 9, 10
    exercise and, 246
    factors influencing, 12–14
    geographic location and, 9
    health care reform and, 10, 11
    Healthy People initiative and, 6–7
    income/education and, 9, 10
    information resources on, 21–22
    lifestyle management and, 14–20

wellness (*Cont.*)
    marriage and, 84
    qualities/behaviors, 2
    sex/gender and, 7–9
    summary points about, 21
    tips for choosing, 20
Western blot test, 333
Western medicine. *See* conventional medicine
West Nile virus, 328
white blood cells, 318–319
WHO. *See* World Health Organization
whole grains, **210**–211, 212
Williams, Redford, 288
wills, **417**–418
wind power, 352
windy weather safety, 387
wine, 178
withdrawal, **156**
    alcohol, 187
    drug, 156
    tobacco, 191
withdrawal method of contraception, **136**

womb, 92
women
    alcohol abuse by, 189
    cardiovascular disease and, 289
    communication advice for, 77
    contraceptive use by American, 140
    health issues for, 8
    life expectancy of, 414
    nutritional needs of, 225
    STDs and, 337
    stress and, 29
    See also females
Women Organized Against Rape (WOAR), 401
Woods, Tiger, 106
Worden, William, 423
work addiction, 154
workaholics, 154
work injuries, **392**–393
workplace
    drug testing in, 170, 172
    injuries in, 392–393
    violence in, 396

World Health Organization (WHO), 5, 94, 199, 372, 397
writing, 38, 364

X
X ray exposure, 359

Y
yoga, 41–42
young people
    antidepressant use in, 60
    dietary challenges for, 225–226
    leading causes of death among, 5, 61
    male injury rate for, 386
    See also adolescents; children

Z
zygote, 107
zygote intrafallopian transfer (ZIFT), **109**

ome KEY INDINGS from ur Personal ealth Course urvey

5% of Personal Health structors are teaching ther a hybrid or a fully nline course.

0% of Personal ealth instructors say at promoting behavior ange through the use of havior change tools is important goal of their urse.

> McGraw-Hill *Connect* connects students with their coursework and with their instructors. With *Connect Personal Health*, students gain access to a wealth of online content, including self-assessments, video activities, quizzes with immediate feedback, and a media-rich eBook. *Connect Personal Health* now includes an adaptive diagnostic tool that assesses students' knowledge and creates individual learning plans to help them master the material. *Connect Personal Health* enables instructors to teach the course in a more efficient and effective way.

Ask Yourself

QUESTIONS FOR CRITICAL THINKING AND REFLECTION

Think of the last time you faced a significant stressor. How did you respond? List the physical, emotional, and behavioral reactions you experienced. Did these responses help you deal with the stress, or did they interfere with your efforts to handle it?

> *Connect Personal Health* equips students with an online toolkit of interactive behavior change tools, tips, and strategies. Features like Take Charge, Tips for Today and the Future, Connect to Your Choices, and Ask Yourself focus on students' awareness, motivations, and goals and help them put personal responsibility into practice.

EMERGENCY CARE FOR CHOKING

- If the victim is coughing, encourage the coughing to clear the object from the airway.
- If the victim is not coughing, follow the steps in "Choking Care for Responsive Adult or Child."

Choking Care for Responsive Adult or Child

 1 Stand behind an adult victim with one leg forward between the victim's legs. (With a child, kneel behind the victim.) Keep your head slightly to one side. Reach around the abdomen with both arms. Make a fist with one hand and place the thumb side of the fist against the abdomen just above the navel.

 2 Grasp your fist with your other hand and thrust inward and upward into the victim's abdomen with quick jerks. Continue abdominal thrusts until the victim expels the object or becomes unresponsive. If the victim becomes unresponsive while you are administering abdominal thrusts, lower the victim to the floor onto his or her back, and follow the steps in "Choking Care for Unresponsive Adult or Child."

Choking Care for Unresponsive Adult or Child: CPR

 1 Call 911 and begin CPR.

 2 Open the airway to see if the victim is breathing. Use the "head tilt–chin lift" maneuver to open the airway: Push down on the forehead and lift the chin.

 3 If the victim is not breathing, give two rescue breaths, each lasting 1 second. Pinch the victim's nose shut and blow a normal breath into the victim's mouth. If the first breath does not go in (the chest does not rise), reposition the head to open the airway and try again. Each time you give a rescue breath, look for an object in the victim's mouth and remove it if present.

 4 If the obstruction remains, begin chest compressions. Place the heel of one hand in the center of the chest between the nipples and the other hand on top of the first. Position your shoulders over your hands and lock your elbows. Give 30 chest compressions at a rate of 100 per minute. The chest should go down by 1½ to 2 inches. Then give two breaths, looking in the mouth for an expelled object. Continue chest compressions until help arrives. **Remember: Push hard and push fast at a rate of 100 compressions per minute.**

EMERGENCY CARE FOR CARDIAC ARREST

For cardiac arrest, the American Heart Association's revised (2005) Emergency Cardiac Care guidelines are as follows:

1 Call 911.

2 Start CPR (100 compressions per minute, stopping every 30 to 60 seconds to give two rescue breaths).

3 If an automated external defibrillator (AED) is available, or when one arrives, give one shock to restart the victim's heart.

4 Go back to CPR immediately after the shock.

Hands-Only CPR

In 2008, the American Heart Association reported that hands-only (compression-only) CPR can be as effective as conventional CPR. There are only two steps:

 1 Call 911.

 2 Push hard and fast in the center of the chest.

Don't wait for an emergency to learn how to use an AED or perform CPR.
To find a course in your area, contact the American Heart Association (800 242-8721) or the American Red Cross (202 303-4498).

Sources: Adapted from American Heart Association. 2010. Hands-only CPR (www.handsonlycpr.org; retrieved August 10, 2010); *Circulation* 117, 2162–2167; National Safety Council. 2007. *First Aid: Taking Action.* New York: McGraw-Hill; American Heart Association. 2005. Adult basic life support. *Circulation* 112, 19–34.